James A. DiSario, M.D.

DIGESTIVE ENDOSCOPY
IN THE
SECOND MILLENIUM
From the Lichtleiter to Echoendoscopy

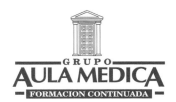

GRUPO
AULA MEDICA
- FORMACION CONTINUADA -

DIGESTIVE ENDOSCOPY
IN THE
SECOND MILLENIUM
From the Lichtleiter to Echoendoscopy

FRANCISCO VILARDELL

MD DSc (Barc.) DSc Med (Penn.)
FRCP FRCP (Ed.) FACP FACG
Director Emeritus,
Postgraduate School of Gastroenterology,
Hospital de Sant Pau, Barcelona

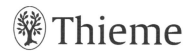

In this work readers will find guidelines on handling patients, dosage and side effects of various drugs, as well as instructions for performing tests, experiments, etc. for various substances and/or devices. The author and the publisher have made every effort to ensure these are in line with current normal practice. Nonetheless, it is up to readers to consult the information provided by pharmaceutical laboratories and the manufacturers of machinery and apparatus and to abide by the current state of the art in this area. The author and the publishing company decline any and all liability arising out of any harm or injury produced as a result of the material published in this work.

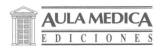

Index

Foreword

Basil I. Hirschowitz MD, FRCP, MACP
Professor Emeritus of Medicine University of Alabama at Birmingham,
School of Medicine.

Francisco Vilardell, a distinguished, internationally recognized gastroenterologist, has produced a labor of love in the form of a meticulously researched and elaborately documented book on the evolution and impact of endoscopy on the digestive tract in the last 100 years.

His credentials for this undertaking show him eminently prepared for the large task he set himself in writing this book. While directing the gastroenterology department of the Hospital de Sant Pau in Barcelona for 33 years until 1996, he found time on the international stage to establish and be the first president of the Spanish Digestive Endoscopy Association, to be President of the European Society for Gastrointestinal Endoscopy, to be Secretary-General and President of the World Organization of Gastroenterology and to be inducted as a member of 10 national gastroenterology societies. He is no stranger to medical writing, with 6 books and over 200 published articles to his credit.

What is striking about this informative and artistic book is not only the broad brush with which he paints the picture of the medical professions' quest to examine body cavities since the early 19th Century work of Bozzini, but the meticulous, fine detail incorporated in this large picture. These details are illustrated by visuals of persons, publications, instruments, procedures, pathology and patients, representing a collector's obsession with completeness, and testimony to his wide international network of gastroenterology in which he has played such an important role for over 40 years.

It must give Professor Vilardell great existential pleasure, as it has for me, to have seen the revolution in endoscopy and its influence on the practice of gastroenterology that followed the introduction of fiberoptic flexible endoscopy forty-five years ago, at the start of his own career in this field. He has repaid it handsomely with this work of fine scholarship, now available in this English edition as well as in the original Spanish. This book will bring pleasure to its many readers.

Introductions

Prof. Meinhard Classen

President of the World Organisation of Gastroenterology (1998-2002)

Francisco Vilardell has done it. He has done what the world of endoscopy expected him to do; to write a book on the history of endoscopy on the basis of his life-long practice and profound studies on this topic in the past years. This book has it all: from the preliminaries of endoscopy ("in the beginning there was a tube"..) to the endoscopy of the narrow channels, endoscopic ultrasound and therapeutic measures like tumor ablation and endoscopic papillotomy. The author concentrates the enormous material in 14 chapters and 316 pages. The result is a concise, highly informative text whose literary quality makes reading a pleasure. An outstanding feature at difference from all other books and book chapters on this subject is the quantity and quality of the picture material hitherto unpublished. I confess that many of these pictures depicting pioneer personalities, tools, endoscopic images, techniques and graphs I had never seen before. We can only guess how much time Francisco Vilardell spent in university libraries and state archives to trace these treasures.

"Habent sua fata libelli". It is easy to forecast that F. Vilardell's work will be published in several world languages because it should be in the hands of every endoscopist. This book could only be written by Francisco Vilardell, honorary president of the World Organisations of Gastroenterology and Endoscopy, a distinguished and admired colleague with a truly global perspective of our speciality. This explains why this book shows no European or American partiality. It is a book by a true world citizen written for all of us.

Prof. Hirohumi Niwa

President, World Organization for Digestive Endoscopy (OMED).
President, Japan Gastroenterological Endoscopy Society.
Professor of Medicine. St Marianna University School of Medicine.

The long awaited English version of "Digestive Endoscopy in the Second Millenium" has been completed by Professor Francisco Vilardell. The book was originally written in Spanish, his native language, and it is a great pleasure and indeed an honour to preface a publication which will bring significant benefits to all those who engage in endoscopy across the world. I would like to express my deepest gratitude and congratulations to Professor Vilardell for his great achievement.

As is well known, Professor Vilardell is a most renowned Spanish gastroenterologist who has a deep knowledge and experience of gastrointestinal disease and who has made brilliant accomplishments in endoscopy. As President of the World Organisation of Gastroenterology (OMGE), as one of the Councillors representing the European Zone on the occasion of the reorganisation of the World Organisation for Digestive Endoscopy (OMED) and as a board member of many other international societies, he has played an important role in domestic and international gastroenterology events. Furthermore, he was one of the associate editors and a consultant of "Bockus Gastroenterology", a treatise which has been a major landmark in the development of academic gastroenterology and of endoscopy.

An attempt to compile the history of endoscopy of all periods and cultures requires such a broad range of knowledge of gastrointestinal endoscopy that could only have been fulfilled by some- one like Professor Vilardell. Such an enormous effort to collect all these documents and pictures from the earliest medical literature deserves our loudest applause. The book is organized into 14 chapters that give extensive and detailed descriptions on the development of various kinds of endoscopes, including early tubes and catheters which anteceded modern instruments, such as Bozzini's Lichleiter, Kussmaul's rigid endoscopes, the semiflexible gastroscopes, the rigid oesophagoscopes, the endoscopic documentation, biopsy and cytology, endoscopic ultrasonog- raphy, the endoscopic treatment of bleeding lesions, rectosigmoidoscopy, fibrecolonoscopy, pan- creatic and biliary endoscopy, diagnostic and therapeutic laparoscopy and other techniques.

It is simply amazing that the author has been able to utilize sources not only in English and Spanish but also in several other languages, giving them a thorough scrutiny and then pro- viding detailed descriptions. Abover all, it is very flattering to us that he extensively refers to Japanese literature, not always properly quoted outside Japan. The book indisputably provides the most comprehensive integration of the global history of endoscopy ever pub- lished. Large numbers of works on gastrointestinal endoscopy are now available, but this book conspicuously distinguishes itself from others by its truly global perspective based on a broad and international range of reference sources plus a great number of valuable pic- tures that have not been made public before. Moreover, many pictures of our great prede- cessors who dedicated themselves to the development of endoscopy will inspire and encour- age young readers to advance their research in the techniques of endoscopy.

This great achievement reminds me of a highly edifying phrase in the Analecta of Confucious, one of the greatest philosophers of ancient China (BC 551-479?), which is often quoted in Japan today; it teaches us the importance of consulting the past when we want to learn new things. History has a lot to teach us! For the further development of endoscopy, I sincerely hope that the younger generations of endoscopists will learn much and obtain guidance for their future endeavours from the historical insights of this book.

As President of the World Organization of Digestive Endoscopy (OMED), I would like to strongly recommend all endoscopists, especially the young, to keep this book on hand and learn from it.

José Ramón Armengol Miró

Director of International Relations and former President,
Spanish Association of Digestive Endoscopy.
President, European Society for Gastrointestinal Endoscopy (1994-1996).

It is a great pleasure for me to preface this outstanding history of digestive endoscopy written by my old friend and mentor, Professor Francisco Vilardell, Director Emeritus of the prestigious Postgraduate School of Gastroenterology at the Hospital de Santa Creu i Sant Pau in Barcelona. His achievements in the field of gastroenterology are well known to all his colleagues due in part to his terms as President of the European Society for Gastrointestinal Endoscopy and as Secretary General and later President of the World Organisation of Gastroenterology.

His book on the development of digestive endoscopy during the second millenium starts with the use and introduction of tubes and probes into the gastrointestinal tract to extract foreign bodies and then follows in great detail the invention and use of instruments from Bozzini's Lichleiter up to the advent of echo endoscopy and other novel techniques. I believe that this is the fairest and most impartial book on the subject; it gives its due to all the pioneers of endoscopy, trying always to find the earliest piece of evidence for each instrument and for each technique.

His personal friendship with many leading endoscopists has enabled him to include documents which until now were practically unknown to most of us. On the other hand, I am aware of the countless hours that Francisco Vilardell has spent in archives and libraries all over the world trying to check and verify his information, as can be readily seen by perusing the long list of ackowledgements that follows his introduction.

The author has dedicated his book to the Spanish Association for Digestive Endoscopy of which he was a founder and its first president, and of which he is now an honorary member. The book was edited in Spanish for the members of our Society presided in succession by Drs Juan Manuel Montero and Juan M. Pou, with the help of Dr. Jaume Boix, chairman of the education committee of the association. Francisco Vilardell offers now an English version, which we hope will reach the wide audience that his efforts deserve. In the name of all Spanish endoscopists may I most warmly thank Professor Vilardell for his outstanding contribution, a gift which should be in the hands of every gastroenterologist.

Preface

· ·

Francisco Vilardell

"Oculi tanquam speculatores altissimum locum obtinent"
(Cicero).

DIGESTIVE ENDOSCOPY AT THE START
OF THE THIRD MILLENIUM

Over the past fifty years, digestive endoscopy has become the most powerful diagnostic and therapeutic tool available to the gastroenterologist. In the late 1990s, a survey in the United States asked specialists what they considered were the most important breakthroughs in gastroenterology in the last decades. The majority ranked the discovery of fibreoptics in first or second place, alternatively with the discovery of Helicobacter pylori and its role in the pathogenesis of gastric diseases[1].

With the rapid diffusion of technological advances and the creation of new endoscopic societies and international organisations, interest in digestive endoscopy has grown far beyond early expectations.

MY INITIAL INTEREST IN DIGESTIVE ENDOSCOPY

My own curiosity in endoscopy was kindled at a very early stage in my career when I was admitted as an assistant at the Postgraduate School of Gastroenterology at the Hospital de Sant Pau in Barcelona. The school was founded in the early 20th century by Dr. Francisco Gallart-Monés and was renowned for its role in the development of diagnostic techniques. In spite of the sophisticated radiological examinations being carried out in our midst by Drs T.A. Pinós and J. Valls Colomer, even as far back as the late 1930s Schindler's gastroscope was being used routinely by Drs E. Vidal Colomer and J. Badosa Gaspar, the pioneers of semi-rigid gastroscopy in Spain. Soon after the Second World War, Dr Pinós, with the help of Drs I. Serés and A. Marti-Vicente, established laparoscopy as a routine diagnostic procedure in the centre. In the 1960s, Dr. E Sala-Cladera was probably the first to employ a fibrescope in Spain, and Dr.V.Cabre Fiol developed ancillary techniques —such as endoscopic cytology— with great accuracy. He soon received well-deserved international recognition for his contributions.

The great masters of endoscopy at the Saint-Antoine Hospital in Paris undeniably played a determinant role in my becoming a clinical gastroenterologist; Drs François Moutier and Charles Debray came to Dr. René A. Gutmann's service to perform gastroscopies, and Drs Paulette Ricordeau and André Fourès performed laparoscopy in Professor Caroli's Service at the same hospital. As foreign fellows, we closely observed their methods and techniques. Some years later, during my initial stay at the University of Pennsylvania Graduate Hospital in Philadelphia in the early 1950s, Gabriel Tucker and Joseph Atkins, Chevalier Jackson's successors, awed me with their skill in oesophagoscopy. Ten years on, during my term as research fellow in the same institution, we were privileged to assist the great gastroenterologic endoscopist Ben Sullivan in his first fibrescopies. It was there that I also developed cytologic diagnostic techniques and together with my mentor, Dr. V. Cabré Fiol, we adapted these to the new fibrescopic instruments on my return to Barcelona.

THE IDEA FOR THE BOOK

The idea to write a monograph on the history of digestive endoscopy arose from a very kind invitation by Professor Michel Cremer, the distinguished gastroenterologist from Brussels, to give a lecture at the United European Digestive Disease meeting held in his city late in 2000[2].

In preparing for this assignment I was fortunate to be helped in the collection of numerous documents by a large number of individuals and institutions whose names appear on the list of acknowledgements. After the congress, I thought that perhaps it would be useful to offer all the information which I had compiled to colleagues who might be interested in the development and evolution of gastrointestinal endoscopy. Although some of the data which I presented in Brussels were well-known to many in the audience, other publications which I quoted were found by serendipity, while on the track of an author, an instrument or another publication.

This monograph, then, is simply an attempt to present the lecture I gave in Brussels in a fuller format, including a greatly expanded iconography as well as a list, as accurate as possible, of the pertinent bibliographic sources which I believe may be of further help to the interested reader. At this point, I would like to emphasise that this book does not pretend to be exhaustive, nor is it in any way a definitive work on the subject.

ON BIBLIOGRAPHICAL SOURCES

Any physician interested in academic medicine will admire the outstanding personality of John Shaw Billings (1838-1913), a physician in the American Medical Corps who started the library of the Department of Health of the American Government in Washington, later to become the prestigious National Institute of Health (N.I.H.). As of 1865, Billings began to catalogue international medical literature[3]. The first volume of the "Index Catalogue" of the

"Library of the Surgeon's General Office" was published in 1880, and by 1895, 16 volumes had appeared. These contained the astonishing figure of 680,000 bibliographic references! The "Index Medicus" appeared for the first time in 1879 as a complement to the "Index Catalogue", and with the exception of a few specific bibliographical indexes and some hand-written catalogues which can still be consulted in some libraries, it is today the only reliable source for old medical literature.

Digital recording of these bibliographies is still very incomplete. Moreover, as the result of wars, and particularly World War Two, many archives and libraries have disappeared. Despite the easy access to current references through computer databases, consulting old medical books remains difficult. As new journals are constantly appearing, old periodicals and books are often taken off their shelves, possibly to be relocated in other buildings quite some distance away. As a result, one may have to wait, sometimes for several days, before the desired publication appears in the reading room. Furthermore, many libraries presently restrict photocopying of old journals for fear of damaging the paper; the advent of digital cameras has palliated some of these difficulties.

Old books, as a rule, do not include detailed references, but just occasionally, one may stumble across a totally unexpected article. Complete references are the exception as 19th century authors generally included only footnotes with very fragmentary information. Moreover, searching the early volumes of the Index Catalogue may be difficult as, unfortunately, they do not always provide a full list of issues of a given journal.

Thanks to Dr. James Gallagher, consultant to C.I.O.M.S., on more than one occasion I was able to consult the complete collections of the "Index Catalogue" and the "Index Medicus". Now filed in the library of the World Health Organisation in Geneva, they were apparently donated by the original owner, the Society of Nations. These old bibliographies were of crucial help in completing many references.

SOME INDISPENSABLE REFERENCES

This monograph does not pretend to compete with the excellent publications on the history of endoscopy which have appeared in recent years and which have been of great help to me. I refer to the splendid book by Irvin Modlin[4], the well-referenced monograph by Herbert Neumann and Andreas Hellwig[5], the interesting and very personal book "Laterna Magica" by the late Laurits Lauridsen[6], whom I can no longer thank personally, and above all, the monumental history of endoscopy by Drs Michael and Hans Joachim Reuter from Stuttgart[7]. I must also mention the excellent chapter on the history of endoscopy written by William S. Haubrich and James Edmonson in the endoscopy treatise by Michael Sivak, as well as that signed by B.Hirschowitz, I.Modlin, A.Elewaut, M.Cremer, K.Kawai, H. Niwa, R.Fujita and S.Shimizu in the outstanding book "Gastroenterological Endoscopy", recently edited by M.Classen, G.N.J. Tytgat and Ch. Lightdale[9].

Special mention should also be made to the "History of Digestive Endoscopy" by Professor Hirohumi Niwa (Nihon Medical Centre, Tokyo, 1997). As far as I know, the only version available is in Japanese and although this may make it difficult for many of us, it contains many graphic documents of considerable interest.

Other indispensable references are the survey on the first rigid endoscopic instruments written in 1875 by Grünfeld, a Viennese dermatologist who was also an endoscopist[10], and the investigations and the study of the first gastroscopes made in 1901 by Gustav Killian, a well-known laryngologist from Freiburg-im-Breisgau[11]. The superb chapters on oesophagoscopy, gastroscopy and rectoscopy written by the eminent clinician Adolf Gottstein from Breslau in the large "Handbuch" edited by Abderhalden (1920-1926) are authentic milestones in the history of digestive endoscopy and an extraordinary source of information[12].

I would also like to mention recent works, such as the excellent review on gastrointestinal endoscopy by James Edmonson of the Cleveland Medical Association Library, published a decade ago[13], as well as the monographs edited by the Institute for the History of Medicine at Vienna University headed by Dr. Manfred Skopec; these are invaluable sources of information on the early endoscopic instruments[14].

ON MEDICAL LIBRARIES

All the libraries which I have visited have unfailingly provided outstanding help. I should like first to mention the Library Josep Laporte at the Hospital de Sant Pau in Barcelona and its chief librarian, Ms. Teresa Mas, who somehow managed to obtain printed material which initially seemed impossible to locate. The medical school library at the Universitat Central in Barcelona and that of the Universidad Complutense in Madrid were also able to locate books which I was unable to find elsewhere.

Of the libraries abroad, I would like to mention firstly, the Archives of the Institute of the History of Medicine of Vienna University and the Library of the Society of Physicians (Verein der Ärtze) in the same city. Other important sources of bibliographic information were the Bayerische Staatsbibliothek as well as the library of the Medical Faculty at Munich University.

Yet another extremely valuable source of old journals, especially in German, was the German Central Medical Library in Cologne (Germany) (Deutsche Zentralbibliothek für Medizin) which, in the same way as N.L.M., can quickly provide iconographic material of great quality.

In Paris, the central library of the old Faculté de Medecine as well as that of the Faculté de Pharmacie provided books and theses which I was able to consult without any difficulties. I have already mentioned the library at W.H.O., but I must also include the splendid library at the University of Geneva Medical School. The librarians at the Wellcome Institute in London and at the marvellous British Library were extremely helpful, as were the personnel at both the Central Library of Amsterdam University and at the University of Amsterdam Medical Centre.

I would also like to mention other fine libraries, perhaps more limited in the field of medicine but with reference rooms and catalogues of tremendous value, such as those at the Salzburg University and even, to my delight, at the smaller Bayreuth University.

Among the institutions contacted electronically in the United States, the outstanding National Library of Medicine (N.L.M.) was of such value that any further comment is unnecessary. Special thanks should also go to the Library of the Philadelphia College of Physicians where I spent many long hours in my American years and which still boasts the most complete department that I know of for 19th century journals, theses and books.

THE PROBLEM OF PRIORITIES

During my research, it was rather disquieting to encounter such a degree of dogmatism and rivalry between colleagues, often hindering the promising development of instruments and techniques. We have seen this occur since the first endoscopist, Bozzini and his "Lichtleiter", at the end of the 18th century, up until the recent controversy over the first laparoscopic appendectomies and cholecystectomies, repudiated by the majority of surgeons. The contempt with which many innovators have been treated by their contemporaries demonstrates how envy and pride have sometimes been the culprits for the delay in adopting invaluable new technologies.

I found it difficult, if not impossible, to guarantee the legitimacy of some priority claims. I have done all I could to find the origin of instruments and techniques by documenting the data as far as possible with bibliographic references, but I must confess that quite often I have remained unsatisfied with the results. This book describes several controversial claims from individuals who considered they were the first to invent an instrument or to perform some examination. I have often been unable to confirm or negate their claims.

One of the most universal gastroenterologists I have known, Franz Ingelfinger from Boston, used to say that during his tenure as editor of the New England Journal of Medicine, he always avoided publishing papers in which the author claimed to be the first to describe a medical entity (or a procedure) which had not been published previously. He based his rejection not on any moral grounds but simply to protect himself against the deluge of letters that would follow from readers who contested such a priority, from correspondents who wanted to establish their own priority, from those who simply desired respect for what they believed to be the truth and finally, from the few who would seize the opportunity to criticise an editor who had allowed an erroneous claim to pass through.

The point I wish to make here is that more comprehensive research in the future may reveal that some priorities cited in this book should be replaced by claims from other clinicians. As

Ingelfinger stated, "Whatever the reason, to show that the one first is just a second or a third is not too difficult"[15]. Misguided patriotism, which may exaggerate the contributions of an author of the same nationality, or the desire to give due recognition to a little known personality, may also be contributing factors. Moreover, there are many examples of original articles that remained unknown because they were published in journals perhaps in a remote country or in an uncommon language. The Second World War disrupted medical communications for many years to come. In spite of the fact that many papers appeared in the "Index Medicus", the same did not occur with published books. Many of those which were published in Europe between 1938 and 1945 have remained in the dark.

A NOTE ON THE ICONOGRAPHY

In the list of acknowledgements that follows I have tried to express my gratitude to all those people who helped me in obtaining articles and books and also in contacting other institutions and colleagues. Many have provided invaluable illustrations for this book. Whenever possible, I have tried to cite the origin of the figures. Several are from the collection gathered by my father, Dr. Jacinto Vilardell, a gastroenterologist in Barcelona who was trained in Germany, Austria and France. From his different sojourns in foreign countries he returned with large numbers of photographs of teachers, colleagues and instruments in the field of medical and surgical gastroenterology. I have also built up my own collection of photos through the years; some given to me by friends, others from professors and fellow students. I must sincerely apologise for reproducing some pictures whose origin I have been unable to find and which might unintentionally infringe upon publishing rights.

LIMITS OF THIS WORK

Which events are to be considered "historical"? As a rule, I have tried to limit my comments and descriptions to those techniques or instruments which are, or were, in existence for at least 25 years. Unarguably, new applications of endoscopy and new instruments are described every day. We can only speculate about the future; the giant step from Bozzini's modest candle to the videoendoscopic microchip has taken two centuries, but in actual fact, very little changed between the late 18th century and the end of World War Two. True progress began in the mid-20th century, since when it has flourished at a tremendous speed with the introduction of fibreoptics, computerised technologies and greater uniformity of teaching programmes for endoscopists.

There are several current techniques which I have not included in this monograph as I do not consider they are yet "historical" as such. I refer to several novelties and recently introduced procedures which do not seem quite relevant in a historical context, such as endoscopic gastrostomy, which started in the United States in 1980[16]. However, I have included more detailed references to endoscopic ultrasonography, which started around the same time in the USA[17] and in Germany[18]. I have not reviewed other currently used techniques such as image magnification systems with the dissecting microscope, in spite of the fact that they had been tried in Germany as far back as 1954[19] and in the United Kingdom in 1964[20], or chromoscopy –much used today– the first report on which seems to have been presented at the First World Congress of Endoscopy in 1966[21].

The monograph ends by relating how endoscopists first started to meet to exchange experiences, to organise congresses and to create societies, first at national and then at international levels, culminating in what is today the prestigious World Organisation of Digestive Endoscopy (OMED).

It is with deep satisfaction that I dedicate this work to the Spanish Association for Digestive Endoscopy, founded in 1969.

REFERENCES

1. Janowitz H.D., Abittan C.S., Fiedler I.M. A gastroenterological list for the Millenium. J.Clin Gastroenterol 1999; 29: 336-338.
2. Vilardell F. The history of digestive endoscopy in the last century of the second millenium. Acta Gastroenterologica Belgica 2002; 45: 13-16.
3. Pulido M. Index Medicus: cobertura y manejo. Med Clin (Barc) 1987; 88: 500-504.
4. Modlin I. A brief history of endoscopy. ASGE Milano, Multimedia, 1999-2000.
5. Neumann H.A., Hellwig A. Vom Schwertschlucker zur Glasfiberoptik. Die Geschichte der Gastroskopie. München, Urban & Vogel, 2001.
6. Lauridsen L. Laterna Magica in Corpore Humano. Svendborg. Isager Boktryk 1998.
7. Reuter M.A., Reuter H.J. Geschichte der Endoskopie. Band 1-4. Stuttgart-Zürich, Karl Kramer Verlag, 1998.
8. Haubrich W., Edmonson J.H. History of endoscopy in Gastroenterologic Endoscopy, (M. Sivak Ed.) 2nd edition. Philadelphia, W.B.Saunders, 2000: 2-15.
9. Hirschowitz B.J., Modlin I.M. The history of endoscopy - The American perspective. Elewaut A., Cremer M.- The European perspective. Kawai K, Niwa H, Fujita R. - The Japanese perspective. in Gastroenterological Endoscopy. M.Classen, G.N.J. Tytgat, C.J. Lightdale (eds.) Stuttgart, Georg Thieme, 2002: 1-41.
10. Grünfeld J. Zur Geschichte der Endoskopie und der endoskopische Apparate. Allgem. Wien med Zeit 1875; 20: 237-259.
11. Killian G. Zur Geschichte der Oesophago- und Gastroskopie. Deutsch Zschr Chir 1901; 58:499-312.
12. Gottstein A. Die Oesophagoskopie. Die Gastroskopie. Die Rektosigmoidoskopie. Handbuch der biologischen Arbeitsmethoden, Abderhalden E. (ed.) Abt IV, Teil /1, Julius Springer, Berlin, 1926.
13. Edmonson J.M. History of the instruments for gastrointestinal endoscopy. Gastrointest Endosc 1991; 37: S27-S56.
14. Meilsteinen der Endoskopie. 2. Symposium der Internationalen Nitze-Leiter-Forschunggesellschaft für Endoskopie. Literas Universitätsverlag. Wien, 2000.
15. Ingelfinger F. Tubes. Gastroenterology 1978;74: 310-318.
16. Gauderer M.W.L., Ponsky J.L., Izant R.J. Jr. Gastrostomy without laparotomy: a percutaneous endoscopic technique. J Pediatr Surg 1980; 15: 872-875.
17. DiMagno E.P., Buxton J.L., Regan F.T. et al. Ultrasonic endoscope. Lancet 1980 1: 629-631.
18. Strohm W.D., Phillip J., Hagenmüller F., Classen M. Ultrasonic tomography by means of an ultrasound fiber endoscope. Endoscopy 1980; 12: 241-244.
19. Gutzeit H., Teige H. Die Gastroskopie, Lehrbuch und Atlas, München, Urban & Schwarzenberg, 1954
20. Salem S.N., Truelove S.C. Dissection microscope appearances of the gastric mucosa. Brit Med J. 1964; 2: 503-504.
21. Yamakawa J., Naito S., Kanai J. Superficial staining of gastric lesions by fiberscopy. Proceedings 1st World Congress International Society of Endoscopy, Tokyo 1966.:586-590.

Acknowledgements

Carolyn V. Newey IOL. Dip. Trans. for invaluable editorial assistance.

COLLEAGUES

My special thanks for their crucial help to Profs. Meinhard Classen (Munich) and Michel Cremer (Brussels) for many unusual pictures, Joseph Kirsner (Chicago), who sent me the complete references of Dr. Schindler's book, Hans J. Reuter (Stuttgart)for his great kindness in providing images and Günther Seydl (Vienna) for invaluable documents from the Vienna University Archives.

Together with: Heinz Affolter (Basel), Sandro Alessandrini (Rome), Jacinto Arán (+) (Barcelona), J.R. Armengol-Miró (Barcelona), Sir Francis Avery-Jones (+) (London), Joaquín Balanzó, (Barcelona), Michel Cremer (Brussels), Michele Cicala (Rome), Aksel Cruse, (Aarhus), Josep Danón (Barcelona), Jean Pierre Delmont (Nice), Jean Delmont (Marseille), Manuel Diaz Rubio (Madrid), Wolfram Domschke (Münster), André Elewaut (Ghent), James Gallagher (Geneva), Alfred Gangl (Vienna), Joseph Geenen (Milwaukee), Keith S. Henley (Ann Arbor), Harald Henning (Mölln, Ger.), M.Hernández-Bronchud (Barcelona), Basil Hirschowitz (Birmingham, Ala), Edouard Jacobs (Brussels), Keiichi Kawai (Osaka), Gunther Krejs (Graz), Enric Laporte (Barcelona), Laurits Lauridsen (+), (Svendborg, Dk), Gregorz S. Litynski (Wroclaw), Armando Martí-Vicente (Barcelona), Irvin Modlin (Yale), Gabriel Nagy (Roseville, Australia), Hirohumi Niwa (Tokyo), Francesco Orlandi (Ancona), Bergein Overholt (Knoxville,Tenn), Eddie Palmer (New Jersey), Eamonn Quigley (Cork), F.J. Sancho (Barcelona), Alain Segal (Reims), Sacha Segal (Reims), Ludovic Standaert (Ghent), Olaf Stanger (Salzburg), Ramón Trias Rubies (Barcelona), Guido Tytgat (Amsterdam), Christopher Williams (London).

LIBRARIES, INSTITUTES, MUSEUMS

Isabel Astals, Library of the Academy of Medical Sciences, Barcelona. Pablo Ayesta, Audiovisual Department, Research Institute, Hospital de Sant Pau, Barcelona. Coral Bacchetta, Director, Library, Medical Faculty, Universidad Central, Barcelona. Vlatko Bungic, Erich Müller, Bodo-Markus Pregler, Medizinische Lesehalle der Universität, Munich. Ramona Casas, Library of the

Academy of Medical Sciences, Barcelona. Marie Veronique Clin, Directeur, Musée d' Histoire de la Médecine, Université René Descartes, Paris. Dra Maria Crapulli, bibliotecaria Universitá Campus Bio Medico, Rome. Heleen Dyserinck, Director, Library of the Academic Medical Centre, Amsterdam. Fabiola Fernandez, Secretary, Institut de Recerca, Hospital de Sant Pau, Barcelona. Elke Golubew, Secretary to Prof.Classen, Technische Universität Munich. Eugenia Lamont, Secretary, Medizinische Universitätsklinik, Graz. Janice Marohl, Secretary to Dr. J.Geenen. Kathy Marquis, Bentley Historical Library, University of Michigan. Teresa Mas, Head Librarian, Biblioteca Josep Laporte Hospital de Sant Pau, Barcelona. Robert Mills, Royal College of Physicians, Dublin. Bernadette Molitor, Directeur, Departament des Livres Anciens, Bibliothèque de la Faculté de Médecine, Paris. Marie Ange Pompignoli, Directeur, Bibliothèque de la Faculté de Pharmacie, Université de Paris. M. Angels Rodriguez, Secretary, Escuela de Patología Digestiva, Hospital de Sant Pau, Barcelona. Julia Sheppard, Wellcome Institute for the History of Medicine, London. Manfred Skopec, Director, Institute for the History of Medicine, Vienna. Michaela Zykan, Institute for the History of Medicine, Vienna.

OTHER IMPORTANT ACKNOWLEDGEMENTS

José María Cabané, Olympus S.A. Spain, (Barcelona), Lawrence (Larry) Curtiss, former Vicepresident, ACMI, (Concord, MA). Jeff Hecht, (Auburndale MD) author of "City of Light". Michael Lamm, (son of Heinrich Lamm). Enrico Lorenzatto, M.G. Lorenzatto, (Grugliasco, Italy). Haruhito Morishima, Olympus Inc. (Tokyo). Karl Storz S.A. (Tuttlingen, Ger.). Reinhold Wappler Jr. (New Canaan, Conn).

OMGE AND CONGREX

The English edition of this book would not have been possible without the patronage of the World Organisation of Gastroenterology (O.M.G.E.) and of Congrex. I am particulary indebted to Professors Joseph Geenen and Meinhard Classen (O.M.G.E.) to Mrs. Ellen de Ranitz (Congrex) and to the International Digestive Cancer Alliance for their invaluable advice and support.

AULA MÉDICA

My deep gratitude to Mr. José Antonio Ruiz and to Mr. Javier Coello for the outstanding technical quality of the Spanish edition of this book.

DEDICATION

Last but not least, I would like to thank my wife Leonor, my daughters Mercedes and Carmen, my son Javier and my grandchildren Leonor, Ana, Lucia, Nicolas, Carmen and Clara for their endless patience and understanding.

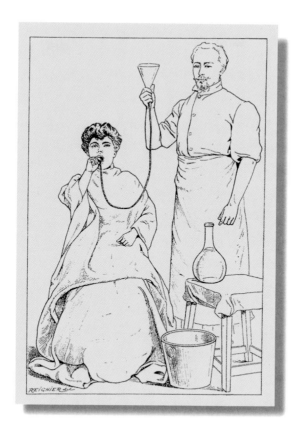

CHAPTER 1

The Forerunners of Endoscopy: tubes and catheters

THERE IS LITTLE DOUBT THAT THE INSERTION OF ANY SORT OF artefacts inside the body orifices for medical reasons emerged in the most remote antiquity.

In his splendid review on the subject, Ralph Major[36] described how tubes, rods, hollow canes and other objects were used for examination purposes, for the extraction of foreign bodies or even perhaps for pleasure. It is possible that the practice of gastric intubation to empty the stomach as a therapeutic procedure might be older than the Christian Era[48].

In 1962, Stöcklin, a Swiss physician[45], visited several primitive indigenous tribes in New Guinea and saw how they used the bent stem of a vine, which was introduced as a probe into the stomach to provoke retching and vomiting and in this fashion empty its contents. He believed that in the Stone Age similar devices were already employed.

In his history of the gastric tube, Major[36] described an artefact made by Oribasius in the fourth century, consisting of ten to twelve leather glove fingers stitched together, most of them filled with wool. This "tube", possibly the first, was pushed into the stomach to induce vomiting. This mechanical stimulus was perhaps more efficient than the feathers used for this purpose by the Romans. According to Maurice Loeper, a professor in Paris, author of an excellent history of gastric secretion[35], it is difficult to decide to whom we should attribute the paternity of gastric tubes and Ingelfinger later agreed with him[30]. In the sixteenth century gastric intubation was known and used to empty the stomach and also for therapeutic purposes by Johannes Arculanus, Hyeronimus Capivacceus and Fabrizio d'Acquapendente.

FABRIZIO D'ACQUAPENDENTE (1537-1619)

Fabrizio was born in the village of that name and died in Padua. He was famous for the discovery of vein valves and for his work on embriology[32] *(Fig. 1)*. This great anatomist designed instruments either to

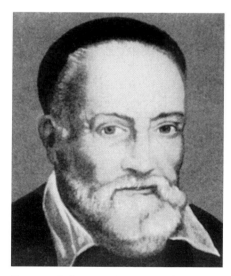

Fig. 1. Fabrizio D'Acquapendente. The great anatomist from Padua (Italy) designed several tools to extract foreign bodies from the oesophagus as well as tubes for feeding (courtesy Dr. F. J. Cortada, Buenos Aires).

extract foreign bodies from the oesophagus or to push them inside the stomach. He also devised a tube for feeding patients who had swallowing disorders. He used a silver tube covered with sheep intestine to ease its introduction into the stomach. The proximal end was wider and funnel-like so that liquids were easily poured into it. Among his various books, one called "De Gula, Ventriculo, Intestinis" (Padua 1617) seems to be the best related to these early forerunners of gastric intubation in which we are interested[35].

GUILHELMUS FABRICIUS HILDANUS (1560-1634)

Hildanus was born in Hilden, Germany (hence Hildanus). Called the father of German surgery, he worked most of his life

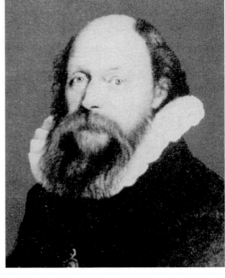

Fig. 2. Fabritius Hildanus. He designed a tube for the extraction of foreign bodies from the oesophagus. (in 100 Portraits de Médecins Illustres, Academia S.P.R.L.) (1960).

in Switzerland and died in Berne[32] *(Fig. 2)*. He designed a gastric tube to extract foreign bodies from the oesophagus which he described in "Observationum et curationum chirurgicarum Centuriae I-IV" as a hollow curved tube made of silver or copper about one foot and a half long, provided with a sponge attached at its distal end. The tube featured multiple perforations which helped in pulling out foreign bodies such as fish bones which might also stick to the sponge. Alternatively, Hildanus would push the foreign body into the stomach *(Fig. 3)*.

THE STOMACH BRUSH

According to Modlin, in the 17th century some physicians already had the idea of "cleaning" the stomach by means of a brush ("Magenkratzer"). Modlin, in his splendid book[39], shows a picture of such an instrument. Usually it consisted of a whalebone, two or three feet long, somewhat curved and provided with a mesh of silk thread firmly attached to its distal end which was rubbed inside the stomach. In some instances, physicians apparently achieved a cure with this method, as they were able to pull residues, pus and necrotic material out of the stomach. According to Stöcklin[45], the indigenous tribes from New Guinea still use vine stems enveloped with hard dried leaves for the same purpose *(Fig. 4)*.

Thomas Willis was apparently the first to dilate the oesophagus in a patient with stenosing oesophagitis using a tube with a sponge fixed at its distal end. Others followed his example[36].

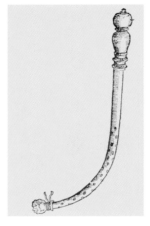

Fig. 3. The Hildanus instrument. A metal tube provided with perforations to pull fishbones and other foreign bodies outside the oesophagus. A sponge was attached to its distal end (ref. 32).

JOHN HUNTER (1728-1793)

The invention of "modern" gastric tubes is often attributed to John Hunter, who used them to withdraw toxic substances from the stomach and also to obtain gastric juice for diagnostic purposes *(Fig. 5)*. Hunter was the youngest of ten brothers and started his surgical training under the supervision of his elder brother William, an anatomist and obstetrician; he was appointed surgeon to the Royal Navy and later to St George's Hospital in London[3]. Hunter observed that gastric secretion discolored "the syrup of violets", a finding which opened the way to chemical techniques for titrating gastric acid using indicators[35]. Hunter used open tubes for feeding patients with oesophageal stenoses. He used flexible tubes made of eel's skin which he introduced using a whalebone as a guide. In the proximal end, which was closed, he attached a pear-shaped rubber bulb as a device for suction or injection.

RENAUD, LARREY, DUPUYTREN, CADET, PHYSICK

Other physicians claimed the paternity of the gastric tube, especially of its rubber version. Casimir Renaud (1802)[42] was one of the first to use a tube to empty the stomach in cases of poisoning. Already in 1801, Larrey (1766-1842) had employed flexible tubes to feed a patient with severe oesophageal wounds, and later on, to empty the stomach. He worked in the service of Dupuytren (1777-1835), the famous Paris surgeon. Larrey used a large syringe full of hot water which he injected in the stomach and then withdrew with the gastric contents, achieving a gastric lavage. Larrey was born in a little village in the Pyrenees (Baudéau, Bagnères de Bigorre) *(Fig. 6)*; he finished his medical training in Toulouse in 1787 and worked thereafter as a ship's surgeon and later on as a military officer. He met Napoleon during the Italian campaign and he followed him in his military adventures. He was appointed personal physician to the Emperor, Surgeon in Chief of La Grande Armée and made Baron Larrey. He was disgraced after the battle of Waterloo where he was made prisoner, but some time later he continued his surgical careeer at the Military Hospital Val de Grâce in Paris[13].

Specific publications of this period are those of Félix Cadet fils[9] who had also worked in Dupuytren's service (Cadet writes his name as Dupuytrein) *(Fig. 7)*. Cadet was probably a pharmacist as in his paper published in the Bulletin de Pharmacie of Paris he states that, "in case of an emergency people run searching for either a practitioner of the art

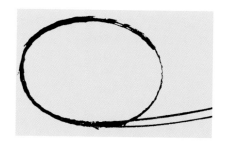

Fig. 4. New Guinea brush made of bent vine stems designed to induce vomiting and to extract foreign bodies (ref. 45).

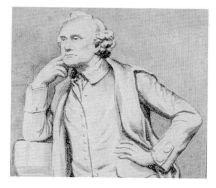

Fig. 5. John Hunter: the famous British anatomist who devised a tube to withdraw gastric contents and to analyze gastric juice (ref. 35).

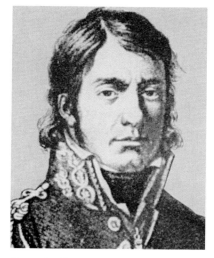

Fig. 6. Baron Dominique Larrey. Napoleon's personal surgeon, he treated patients with severe thoracic wounds by feeding them through a gastric tube (courtesy Dr. F.J.Cortada, Buenos Aires).

or preferably a pharmacy because there one goes directly to the remedy".

Cadet described the technique of Dupuytren and Larrey in great detail. He used a large syringe attached to a rubber tube about 60 cm in length and 2 cm in diameter in its proximal end. It was progressively reduced in caliber down to 6 mm at the distal end which was tapered to avoid injury and was provided with a distal and a lateral hole. The tube was about 2 mm thick. The technique consisted of injecting water and repeatedly aspirating the gastric contents until the toxic substance was presumably removed. Cadet recommended purging the patient afterwards.

Physick, a surgeon from Philadelphia, introduced the gastric tube in the United States[41]. John Syng Physick (1768-1837) *(Fig. 8)* studied medicine at the University of Pennsylvania and then went to London where he trained under John Hunter who had him appointed surgeon at St George's Hospital. He then read a doctoral thesis in Edinburgh and returned to the United States in 1792. He worked at the Pennsylvania Hospital in Philadelphia which had been founded by Benjamin Franklin and in 1805 he was appointed professor of surgery[11]. In 1805, Physick did gastric intubations to treat poisoning using rubber devices made in Paris. Later on he devised a suction pump by modifying a syringe. An improvement of this instrument was made by Weiss in London in 1825 which was further developed by Kussmaul[31].

In conclusion, at the beginning of the 19th century in many hospitals flexible rubber tubes were employed to withdraw poisonous substances from the stomach and to inject antidotes using large syringes. Most of these tubes were made for the Paris hospitals *(Fig. 9)*, particularly by the firm of Joseph Charrière (later Collin)[10]. Rubber was already available but it was uncommon and vulcanization, which would harden it, was not discovered until 1839.

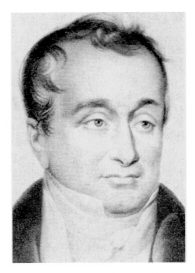

Fig. 7. Baron Guillaume de Dupuytren. (1777-1835) Distinguished surgeon of the Paris Hôtel-Dieu, teacher of Larrey. In his service gastric tubes were used for feeding (courtesy Dr. F. J. Cortada, Buenos Aires).

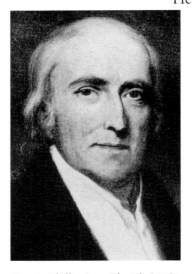

Fig. 8. Phillip Syng Physick (1768-1837). Professor of surgery in Philadelphia, he studied with John Hunter. He was the first to introduce gastric tubes in the United States. Portrait at the University of Pennsylvania (copyright unknown).

CHARRIÈRE AND THE STANDARDIZATION OF TUBE SIZES

Joseph Fréderic Benoît Charrière *(Fig. 10)* deserves a special mention. He was born in 1803 in Cerniat, a small village near La Gruyère

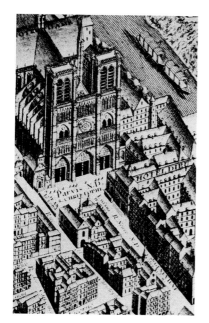

Fig. 9. The famous hospital Hôtel-Dieu in Paris, at the lower right end of the figure, facing Notre Dame Cathedral.

(Switzerland) and died in 1876. In a few years he became the most important maker of surgical instruments in France, under the patronage of Dupuytren, surgeon-in-chief of the Hôtel-Dieu in Paris[6]. At the peak of his career he had 150 employees in his factory, an astonishing figure. He designed lythotryptors, forceps, saws, hypodermic syringes, haemostatic clamps, etc. He was honoured with several distinctions, among them that of Officer of the Legion of Honour.

Along with the many surgical instruments which he devised, were gastric tubes which he manufactured in many diameters. He standardised their size by measuring their diameter using a progressive scale (in thirds of a milimeter, in his own words), printed on cardboard and featuring a series of thirty holes of progressive diameters through which the tubes could be passed[14]. He started with vey thin bougies and ended with large bore tubes for gastric washings. He called the scales "La Filière Charrière". They are still being used to gauge the diameter of sounds, tubes, catheters and fiberoptic bundles[14]; each tube has a number followed by the initial F (French). Thus a 16F tube has an external diameter of 5,33 mm.

According to Boschung[6], Charrière had already introduced his device in 1842. In 1848 he published a catalogue in which he described his gastric tubes as well as the scale which he had invented. The firm Charrière was led later by his son, who died young, and then by some of his former pupils. One of them, Collin, managed to take control of the firm in 1870 continuing the business under the name Maison Charrière-Collin until 1930 when it was bought by the firm Gentile. It finally disappeared in 1978.

Thanks to Charrière's work it has been easy everywhere to compare techniques for the introduction of tubes into the stomach. The Collin catalogue of 1903 features many different types of tubes[10]. Around 1900, a Spanish firm based in Barcelona, Vicente

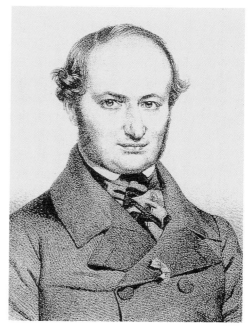

Fig. 10. Joseph Charrière. Of Swiss origin, he was the most important manufacturer of surgical instruments in Paris. He standardised the diameters of gastric tubes by means of a scale which is still used (ref. 6).

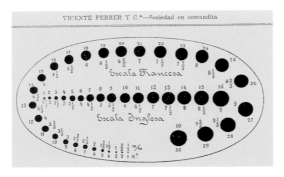

Fig. 11. The Charrière gauge for measuring gastric tubes (from the catalogue of the firm Vicente Ferrer in Barcelona, around 1900).

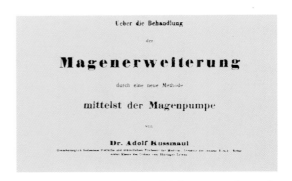

Fig. 12. Monograph by Adolph Kussmaul on the "Treatment of gastric dilatation by means of a gastric pump" (1869).

Ferrer, published its own catalogue featuring Charrière's cardboard gauges and also including the corresponding English measures *(Fig. 11)*.

KUSSMAUL, EWALD, LEUBE, BOAS, FAUCHER

Kussmaul's pump: Kussmaul, whom some authors have named "the father of gastroenterology" was the first to use gastric tubes for therapeutic purposes in diseases of the stomach[29, 36] *(Fig. 12)*. After 1867, Kussmaul used the gastric tube not only for gastric lavage but also for the treatment of oesophageal stenoses. For that purpose he employed rigid hard rubber tubes[31]. He also fitted his tubes to the suction pump devised by Weiss[26] to treat gastric dilatation secondary to pyloric stenosis *(Fig. 13)*. He demonstrated his modified pump at the Congress of Naturalist Physicians in Freiburg where he also presented an oral communication on gastroscopy which we will discuss in another chapter of this book. In 1869, Kussmaul published a long paper on gastric stasis and his treatment became popular around the world[31]. Kussmaul tried to convince patients to do their own gastric washings, which were usually accepted willingly. For that particular purpose he recommended soft tubes and simple siphonage instead of the rigid tubes and the pump which could cause tears in the gastric mucosa if they were not properly monitored[2]. Around 1870 Dieulafoy in Paris began to use Kussmaul's method extensively.

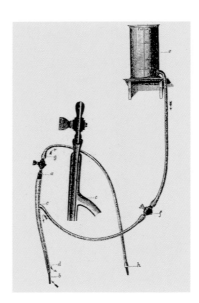

Fig. 13. Kussmaul's tube and pump used for gastric suction and lavage in cases of stomach dilatation (ref. 31).

Leube, Ewald, Boas and the test meal: In 1871 Wilhelm Olivier Leube (1842-1922) *(Fig. 14)* was the first to use gastric intubation as a scientific diagnostic method[33]. Leube was born in Ulm in 1842 and died near the Bodensee in 1922. He studied medicine in Tübingen, Zürich and in 1872 at the University in Erlangen where he organised a gastroenterology service which was to stay in the front line of German gastroenterology under his successors Norbert Henning and Ludwig Demling. He quit Erlangen for Iena and ended his career as Rector of the University of Würzburg. Leube used a relatively soft gastric tube made of red rubber, including a whalebone as a guide for insertion. If the stomach emptied within seven hours after a meal and gastric juice appeared to have normal characteristics, Leube concluded that the patient had no organic disease and classified him as a case of nervous dyspepsia.

Gastric intubation became the standard method for the study of gastric motility and gastric emptying. Leube later used a thinner rubber tube, more acceptable to the patient, to aspirate gastric juice and implement techniques for the fractional analysis of gastric juice. He started using a variety of stimuli which became more and more popular in Germany, the so-called "test meals" devised by Leube, Ewald and particularly by his pupil Boas[4] *(Figs. 15 and 16)* who put an end to his life after being persecuted by the Nazis[46].

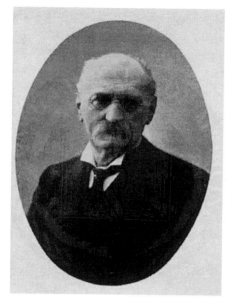

Fig. 14. Wilhelm Leube was the first to use test meals for the study of gastric physiology (courtesy National Library of medicine, copyright unknown).

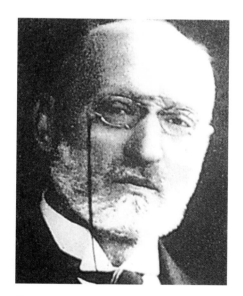

Fig. 15. Istmar Boas, the great clinician from Berlin, a pupil of Ewald. Portrait of his Berlin years. He had to leave Germany persecuted by the Nazis because of his Jewish origin. He went to Vienna but he committed suicide because of the German occupation of Austria (courtesy Falk Foundation).

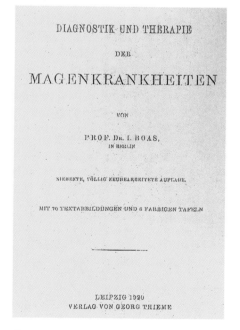

Fig. 16. Istmar Boas was a keen student of gastric secretion. His book "Magen Krankheiten" made him famous all over the world.

Leube gave the patients a standard meal including soup, meat, potatoes and vegetables which was used in many centres until the 1920s, when it was replaced by a simple Ewald meal consisting of two slices of bread and two glasses of water. I saw this Ewald test performed at the University of Pennsylvania until the mid-fifties.

Carl Ewald, the eldest of two brother physicians, was born in Berlin in 1845 and died in the same city in 1915 *(Fig. 17)*. He was the mentor of Boas, Katsch and many other investigators of gastric secretion[20]. In 1874 Ewald sampled gastric contents using flexible pieces of rubber gas pipes in which he cut lateral holes. He introduced them into the stomach after lubrication with olive oil. The large bore Ewald tube was used mostly in Germany but also in the United States. It became a very useful instrument to empty the stomach before gastroscopy[12]. Possibly the best indication for its use was gastric lavage in cases of pyloric stenosis due to peptic ulcer, a syndrome which nowadays has practically disappeared from the gastroenterology wards.

Rosenows' suction pump, which was connected to a vacuum bottle, became popular around that time *(Fig. 18)*. Many surgeons like Péan (1879), Billroth (1881) and Tuffier (1911) used stomach pumps for gastric suction after gastrectomy.[37]

After that time, many devices for intubation became available. Einhorn, Rehfuss, Debove, Ryle, Wilkins, Hess, Pawlesky, Hemmeter, Diamond, Lagerlof and Wangensteen described their own tubes. With veiled irony, Franz Ingelfinger commented *(Fig. 19)*, "By using a knob with five

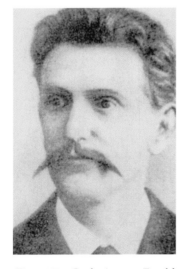

Fig. 17. Carl Anton Ewald. Professor in Berlin, teacher of Boas, Katsch and many other great German clinicians. He devised a gastric tube to withdraw gastric juice for diagnostic purposes. The Ewald test meal (bread and water) was still used around 1950 (ref. 47).

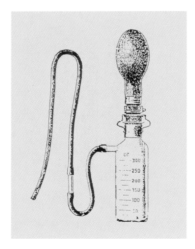

Fig. 18. Rosenow's pump, used to withdraw the gastric contents by means of a tube connected with a vacuum bottle (1908) (ref. 26).

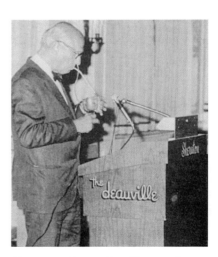

Fig. 19. Franz Ingelfinger, famous American physiologist and gastroenterologist, swallowing a gastric tube and lecturing at the same time. (courtesy Dr. F. Ingelfinger).

instead of four perforations or by cutting elyptical rather than round holes in a catheter type tip, one could proudly invent and name after himself a new gastric or duodenal tube...".[30].

Secretory stimuli also proliferated: tea, alcohol, bread and water, meat broth, etc. Until at least 1950, gastric analysis was done at the University of Pennsylvania using stimuli of that sort, to be replaced by histamine injections and synthetic gastrin analogues around 1960[47]. Little by little a semiology of gastric secretion was created: hyperacidity suggested duodenal ulcer, while achlorhydria indicated gastric atrophy or carcinoma[4, 20, 28, 47].

THE FAUCHER'S TUBE

In France and Spain the most popular gastric tube was the one designed by Faucher which was similar to Leube's tube but of a larger bore. It was attached to a glass funnel for the introduction of fluids for lavage. It was manufactured by the firm Galante and later on also by Collin *(Fig. 20)*.

Possibly the most comprehensive study on gastric lavage was done in 1882 by a physician from Barcelona, José Armangué who wrote a series of 18 articles on the subject which were published in two different journals. Armangué minutiously described oesophageal bougienage, oesophageal tubes for feeding, stomach lavage and aspiration for gastric dilatation. The papers comprised a series of illustrative case reports observed in the Hospital Santa Creu in Barcelona and included a huge list of references[2] *(Fig. 21)*.

According to Armangué, in 1879 Faucher presented his "undeservedly praised" oral communication on his tube at the Académie de Médecine in Paris. Although he was not the first to use gastric lavage in France, his method was readily adopted as it was easy to perform and devoid of danger *(Fig. 22)*.

Henry Faucher was born in Paris in 1848, studied medicine there and received the Barbier prize of the Medical Faculty upon graduation in 1875. He was an intern at several hospitals in Paris (Beaujon, Saint Louis and Hôtel-Dieu). He employed a soft red rubber tube (British rubber) 8 to 12 mm in diameter. The 10 mm model was the most popular; it was

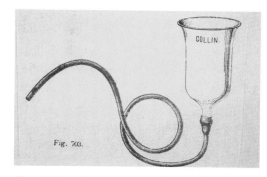

Fig. 20. Faucher's tube manufactured by the firms Galante et fils and Collin from Paris (1900). It was used extensively for stomach lavage in France and in Spain. (Catalogue of the firm Collin, courtesy Dr. J.Danón, Fundación Uriach).

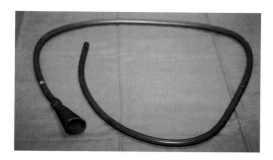

Fig. 21. One of Faucher's tubes, used at the Hospital de Sant Pau in Barcelona around 1930.

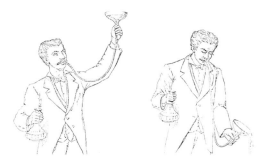

Fig. 22. A demonstration of a self-administered gastric lavage with Faucher's tube (Faucher's doctoral thesis 1881, page 13) (ref. 13).

1.50 meters in length with both ends open, to one of which the funnel, made either of glass or metal, was attached. Faucher recommended the glass funnel which allowed the physician to assess the amount of fluid entering the stomach.

The tube had a mark to indicate the depth required to enter the stomach. The emptying of the gastric contents was done by simple siphonage. Some patients succeeded in lavaging the stomach themselves. According to Armangué, the tube was very cheap and cost only the equivalent of a few pennies in 1882. Faucher published several papers and in 1881 he wrote a doctoral thesis on his device. The President of the Jury was the famous cardiologist Potain, to whom Faucher dedicated his thesis[22].

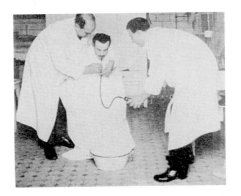

Fig. 23. Gastric lavage performed in Dr. F. Gallart-Mones's service at the Hospital de Sant Pau (Barcelona) (around 1920).

Faucher's method was used in Spain for the first time in 1877[19]. He recommended its use for the treatment of dyspepsia, gastric dilatation, chronic gastric ulcer and in some cases of hysteria. The palliative treatment of gastric cancer was another indication (Fig. 23).

Other instruments, manufactured by Collin such as the one designed by Tuffier, a well-known surgeon from Paris (Figs. 24-25), included double lumen tubes which allowed injection of water through one and suction through the other. The Audhouy tube consisted of two separate tubes glued together. Collin also made curved tubes provided with wire guides to render their introduction less difficult[2]. Einhorn's double lumen tube was similar; the stomach was emptied by gravity. A water container was previously placed above the patient's head. (Fig. 26). Its rubber distal end featured several holes to improve suction.

In Germany and in the United States the Ewald tube became the most popular. Schindler recommended gastric lavage before gastroscopy by using an Ewald tube number 11 or 12 of the German scale, corresponding to Charrière French 33 to 36. (10.7 - 11.7 mm). According to Schindler, the tube should have lateral holes but the distal end should be closed[43]. Schindler also used Ewald's tube to detect an obstruction at the cardia

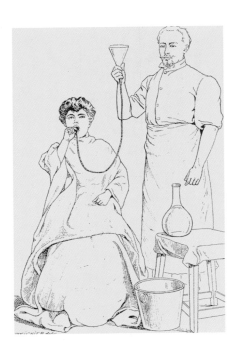

Fig. 24. Gastric lavage performed with Tuffier's tube (ref. 37).

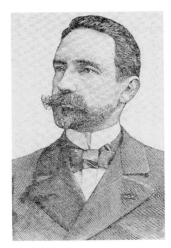

Fig. 25. Théodore Tuffier, famous Paris surgeon (1857-1921) specialised in digestive and thoracic surgery. He introduced enemas with bismuth for radiological studies of the colon in France (ref. 40).

which would have prevented the gastroscope from entering the stomach. He also recommended that the lavage should be done several hours before the examination as the gastric mucosa may change its colour after recent washings and "make a diagnosis of mucosal atrophy difficult".

The introduction of tubes into the stomach was not entirely devoid of danger and already in 1884 the death of a patient after gastric intubation was reported[8]. Armangué also published two cases of pneumonia apparently due to washing the stomach with "excessively cold water"[2].

Until the mid-twentieth century, gastric aspiration and lavage before retiring were standard procedures in patients who vomited because of gastric retention due to pyloric ulcers with stenosis. It was a relevant activity for all of us who were on duty as intern and resident physicians in most gastroenterology services around the world.

Quoting Kussmaul, "I often had the thought, when I observed unfortunate patients in the wretched prodromal phase of a protracted period of vomiting that I might relieve their suffering by using a stomach pump because the withdrawal from the stomach of large amounts of putrescent acid contents should readily alleviate unbearable retching and heartburn".

Gastrodiaphanoscopy

Apart from the use of tubes for the study of gastric contents and the therapeutic attempts to empty the stomach in cases of poisoning or pyloric stenosis, there was little that the physician could do to identify diseases of the upper gastrointestinal tract. Thus clinicians greatly developed their sensory ability: auscultation, percussion and palpation were practiced with refined techniques, as shown by the second edition of a 389-page book[27] dealing exclusively with abdominal palpation which its author, Th. Hausmann, described in painstaking detail. In his preface to the work, his teacher Ewald, says, "The researcher should in some way be able to look into the abdominal cavity with the tips of his fingers" (Fig. 27).

However, clinicians were not satisfied with just the physical examination and taking advantage of the invention of the gastric tube, tried other diagnostic techniques, such as diaphanoscopy.

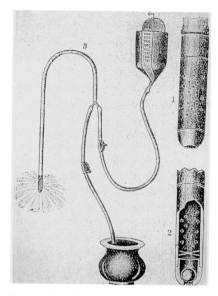

Fig. 26. Einhorn's pump for gastric irrigation and lavage (ref. 16).

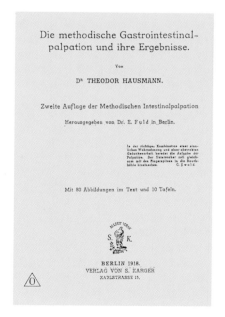

Fig. 27. Title page of the large book that the German clinician Theodor Hausmann, a pupil of Ewald, wrote on abdominal palpation. A second edition was published in 1918.

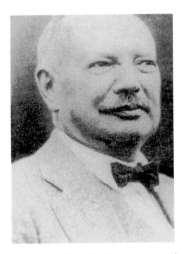

Fig. 28. Max Einhorn practiced gastroenterology in New York. He was the teacher of Henry Bockus. He designed several kinds of gastric and duodenal tubes as well as the diaphanoscope. (Dr. H. L. Bockus' archive).

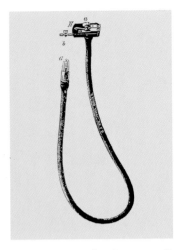

Fig. 29. Einhorn's gastrodiaphanoscope which lit the stomach by transillumination. In a dark room, the glow of the lamp through the abdominal wall allowed to roughly assess the size and contour of the stomach (ref. 17).

Gastrodiaphanoscopy was based on the introduction of an electrical source of light into the stomach which would produce such brightness inside the abdominal cavity that the shape and configuration of the stomach could be roughly assessed by transillumination. Apparently, diaphanoscopy was first tried by P.L.A. Cazelave in 1845[13]. Max Einhorn, the mentor of Henry L. Bockus, was the first to devise an instrument which consisted of a rather thin gastric tube with an incandescent Edison lamp attached to its distal end and connected through wires to a battery and an external switch. The instrument was named "gastrodiaphane" and was employed extensively before the advent of x-rays around 1908[17] (Figs. 28, 29 and 30).

The patient was ordered to drink one or two glasses of cold water to prevent the lamp from excessively heating the gastric wall and the examining room had to be darkened to be able to perceive the shadow of the stomach through the abdominal wall. The examination was carried out with the patient in the standing position. The greatest usefulness of the method apparently was the diagnosis of gastric dilatation secondary to pyloric stenosis. However, both Einhorn and Meltzing[30] were able to diagnose gastric carcinomas (obviously of large size) (Figs. 31 and 32).

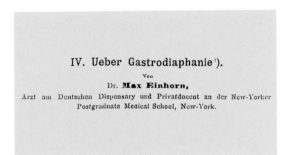

IV. Ueber Gastrodiaphanie¹).

Von

Dr. Max Einhorn,

Arzt am Deutschen Dispensary und Privatdocent an der New-Yorker Postgraduate Medical School, New-York.

Fig. 30. The original article by Einhorn describing diaphanoscopy of the stomach. It was published in a German journal (ref. 17).

XVI.

(Aus der medicinischen Poliklinik in Rostock.)

Magendurchleuchtungen.

Untersuchungen über Grösse, Lage und Beweglichkeit des gesunden und des kranken menschlichen Magens.

Von

C. A. Meltzing,

Cand. med.

(Fortsetzung.)

B. Pathologischer Theil.

Fig. 31. Meltzing, a medical student (Medizin Candidat) who became known later because of the invention of the gastrocamera, was also a pioneer of diaphanoscopy.

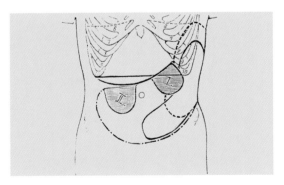

Fig. 32. Transillumination with the diaphanoscope of a gastric cancer. Drawings made by Meltzing showing the displacement of the tumoral mass when the stomach, previously empty, was filled with air (ref. 38).

Mas Einhorn[5] was born in Suchowol (Poland), studied in Riga and went to medical school in Berlin where he graduated in 1884. There he was one of Ewald's pupils. He emigrated to the United States, became an American citizen and took part in World War 1914-1918 as an officer in the Medical Corps. For many years he was chief of medicine at the Lennox Hill Hospital in New York, where among others, he trained Henry Bockus from Philadelphia. According to Bockus[5] he was a very ingenious person; besides the diaphanoscope, he designed the first duodenal tube with which he studied gallbladder emptying and pancreatic secretion. Later on he experimented with oral cholecystography. In 1897, he was one of the founders of the A.G.A. (American Gastroenterological Association).

In accord with his Germanic education, Einhorn was very authoritarian and did not easily tolerate contradiction. Bockus tells that on one occasion while making rounds with him in the hospital he told a patient that she looked better, to which the lady answered, "On the contrary, Dr. Einhorn, today I am much worse!" Einhorn replied curtly, "Professor Einhorn says that you are better. Have a good day!" leaving the patient and Dr. Bockus bemused. He died at the age of 91 at the Lennox Hill Hospital where he had spent the greatest part of his professional life[5].

Diaphanoscopy did not have the expected success. Hemmeter thought that transillumination could provide images compatible with the existence of a tumour only in lesions localised in the anterior wall of the stomach. He quotes a review by W.H. Welch of 1300 cases of gastric cancer of which only 30 had grown in the anterior gastric wall, somewhat more than 2.3 per cent. On the other hand, according to Hemmeter's observations, a significant shadow could be provided only by tumours at least 1.5 to 2 cm in thickness, a relatively rare occurrence.

Enemas, rectal tubes and bougies for dilation.

In the same vein that tubes and catheters in their different modalities were the forerunners of endoscopic examinations of the upper gastrointestinal tract, similar events occurred at the other end of the gut. Tubes, sounds and bougies were inserted into the rectum[14]. The main difference between the two techniques was the fact that faecal material was often present in the bowel and required the previous practice of enemas, as is still done today.[24]

The introduction of tubes through the anus as a diagnostic or therapeutic method dates also from very ancient times. Solid rectal tubes were described in Hindu manuscripts before the Christian era and the practice of enemas using hollow tubes was known to the Egyptians and was of current use among

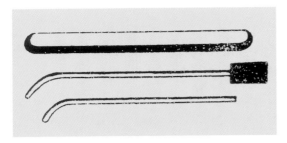

Fig. 33. Artefacts made in India before the Christian Era to examine the rectum (ref. 32).

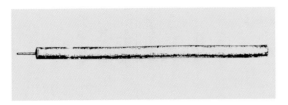

Fig. 34. Tube used by the Choco Indians from the Amazonic region to practice enemas (ref. 32).

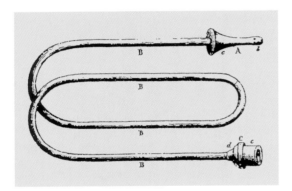

Fig. 35. Clyster for rectal irrigations designed by Regnier de Graaf. In De Graaf R. "De virorum organis generationi inservientibus, de clysteribus et de usu siphonis in anatomia" Leyden and Rotterdam, 1668.

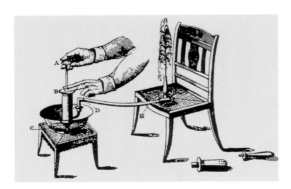

Fig. 36. The Jukes device for rectal irrigations (1831) (ref. 40).

primitive tribes, such as some indigenous inhabitants of the Amazonic region[32] (Figs. 33 and 34). The introduction in Europe of rubber from South America helped a great deal as adequately flexible tubes were less dangerous than previous devices made of wood or metal.[32]

Colonic lavage was done for therapeutic purposes in cases of severe constipation and faecal impaction, but also among some populations for religious reasons, mainly to achieve the "purity" of the person[24]. It is perhaps fitting to comment here on the boom of colonic lavage in some European spas where until recently, total irrigation of the colon was performed with double lumen tubes which allowed injection and withdrawal of water in amounts of at least 10 liters. These methods are still used in so-called "natural" medicine[24, 32].

Besides the enema apparatus devised in the sixteenth century[40] by the Dutch physician De Graaf (Fig. 35), best known for his description of ovarian follicles, one of the first "modern" bowel irrigators was that of Jukes (1831) (Fig. 36) in England. It was followed by that of Eguisier[15] in Paris (1848) (Fig. 37) and the rubber syringe designed by Higginson which could produce a vacuum by squeezing a rubber ball (Fig. 38).

One of the best known colonic lavage tubes in 1920-1930 was designed by the American proctologist Pennington. It was provided with a valve to facilitate the entrance of water at 37-38 C. The patient was supine with flexed knees. The valve was shut once in a while to let the washing fluid leave the colon. Patients received series of lavages and some of them got so used to them that cases of addiction to enemas have been described[18] (Fig. 39). Pennington's tubes were made by the firm Sharp and Smith. The firm Collin from Paris also made several models of rectal tubes.

Constipation was treated by several physicians with olive oil enemas in smaller containers. Pennington also designed a curved aluminum tube with a bulbous enlargement at its distal end which prevented the tube from slipping out during rectal contractions[40]. Insertion of rectal tubes to ease the passage of excessive flatus is still used today.

REFERENCES

1 Acquapendente, Fabricius G. di. Opera chirurgica in duas partes divisa. Padua 1617.

2 a) Armangué J. Apuntes históricos sobre el lavado gástrico y cateterismo del estómago Rev Ciencias Médicas Barcelona 1882; año VIII: 196-198, 235-239, 292-296, 355-360, 423-428, 488-492, 549-554, 614-619. b) Armangué y Tuset J. Del Cateterismo y del lavado del estómago. Rev. de Clin Medica. 1882; 1:26-29, 109-112, 148-152, 163-166, 235-236, 240-251.

3 Bailey H., Bishop WJ. Notable names in medicine and surgery. Second edition. London, H. K. Lewis, 1946.

4 Boas I. Diagnostik und Therapie der Magenkrankheiten. 8. Aufl. Leipzig, Thieme, 1925.

5 Bockus H. L. The Einhorn story. Gastroenterology 1978; 74: 949-950.

6 Boschung U. Joseph-Frédéric-Benoît Charrière (1803-1876): París surgical instrument maker from Switzerland. Caduceus 1988; 4: 34-46.

7 Brunn W., von. Von Katheter und Bougie bis zur Wende des 19 Jahrhunderts Dermat Wschr 1927; 84:107.

8 Bundy A. D. Death from the introduction of a stomach tube. Med Record 1884; 26: 504-505.

9 Cadet F. Fils. Secours à administrer dans les empoisonnements, d'après la méthode de M. Dupuytrein. Bulletin de Pharmacie, tome 2, 2ème année, (feb.) Paris, D. Colas imprimeur 1810: 62-65.

10 Collin fabricant d'instruments de chirurgie. (Maison Charrière, catálogo, París 1903.

11 Corner G. W. Two centuries of medicine. A history of the school of medicine, University of Pennsylvania. Philadelphia, J. B. Lipincott, 1965.

12 Dagradi A. E., Stempien S. The Ewald tube, an important adjunct to gastroscopy Gastrointest Endosc 1967; 13: 36-38.

13 Dechambre A., Lereboullet L. Dictionnaire encyclopédique des Sciences Médicales, París, Asselin-Masson, 1866-1889.

14 Edmonson J. M. Joseph-Frédéric-Benoît Charrière and the French scale. Gastrointest Endosc 2001; 53: 19-20A.

15 Eguisier C. Rapport sur un appareil nommé irrigateur inventé par Eguisier. Séance du 21 Novembre . Bull Acad Nat Med 1848-1849; 14.

16 Einhorn Max. Diseases of the Stomach. New York, William Wood, 1896.

17 Einhorn Max. Ueber Gastrodiaphanie, Berliner Klin Wschr. 1893; 51:1307-1309.

18 Engel G. L. Psychological processes and gastrointestinal disorders: laxative and enema addiction. en Gastroenterologic Medicine (M. Paulson (ed) Philadelphia, Lea & Febiger, 1969: 1433.

19 Esquerdo P. Estudios de Clínica Médica. Gac med Catalana 1881; 1: 471-477.

20 Ewald G. A. , Boas I. Beitrage zur Physiologie und Pathologie der Verdauung. Virchows Arch f. Path. Anat 1885; 51: 325-345.

21 Faucher H. Du traitement des maladies de l'estomac par les lavages. Jour de Thér (Paris) 1880; 7: 568-570.

22 Faucher H. Du lavage de l'estomac, procedé opératoire, indications, résultats. Thèse pour le Doctorat en Médecine, n° 167, (tome 8), Paris, F. Pichonet, A. Cotillon imprimeurs, 1881:1-52.

23 Friedenwald J., Morrison S. The history of the development of the stomach tube with some notes on the duodenal tube. Bull Hist Med 1936; 4 425-454.

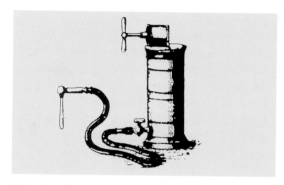

Fig. 37. Eguisier's rectal irrigation device (Paris, 1848) (ref. 15).

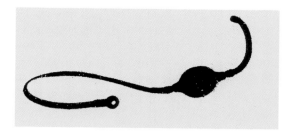

Fig. 38. Higginson's syringe for colonic lavage. The rubber ball created a vacuum which allowed suction of the colonic contents (ref. 40).

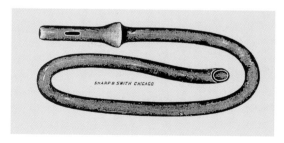

Fig. 39. Pennington's rectal tube used to treat meteorism by easing the passage of flatus. The manufacturers were Sharp & Smith (ref. 40).

[24] Friedenwald J., Morrison S. The history of the enema with some notes on related procedures. Bull Hist Med 1940;8: 68-114, 239-276.

[25] Gurlt E. Biographisches Lexicon der hervorragender Ärzte aller Zeiten und Völker. Berlin-Wien, V. V. 1934.

[26] Gumprecht F. Die Technik der speziellen Therapie. Vierte Aufgabe. Jena, Gustav Fischer, 1906.

[27] Hausmann Th. Die methodische Gastrointestinale Palpation und ihre Ergebnisse. 2. Auflage. Berlin, Karger, 1918.

[28] Hemmeter J. C. The early diagnosis of cancer of the stomach. Medical Record N. Y. 1899; 56:577-583.

[29] Hollander F., Penner A. History and development of gastric analysis procedure Am J Dig Dis 1939; 6: 739-743.

[30] Ingelfinger F. J. Tubes. Gastroenterology 1978;74:310-318.

[31] Kussmaul A. Uber die Behandlung der Magenweiterung durch eine neue Methode mittelst der Magenpumpe. Dtsch Arch Klin Med 1869; 6: 455-500.

[32] Lain Entralgo P. Historia Universal de la Medicina, Barcelona, Salvat editores, 1975.

[33] Leube W. O. Beiträge zur Diagnostik der Magenkrankheiten. Deutsch Archiv f. klin Medicin. 1883;33: 1-21.

[34] Lockhart-Mummery J. P. Modified rectal bougie. Lancet 1937; 1: 874.

[35] Loeper M. Histoire de la sécrétion gastrique. Paris, Masson, 1924.

[36] Major, A. R. History of the stomach tube. Ann Med Hist 1934; 6: 500-509.

[37] Mathieu A, Sencert I, Tuffier Th. Traité Medico-chirurgical des maladies de l'estomac et de l'oesophage. Paris, Masson, 1913.

[38] Meltzing C. A. Magendurchleuchtungen. Zeitschrift f. Klin Med 1893; 27: 411-445.

[39] Modlin I. M. A brief history of endoscopy. Milano, Multimed, 2000.

[40] Pennington J. R. A treatise in the diseases and injuries of the rectum, anus and pelvic colon. Philadelphia, P. Blakiston, 1923.

[41] Physick, P. S. Account of a new mode of extracting poisonous substances from the stomach. Eclectic Repertory 1813; 3: 111-113.

[42] Renaud, C. Essai sur les contrepoisons de l'arsenic. Paris, an X, Thèse de París n. 39, 1802.

[43] Schindler R. Gastroscopy. The endoscopic study of gastric pathology 2 ed. New York. Hafner, 1966. p. 76, 81, 82.

[44] Shepard W. L. Two new forms of enema apparatus Brit Med J 1872, 1, 670.

[45] Stöcklin W. H. Die Erfindung der Magensonde. Gesnerus 1981; 1/2: 237-246.

[46] Teichmann W. Istmar Boas (1858-1939) Freiburg i. Br. Falk Foundation, 1992.

[47] Vilardell F. Notas para una historia de la secreción gástrica Rev Esp Enf Apar Digest 1969; 28: 455-466.

[48] Wilbur D. L. The history of diseases of the stomach and duodenum with reference also to their etiology. Eusterman GB, Balfour DC (eds.) The stomach and duodenum, Philadelphia, WB Saunders, 1936.

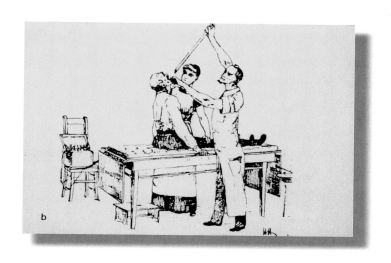

CHAPTER 2

Endoscopy from Bozzini to Kussmaul

PHILLIP BOZZINI (1773-1809) AND HIS "LICHLEITER»

EXAMINING GREEK AND ROMAN VASES AND BAS-RELIEFS, columns with Romanesque capitals or medieval manuscripts, the historian can readily identify medical devices such as specula or pincers and observe scenes in which physicians from all parts of the antique world perform procedures which may be interpreted as attempts to endoscopy.

The word "speculum", which is used to define the majority of these very old instruments, differs somewhat in meaning from one dictionary to another. In some (Littré, Dorland, Oxford), a speculum is "an instrument for dilating cavities of the human body for inspection". Other dictionaries, such as that of the Spanish Royal Academy or the French Larousse, are more specific and state that a speculum "allows examination of body cavities by means of the reflection of light", which implies the use of a light source. Still other dictionaries (Webster) add that a speculum should have a tubular shape. A speculum may also be a "reflector of polished metal or glass".

However, although these definitions are somewhat different, the majority of medical historians agree that the first formal attempt to inspect the natural orifices of the body with a kind of tubular speculum using a lighting system other than sunlight, was made by Phillip Bozzini. In 1806 he invented the "Lichtleiter" ("Light conductor"), an instrument which consisted of a metal tube lit by a candle and provided with a mirror that could reflect the candle light to the body cavities (Fig. 1).

The "Light conductor" was the first endoscopic instrument and the forerunner of all successive attempts by other physicians, mainly French, to visualise the inside of the body. I am greatly indebted to Professor Hans Joachim Reuter from Stuttgart for his detailed investigations on Bozzini and for his outstanding contributions to the his-

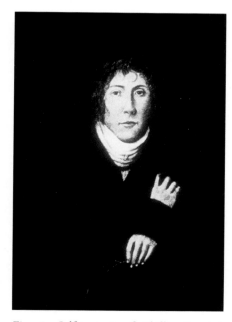

Fig. 1. Self-portrait of Phillip Bozzini, inventor of the first useful instrument for endoscopy, the "Lichtleiter" (light conductor). The original painting is in the Archives of the city of Frankfurt.

tory of endoscopy, such as the organisation of the Nitze-Leiter Endoscopy Museum currenty located at the Josephinum in Vienna, as well as for his magnum opus on the History of Endoscopy which he wrote together with his son, Dr. Mathias Reuter[33, 34].

Bozzini, whose father came from a family of Italian nobility, was born in Mainz. He began his medical training in the city of his birth and later in Jena. He graduated from Jena University in 1796 and started to practice general medicine and obstetrics in 1803 in Frankfurt after several years as an army physician. His interest in endoscopy developed from his work in gynaecology. A similar path was followed in years to come by other endoscopists.

In 1805 Bozzini wrote a letter to the Archduke Karl, brother of the Emperor Franz I who lived in Vienna, explaining that he had invented an instrument which allowed the examination of natural cavities of the body[29]. Bozzini published his invention in a medical journal in 1806 and one year later he wrote a monograph illustrated with his own drawings in which he described his instrument in detail. With the device, rays of light were directed into the inner cavities and an image was reflected in the eye of the observer[27] *(Figs. 2 and 3)*.

The "Lichleiter" consisted of two parts. The light source was a leather covered metal container provided with a large round opening divided by a vertical partition. A wax candle was placed on one side and fixed with springs so that the flame was always

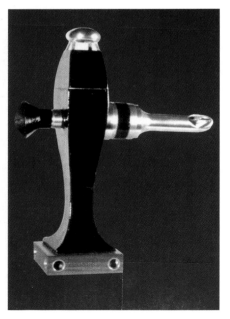

Fig. 2. Bozzini's "Lichtleiter", a reproduction made according to the inventor's original drawings. (Steno Museum, Aarhus, courtesy Dr. Laurits Lauridsen)

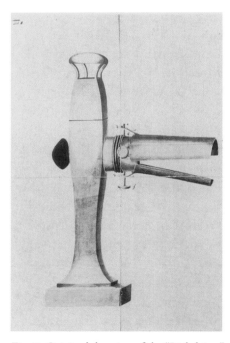

Fig. 3. Original drawing of the "Lichtleiter" by Bozzini (courtesy of Prof. H.J.Reuter).

in the same position. The second part consisted of a concave mirror behind the candle which reflected its light through an examining tube fitted in the round opening, facing the cavity to be examined. A collimating lens was attached on the side facing the light source. Bozzini constructed various tubes of several sizes for the inspection of the auditory canal, the urethra and the rectum[16]. He also made an "angle conductor" provided with two mirrors, a concave one placed on one side and a plane mirror on the other side which apparently helped him inspect the pharynx, the larynx and the oesophagus[4, 5].

Although Bozzini did not publish any results of examinations in human beings, he suggested that his instrument could visualise urethral inflammation, fistulae from necrotic bone lesions, tumours in the rectum and abdominal cavity after paracentesis for ascites (possibly the first attempt to perform laparoscopy). The "Lichleiter" was used to examine cadavers and also some healthy persons in Vienna and the protocols are still available[36]. The favourable report written by the surgeons of the Josephs Akademie, the so-called Josephinum, a teaching centre for military physicians, where the instrument was tried on the 17th of January 1807, was contradicted by the overwhelmingly negative opinion of the Medical Faculty of the traditional university. Apparently, the professors of the Medical Faculty were displeased because the "Lichleiter" had not been shown to them before its presentation to the military surgeons of the Josephinum *(Fig. 4)*.

The members of the Medical Faculty therefore made a report to Emperor Franz II in which they expressed the view that the "Lichleiter" would always be "a toy" even if it could be perfected and that diagnoses should be based on common sense and skill with the digital examination ("Das Urtheil des rationelles Arztes und der Finger des Erfahrenen")[44]. In their statement they mentioned the drawbacks of the instrument: the small visual field (one inch in diameter) and its painful introduction when there were lesions in the cavity to be examined. In spite of the protection offered by Archduke Karl, under whom Bozzini had served, and the support of other friends, the work of Bozzini was never recognised officially and his contribution, although very relevant, was practically forgotten *(Figs. 5 A - B)*.

There is no doubt, however, that the "Lichleiter", a sort of polyscope, contributed decisively to the progress of medical diagnosis. Bozzini was the first to show that one could illuminate the inside of the body cavities introducing a ray of light which could be directed by means of mirrors and that the image could be magnified by lenses, as shown in his own drawings of the "Lichleiter" made on copper plates. His followers took

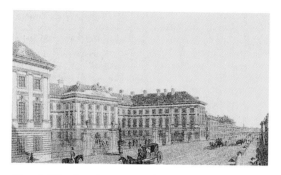

Fig. 4. The Josephinum, Military Medical Academy founded by Emperor Joseph II where Bozzini's instrument was tried and reported on favourably. Currently the site of the Institute for the History of Medicine and the Endoscopy Museum of Vienna University. (courtesy of the Institute for the History of Medicine, Vienna).

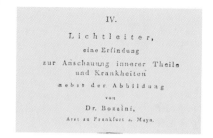

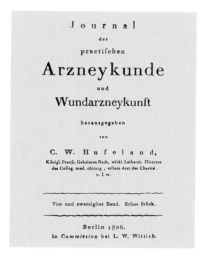

Fig. 5. A. Reproduction of the original article by Bozzini, on his "Lichleiter" published in the "Journal von praktische Arzneykunde", Berlin 1806.
5. B. Title page of the "Journal der praktische Arzneykunde" in which it was published. (courtesy of Prof. H.J.Reuter).

advantage of his various designs, but Bozzini had no luck; he died from typhoid fever at the age of 35, a pauper.

AN ENDOSCOPY MYTH: DID "BOMBOLZINI" EXIST?

As the successor of Bozzini, several medical historians cite another Italian named "Bombolzini" (also mentioned as "Bombalgini"). His name appears in several publications as the author of an instrument similar to the "Lichleiter". The first mention of "Bombalgini" can be found in an article by Isaac Hays in 1827 on the endoscope devised by Fisher, in which he quotes a paper by "Bombalgini" which had apparently been published in the journal "Archives Générales" in 1827. According to an admirable review of endoscopic instruments made by Josef Grünfeld in 1879[16], "Bombalgini" had invented a speculum for the examination of the stomach, the bladder, the uterus and the rectum . Grünfeld also quoted the article in "Archives Générales", stating however, that he had been unable to locate the paper. "Bombalgini" was also cited by Cruise from Dublin in his publications and even very recently (1998) by Reuter in his History of Endoscopy.

Two medical historians have reexamined the fate of "Bombalgini", Peter Paul Figdor[14] from Vienna and Alain Segal from Reims[38]. Both have reached the conclusion, which they have kindly advanced to me, that a curious myth has developed around the name "Bombalgini" (also quoted as "Bombolzini") as a result of several mispellings of Bozzini's name, and that the man in fact never existed. Bozzini was called "Barrini" by Cruise[7] and "Borrini"[18] by Hays!

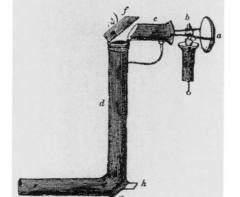

Fig. 6. The endoscope described by John Fisher of Boston (from the paper by I. Hays, 1827). Fisher was the first to use a lens and a mirror to reflect the image. The light ray "b" is reflected in the mirror "a", then on the mirror "f" and through tube "d". It is reflected again in the mirror "g" and onto tube "e" where it reaches the visual field (ref. 18).

ENDOSCOPES BY FISCHER, AVERY, SEGALAS, BONNAFONT

The endoscope of John D. Fisher (1797-1850)

Among the pioneers of endoscopy a special mention should be made to a physician from Boston, Dr. John Fisher, about whom there is little information. In a paper published in a medical journal of Philadelphia in 1827, Dr. Isaac Hays, a well known ophthalmologist and editor[18] who was apparently aware of the work of Bozzini and Ségalas, reported on the instrument devised by Fisher, including an excellent drawing which clearly shows the instrument. It consisted of a tube bent at a right angle, somewhat similar to a marine periscope, provided with a candle, reflecting mirrors and a double convex lens for image magnifying. *(Fig. 6)* By means of his endoscope, Fisher had been able to inspect the uterine cervix of a woman who had shyly refused the standard gynaecological examination. Fisher stated that he had designed his instrument three years earlier, while still in medical school. He made drawings of several versions of his endoscope which he sent to William Horner, professor of anatomy in Philadelphia[6]. Possibly Fisher's greatest merit was the successful transmission of an image through an angled instrument and its magnification by means of a lens. Fisher was a true precursor of endoscopy; he also attempted to use galvanic current to provide more light for his instrument[32].

John Avery (1807-1855)

All instruments designed at this time were based on the principle of the "Lichtleiter", that is, an external source of light and a system of mirrors to guide the light rays inside the body cavities through a tube. Most pioneers in these primitive endeavors were physicians who examined easily accessible cavities: otologists, gynaecologists and urologists. Instruments made to examine one cavity were then adapted to the inspection of other orifices in the body. In 1843, a London physician, John Avery[1], asked the firm Weiss and Son to manufacture an instrument for urethroscopy and laryngoscopy *(Fig. 7)* which consisted of a large reflector placed on the forehead of the examiner and lit by a small Palmer lamp. This apparently allowed him to examine the urethra, the bladder, the vocal cords and the oesophagus. Unfortunately, no publication by Avery can be found, and his instruments are only known owing to the descriptions and drawings published by Sir Morrell Mackenzie in his treatise of laryngoscopy[31]. Mackenzie considered them to be of little use. However, other laryngologists such as Türck[41], also mentioned Avery's laryngoscopes. Some of Avery's achievements may be found in an anonymous obituary published in "the Lancet" in 1855[1].

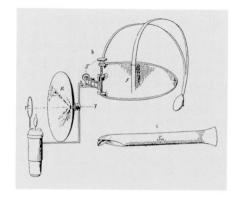

Fig. 7. John Avery's laryngoscope. Light is reflected on a large concave frontal mirror. At the right lower end, the tube used for laryngoscopy provided with a small oblique mirror. (from Morrell MacKenzie, "The uses of the laryngoscope in diseases of the throat", London, R.Hardwicke, 1865).

The speculum of Pierre Salomon Segalas d'Etchepare (1792-1875)

In 1826, at the "Académie des Sciences of Paris, the French surgeon Segalas presented his "spéculum urethro-cystique" which he used to inspect the urethra and the bladder and as an aid to fragment bladder stones. With this instrument he was able to identify a stone in a 3-year-old girl[41]. *(Fig. 8)*.

Segalas' instrument consisted of two silver tubes, two metal mirrors, two candles and an elastic tube. One of the tubes was introduced in the urethra and its prox-

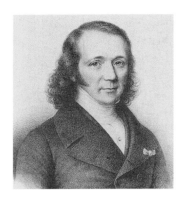

Fig. 8. Pierre Salomon Ségalas d'Etchepare, famous Parisian urologist, inventor of the "spéculum urethro-cystique" (courtesy Dr. Alain Ségal).

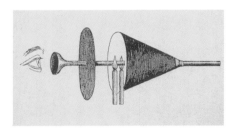

Fig. 9. The urethro-cystic speculum of Ségalas lit by two candles. (from Grünfeld, ref. 16).

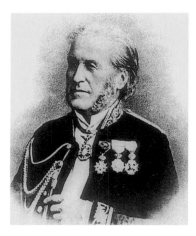

Fig. 10. Portrait of J.P. Bonnafont from "Ma Biographie", Paris, Oudin et Cie, 1892. Bibliothèque Universitaire de Médecine (Paris) (courtesy of Mme Marie Véronique Clin-Meyer, Conservateur, Musée d'Historie de la Médecine, University René Descartes, Paris).

imal end was attached to a large conical mirror about 9 cm in diameter. The examiner held the two candles with his left hand in front of the mirror. Between the candles, a second tube, blackened internally and expanded funnel-like to be used as an ocular, was aligned with the urethral tube. A round concave mirror reflected the light of the candles into the conical mirror, and through it, to the urethra. Segalas' speculum was probably the first useful instrument for endoscopic diagnosis and treatment[40] *(Fig. 9)*.

Segalas was born in Saint-Palais (Basses Pyrenées) in 1792 and he died in Paris in 1875. He took his medical degree in Paris in 1817 and he became an assistant professor at the medical school at La Sorbonne, the university of Paris. He specialised in urology and was one of the first to perform lithotrypsy and pelvic incisions, and he treated a huge number of private patients[12].

He published numerous papers on subjects as heterogenous as intestinal absorption, diabetes, blood dyscrasias and the chemical composition of urine in collaboration with the well-known chemist Vauquelin, but mostly on urological diseases. He was a member of the Royal Academy of Medicine, of the Paris City Council and of the General Council of the Department of the Seine.

The otoscope of Jean-Pierre Bonnafont (1805-1891)

The "First Class Principal Physician" (Médecin Principal de Première Classe), Jean-Pierre Bonnafont, studied medicine at the Military Medical School Val-de-Grâce in Paris and specialised in otology, becoming an indisputed master of the art[37]. Bonnafont devised an otoscope which consisted of a so-called "autostatic" bivalve speculum. A lateral light source allowed vision through an opening in the mirror that reflected the light *(Fig. 10)*. When the light source was adapted to the speculum, the instrument became very similar to the one devised subsequently by Désormeaux. When the latter presented his endoscope in 1851 at the Académie de Médecine of Paris, Bonnafont claimed, "I have been using a similar instrument for twenty years to examine the acoustic canal". Bonnafont was upset because Désormeaux was awarded the Académie's Argenteuil prize for his work in endoscopy, but his priority claim (which went on record in the proceedings of the Académie) was not considered. This drawback was not an obstacle to Bonnafont's brilliant career as an otolaryngologist. He received many distinctions, among them that of Officer of the Legion d'Honneur which helped him in getting a chair after writing a treatise of otology, for which he became famous[3] *(Fig. 11).*

The "endoscope" of Antonin Jean Désormeaux (1815-1894)

In 1853, Antonin Jean Désormeaux, surgeon of the Hôpital Necker in Paris, demonstrated his "endoscope" at the "Académie Impériale de Médecine". The instrument was devised to examine the urethra, the vagina and the rectum as well as fistulae originating from wounds[20]. *(Fig. 12).*

Until 1862, year in which he was appointed surgeon at the Hôpital Necker in Paris, an institution which still follows its long tradition in the field of renal and urological diseases, Désormeaux did not pursue his investigations on the endoscope. These were obviously influenced by the contributions of Ségalas[10]. In 1865, Désormeaux published his famous book "De l'endoscope et de ses applications au diagnostic and au traitement des affections de l'urèthre et de la vessie", a compilation of his lectures to the students at the hospital and considered one of the classic works in urology[11].

The crucial contribution of Désormeaux was the lighting system of his instrument. He used a much more potent source of light than the available candles; he first experimented with alcohol alone and later with a mixture of alcohol and turpentine in a proportion of four to one which he called "gazogène". The fumes resulting from burning this mixture dissipated through a sort of chimney tube placed at the top of the instrument. The light source was located between the lens and the reflector, made of a concave mirror with a central opening placed at an angle of 45 degrees. The lens focused the ray of light onto a flat mirror from where it reflected the light right through the tube inserted in the urethra. Désormeaux designed various models of catheters according to the shape of the orifice to be explored, including a bent one for insertion in the urethra. The endoscope was manufactured by the well-known firm of Charrière which specialised in many models of tubes. One of Désormeaux's endoscopes can be seen in the Museum for the History of Medicine at the University of Paris; visitors are often impressed by its relatively large size *(Figs. 13 and 14).*

With his endoscope, Désormeaux was able to identify bladder stones and bladder vascularisation, this being the first example of "contact" endoscopy. Désormeaux even performed endoscopic surgery (urethrotomy, section of a papilloma). There are good reasons for calling Désormeaux the father of endoscopy as he is responsible for coining the term "endoscope". His instrument, which had a relatively acceptable light-

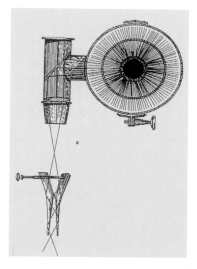

Fig. 11. Bonnafont's otoscope. The speculum is seen in the lower left part of the drawing. It is independent from the lighting system which consists of a tube that collects the light rays reflected on an oblique mirror and transmitted through a lens. The light source is located at the upper right end. The instrument resembles that of Désormeaux, differing only in that the speculum is not a direct part of the instrument. (Bonnafont, Traité pratique des maladies de l'oreille et des organes de l'audition, Paris, J.F.Baillière et fils, 2ème édition, 1873).

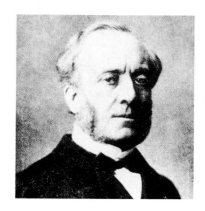

Fig. 12. Antonin Jean Désormeaux, inventor of the first useful multiple-use endoscope, but mostly employed for urological examinations. He created the term "endoscope" (courtesy of Fundación A. Puigvert, Barcelona).

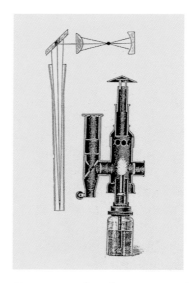

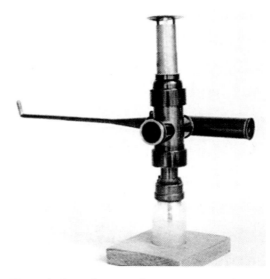

Fig. 13. The functioning of Désormeaux's endoscope. The light ray provided by the "gazogène" lamp is reflected on an oblique mirror and onto the endoscopy tube (ref. 16).

Fig. 14. Reproduction of Désormeaux endoscope, (Steno Museum, Aarhus, courtesy Dr. L.Lauridsen). An original instrument can be seen at the Museum of the History of Medicine, University René Descartes, Paris; there are other models at the Museums of the History of Medicine in Vienna and in Rome.

ing system, was used in many countries, although successive modifications were made by others until the advent of electric light (Fig. 15).

Désormeaux and his associates, in particular Edouard Labarraque who was an intern of the Paris Hospitals, also examined the naso-pharyngeal cavity and the oesophagus[26] (Fig. 16). Labarraque described in detail two cases of fibrotic oesophageal stenosis due to the ingestion of lye. He succeeded in dilating these after performing radial incisions through the endoscope. In another case, endoscopy was performed to confirm the suspicion of cancer of the oesophagus, but as the examination results were completely normal, Labarraque concluded that he was dealing with a case of "spasmodic stenosis". Désormeaux considered using voltaic current to illuminate his instrument, but he discarded the idea as it required not only a large rheostat but also the presence of an assistant who would control the brightness of the light.

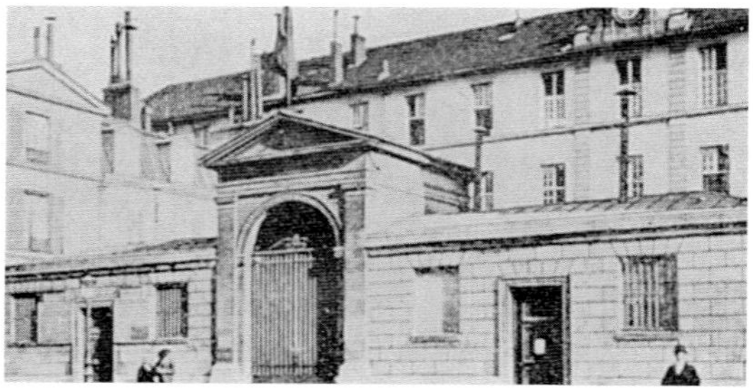

Fig. 15. The Hospital Necker in Paris where Désormeaux practiced urology. (photographed at the end of the 19th century).

Labarraque was well aware of Kussmaul's work on gastric endoscopy but was sceptical about his accomplishments as he stated that "deep in the stomach, the endoscope could not be moved freely and the field of vision would be very reduced". Here are his own words on the subject: "Nous ne mentionnerons que pour mémoire le fait que Monsieur le professeur Kussmaul de Fribourg qui prétend avoir pénétré avec l'endoscope jusqu'à dans la cavité estomacale... on ne doit pas oublier que l'instrument a une pareille profondeur ne jouit plus d'aucune liberté de mouvements et que par la suite le champ d'exploration se trouve singulièrement limité..."

Cruise (1834-1912) and his polyvalent endoscope

The Irish urologist Sir Francis Richard Cruise was the first to modify Désormeaux endoscope. His description dates back to 1865[7]. Cruise was born and educated in Dublin. He was interested in many aspects of medicine but his main contribution was the design of a cystoscope inspired by the Désormeaux's instrument which he considered poorly lit. His improvements were mainly on the light source, substituting the "gazogène", which gave rise to unpleasant fumes, for a lamp which contained petrol and camphor. Cruise described his instrument in the following way, "In the first place there is a tube or speculum, which is introduced into the cavity to be examined; and at one extremity of this, a mirror of polished silver, perforated in the centre, is placed at an angle of 45 degrees. The function of the mirror is to reflect the light, which is placed laterally, into the tube, so as to illuminate it to the end. As the calibre of the tube is very small, a most brilliant light is required and in order to obtain the best effects, it should be made to converge slightly upon the mirror. This convergence is attained by interposing between the light and mirror a plano-convex lens of suitable focal length. The light being sufficient, the lens properly adjusted, the mirror bright and correctly placed with respect to the tube, it becomes a matter of facility for the eye of the observer, looking through the perforation in the mirror, to see clearly to the bottom of the speculum" *(Fig. 17)*.

At that stage, instead of petrol and camphor, Cruise used a mixture of paraffin and camphor which produced a brighter light, but generated such heat that the instrument had to be isolated in a mahogany wooden casing, which made the instrument rather cumbersome[27].

Cruise adjusted a series of tubes of different shapes to his instrument, which allowed him to examine not only the urethra and the bladder but also the external ear, the vagina and the rectum. Both the firm Thompson and O'Neill in Dublin and Charrière in Paris manufactured the entire set of instruments developed by Cruise. This became very popular until the advent of the Nitze-Leiter cystoscope[28].

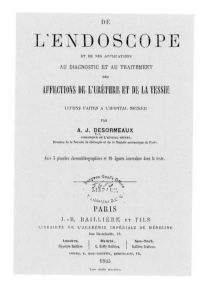

Fig. 16. The classical treatise by Désormeaux, "L'Endoscope" published in Paris in 1865 (courtesy of the National Library of Medicine, Washington D.C.).

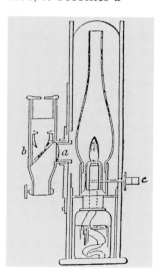

Fig. 17. Drawing of Cruise's endoscope, similar to that of Désormeaux but with better lighting due to the lateral position of the light source (ref. 7).

Sir Francis Cruise had a distinguished career: he was knighted by Queen Victoria in 1896, and in 1901 he was appointed physician to King Edward VII. He was a man of many interests; he played the cello and translated religious books from Latin. He was also a very good shot with a rifle[28] *(Fig. 18)*.

FROM LARYNGOSCOPY TO OESOPHAGOSCOPY

Manuel García, inventor of the laryngoscope

Among the great variety of instruments that were devised at that time, a special place should be given to the first laryngoscope, designed by a famous Spanish singer and teacher, Manuel García, who was born in 1805 in Madrid and died 101 years later in London. He was the son of another singer of the same name, the baritone Manuel García, and brother of two popular operatic stars, Pauline Viardot and Maria Malibran. García studied singing with his father and pursued a short international career in Paris, New York and London. *(Fig. 19)* He retired young and in 1829 he began to study medicine and public health in Paris. He devoted much time to the study of the physiological basis of singing and presented a memoir at the Paris Académie des Sciences, "Mémoire sur la voix humaine" which became the foundation of all subsequent investigation on the voice and the art of singing. He was a professor at the Conservatoire de Musique

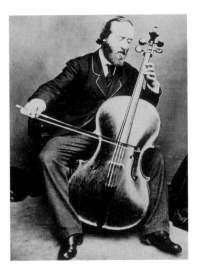

Fig. 18. Photograph of an inspired Sir Francis R. Cruise playing the cello in Dublin. Cruise performed cystoscopies but also rectoscopies and laryngoscopies with his invention (courtesy of Mr. Robert Mills, Librarian, Royal College of Physicians of Ireland and Prof. Eamonn Quigley, Cork).

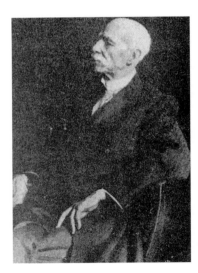

Fig. 19. Manuel García (1805-1906), famous Spanish singer, later a teacher in Paris and London. He invented the laryngoscope, which he used on himself to observe the movements of his vocal cords (portrait by John Singer Sargent).

in Paris and at the Royal Academy of Music in London. In 1855, he demonstrated the first laryngoscope, which brought him international acclaim[13].

García's laryngoscope was a very simple device. The light source originally consisted of a petrol lamp and nothing else, but later he used a mixture similar to that used by Désormeaux (the "gazogène"). and finally an electrical lamp. The equipment included a laryngeal mirror and another reflective mirror to concentrate the light rays. The reflector had a central round opening, about 6-7 mm in diameter, placed in front of the eyes of the physician. The reflector mirror was 8 to 12 cm in diameter with a focal distance of 20 to 25 cm. The laryngeal mirror was 13 to 30 mm in diameter and it was fitted to a handle making an angle of 120 degrees. It consisted of white glass which provided a clearer image than other colours. The examination was done with the patient seated facing the examiner and García recommended that the physician should support the knees of the patient between his own. This very simple instrument was the precursor of the oesophagoscope *(Fig. 20)*.

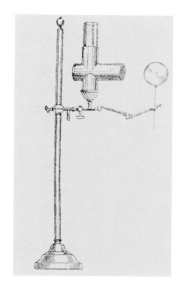

Fig. 20. Manuel García's laryngoscope. The light source in the centre. He first used a petrol lamp, later the Désormeaux "gazogène" lamp (ref. 13).

Other laryngoscopes: Czermak, Türck, Semeleder, Voltolini.

Laryngoscopy flourished in Vienna, preceeding the attempts to oesophagoscopy; around 1858, the Czech physician Johann Nepomuk Czermak (1828-1873) presented a laryngoscope which was quite similar to that devised by García, but he used sunlight instead of a lamp. By manipulating a mirror, he was able to visualise his own larynx and to take photographs of it! (these photos are in the archives of the Academy of Sciences in Vienna)[8, 9]. *(Figs. 21 and 22)*. Czermak was born in Prague and after graduation there, he became professor at the universities of Graz, Krakow, Pest and finally in Leipzig where he founded a large physiology laboratory[17].

In 1866, Ludwig Türck from Vienna (1810-1868)[15] devised another laryngo-

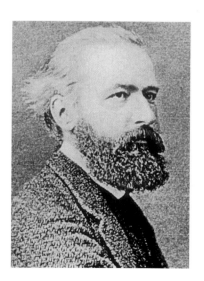

Fig. 21. Johann Nepomuk Czermak. With an instrument similar to that of García, he succeeded in photographing his own larynx. (Semmelweis Museum of the History of Medicine, Budapest).

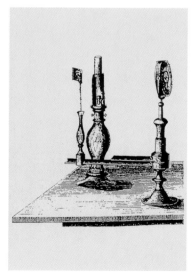

Fig. 22. Czermak's laryngoscope, arranged in the same way as García's instrument. (Semmelweis Museum of the History of Medicine, Budapest).

scope which helped him in diagnosing neurological disorders of the vocal cords for the first time[45].

In 1859, Friedrich Semmeleder (1832-1901), a Viennese like Türck, designed illuminated goggles for laryngoscopy[15]. He also made the first attempts to visualise the pharynx and the higher oesophagus by means of a curved tongue depressor that could be lit. In 1862 he wrote on oesophagoscopy and predicted that in the future "someone would devise tubes that could visualise the inside of the stomach"[43]. Semmeleder went to México as a personal physician to Emperor Maximilian, thus interrupting his academic career[16, 30].

Friedrich Rudolph Voltolini (1819-1889), from Breslau, also devised a more perfected instrument in 1879, consisting of a concave mirror 20 cm in diameter made of nickel and provided with a useful magnifying lens. However, other researchers, such as Julius Bruck[16] in Germany and Gustave Trouvé in France[2, 39] were the first to apply electricity to the illumination of endoscopes and in this way, they established the basis of modern endoscopy.

KUSSMAUL AND GASTROSCOPY

Kussmaul's gastroscope

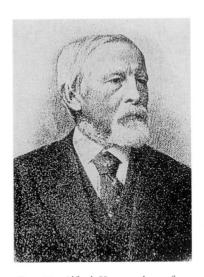

Fig. 23. Alfred Kussmaul, professor of medicine in several German universities, known as "the father of gastroscopy". He devised his first instrument after observing a professional sword swallower in action (courtesy Falk Foundation).

The first attempts at oesophagoscopy and gastroscopy were made using hollow tubes longer than a laryngoscope, which could rarely be introduced beyond the cricopharyngeal sphincter. In 1901, Killian, an otolaryngologist[22], endeavored to publish a history of digestive endoscopy. He was interested in Adolf Kussmaul and his achievements during his term as professor of medicine in Freiburg. Killian got in touch with Kussmaul who was living in retirement in Heidelberg. There followed some interesting correspondence between Killian, Kussmaul and some of his former assistants, mainly with Müller, but also with Joseph Leiter, the instrument maker who had manufactured Nitze's cystoscopes and later Kussmaul's gastroscope[23].

Adolf Kussmaul *(Fig. 23)* was born in Graben, near Karlsruhe, in 1822[17, 24]. After brilliant academic studies and graduation, he was appointed professor in Heidelberg (1855) and later in Erlangen (1859). He successively chaired departments of medicine in Freiburg (1863), and in Strasbourg (1876), then under German rule. He retired in Heidelberg in 1888, where he died in 1902.

Kussmaul was best known for his observations on diabetic acidosis (Kussmaul's respiration), the invention of the gastric pump and the first clinical description of polyarteritis nodosa.

Practically all historians have attributed the performance of the first oesophagoscopies and gastroscopies to Kussmaul, after his well-known observations on the technique of a professional sword swallower. His assistant, Müller, had introduced the performer to Kussmaul through another colleague, a Dr. Keller who was his neighbour[24].

The sword swallower had clearly shown that one could pass a rigid tube into the stomach if head and neck were well hyperextended. One hundred years later, sword swallowers may still be seen in fairs and public places as they continue to practice their "profession" *(Figs. 24, 25, 26 and 27).*

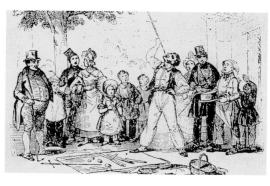

Fig. 24. Professional sword swallowing may be traced to the Greeks and the Romans. In his "Metamorphoses" Apuleius described one who performed his act in the Acropolis market in Athens. Sword swallowing requires a long-term conditioning of the pharynx, the oesophagus and the stomach. The scene shows a sword swallower in the midst of a crowd of onlookers.

Leiter, the instrument manufacturer from Vienna, also took advantage of the sword swallower's demonstrations and induced several young volunteers to swallow hard rubber rods and pass them into their stomachs. In many instances they were successful[21]. Professional sword swallowers can be traced as far back as the Romans, and Apuleius writes, "At the Stoa Poikile in Athens I saw a man who swallowed a sword to the hilt and then asked for an obolus". Several such people were studied at different clinics in Kussmaul's time, one interested physician being von Mikulicz. In 1968, Huizenga published his observations on a professional sword swallower whom he could examine in detail, making radiographic studies during his act[21].

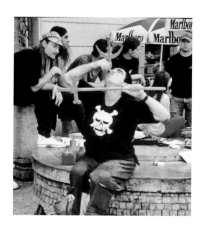

Fig. 25. Sword swallowing continues to be a popular form of entertainment as shown by this performer photographed in Prague in 2001 (courtesy of Dr. Tomás Pinós Desplat).

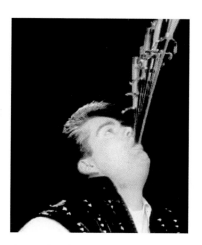

Fig. 26. The American professional sword swallower Brad Byers, swallowing several swords simultaneously (courtesy Mr.Brad Byers).

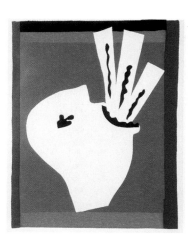

Fig. 27. Sword swallowing has attracted the attention of famous artists. Here "L'avaleur de sabres" by Henri Matisse.

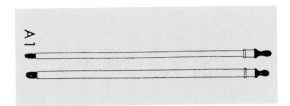

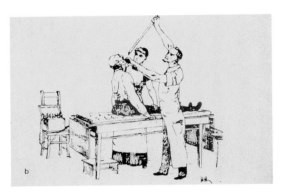

Fig. 28. Two prototypes of Kussmaul's gastroscope with their obturator. (from H.Elsner "Die Gastroskopie", Leipzig, G.Thieme, 1911).

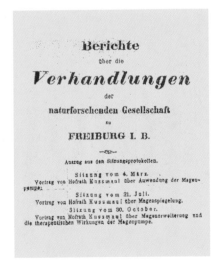

Fig. 29. Introducing Kussmaul's rigid gastroscope, a rather formidable procedure. The patient was first seated but later had to lie down during the examination (ref. 16).

Fig. 30. The announcement of Kussmaul's report on gastroscopy, presented in 1879 at the Society of Natural Sciences in Freiburg. Although it is often quoted in some historical publications as the first paper on the procedure, only the title was published (courtesy of Prof. Wolfram Domschke, Münster).

Kussmaul knew of Désormeaux endoscopes and sent his assistant Adolf Honsell to Paris to study them. When he returned with his report, Kussmaul had made a hollow metal tube, rigid and straight, 47 cm in length and 1.5 cm in diameter provided with a mandrel. The main problem was to carry enough light to the distal end of a long tube introduced into a dark cavity. The illumination system, which he had made by Fischer in Freiburg, was very similar to that of the French clinician. Unfortunately, the light which was reflected into the tube was very weak. It consisted at first of a paraffin lamp, later replaced by petrol and finally, by Désormeaux "gazogène". With these devices it was practically impossible to provide enough light to examine the stomach through such a long tube. Apparently, Kussmaul was only able to observe part of the gastric mucosa and moreover, the vision was obscured by mucous secretions and by gastric contents, as Müller explained later to Killian. In Paris, as we have already mentioned, Labarraque was very sceptical about Kussmaul's results. However, in 1868, Kussmaul, with a shorter instrument, performed oesophagoscopies and was able to diagnose a carcinoma of the oesophagus. *(Fig. 28).*

The instruments used by Kussmaul and his associates remained forgotten in the medical department of the Freiburg University many years after their departure and Killian was able to examine them thirty years later. He personally realised the deficiencies of their lighting system[22].

In 1876, Kussmaul moved to Strasbourg and asked his assistants Arnold, Cahn amd Eugen Pönsgen to start gastroscopies again. According to Cahn, the oesophagoscope which they used was a totally straight tube, while the gastroscope manufactured in 1881-1882 was slightly bent and contained a prism for the direction of the light *(Fig. 29).*

Kussmaul never published his endoscopic experiences, although he presented an oral report to the Naturforschenden Gesellschaft (Society for Nature Research) in Freiburg in 1870, which he called "Über Magenspiegelung" (on the inspection of the stomach). It is usually quoted in the medical literature as the first publication on gastroscopy *(Fig. 30).*

However, only the title was printed and the text was never published. According to Killian, Kussmaul remembered that the sword swallower was invited to attend the meeting and that he performed a gastroscopic demonstration on him. Together with this report he presented two other communications on the treatment of gastric dilatation by aspiration of the stomach with his suction pump (see Chapter 1).

Professor Edmund Rose, chairman of the surgical clinic at Zurich University from 1857 to 1881, did some examinations with Kussmaul's instrument. He presented the gastroscope to his associates in the hospital accompanied by the sword swallower whom he had brought from Germany. He wrote, "The audience looked with great interest at the bulging of the gallbladder on the red background of the gastric wall that the sword swallower made more prominent by contracting his abdominal muscles. Some time later I invited Désormeaux and told him how pleased I was using this new examining tool". According to Kussmaul, the sword swallower travelled even to Berlin, where he was examined by Wirchov, who took measurements of him[24].

From the extensive correspondence between Kussmaul, his associates and Joseph Leiter, one can deduct that Kussmaul became less interested in endoscopy when he moved to Strasbourg.

Kussmaul even said that, "In ganzen, schien mir die Spiegelungsmethode deren ich mich bediente, praktisch wenig Wert zu besitzen" ("in conclusion, it seems to me that the method of endoscopic examination of the stomach which I have used has little practical value"). He thus acknowledged the criticisms of Labarraque who objected that it would be very difficult to introduce a rigid instrument so deeply, unless the patient was a sword swallower and that once in the stomach, the insufficient light and the limitations in handling the instrument would considerably reduce the visual field. However, Kussmaul's pupils continued using the instrument, and Müller even designed a sort of metal harpoon to extract polyps and foreign bodies from the oesophagus[16].

The advent of electric light totally changed the outlook of endoscopy; in 1882 Joseph Leiter visited Kussmaul in Freiburg and showed him several prototypes of oesophagoscopes and gastroscopes which he was developing in Vienna together with the surgeon von Mikulicz. Later on he manufactured the Mikulicz gastroscope of which Kussmaul made very appreciative comments.

Possibly Kussmaul's main contribution was the demonstration that a rigid straight tube could be introduced into the stomach without excessive difficulty. He made several technical remarks to Leiter about the instruments that he was showing him but Leiter did not tell Mikulicz about them. Afterwards Kussmaul complained about this in his letters to Killian, "I have it in "black in white" that I was the first to insert a rigid tube into the stomach, although I only was able to see bubbles and mucus and a tumour of the oesophagus near the tracheal bifurcation. Unfortunately, the comments that you made to Mikulicz about my complaints have greatly distressed him because he believes that we are accusing him of appropriating my ideas for his gastroscope. I have tried to reassure him, telling him that the entire fault is Leiter's as he did not tell him about the conversations which we had had before"[23].

According to Seydl[43], who has studied this controversy, Kussmaul should only be considered as the father of oesophagoscopy. Since there is no indisputable proof that his instrument made true gastroscopies, the paternity of gastroscopy should be attributed to Mikulicz, who opened the way to gastric endoscopy with optic instruments.

REFERENCES

[1] Avery J. Obituary. Lancet 1855;1:331-333.

[2] Baratoux J. De l'oesophagoscopie et de la gastroscopie. Rev Mens. Laryngol Otol Rhinol (Bordeaux) 1882; 3: 97-107.

[3] Bonnafont J. P. Traité théorique et pratique des maladies de l'oreille et des organes de l'audition. París, J.-F. Baillière et fils, 2ème édition, 1873.

[4] Bozzini Ph. Der Lichleiter oder Beschreibung einer Einfachen Vorrichtung und ihrer Anwendung zur Erleuchtung inneren Höhle und Zwischenräume des lebenden animalisches Körpers, Weimar 1807.

[5] Bozzini Ph. Lichleiter, eine Erfindung zur Anschauung innere Theile und Krankheiten nebst der Abbildung Journal der praktische Arzneykunst, Berlin, 1806.

[6] Corner G. W. Two Centuries of Medicine. A History of the School of Medicine, University of Pennsylvania. Philadelphia, J. B. Lipincott, 1965.

[7] Cruise F. R. The endoscope as an aid in the diagnosis and treatment of disease Brit Med J 1865; 39: 345-347.

[8] Czermak J. N. Über den Kehlkopfspiegel. Wien med Wschr 1958;8: 196-198.

[9] Czermak J. N. Der Kehlkopfspiegel und seine Verwerthung für Physiologie und Medizin Leipzig, Engelmann 1863.

[10] Dechambre A., Lereboullet L. Dictionnaire encyclopédique des Sciences Médicales. París, Asselin-Masson, 1866-1889.

[11] Désormeaux A. J. De l'endoscope, instrument propre à éclairer certaines cavités intérieures de l'économie. Comptes Rendus Acad Sci París 1855; 40: 692.

[12] Désormeaux A. J. De l'endoscope et de ses applications au diagnostic et au traitement des affections de l'urèthre et de la vessie. París, J.-F. Baillière et fils, 1865.

[13] Enciclopedia Universal Ilustrada. Manuel García. Barcelona, Tomo 25. Hijos de J. Espasa editores, 1924.

[14] Figdor P. P. A reinvestigation on the significance of "Bombolzini" in the history of endoscopy. Historical Committee European Association of Urology. de Historia Urologiae Europeae. Vol 8. 2000 109-116.

[15] Gröger H. Die Entwicklung der Endoskopie in der Wiener Schule der Laryngologie. Das Wiener Endoskopie Museum. Eröffnungssymposium 1996. Wien, Literas Universitätsverlag. 1997: 34-42.

[16] Grünfeld J. Zur Geschichte der Endoskopie und der endoskopischen Apparate Mediz Jahrbücher Wien III n. IV 1879: 237-291.

[17] Gurlt E. Biographisches Lexicon der hervorragenden Ärzte aller Zeiten und Völker. VC. Berlin-Wien, 1934.

[18] Hays I. Instruments for illuminating dark cavities. Philadelphia J Med Phys Sci 1827;14: 409-411.

[19] Henning N. Lehrbuch der Gastroskopie, Leipzig, Johann Ambrosius Barth, 1935.

[20] Hillemand P., Gilbrin E. Antonin-Jean Désormeaux (1815-1894) le créateur de l'endoscopie. Bull Acad Med 1976;160: 95-100.

[21] Huizenga E. On esophagoscopy and sword swallowing. Ann Otology 1969; 78: 32-39.

[22] Killian G. Zur Geschichte der Oesophago und Gastroskopie. Deutsch Zeitschrift für Chirurgie 1901; 58: 499-512.

[23] Kluge F., Seidler E. Zur Erstanwendung der Ösophago-und Gastroskopie. Briefe von Adolf Kussmaul und seinen Mitarbeitern. Medizin Historisches J. 1986; 21: 288-307.

[24] Kluge F. Adolf Kussmaul (1822-1902). Eine biographische Skizze. Freiburg, Falk Foundation, 5 Auflage, 1996.

[25] Kussmaul A. Ueber Magenspiegelung. Berichte der Verhandlungen der Naturforschendes Gesellschaft zu Freiburg I. B. 1870;5:112.

[26] Labarraque E. Des applications de l'endoscope. Son utilité dans le traitement des affections de certains organes. Bull Thérap. Med. Chir. (París) (15 avril) 1871; 24: 297-313.

[27] Lauridsen L. Laterna Magica in Corpore Humano. From the History of Endoscopy. Svendborg, Isager Bogstryk, 1998.

[28] Leader M., Benson D. Cruise's contribution to endoscopy. Das Wiener Endoskopie Museum. Eröffnungssymposium 1996. Wien, Literas Universitätsverlag. 1997: 73-80.

[29] Lesky E. Die Wiener Experimente mit dem Lichtleiter Bozzinis (1806/1807) Clio Medica 1970; 5: 327-350.

[30] Lesky E. Die Wiener Medizinische Schule im 19 Iahrhundert. Studien zur Geschichte der Universität Wien, vol. VI, 1965.

[31] MacKenzie M. The use of the laryngoscope in diseases of the throat. London, R. Hardwicke, 3rd edition, 1871: 24.

[32] Modlin I. M. A brief history of endoscopy. Milano, MultiMed, 2000.

[33] Reuter H. J. , Reuter M. A. Phillip Bozzini and Endoscopy in the 19th Century Stuttgart, Max Nitze Museum, 1988.

[34] Reuter M. A. Geschichte der Endoskopie, Stuttgart-Zürich, Karl Krämer Verlag, 1998.

[35] Ringleb O. Zur Erinnerung Philip Bozzini und seine Lichtleiter. Zeitschr f. Urol Leipzig 1923; 2: 321-330.

[36] Roediger L. Der Frankfurter Arzt Phillipp Bozzini der Erfinder des Lichleiters (1773-1809). Medizinhist 1972; 7: 204-217.

[37] Segal A. Le Médecin principal de 1ere classe JP Bonnafont (1805-1891) Hist Sciences Med París 1983; 17: 63-70.

[38] Segal A. Les tribulations du mystérieux Dr. B.....i, précurseur de l'endoscopie. Vesalius 1999;5: 85-90.

[39] Ségal A. Place de l'ingénieur Gustave Trouvé (1839-1902) dans l'histoire de l'endoscopie. Hist Sciences Méd 1995; 29 123-132.

[40] Segal A. Pierre-Salomon Ségalas d'Etchepare, précurseur de l'endoscopie moderne. Bull Acad Nat Med 1978; 162: 709-714.

[41] Segalas P. S. Traité des retentions d'urine et des maladies qu'elles produisent. Méquignon-Marvis, París 1828. 634 pp ill. page 88-90.

[42] Semeleder F. Über Oesophagoskopie. Wien Medicinal Halle 1862; 3: 319.

[43] Seydl G. Mikulicz und die Gastroskopie. Referat gehalten am 5 Symposium der Internationalen Nitze-Leiter Forschunggesellschaft für Endoskopie "150 Geburtstag von Mikulicz-Radecki" 21-22 Jan 2000, Josephinum, Viena.

[44] Skopec M. Die Versuche mit Bozzini's Lichtleiter in Josephinum. Das Wiener Endoskopie Museum. Eröffnungs Symposium 1996. Wien, Literas Universitätsverlag. 1997:34-42.

[45] Türck L. Der Kehlkopfspiegel und die Methode seines Gebrauches. Zeitschr Ges Ärzte Wien 1858; 14: 401-409.

[46] Voltolini F. E. Über die Durchleutung des Kehlkopfes und anderer Höhlen des menschlichen Körpers. Allgm. Wien med Zeitung 1888; 33: 569, 581, 594.

[47] Walk L. The history of gastroscopy. Clio Medica 1966;1:209-222.

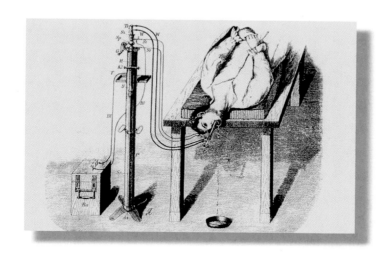

CHAPTER 3

Rigid
gastroscopes

FROM THE NITZE-LEITER CYSTOSCOPE TO THE GASTROSCOPE

I is to Max Nitze, the famous urologist from Dresden (1848-1906), that we owe the design of the first practical cystoscope. The instrument was provided with an optical system made of lenses, an idea which came to him while cleaning the eye piece of his microscope; looking through the clean lens he saw the reduced image of a nearby building[40]. Nitze´s first endoscope included part of the optical system from his own microscope *(Fig. 1)*. After beginning his urology practice in Dresden, Nitze moved to Vienna to the surgical department of Von Dittel where for many years he closely collaborated with Joseph Leiter (1830-1892), a medical instrument maker. In 1879 they presented their instrument to the Imperial and Royal Society of Physicians of Vienna[35], introduced by the eminent surgeon Leopold von Dittel. The cystoscope was lit with platinum filaments by means of an electric current which was strictly controlled with a rheostat similar to that used by Trouvé and a water-cooling system. Although the instrument was somewhat bulky and cumbersome, a few specialists managed to perform ambulant endoscopy, as described by Leiter in his catalogue of medical instruments[24].

The cystoscope caused quite a revolution and Nitze became internationally known as the creator of cystoscopy. In honour of his accomplishments, the Max Nitze Museum was founded in Stuttgart by Professor Hans Joachim Reuter. It was recently moved to the Institute for the History of Medicine at the Josephinum, part of the University of Vienna.

Apart from Kussmaul's efforts, already described in chapter 2[19, 50], the first instrument manufactured for the specific task of examining the oesophagus and the stomach was made by Max Nitze and Joseph Leiter[31, 34, 59] *(Fig. 2)*.

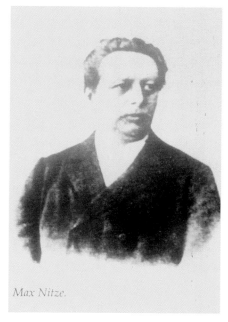

Max Nitze.

Fig. 1- Maximilian Nitze. Famous German urologist who in 1877 designed the first optical cystoscope, a forerunner of all optical instruments for endoscopy (courtesy Prof. H.J.Reuter).

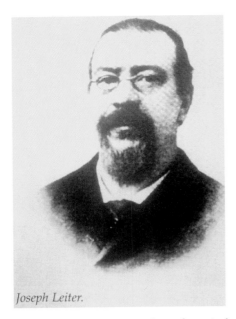

Joseph Leiter.

Fig. 2. Joseph Leiter, maker of surgical instruments. He founded the most important firm of his time in Vienna. He contributed decisively with Nitze in the design and manufacture of the first cystoscopes and urethroscopes and later of other tools, such as the Mikulicz gastroscope (Institute for the History of Medicine, Vienna).

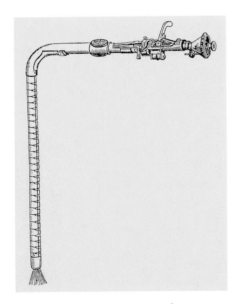

Fig. 3. The Nitze-Leiter oesophago-gastroscope. The right angle design and semiflexible distal end together with the poor illumination and the limited mobility prevented its practical use (ref. 24).

Although Gustave Trouvé from Paris had exhibited his polyscope in 1870[1, 28, 49] it was Leiter who, as of 1879, manufactured an oesophago-gastroscope based on an optical lens system tested by Nitze[40]. The instrument was bent at a right angle and consisted of two parts; a flexible distal portion and a proximal rigid tube. The distal part was made of metal segments ("lobster tail") and was fitted to the proximal tube which, once inserted, rested on the pharynx *(Fig. 3)*. The right angle of the instrument made illumination very difficult. Although some reports appeared and these can be inspected at the Museum of Endoscopy in Vienna, the instrument was virtually never employed and quickly fell into disrepute[48]. None of these instruments, such as Kussmaul's[22], Trouvé's[57] or Nitze-Leiter's[24], were sufficiently practical; the lighting system was very poor, there was no provision for insufflation, and the light source required large batteries to activate the platinum filaments. Moreover, the instrument had to be cooled by means of an irrigation system.

Leiter took his endoscope to Kussmaul who, years later, told Killian[18] that he had suggested to the manufacturer that he should design straight rigid instruments that would be handled more easily than the ones that he was showing. Leiter then got in touch with von Mikulicz, who was working as a surgeon in Vienna, and started to manufacture a new rigid endoscope. Apparently, as previously mentioned, (Chapter 2), Leiter never told Mikulicz about Kussmaul's suggestions, and this accounted for the animosity which later developed between Mikulicz and Kussmaul. Neither did Leiter ever mention Trouvé's contributions, which he must have been aware of, as the French inventor had presented his polyscope at a congress in Vienna.

Born in Vienna, the son of a hard-up shoemaker, Leiter[39] decided early on to become a medical instrument maker and he travelled, mainly on foot, to Belgium and France where he visited the factories of Lüer and Charrière. He studied electricity and especially the properties of galvanic current. He later made an electric clock which won a prize at an exhibition in Munich. He returned to Vienna and started the Leiter firm in 1855 with two employees near the University Hospital. Soon he started manufacturing instruments for the famous surgeon Billroth. By 1861 the firm had as many as 15 workers. He continued making instruments for the surgical clinic of Professor von Dittel and in 1887 he designed the first cystoscope featuring an incandescent lamp which was then adapted to other endoscopes.

Leiter was a man with a complex and difficult personality, perhaps a consequence of his unfortunate family life; all six of his children died, the eldest at the age of 18. He fell out with Nitze and also with Trouvé who he never quoted in his publications. This caused violent disagreements between them. He also quarrelled with Mikulicz.

THOMAS ALVA EDISON (1847-1931) AND THE INCANDESCENT LAMP

Little by little, several instrument makers succeeded in providing a brighter illumination using either magnesium or platinum filaments, but these generated much heat and could cause burns[31]. Julius Bruck, a Breslau dentist, had the idea of isolating the platinum filaments inside a double walled glass tube. Between the two glass walls a water irrigation device was arranged, partly solving the problem[7].

The invention of the first incandescent light bulb by Thomas Alva Edison in 1879 was a giant step in the right direction. The lamp consisted of a glass bulb in which a vacuum had been created *(Fig. 4)*.

Quite rapidly, a miniature lamp was manufactured, the so-called "Mignon lamp". It could be screwed to the tip of the endoscope, so that water cooling devices became superfluous[34]. In 1887, Nitze and Leiter separately presented their cystoscopes, each incorporating incandescent bulbs[24] *(Fig. 5)*.

Nitze later ordered an oesophagoscope and a gastroscope with Mignon lamps from another manufacturer and Leiter also produced his own version[25]. The proximal right angle bend of the Nitze-Leiter gastroscope greatly limited its use. For the first time Nitze used the term "gastroscope" for his instrument which he tested in cadavers and in some patients, but he remained unsatisfied with Leiter's prototype and never published his findings. Nitze devoted his time exclusively to his Berlin chair of urology and lost interest in digestive endoscopy.

As of this point, the paths of oesophagoscopy and gastroscopy diverged. Oesophagoscopy, frequently employed for the extraction of foreign bodies or to dilate stenotic lesions, required a hollow instrument while the gastroscope, which was essentially a diagnostic tool, generally consisted of a closed optical system. The endoscope was also used for different purposes; the open rigid oesophagoscope was used as an extension of the laryngoscope by otolaryngologists, while from

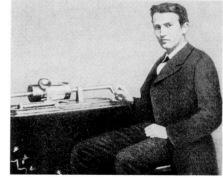

Fig. 4. Thomas Alva Edison. Inventor of the electric incandescent lamp. The use of small electrical bulbs ("Mignon lamps") was a very important step in the development of endoscopy.

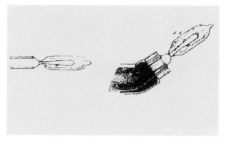

Fig. 5. The "Mignon" lamp. (from Gottstein, ref. 7).

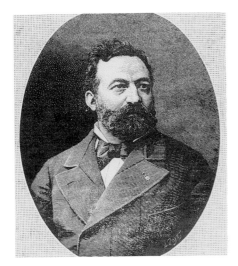

Fig. 6. Gustave Trouvé. French inventor, author of various electromedical instruments. He was the first to apply electrical illumination to an endoscope. A violent controversy with Joseph Leiter on the priority of the electroscope ended finally in favour of Trouvé, although the diffusion and manufacturing of endoscopes owes a great deal to Leiter (courtesy Dr. Alain Segal).

its early days, gastroscopy became the domain of the digestive surgeon and the gastroenterologist.

THE POLYSCOPE OF GUSTAVE TROUVÉ (1838-1902)

Priority for using Edison's invention in endoscopy should be attributed to Gustave Trouvé, a Parisian engineer with many scientific interests, for his "polyscope"[49] *(Fig. 6)*. Trouvé made his instrument in 1869 and displayed it in 1873 at the Universal Exhibition in Vienna. Very probably Leiter saw the endoscope there and was influenced by it. Trouvé was the first to fit an electric light at the distal tip of his instrument. It consisted of thin filaments of platinum, isolated in a glass tube, and activated by an electric current generated by a battery devised by the physicist Gastón Planté[58]. Trouvé also designed a rheostat so that the intensity of the current could be adjusted in order to avoid excessive heating. Thus he was the first *(Figs. 7, 8 and 9)* to achieve illumination inside the human body. He also introduced a prism to deflect the visual field about 90 degrees laterally, and he later used Edison's incandescent lamp. However, the polyscope also generated excessive heat and large cavities could be inspected only for very brief periods of time[57]. Several polyscopes

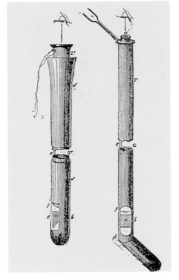

Fig. 7. Trouvé's polyscope. It was used by several physicians, mainly in France but also in Germany, for many kinds of endoscopic procedures (ref. 1).

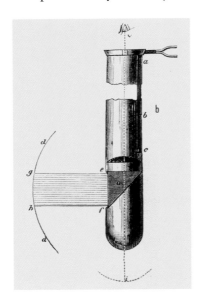

Fig. 8. Distal prism of Trouvé's polyscope which allowed the reflection of the image and better visibility (ref. 1)

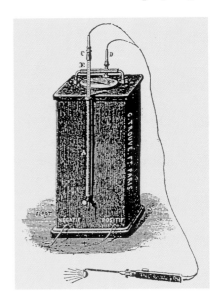

Fig. 9. Rheostat and battery devised by Gastón Planté, a French physicist, for Trouvé's polyscope. They were very cumbersome but allowed the control of the light power and the reduction of excessive heat caused by the light sources (ref. 49).

designed by Trouvé were used in otology, laryngology, urology and proctology.

In 1876, Professor Collin d'Alfort from Paris examined the stomach of an ox with Trouvé's "gasteroscope". The polyscope was used by several physicians, among them the famous surgeon Péan. Another surgeon, Le Dentu, and the clinician Raynaud, working at the Hospital Lariboisière, diagnosed a syphilitic stenosis of the oesophagus by means of the polyscope[49]. The instrument was also employed in Germany by Theodor Stein from Frankfurt (perhaps the first to take endoscopic photographs)[52]. Stein sided with Trouvé in his controversy with Leiter on the priority of the electric endoscope. As already mentioned in relation to the diaphanoscope (see Chapter 1), Trouvé boasted that his gastroscope left Einhorn's diaphanoscopy "twenty years behind". It certainly was the forerunner of the instruments which Leiter manufactured for Nitze.

In 1880, Trouvé, a man of great genius, together with three friends (Charles Jeantaud, Camille Faure and Nicolas Raffard) designed a rather aerodynamic electric automobile, propelled by means of a battery, with a rheostat and a transformer which would change the DC current generated by the battery into the alternating current needed to start the engine. Trouvé had a peculiar sense of humour and as Alain Segal has shown, as a trade-mark for his instruments he used the Greek word "Eureka" (I have found: in French, j'ai trouvé, a pun on his own name, G.Trouvé) *(Figs. 10 and 11).*

THE MIKULICZ GASTROSCOPE

On the 29th of October, 1881, in one of the most prestigious journals of that time, the Centralblatt für Chirurgie, an article was published on gastroscopy and oesophagoscopy which had been written by von Mikulicz[29]. In this seminal paper, the author described the results of gastroscopic examinations in human beings for the first time. *(Fig. 12).*

Mikulicz had instructed Leiter to follow the principles of the Nitze-Leiter cystoscope, and to make a gastroscope which should include an optical system with indirect vision, a lamp at its distal end and a mechanism for insufflation of the stomach. The instrument was rigid with a 150 degree angle at its distal end. This was the first endoscope which tried to adapt its design to the anatomic structures and to the technical problems related to its introduction. The instrument was fitted with a small platinum filament lamp which required cooling by means of a water irrigator.

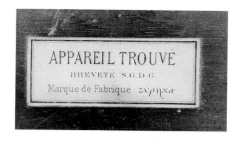

Fig. 10. The logo of Trouvé's firm, «Eureka» (I have found!) in French: "J'ai trouvé!", (a pun on his name) (courtesy Dr. Alain Segal).

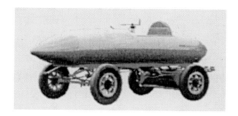

Fig. 11. Automobile invented by Trouvé with Jeantaud, Faure and Raffard in 1880.

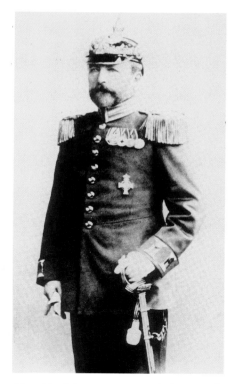

Fig. 12. Johannes von Mickulicz in the uniform of an Army general (courtesy Prof. M.Classen).

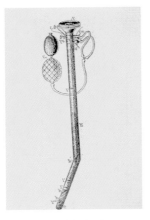

Fig. 13. Mikulicz's gastroscope made by Leiter in Vienna. (Described by some as a "gigantic" cystoscope) (ref. 7).

Mikulicz also studied the performance of a sword swallower and tested several prototypes of gastroscopes on cadavers. In April 1881, Mikulicz performed his first gastroscopy on a living person[30].

The gastroscope, which can be viewed at the Endoscopy Museum in Vienna, is 65 cm long and 14 mm in diameter, and it very much resembles the Nitze-Leiter cystoscope, although obviously much bulkier. It was coupled to an insulated current generator ("Stromleitung"). The tube of the endoscope included a channel for cooling by water irrigation and another thin one for air insufflation. A third channel was used to introduce the wires of the lighting system. In its distal angular piece the tube had a glass window for the platinum filament and a smaller one for a prism for the optical system, as well as an opening for the entrance of air. A detailed description of the instrument can be found in the Leiter catalogue "Elektrooptische Instrumente" printed in Vienna in 1880 *(Fig. 13)*.

The distal angle of the endoscope was adapted to the concavity of the thoracic vertebral column. Mikulicz believed that an entirely straight tube could not pass through the cardia and after studies on cadavers he concluded that when the instrument was inserted, the distal angle would conform to the shape of the oesophago-gastric junction[13]. Rotating, pushing and pulling the endoscope he could visualise a great part of the stomach. However, as the endoscope could only be rotated 180 degrees, Leiter was obliged to manufacture twin endoscopes to enable inspection of the entire circumference of the stomach; one instrument was used for the right part of the stomach and the other for the left[7]. Mikulicz started by examining his patients in the upright position but retching and salivation made the examination rather cumbersome. After testing several positions, Mikulicz decided that the best results were obtained with the patient lying down in the supine position, with the head hyperextended as for oesophagoscopy. *(Figs. 14 and 15)*.

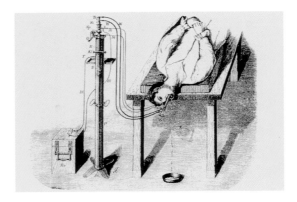

Fig. 14. Position of the patient for gastroscopy with the Mikulicz instrument. The patient is lying on his back and the head is hyperextended.(ref. 7).

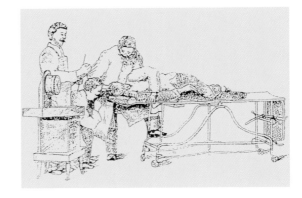

Fig. 15. The patient in the left lateral position used later by Mickulicz. It was less uncomfortable for the patient (ref. 7).

Mikulicz prescribed a gastric lavage prior to the examination. Attempts to distend the stomach walls with water were unsuccessful as the patient quickly vomited the water. However, air insufflation was well tolerated and has been carried out ever since. Mikulicz considered that general anaesthesia with chloroform was dangerous and he used morphine for sedation; this was sufficient for an examination of some 15 minutes. He used a four per cent solution of the drug. The same premedication was used for oesophagoscopy[7]. "Everything needs practice and skilled hands" said Mikulicz.

Johannes von Mikulicz was born in 1850 in Czernovitz, the capital of Northern Bucovina, nowadays part of the Ukraine, but included at that time in the Austro-Hungarian Empire[8]. When he died in 1905, he had become one of most famous surgeons of his time, due at least in part to the teachings that he received from his mentor Billroth, with whom he worked for many years. He was the first to operate with cotton gloves, and the first with Sauerbruch to resect a cancer of the oesophagus by the transpleural route (1886). His name is attached to 18 eponyms of diseases, operations and instruments[10]. Perhaps the best known of them has been the "Mikulicz syndrome" (chronic hypertrophy of the salivary and lacrimal glands)[31]. Mikulicz devised an operation to treat achalasia and he developed the technique of pyloroplasty. In early days he was sceptical about the value of gastroscopy and it was Leiter who, with his ingenuity and enthusiasm, convinced him to continue his endoscopic research.

As already stated in the previous chapter (Chapter 2), Mikulicz hired a professional sword swallower to test the field of vision of his endoscopes. He left Vienna for a chair in Krakow, then for another in Koenigsberg and finally he settled in Breslau where he lived until his death from cancer of the stomach in 1905. With the many teaching and administrative duties of his academic career he lost interest in endoscopy and concentrated on abdominal surgery.

Gastroscopy was pursued by his disciple Georg Kelling[17] who would become famous for his performance of laparoscopy. Using the Mikulicz-Leiter gastroscope, Kelling examined twenty patients and succeeded in identifying a gastric carcinoma which was not palpable. He modified the optical window of the endoscope so that it could also be rotated. However, in spite of the fact that the Mikulicz gastroscope was the first useful instrument to inspect the stomach and that Kussmaul had praised it[50], the tool did not become popular because of the tecnical difficulties related to its introduction and the need to inject morphine for sedation. Leiter improved the lighting system of his endoscopes by using a Bunsen battery as the light source. This enabled ambulant endoscopy and he later devised his electroscope, a light source that could be adapted to various instruments, such as oesophago-gastroscopes, rectoscopes and cystoscopes (*Figs. 16, 17 and 18*).

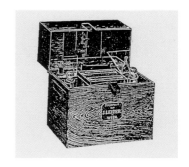

Fig. 16. Bunsen's battery made for the firm Leiter. Its smaller size allowed illumination of the endoscopes for ambulant purposes (ref. 7).

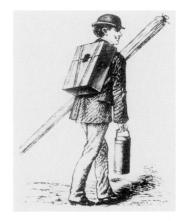

Fig. 17. Portable equipment for endoscopy (J.Leiter's catalogue).

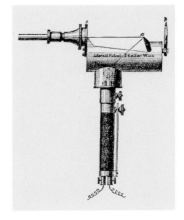

Fig. 18. Leiter's panendoscope included the light source which could be adapted to various types of endoscopes by means of a battery (ref. 7).

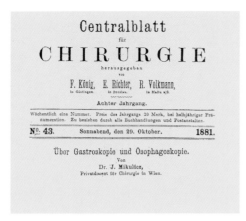

Centralblatt
für
CHIRURGIE
herausgegeben
von
F. König, E. Richter, R. Volkmann,
in Göttingen. in Breslau. in Halle a/S.

Achter Jahrgang.

Wöchentlich eine Nummer. Preis des Jahrganges 20 Mark, bei halbjähriger Prä-
numeration. Zu beziehen durch alle Buchhandlungen und Postanstalten.

No. 43. Sonnabend, den 29. Oktober. 1881.

Über Gastroskopie und Ösophagoskopie.
Von
Dr. J. Mikulicz,
Privatdocent für Chirurgie in Wien.

Fig. 19. The well-known article by Mikulicz on oesophagoscopy and gastroscopy (1881). Its conclusions are still valid today.

THE EVOLUTION OF THE GASTROSCOPE

According to Schindler[48], the development of the gastroscope followed three different paths:

1) rigid gastroscopes with a closed optical system, derived from the Nitze-Leiter cystoscope.
2) rigid gastroscopes, with open hollow tubes such as Kussmaul's instrument and which would be used many years later as rigid oesophagoscopes until the advent of the fiberscope.
3) flexible gastroscopes which could be straightened by some spring mechanism after their insertion into the stomach, forerunners of Wolf-Schindler's semi-flexible gastroscope[47] *(Fig. 19)*.

GASTROSCOPES FEATURING A CLOSED OPTICAL SYSTEM

The Rosenheim gastroscope

Fifteen years later, around 1895, Rosenheim renewed clinicians' interest in gastroscopy[42]. He devised an instrument, again based on Nitze's cystoscope[43], but it differed from the Mikulicz endoscope in two essential points: it was much thinner and therefore easier to introduce, and it was straight; being free of angles allowed a better positioning of the optical system *(Fig. 20)*.

Theodor Rosenheim was born in Bromberg in 1868 and he died in Berlin in 1939[8]. He graduated in Berlin and worked at the University Medical Clinic where he was appointed professor in 1921. He was a physician at the Jewish Hospital in Berlin until 1933, the year when the Nazis began their rule in Germany. I have been unable to find further data about him.

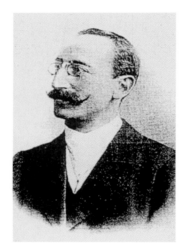

Fig. 20. Theodor Rosenheim. Photograph taken at the end of the nineteenth century. (courtesy Dr. I. Modlin).

The instrument, described by Rosenheim in the Berlin Klinische Wochenschrift[49], had been tested both in cadavers and in volunteer patients and was quite ingenious; it consisted of three concentric tubes. The external tube measured 12 mm in diameter. The inner tube included the optical system, an ocular lens and a rectangular prism which enabled lateral vision. This was protected by a second tube which had a distal opening that could be rotated 180 degrees to face the window of the inner tube, so that the optical lenses would *(Figs. 21 and 22)* not be soiled during the introduction of the gastroscope. The external tube was provided with an incandescent Edison lamp. Two channels allowed irrigation with water to prevent excessive heating. A third channel included wires for connecting the lamp to a 16 volt electricity source. A fourth channel was used for air insufflation. The distal end of the instrument, manufactured by Hirschmann in Berlin, was covered with a hard rubber tip devised to avoid damage to the mucosa during the introduction.

The stomach was emptied before the examination and Rosenheim first introduced a probe to make sure that the oesophagus was permeable. The pharynx was brushed with cocaine and the gastroscope was then introduced, while in a supine position, with the patient's head dropping back over the edge of the examining table. In spite of the improvements made by Rosenheim, there were still blind areas in the gastric cavity, such as part of the greater curve and the posterior wall as well as the cardia.

Rosenheim listed a series of contraindications to gastroscopy; heart disease, lung emphysema, liver cirrhosis and an ulcer high in the lesser curve of the stomach or at the cardia. His gastroscope was little used. A few years later at an International Congress of Internal Medicine in Moscow in 1899, a Russian physician, P. Redwizov[41], showed a modification of Rosenheim's gastroscope, substituting the external metal tube with a hollow one made of rubber. This was introduced first to ease the passage of the optical tube, thus diminishing the danger of perforation. Rosenheim, who attended the meeting, stated that he had had no special difficulties with his own instrument and that this new modification avoided perhaps some risks but that it lengthened the time required for the procedure. According to Walk[59] and Modlin[31], Rosenheim had some unfortunate experiences with his gastroscope and did not attempt further improvements. Redwizov's instrument fared no better.

Elsner's gastroscope

Between 1908 and 1911 Elsner devised another straight rigid gastroscope provided with an elastic rubber tip which stretched the last centimeters of the oesophagus, easing its introduction down to the posterior wall of the stomach[5]. This *(Fig. 23)* instrument prevailed over all other rigid endoscopes. Like a cystoscope, the optical system would slide inside an external sheath provided with a lamp. The optics were rather good as far as one can judge from the watercolours published

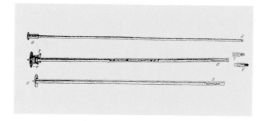

Fig. 21. The straight rigid gastroscope designed by Rosenheim, presented by the author at the Berlin Medical Society (1895) (ref. 43).

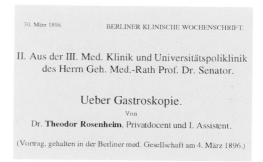

Fig. 22. Rosenheim's article in which he described his gastroscope (1896).

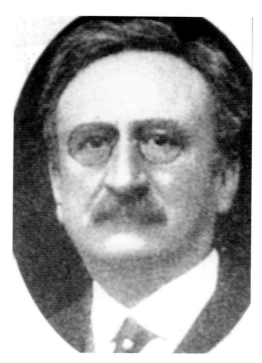

Fig. 23. Hans Elsner. Author of numerous books on gastroenterology, among them his treatise on "Diseases of the Stomach". (courtesy Prof. M. Classen).

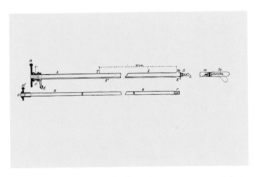

Fig. 24. Diagram of Elsner's gastroscope with its system of lenses (ref. 4).

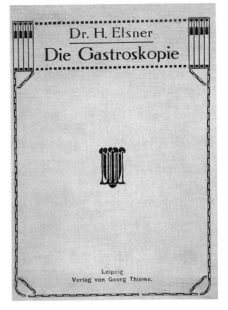

Fig. 25. Front page of Elsner's book on "gastroscopy" that made him famous.

in Elsner's book[4]. The window of the optical system, as in Rosenheim's gastroscope, was protected from soiling by rotating the inner tube. However, soiling could not always be prevented and until *(Fig. 24)* 1923, a channel for air insufflation which would have helped in cleaning the lenses, was not provided by the manufacturer. Elsner published his wide experience in a book which became very popular and was based on a large number of gastroscopies. A Danish physician, Maaloe, performed 500 gastroscopies with Elsner's instrument without complications[48]; however, some time later a case report on a perforation was published. Elsner's gastroscope was widely employed until 1932. Schindler[45] made his first gastroscopies with a gastroscope of this kind which had been stacked away and forgotten about for ten years in the storeroom at his hospital. Elsner also tried to take photographs[6]. These were greatly improved by Henning who used a better instrument. (see Chapter 7) *(Figs. 25, 26 and 27).*

More gastroscopes: Schindler, Sternberg, Bensaude and Korbsch

In order to ease insertion manoeuvres, thinner gastroscopes were designed. Some of these were only 8 mm in diameter, and one gastroscope measuring just over 6 mm was even made[3]. Schindler himself designed an instrument modified from that of Elsner. Like Rosenheim's gastroscope, it consisted of three concentric tubes. The outer tube included a channel for insufflation. The second

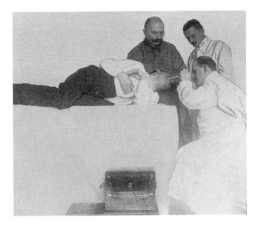

Fig. 26. Elsner performing a gastroscopy (from his own book).

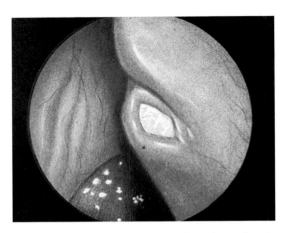

Fig. 27. Watercolour of a gastric ulcer (from Elsner's book).

tube was provided with an obturator ending in a rubber *(Fig. 28)* finger somewhat longer than that of Elsner's but designed with the same purpose in mind: to straighten the distal angle of the cardia and to keep it in line with the rest of the oesophagus. The inner tube was introduced after withdrawing the obturator, and it contained an optical system whose lighting was better than that of Elsner's. The instrument was introduced in the left lateral decubitus.[45].

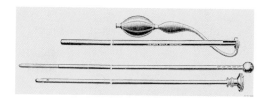

Fig. 28. Schindler's rigid gastroscope, a modification of Elsner's instrument, used by the author until he designed the first semiflexible gastroscope together with Georg Wolf (ref. 9).

At the Medical Society of Munich in 1922 (Aertzlicher Verein), Schindler presented the results of 120 gastroscopies performed with his own modification of Elsner's instrument[46]. The report was illustrated by the projection of 60 watercolour illustrations made by an artist who worked as a technician in the Pathology Department at the hospital in Schwabing, a district of Munich.

At that time, Schindler had already identified three different types of gastritis: superficial, atrophic and hypertrophic. He also observed the contractions of the pylorus. Schindler stated, "the gastroscopic examination enables differential diagnoses that cannot be made by any other means, and images of various lesions which were never diagnosed previously can be interpreted. Various types of gastritis and gastric polyposis belong to this group of lesions".

In a short time Schindler had performed over 400 gastroscopies with his instrument without mishaps and he even took photographs[46]. Shortly afterwards however, he had a severe accident: perforation of an oesophagus. Gutzeit and Henning continued to perform gastroscopies with this instrument, apparently without major complications.

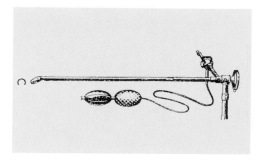

Fig. 29. Sternberg's gastroscope. The angle at the distal end is very similar to that of a cystoscope. Schindler believed this instrument to be dangerous (ref. 54).

Sternberg's optical gastroscope[54] featured a short distal angle, similar to that of a cystoscope, as Sternberg believed that this modification was important to negotiate the cardia. However, the blind introduction of the instrument required *(Figs. 29 and 30)* complicated manoeuvres[53]. Schindler[45] and Bensaude[2] believed that the instrument was dangerous. The famous surgeon Sauerbruch invited Schindler to give a demonstration of his instrument in his service, but he refused the invitation, as in the same session Sternberg would also exhibit his own gastroscope and Schindler did not want to have his name associated with that of the designer of a dangerous instrument[48]. Unfortunately, he was right to refuse, as Sternberg's gastroscope caused a perforation of the oesophagus

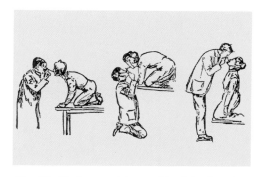

Fig. 30. Various positions utilized by Sternberg for the introduction of his gastroscope (ref. 53).

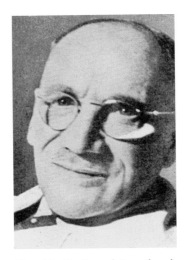

in a young woman who died *(Figs. 31 and 32)* from mediastinitis in spite of several surgical attempts to drain the infected tissues. Sauerbruch published the case in full[44] and ended by condemning gastroscopy and forbidding its performance in his service with the following words, "This death is not the only one. Sternberg as well as Schindler must regret several more".

Bensaude's gastroscope was made by the well-known firm of Collin *(Fig. 33)*. It differed from other endoscopes in that it included a channel through which the operator could slide a wire provided with a metal olive at its tip. This was introduced first as a guide[33]. The distal end of the gastroscope was fitted with a spring 2 cm in length which could be bent during the introduction of the rigid part[32]. The optical window was therefore more distant from the tip of the instrument than in the Elsner-Schindler gastroscope *(Figs. 34, 35, 36)*.

The examination was done with the patient kneeling[37] as in the Sternberg procedure; in the previous three years Bensaude had already been using this position for oesophagoscopy.

All these instruments were criticised by Chevalier Jackson[16] because of their difficult introduction and the poor illumination due to the absorption of light by the optical system which became easily soiled or misted due to lack of an adequate cleansing system.

Fig. 31. Ferdinand Sauerbruch, famous German surgeon. Sternberg performed a gastroscopy in his department in Munich which ended fatally. Sauerbruch then forbade the use of rigid gastroscopes in his service (courtesy Dr. Ramón Trias).

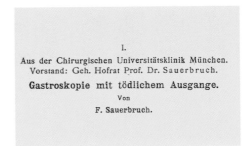

Fig. 32. Report published by Sauerbruch on this ill-fated case.

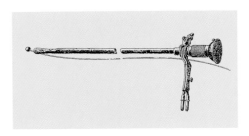

Fig. 33. Bensaude's gastroscope featuring an external metal guide (ref. 33).

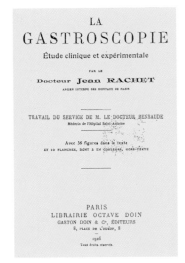

Fig. 34. Frontispiece of a book on gastroscopy by Jean Rachet, depicting Bensaude's assistant using the instrument designed by his teacher. Rachet was recognised in years to come for his work on inflammatory bowel disease.

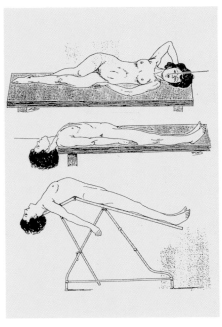

Fig. 35. Positions used by Rachet for the introduction of Bensaude's gastroscope (from his own book).

The gastroscope designed by Roger Korbsch, who was also a prominent laparoscopist, had a smaller diameter and it was somewhat more flexible than other instruments[20, 21]. It included two optical systems, one frontal and prograde and a second which was oblique and retrograde, allowing a very comprehensive view of the gastric cavity. It was also used by Henning[9]. (Fig. 37)

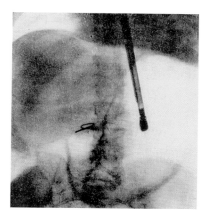

Fig. 36. Radiography of Bensaude's endoscope inside the stomach (from Rachet's book).

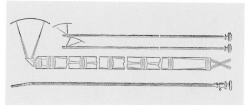

Fig. 37. Korbsch's thin gastroscope was easier to handle than other instruments. It was provided with two optical systems (prograde and retrograde). Henning also used this endoscope (ref. 9).

The Loening-Stieda gastroscope

This instrument was more practical than the others, because the rigid endoscope was introduced through a tube with a flexible distal end[26, 27]. According to Schindler[47], the Loening-Stieda gastroscope was more useful and less dangerous than others and was provided with an improved optical system (Fig. 38). Stieda (1908) published valuable reports using this instrument, which was also used in France by Couraud from Bordeaux[28].

Souttars' gastroscope

(Figs. 39 and 40) In 1909 Souttar and Thompson published the description of an original gastroscope[51]. This new tool, based on the Mikulicz gastroscope, consisted of a rigid tube with two angles: one of 80 degrees in its proximal part and another one of 30 degrees at its distal end. The angles were

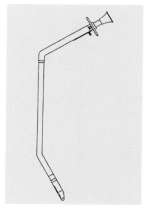

Fig. 39. Gastroscope devised by Souttar and Thompson (1909). It consisted of a rigid tube with two angles, one at the level of the pharynx and the second one at the cardiac area. It was introduced blindly and was deemed dangerous by Hill who, like Chevalier-Jackson, advocated the introduction of all instruments under visual control (ref. 51). Below: Sir Henry Souttar (1875-1964) (copyright unknown).

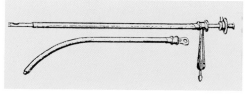

Fig. 38. Gastroscope designed by Loening and Stieda (1908) consisting of an external soft rubber tube which was inserted first into the stomach by means of a metal guide. The guide was then withdrawn and a rigid optical system was introduced (ref. 27).

THE GASTROSCOPE AND ITS USES.

BY

HENRY S. SOUTTAR,   and   THEODORE THOMPSON,
B.M., B.Ch.Oxon.,   M.A., M.D., M.R.C.P., F.R.C.S.,
London Hospital.   Assistant Physician and
                                           Pathologist to the London
                                           Hospital.

[With Special Plate.]

I.—DESCRIPTION OF THE INSTRUMENT.
By Dr. SOUTTAR.

Fig. 40. Front page of an overly optimistic article by Souttar and Thompson on their gastroscope which was not successful.

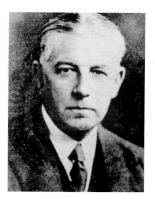

meant to avoid the curvature of the spine at the level of the cardia. After various tests, including some on himself, Souttar ordered a series of prototypes of his instrument. The seventh one was made in Berlin and was very expensive (60 pounds sterling!). Thanks to a grant from the British Research Council, Souttar was able to pursue his research. The gastroscope, like Rosenheim's, included three tubes: an outer sheath of steel provided with a window, a second tube covered with silk thread to carry the electrical current to the distal lamp and an inner tube which could be freely rotated inside the other tubes and was fitted with two mirrors and one lens. The entire gastroscope could be rotated inside the stomach and Souttar claimed that he could observe the whole of the gastric cavity after insufflation with air through the inner tube. The examination was performed after gastric lavage, preferably under general anaesthesia. Souttar's associate, Thompson, managed to identify gastric ulcers, a pyloric carcinoma, foreign bodies and the like with this instrument. Following several accidents, the gastroscope was manufactured with a single distal angle, but this "improvement" was not apparently successful.

Hill[11], who had designed a popular oesophagoscope, criticised all these instruments. He praised the Mikulicz instrument and the remarkable results obtained by Chevalier Jackson with a straight hollow tube. He considered the blind introduction of a gastroscope, as done by Souttar, was dangerous and he even stated that a simple blind oesophageal intubation had caused more than one death.

RIGID HOLLOW GASTROSCOPES

The Chevalier-Jackson gastroscope.

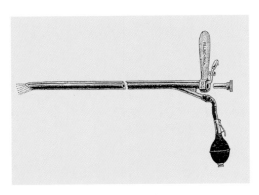

Fig. 41. Chevalier-Jackson's gastroscope (1907). It consisted of an open tube which was introduced under visual control, provided with a simple distal or proximal lamp without any optical lenses. It was similar to an oesophagoscope, although much longer. The stomach was explored without air insufflation. Continuous suction was performed through a thin external tube attached to the endoscope (from the Maison Collin's catalogue).

This distinguished American otolaryngologist was the most effective champion of the hollow rigid gastroscope. His own instrument was quite similar to an oesophagoscope, although more far-reaching. Chevalier-Jackson began working in Pittsburgh around 1904 and rapidly became a world renowned endoscopist. He believed that the great advantage of the hollow tube was that it could be introduced under visual control. Jackson thought that this was essential to avoid accidents and he opposed the blind insertion of endoscopes, as done in all types of closed optical systems. His own gastroscope consisted of a simple hollow metal tube, 9 mm in diameter (Figs. 41 and 42) and provided with a distal lamp for illumination[14]. In reality, he was doing an "extended" oesophagoscopy and Jackson demonstrated in several publications that he could visualise the greatest part of the stomach with the help of an assistant who compressed the abdomen manually so as to draw the gastric walls in close to the tip of the instrument. Jackson published his first paper on gastroscopy in 1907. It was illustrated with numerous coloured drawings and he prophetically stated that "vision is so clear and satisfactory that the next decade will see the internist and the gastroenterologist introduce gastroscopes as frequently as the gynecologist introduces a cystoscope".

All his endoscopies were done under general anaesthesia and the examination required an assistant who would keep the head of the patient firmly but flexibly extended during the examination. In one of his articles he reported the diagnosis of two cases of cancer of the cardia and three instances of pyloric cancer. He was able to take biopsies in two cases. On one occasion he managed to extract a foreign body from the stomach. He stated that his gastroscope could clearly visualise the middle third of the stomach, the inferior aspect of both gastric walls and the lower third of the greater curvature[15]. As already mentioned, the fundus and *(Fig. 43)* the antrum could be examined with the help of a second assistant who, by means of deep palpation, was able to place the instrument near to the gastric mucosa[38]. Jackson presented his findings at a meeting of the laryngology section of the American Medical Association[16]. The German otolaryngologist, Gustav Killian, who was visiting America, was a guest at that session and later commented that he had introduced Jackson's gastroscope easily once it had passed through the cardia, and he also said that one could see gastric ulcers, provided they were not too small[16].

The gastroscope designed by Hill[12], who had made unfavourable commments about Souttars's curved instrument, was based on the same principle as the Chevalier-Jackson gastroscope. It was rigid, straight and hollow and was used frequently in some hospitals in the United Kingdom. *(Fig. 44)*.

Gastroscopes with flexible mechanisms

According to Schindler, the third type of gastroscope comprises those instruments provided with a mechanism to straighten them once introduced into the stomach. The best known were those of Kuttner[23] and Sussman[56], but other prototypes were also made[7, 31, 34]. They are described in the following chapter.

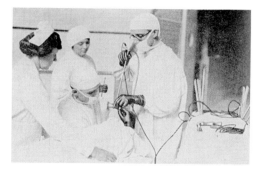

Fig. 42. Chevalier-Jackson and his team starting a gastroscopy examination at the Hospital of the University of Pennsylvania in Philadelphia (1933).

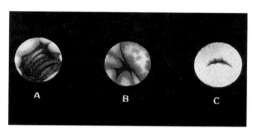

Fig. 43. Original colour drawings from Chevalier-Jackson's archives using his endoscope. A) gastrojejunal anastomosis B) carcinoma of the lesser curve of the stomach. C) healing penetrating gastric ulcer.

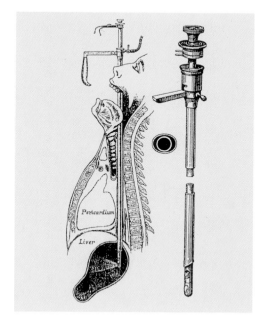

Fig. 44. Hill's open gastroscope, similar to the Chevalier-Jackson instrument, being introduced into the stomach (1912) (ref. 12).

REFERENCES

1 Baratoux J. De l'oesophagoscopie et de la gastroscopie. Rev Mens Laryngol Otol Rhinol (Bordeaux) 1882; 3: 97-107.

2 Bensaude R. Un noveau type de gastroscope. Le gastroscope a fil conducteur. Bull Acad Med Paris 1924; (3 série) 91: 712-716.

3 Edmonson J. M. History of the instruments for gastrointestinal endoscopy. Gastrointest Endosc 1991;37:S27-S56.

4 Elsner H. Die Gastroskopie, G. Thieme, Leipzig, 1911.

5 Elsner H. Mein verbessertes Gastroskop. Deutsche Med Wschr 1923; 49:253-256.

6 Elsner H. Photographie der Magenhöhle. Med Klin 1928; 24:1511-1515.

7 Gottstein G. Gastroskopie. in Abderhalden E. Handbuch der biologischen Arbeitsmethoden. Abt. IV. Teil 6. Verdauungsapparat. Berlin, Urban & Schwarzenberg 1926.

8 Gurlt E Biographisches Lexicon der hervorragender Arzte aller Zeiten und Völker Berlin-Wien, V. C. , 1934.

9 Henning N. Lehrbuch der Gastroskopie. Leipzig, J. A. Barth, 1935.

10 Herrington J. L. Historical aspects of gastric surgery. in Surgery of the Stomach, Duodenum and Small Intestine, H. W. Scott, J. L. Sawyers (eds) Oxford, Blackwell, 1992.

11 Hill W. On gastroscopy: a plea for its routine employment by gastric experts. Brit M J 1911; 2:1704.

12 Hill W. M. On gastroscopy and oesophago-gastroscopy London, Bale sons and Danielson, 1912.

13 Huizenga E. On esophagoscopy and sword swallowing. Ann Otology 1969; 78: 32-39.

14 Jackson, Ch. Gastroscopy. Medical Record (New York) 1907; 71: 549-555.

15 Jackson, Ch. Gastroscopy: report of additional cases. J. A. M. A. 1907; 49: 1425- 1428.

16 Jackson Ch. , Jackson C. L. Peroral gastroscopy. J. A. M. A. 1933; 104: 271.

17 Kelling G. Endoskopie für Speiseröhre und Magen. Gegliedertes Oesophagoskop welches durch Zug und Drehung streckbar ist. München med Wchnschr 1897; 44:934-937.

18 Kluge F. Seidler E. Zur Erstanwendung der Ösophago-und Gastroskopie. Briefe von Adolf Kussmaul und seinen Mitarbeitern. Medizin Historisches J. 1986; 21: 288-307.

19 Kluge F. Adolf Kussmaul (1822-1902). Eine biographische Skizze. Falk Foundation, 5 Auflage, 1996.

20 Korbsch R. Gastroskopische Ergebnisse. München med Wchschr 1924; 71:1498-1501.

21 Korbsch R. Die Gastroskopie, Berlin, S. Karger, 1926.

22 Kussmaul A. Über Magenspiegelung. Ber. d. Naturforsch Gesellschaft, Freiburg 1868; 5:112.

23 Kuttner L. Über Gastroskopie, ein gegliedertes Gastroskop, das durch Rotation gestreckt werden kann. Berliner klin Wchnschr 1897; 45: 912-915.

24 Leiter J. Elektroendoskopische Instrumente. Wien, W. Braumüller und Sohn, 1880. Drs. H. J. Reuter and M. Reuter, Max-Nitze Museum, 1985.

25 Leiter J. Erklärung bezüglich der Priorität in der Frage der jetzigen Cystoskopie. Int Centralbl Physiol Pathol der Harn u. Sexual-organe. 1890;1: 421-422.

26 Loening K., Stieda A. Über Gastroskopie. Zentralblatt f. Chirurgie 1908; 915.

27 Loening K., Stieda A. Die Untersuchung des Magens mit dem Magenspiegel. Mitteilungen Grenzgebieten Med Chir. 1910;21: 181-188.

28 Michon P. Revue critique. La gastroscopie. Ann Med 1924; 16: 146-166.

29 Mikulicz J. Über Gastroskopie und Oesophagoskopie. Centralbl f. Chirurgie 1881; 43:673-676.

30 Mikulicz v. J. Über Gastroskopie. Wien med Presse 1881; 22: 1410, 1439, 1473,1505, 1537, 1629.

31 Modlin I. M. A brief history of endoscopy. Milano, MultiMed 2000.

32 Moure E. J. De l'examen gastroscopique, sa technique et sa valeur clinique . Presse Med 1912; 25: 101-103.

33 Moutier F. Traité de gastroscopie et de pathologie endoscopique de l'estomac. Paris, Masson, 1935.

34 Neumann H. A. , Hellwig A. Von Schwertschlucker zur Glasfiberoptik. Die Geschichte der Gastroscopie. München, Urban & Vogel, 2001.

35 Nitze M. Eine neue Beleuchtungs- und Untersuchungsmethode für Harnröhre, Harnblase und Rektum. Wiener med Wschr 1879; 29: 651-652, 714-716, 780-782.

36 Niwa H. History of Digestive Endoscopy, Tokyo, Nihon Medical Center, 1997.

37 Rachet J. La gastroscopie. Paris, C. Doin, 1926.

38 Rehfuss M. The diagnosis and treatment of diseases of the stomach. Philadelphia, WB Saunders, 1927.

39 Reuter H. J. Biographie von Josef Leiter, Instrumentmacher Nitzes. Eröffnungssymposium, das Wiener Endoskopie Museum 1966, Wien, Literas Universitätsverlag, 1997.

40 Reuter M. A. Geschichte der Endoskopie. Band 1-4,Stuttgart-Zurich, Karl Krämer Verlag, 1998.

41 Redwizov P. Zur Technik der Gastroskopie (Modification des Rosenheim'schem Gastroskop) Congrès International de Medicine, Moscú 1899, III Section 5, pp. 214-218.

42 Rosenheim T. Über die Besichtigung der Kardia nebst Bemerkungen über die Gastroskopie. Deutsch med Wchnschr 1895; 21: 740-744.

43 Rosenheim T. Über Gastroskopie Berliner klin Wchnschr 1896; 33: 275-278.

44 Sauerbruch F. Gastroskopie mit tödlichem Ausgange Zentralbl f. Chir 1924; 38: 2071-2072

45 Schindler R. Bericht über 120 Fälle von Gastroskopie. Ärtzl Verein München 25, Januar 1922. Reported in Deutsch Med Wchnschr 1922; 48: 310.

46 Schindler R. Lehrbuch und Atlas der Gastroskopie, München, I. F. Lehmann, 1923.

47 Schindler R. Gastroscopy: the endoscopic study of gastric pathology. Chicago, University of Chicago Press, 1937.

48 Schindler R. Gastroscopy: the endoscopic study of gastric pathology. (2ª edition) New York, Hafner Publishing Company, 1966.

49 Ségal, A. Place de l'ingénieur Gustave Trouvé (1839-1902) dans l'histoire de l'endoscopie. Histoire Sciences Médicales 1995; 29: 123-132.

50 Seydl G. - Mikulicz und die Gastroskopie. Referat gehalten am 5 Symposium der Internationalen Nitze-Leiter Forschunggesellschaft für Endoskopie "150 Geburtstag von Mikulicz-Radecki" 21-22 Jan. 2000, Josephinum, Viena.

51 Souttar H. S, Thompson Th. The gastroscope and its uses. Brit Med J 1909; 2: 842-845.

52 Stein Th. Das Trouvé'sche Polyskop und Herr Leiter in Wien. Wien med Presse 1880; 10: 304-310.

53 Sternberg W. Eine neue Position zur gastroskopischen Untersuchung. Zentralbl Chir 1922; 49: 1402-1406.

54 Sternberg W. Fortschritte und Ruckschritte der Gastroskopie. Acta Chir Scand 1923;55: 563-576.

55 Stieda A. Der gegenwärtige Stand der Gastroskopie. Ergebn der Chir u. Orthop. 1912: 4: 387-399.

56 Sussmann M. Ein biegsames Gastroskop. Therapie der Gegenwart 1911; 52: 433-441.

57 Trouvé G. das Polyskop, ein neuer galvanischer Universal-Beleuchtungs und Kauterisations Apparat. Illustr. Viertel Jahrschr der ärtzl. Polytech (Bern) 1880; 2, nº 24, 68-72.

58 Trouvé G. Manuel théorique, instrumentale et pratique d'electrologie Médicale. Paris, Doin, 1893.

59 Walk L The history of gastroscopy. Clio Medica 1966; 1:209-222.

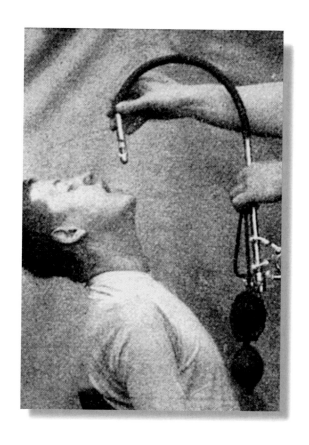

CHAPTER 4

Rudolf Schindler
and the semi-flexible
gastroscope

DEVELOPMENT AND DRAWBACKS
OF RIGID GASTROSCOPY

In 1922 THERE WERE FIVE TYPES OF GASTROSCOPES ON THE MARKET; four rigid ones (Loening-Stieda, Elsner, Schindler and Kausch)[46] and the semi-flexible instrument designed by Sussmann. In 1931 there were at least seven endoscopes available, including those of Elsner, Sternberg, Schindler (with the Hohlweg modification), Korbsch, Hübner and Bensaude[46], all of them of the rigid kind. Georg Wolf, the instrument-maker from Berlin, had manufactured the endoscopes of Elsner, Sternberg and Hohlweg, the semi-flexible gastroscope of Sussmann and the prototype invented by Hoffmann which inspired the later designs by Schindler and Wolf.

The interest in gastroscopy at that time can be judged by the number of patents on instruments, optical systems, light sources, and so on, that were granted to various instrument makers, institutions and private individuals[34]: eighteen patents between 1877-1900, thirty-four between 1901 and 1920 and seventy-seven between 1921 and 1940[16].

The mortality with gastroscopy was substantial. A review made by Hübner in 1926 based on an analysis of 3,627 examinations gave a mortality of 0.1-0.3 per cent. However, after 1931, mortality diminished considerably and hundreds of examinations were performed, most of them in Germany[14, 26, 46].

GASTROSCOPES WITH FLEXIBLE TUBES
AND RIGID OPTICAL SYSTEMS

Having mentioned Schindler's classification in the previous chapter, we will now deal with gastroscopes featuring flexible tubes and rigid optical systems. From 1900 until the late 1930s, endoscopists, influenced by Mikulicz's ideas, believed that in order to provide a straight view and to be able to rotate the gastroscope on its axis to visualise the entire gastric cavity, the instrument should be rigid.

However, it was obvious that introducing a gastroscope with a flexible end, like the first tool designed by Nitze and Leiter, was better tolerated by the patient and probably less dangerous.

The principle of a "flexible" gastroscope that could be straightened once inside the stomach was adopted mainly by Kelling, Kuttner and Sussmann.

Kelling's gastroscope

Georg Kelling, a surgeon from Dresden and Mikulicz's pupil[10], is best known among endoscopists for his publications on laparoscopy *(Fig. 1)*. After using Mikulicz's endoscope and testing the difficulties and risks of its introduction, as well as the limited view it provided which required the use of "twin" endoscopes[21], Kelling[20] designed an original instrument which was manufactured by Eugen Albrecht in Dresden in 1897 *(Figs. 2, 3, 4)*.

The "articulated" instrument was made of several hollow metal segments which could be straightened up, leaving a single angle at the end of the instrument, like that of the gastroscope of his mentor Mikulicz. This straightening was achieved by introducing the instrument with the patient initially seated and then lying down. The instrument was inserted beyond the cardia by means of a system of wires which controlled the position of the metal segments "just as the tendons of a finger control the phalanges" in Schindler's words. Once the tube was straightened, a thinner tube carrying the optical lenses was inserted into its lumen.

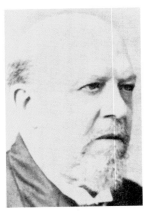

Fig. 1. Georg Kelling, a surgeon and Mikulicz's pupil, a pioneer of digestive endoscopy. He designed ingenious flexible instruments for oesophagoscopy and gastroscopy. He became more famous as the first physician to perform a laparoscopy (courtesy of Dr. Harald Henning).

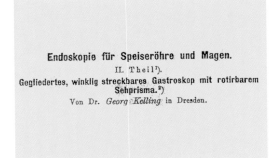

Fig. 2. Title page of Kelling's article describing his instrument which was provided with a distal rotating prism (1898).

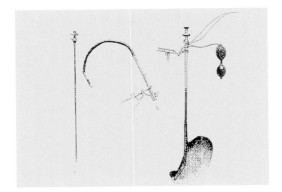

Fig.3 . Kelling's flexible gastroscope.

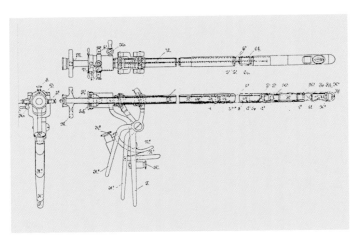

Fig. 4. Cross-section of the instrument showing the construction details, the wire system and its manipulation through the handle of the endoscope. (ref. n. 20).

The proximal end of the external hollow tube was 36 cm long and made of rigid metal. It was connected with the distal flexible part made of articulated segments 14 mm in diameter and provided with a channel through which the wires were passed. The flexible part was entirely covered by a rubber sheath. The distal end could be flexed about 45 degrees, it was 10 cm long and ended in a round tip. It featured a window which contained a miniature lamp and a prism which could be independently rotated 360 degrees. Kelling made moulds of the stomach of cadavers which he studied carefully before giving a definitive design to his instrument.

Kelling's endoscope, however, had many drawbacks and was little used, as the wire mechanism was easily broken and the insertion technique was difficult, especially because of the angular distal portion of the endoscope *(Fig. 5)*. Kelling examined more than 30 patients with his instrument; he strongly believed that to examine the entire stomach it was necessary that the instrument should be straight and rigid because otherwise it could not be properly oriented inside the gastric cavity. The same problem reappeared many years later when clinicians started to use the soft, flexible fiberscope.

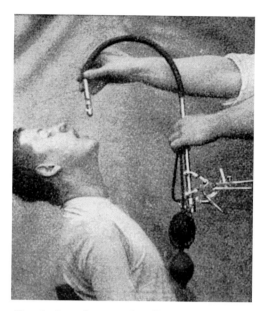

Fig. 5. Introduction of Kelling's flexible endoscope. The patient is seated; the gastroscope was straightened by moving the wires to allow vision (ref. n.20).

Kuttner's gastroscope *(Fig. 6)*

At that time, Kuttner in Berlin described another flexible instrument based on an entirely different principle[22]. His gastroscope consisted of two concentric tubes made of metallic segments of equal length linked by hinges. If the joints were in the same plane, the whole instrument was flexible. If the tubes were turned on their own axes, so that the joints of one tube did not overlie those of the other, the instrument became straight and rigid[22]. The two tubes were introduced, one inside the other; once in the stomach, the instrument was straightened by rotating the inner tube so that the joints of the segments of both tubes were facing each other on the same plane. However, although this instrument was in theory much simpler than that of Kelling and could be introduced and manipulated in a seated patient, it was in practice difficult to use as the rotation manoeuvres were never easy and sometimes required vigorous handling of the tubes. Kuttner's gastroscope received even less acceptance than that of Kelling[2].

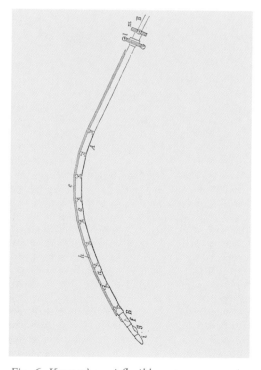

Fig. 6. Kuttner's semi-flexible gastroscope consisting of two concentric tubes made of metal segments that had to align to straighten the instrument. (from Elsner's book "Die Gastroskopie", 1911)

Sussmann's gastroscope *(Figs. 7, 8, 9, 10)*

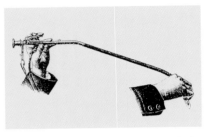

Die Therapie der Gegenwart
1911 herausgegeben von Prof. Dr. G. Klemperer Oktober
in Berlin.
Nachdruck verboten.
Ein biegsames Gastroskop.
Von Dr. Martin Sussmann-Berlin.

Fig. 7. Title page of Martin Sussmann's article (1911) describing his flexible gastroscope. (ref. n.42).

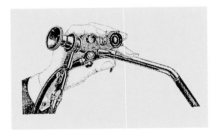

Fig. 8. Sussmann's gastroscope consisting of a proximal rigid portion and a longer distal flexible portion. (ref. n.42).

Some years later, in 1911, Martin Sussmann[42] again tried to design a flexible gastroscope. The concept of the instrument was very ingenious: the endoscope was flexible in its distal two thirds and the proximal rigid segment had an angle which once inserted, lay on the base of the tongue. This angulation did away with the need for the head to be tilted so far back, a requisite with rigid endoscopes. The end of the instrument was fitted with a glass capsule provided with a window so that the optical system could be rotated in several directions. A wire system controlled by a wheel at the handle of the endoscope served to straighten the instrument inside the stomach. The gastroscope was inspired by Kelling's instrument. It was technically outstanding and relatively easy to introduce but unfortunately, it was rather fragile and very expensive. In general, the straightening manoeuvre was simple, but stronger manipulation was occasionally needed and this was painful for the patient. The examination was done with the patient lying on his right side and the stomach was insufflated by means of oxygen or compressed air. Sussmann applied for a patent in Berlin *(Fig. 11)* in June 1911[16]; this was granted with the number 235270, and it was marketed by the firm Georg Wolf. Sussmann's gastroscope was apparently used in several university clinics but I have found no references or statistical data about

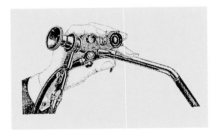

Fig. 9. Detail of the wheel mechanism at the handle of Sussmann's instrument. Vision was made possible by pulling the wires and straightening the endoscope. (ref. n.42).

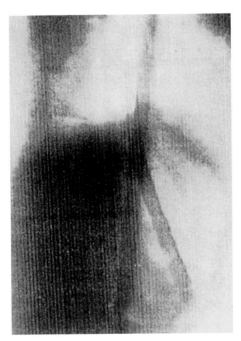

Fig. 10. Radiograph of Sussmann's gastroscope in the stomach once straightened by the wire system. (ref. n. 42).

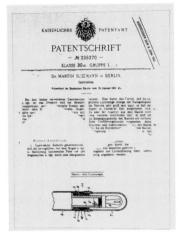

Fig. 11. Drawing of Sussmann's application for a patent for his gastroscope. The instrument was manufactured by Georg Wolf but its extreme fragility prevented its general use. (from Hellwig: Meilensteinen der Endoskopie, Wiener Endoskopie Museum, 2000).

the performance of this instrument in the literature. However, a report on a perforation using this gastroscope was duly published.

Hardt's "flexi-rigid" gastroscope

In 1944, when Schindler's gastroscope, manufactured by the firm Cameron, was being widely used in the United States, Leo Hardt[15] designed a "flexi-rigid" gastroscope which consisted of two parts: a flexible sheath and a removable rigid optical system comprising 25 optical elements. The device was possibly inspired by the Loening and Stieda gastroscope which we have already described. The twelve distal centimeters of the sheath were flexible and after introduction of the optical system, the gastroscope became rigid. The sheath was introduced first and the optical system was inserted into the sheath after this was placed in the stomach. A window at the distal end of the sheath included the lamp and an adjustable mirror which provided up to 80 degrees of vision. The greatest diameter of the metal housing was 10 mm, and that of the flexible portion 10.5 mm, about 2 mm. thinner than that of Schindler-Cameron's gastroscope. The manufacturing of Hardt's gastroscope was aided by a grant from the Research Committee of the American Medical Association. Even so, the instrument had little acceptance.

GASTROSCOPES WITH AN OPTICAL SYSTEM INCORPORATED INTO A FLEXIBLE TUBE

Hoffmann's gastroscope *(Figs. 12, 13)*

In 1911, Michael Hoffmann[18], an assistant physician at the Ophthalmology Department of Munich's University[13], described a new instrument which was to become a direct forerunner of Wolf-Schindler's gastroscope. Hoffmann had shown that "it was possible to transmit images along flexing curves if numerous prisms were placed in a movable tube". The prism system was manufactured for the Zeiss firm by A.Köhler and M. von Rohr, while the other parts of the gastroscope were made by Georg Wolf in Berlin.

Optische Instrumente mit beweglicher Achse und ihre Verwendung für die Gastroskopie.
Von Dr. Michael Hoffmann, Assistenzarzt der Kgl. Universitäts-Augenklinik zu München.

Die Möglichkeit, optische Instrumente mit beweglicher Achse herzustellen, d. h. durch einen beliebig gekrümmten Schlauch zu sehen, ist seitens der Aerzte, die sich mit dem Problem der Gastroskopie beschäftigt haben, mehrfach in

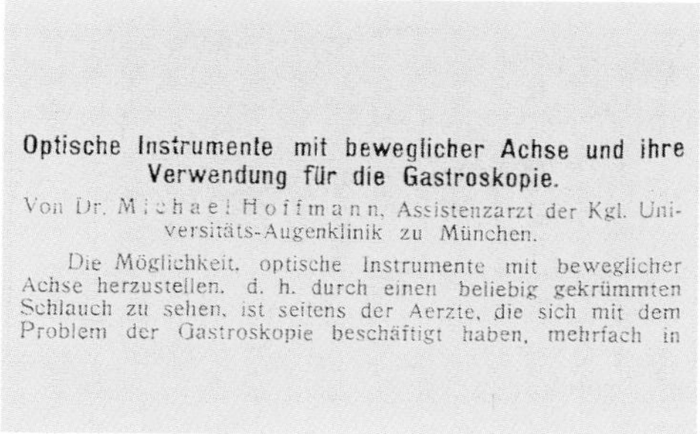

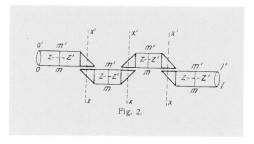

Fig. 12. Title page of Michael Hoffmann's article describing his flexible axis gastroscope. (ref. n.18).

Fig. 13. Drawing of the movable prisms of Hoffmann's instrument. Georg Wolf's firm only made one prototype. (from Hoffmann's paper, ref. n.18).

The instrument was tested in cadavers, and according to Hoffmann, vision was much better than with the rigid gastroscopes. However, a considerable amount of light was lost, absorbed by the optical system, because when the instrument was bent, the movable prisms often changed their orientation

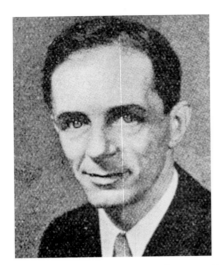

Fig. 14. Rudolf Schindler at the time of his arrival in the United States as an immigrant. (portrait courtesy of Dr. Enrique Sierra, Editorial Científico-Médica).

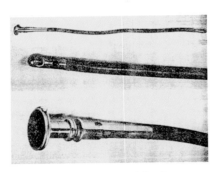

Fig. 15. Various views of the first prototype of the totally flexible gastroscope made by Georg Wolf for Rudolf Schindler. It was unsuccessful due to image distortion. The instrument is on display at the Smithsonian Institution in Washington together with other endoscopes, including the first fibrescope. (composite picture modified from ref. n. 6).

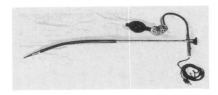

Fig. 16. The standard Wolf-Schindler gastroscope (ref. n. 39).

and image transmission was difficult. Apparently, the results of Hoffmann's prototype were not sufficiently consistent for its use in routine clinical work, but Schindler and Wolf further developed Hofmann's ideas and designed the semi-flexible gastroscope that later made them famous.

The first Schindler-Wolf gastroscopes

In 1916, an optician named Lange, who was employed by the Goertz factory in Berlin, discovered that a tube filled with a series of thick convex lenses with a short focal distance could transmit an image without distortion even when bent on different planes. His designs, however, were never published[39, 46]. Schindler already had vast experience with rigid gastroscopes when he began his close collaboration with Georg Wolf around 1928 and Wolf had manufactured the majority of instruments available on the market. The two carefully studied Hoffmann's paper and had the crucial idea of substituting the prisms for lenses, thus independently reaching the same conclusion as Lange[6] (Figs. 14, 15).

Wolf's first prototype was entirely flexible and very soft. The tip could be moved backward and forward covering an angle of 180 degrees. However, the gastroscope was quite unmanageable and was not marketed. According to François Moutier, the famous French endoscopist[26] who around 1930 was able to test this instrument in Schindler's clinic, the transmitted images were very distorted and the tube could not be oriented properly as it would twist on its own axis. Moreover, in the left lateral position, the distal objective rested on the greater curve and the "mucous lake" of the stomach, making vision even more difficult. Schindler then realised that the instrument had to be flexible from a point about 3 cm. above the cardia to the distal end of the tube[35]. He then asked Wolf to make the flexible part of the instrument more elastic and harder than that of the first model, while the rest of the instrument, including the oesophageal portion, should be entirely rigid. Between 1928 and 1932, Wolf made six different prototypes, until he designed an instrument which Schindler in 1932 qualified as "magnificent" and which became very popular in Germany as well as in other countries[38, 39]. (Fig. 16).

Georg Wolf was awarded two patents for his gastroscopes (#629.590 and #662788) in 1930 and 1932, respectively. Three years later, he succeeded in patenting his instrument in the United States (Fig. 17).

Georg Wolf

Georg Wolf (1873-1938) began his career in the Reiniger, Gebbert and Schall factory in Erlangen[36] where he acquired experience in the manufacturing of cystoscopes. He then moved to Berlin where he set up his own firm. According to Schindler, he started out in 1911 manufacturing Sussmann's flexible gastroscope which was considered as a small technical marvel. He later made rigid instruments like Elsner's. His big opportunity came when he associated with Schindler. Between 1928 and 1932, Wolf made six different prototypes of semi-flexible gastroscopes. From then on, he gained prestige and wealth. After World War Two, his firm was split into two factions: Sass-Wolf, that remained in Berlin, and Richard Wolf, which was established in Knittlingen (then in West Germany) by other members of the firm, including his direct successors.

A few years later, the firm Richard Wolf had become one of the most important factories for medical and surgical endoscopy equipment.

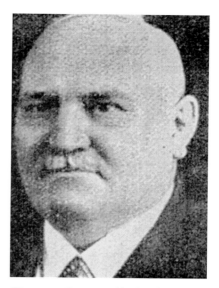

Fig. 17. Georg Wolf, the founder of Wolf's firm in Berlin, nowadays the Richard Wolf GmbH, Knittlingen, Germany) (courtesy of Prof. H.J.Reuter).

The standard Schindler-Wolf instrument

As already mentioned, this revolutionary gastroscope consisted of a proximal rigid part and a distal flexible portion[35]. The flexible portion of the instrument was made of six equal elements, each containing three spacers. Two of the spacers carried double convex lenses and one a single convex lens, making a total of 31 lenses. The spacers were articulated with each other by a ball and socket joint and were placed 15 mm apart. These six elements, totalling twenty-four centimeters, produced a real image in the last focal plane that was unaffected when the flexible distal tube was bent into an arc as wide as thirty-four degrees. The entire instrument was composed of fifty-one optical elements, all firmly secured with a flexible bronze coil (Fig. 18).

The first gastroscope that Wolf made for Schindler had a rigid portion of 11 mm in diameter, although a thinner prototype, 8.5 mm in diameter, was also manufactured. The flexible distal tube was 14.5 cm in length and 12 mm in diameter because of its rubber cover. It was attached to the proximal rigid portion and the junction was protected by a metal sleeve as during a demonstration in Paris in 1932, Schindler broke three instruments, one after the other, at this point[39].

The total length of the instrument was 74 cm. The distal end of the flexible portion, about six cm in length, was made of rigid metal and was provided with a glass window one centimeter from the tip to allow rays from the illuminated gastric wall to enter the optical system. A prism deflected the light

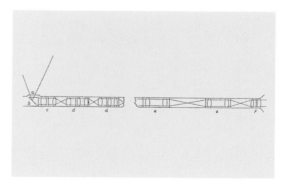

Fig. 18. Cross-section of the spaced lenses included in the flexible part of Schindler's gastroscope (1937). It comprised a total of 51 optical elements. (ref. n. 39).

rays entering the window into the optical axis of the gastroscope. Immediately below the window was a filament lamp which, according to Schindler, was not an ideal source of light as the complicated lens system absorbed much of it. The lamp operated with a current of 8-10 volts and the examination had to be performed in a completely darkened room. A 4.6 cm long solid rubber finger attached to the tip of the gastroscope allowed easy passage into the stomach by stretching the angle of the lower oesophagus.

The outer rubber sheath of the flexible part had three small holes at its gastric end as outlets for the air which was insufflated with a rubber balloon. The inner flexible portion containing the optical system was attached by threads to the distal objective-bearing metal piece. It also included an electric wire which was connected to the distal lamp. Air was insufflated between the outer rubber sheath and the inner rubber tube containing the lenses.

The rigid portion of the instrument remained 1-2 cm above the cardia at all times[26], thus avoiding damage to this area. The eyepiece which contained the last two lenses was 5.5 cm long and was provided with two attachments: a handle with a sliding thumb switch connected to the electric outlet and another attachment in which an air balloon for insufflation was fastened.

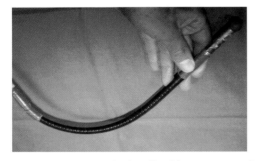

Fig. 19. View of the flexible portion of Schindler's gastroscope. Instrument used at the Postgraduate School of Gastroenterology, Hospital de Sant Pau, Barcelona).

According to Moutier, vision through these first prototypes was not as good as that of rigid instruments and the image was a yellowish colour due to so many lenses.

The angle of vision had to be narrow, because gastroscopy required a deep focal distance so that the antropyloric region could remain at a distance of 10 cm or more from the objective of the instrument. According to Schindler, sharpness of image and magnification were best at an angle of between 46 and 55 degrees.

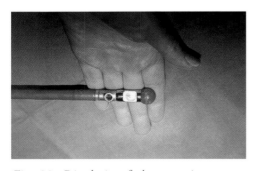

Fig. 20. Distal tip of the same instrument, showing the optical window and the lamp. The distal rubber ball was added according to N.Hennings suggestion.

The rubber finger tip which Schindler deemed necessary to avoid lesions of the hypopharynx and to protect the gastric wall was criticised by Moutier who found it inconvenient because it often bent in the pharynx during insertion[38]. Henning used instead a small rubber sponge, but this caused several accidents[19, 39]; he later employed a solid rubber ball which was adopted by Wolf for his gastroscopes, in spite of Schindler's misgivings. This rubber ball was also used by Moutier and it can be inspected on Moutier's gastroscope donated by his pupil André Cornet to the Museum of the History of Medicine at Paris University. A model of this kind was also used at the Hospital Sant Pau in Barcelona. A smaller rubber ball was later used by Heinkel in the design of gastric suction biopsy instruments which he devised in Henning's department in Erlangen (Figs. 19, 20).

History repeats itself, and in the same way as disputes arose between Leiter, Kussmaul and Mikulicz, Georg Wolf also had trouble with the American gastroenterologist Samuel Weiss who had visited him in 1927 and shown his own designs for a new gastroscope that Wolf considered impractical. However, Weiss later contended that Wolf had used his suggestions in the design of his new models without mentioning his contribution[23].

The flexible gastroscope eliminated the risk of perforating the distal oesophagus where the majority of lesions produced by rigid gastroscopes occurred. Schindler's gastroscope comfortably permitted a wide view of the gastric cavity, particularly the antro-pyloric region which could be visualised in some 89 per cent of cases *(Fig. 21).*

Schindler presented his instrument at a session of the Physician's Association ("Ärtzlichen Verein") in Munich on the sixth of July, 1932. His paper was published in August in the Münchener Medizinische Wochenschrift under the title " A flexible gastroscope totally devoid of danger"[35]. The article was followed in the same issue, by another from Norbert Henning, then in Leipzig, who described his experience with the instrument[17]. In spite of some discrepant views, a long lasting friendship united Schindler with Henning, who after World War Two created a renowned centre for digestive endoscopy at Erlangen University.

The technique of gastroscopy according to Schindler

A pupil of Schindler's, the Spaniard Morales Noriega[25] described the technique of gastroscopy in detail; the patient should be fasting, and sedation with morphine-codeine and 0.5 mg of atropine should be administered 45 minutes before the examination. Local anaesthesia with 2 per cent pantocaine was then administered through a tube with multiple perforations apparently invented by Schindler's son Richard when he was only eleven years old! The stomach was emptied by means of a standard Ewald tube while the patient was lying on a specially designed folding table *(Fig. 22).*

The patient was placed on his left side with his left shoulder right at the edge of the examining table. The head was tilted back but relaxed and supported by an assistant. The instrument was introduced as deeply as possible and was then rotated on its axis and slowly withdrawn, thereby visualising the gastric surface *(Figs. 23, 24).*

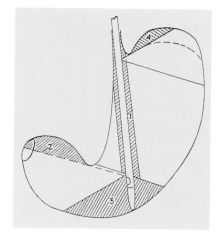

Fig. 21. Drawing of the blind areas of the stomach (shaded) not seen with Schindler's gastroscope (ref. n. 39).

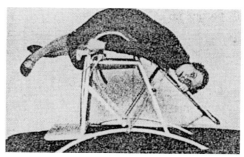

Fig. 22. A patient in the stomach drainage position prior to gastroscopy, she is bent on the folding table designed by Schindler. (from Morales-Noriega, ref. n. 25).

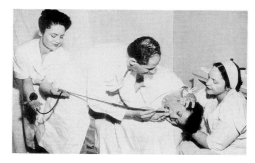

Fig. 23. Rudolf Schindler performing a gastroscopy. His wife Gabriele who helped her husband in most examinations, is seen supporting the patient's head. (courtesy of Prof. Michel Cremer).

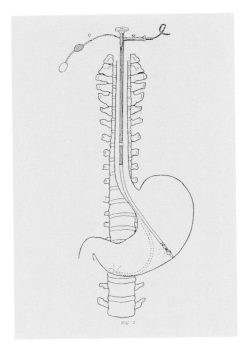

Fig. 24. Drawing by Morales Noriega, a pupil of Schindler's from Spain, showing the position of the gastroscope introduced into the stomach. (ref. n. 25).

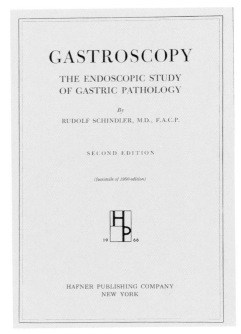

Fig. 25. "Gastroscopy", the famous book by Schindler (2nd edition, 1966).

A few attempts to perform gastroscopy under general anaesthesia with penthotal-curare were made in the following years[41] but the procedure was not readily accepted.

Rudolf Schindler (1888-1968) and his pupils

For those interested in the life of Rudolf Schindler, we recommend reading the excellent biography by Audrey B. Davis[6]. I am greatly indebted to it for many of the following data.

Schindler was born in Berlin. His father, a banker, was Jewish but his mother, the artist Martha Simon, was not. He was educated in Berlin and following the advice of his uncle Richard Simon, an ophthalmologist, he studied medicine and zoology in Freiburg. He started endoscopy with an Elsner's gastroscope in 1929 in a hospital in Schwabing, a district of Munich. Later, he employed a gastroscope of his own device, a modification of Elsner's instrument (see Chapter 3) which was manufactured in Munich by the firm Reiniger, Gebbert und Schall.

In 1922, he married Gabriele Winkler who spent the rest of her life at his side. She was an irreplaceable aide for his gastroscopies, to the point that he met with accidents when she was unable to be present. In 1923 he published his first book "Lehrbuch und Atlas der Gastroskopie" based upon his experience with the rigid gastroscope manufactured by Georg Wolf. As of 1924, Schindler met several American gastroenterologists —who visited him in Munich— in particular, Marie Ortmayer from Chicago. The advent of Hitler and Nazism compelled him to leave Germany along with countless other physicians and scientists who had been classified as Jewish. In 1934, thanks to his American friends, Schindler managed to emigrate to the United States; he was invited by the University of Chicago where two eminent gastroenterologists, Walter Palmer and Joseph B. Kirsner, were running a gastroenterology department.

Schindler trained more than 300 endoscopists and became known all over the world. He founded the American Gastroscopic Club, the first known endoscopy organisation which later became the pre-eminent "American Society for Gastrointestinal Endoscopy" (ASGE) *(Fig. 25)*. In 1943, as a result of disagreements with the head of the Department, Walter Palmer, partly the result of Schindler's dogmatic views on gastritis, he moved to the College of Medical Evangelists in

Los Angeles where he pursued his teaching and clinical tasks. In 1958, nearing retirement, he was invited as professor at the University of Belo Horizonte in Brazil where he lived until 1960. He then returned to the United States where for a period of time he was a consultant at the Long Beach Veterans Hospital in California. There he worked with two well-known endoscopists, Stephen Stempien and Angelo Dagradi[5]. After the death of Gabriele, his devoted wife and assistant, he returned to Munich in 1965 and died there in 1968.

Schindler himself performed over 10,000 gastroscopies, with very few accidents, and he kept careful records of all his observations. He performed his first gastroscopies on his assistants and on his maid! Besides his numerous students, Schindler left a legacy of five books and more than 170 articles. He always insisted that the physician who did endoscopy should not only be a technician but a complete gastroenterology specialist. Schindler spoke six languages: German, English, French, Portuguese, Greek and Latin. He was an accomplished chess player and he was an excellent musician –he conducted an orchestra of physicians in Munich[23].

The advent of fiberscopy relegated his work to a secondary position, but there is no doubt that Schindler was the person who exerted most influence on the endoscopic diagnosis of gastric diseases.

While still working in Munich, at least fifty physicians from all over the World attended Schindler's clinic to learn endoscopy. Table 1 shows a list of his first European pupils whom Schindler cites in his book on gastroscopy. Some of

TABLE I. A LIST OF SCHINDLER'S FOREIGN ALUMNI DURING HIS LATE YEARS IN GERMANY (1932-1934)

Argentina: Keiva Daza, Royer	**Hungary:** von Friedrich
Austria: Moskowicz	**Italy:** Brunetti, Torrigiani
Belgium: Graulich	**Japan:** Kirihara, Okada
Cuba: García	**Mexico:** Ayala Gonzalez
Czechoslovakia: Halmos, Scheiner	**Netherlands:** Bloem
Spain: Morales Noriega	**Switzerland:** Kapp, Oberholzer.
France: Moutier, Chevallier	

(Published in "Gastroscopy", R. Schindler (1966).

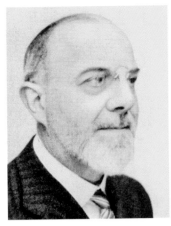

Fig. 26. *François Moutier, the most famous endoscopist of his era after Schindler and pioneer of gastroscopy in France (collection Dr. J. Vilardell).*

them became famous in *(Figs. 26, 27, 28, 29)* their own countries, such as François Moutier in France, Marcelo Royer in Argentina (a pioneer of laparoscopic cholangiography), von Friedrich in Hungary, Graulich and Desneux in Belgium[12], the Italians Camillo Torrigiani from Florence and Federico Brunetti from Venice, both laryngologists, and Morales Noriega, who published a detailed account of his stay in Munich in 1933, in Spain *(Fig. 30).*

Gastroscopy with Schindler's instrument was also performed in Spain by A. Rodriguez Olleros in Madrid and E. Vidal Colomer and J Badosa Gaspar in the Hospital de Sant Pau in Barcelona *(Figs. 31, 32).* In Italy, gastroscopy was particularly developed by Paolo Alessandrini head of the Institute of Digestive Diseases in Rome, and his assistant P. Bonadies.

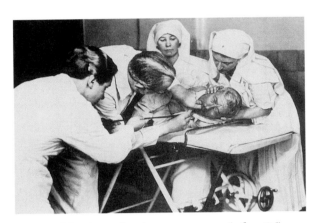

Fig. 27. *Moutier performing a gastroscopy (ref. n. 26).*

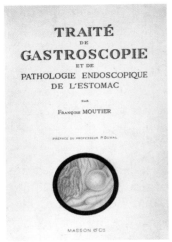

Fig. 29. *Moutier's "Traité de Gastroscopie" (1926). Possibly the most complete and objective book published on the subject. It had a decisive influence on European endoscopy in general.*

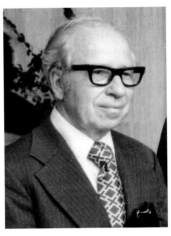

Fig. 31. *Angel Rodriguez Olleros, one of the first Spanish gastroscopists. Following the Spanish Civil War, he went into exile in Puerto Rico, where he introduced gastroscopy. (author's collection).*

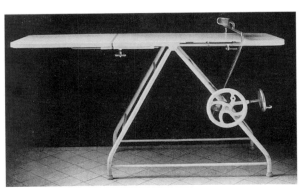

Fig. 28. *Gastroscopy examining table designed by Moutier (ref. n. 26).*

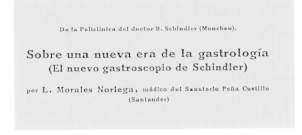

Fig. 30. *First Spanish article on gastroscopy written by L. Morales Noriega, a pupil of Schindler's (1933).*

Schindler's gastroscope was employed extensively in Germany by Henning who made some improvements and designed a special examining table. Later he began using a fiberoptic system as a "cold" light source *(Figs. 33, 34)*.

Semiflexible gastroscopes of Hermon Taylor, Chamberlin and Eder

Four American firms manufactured Schindler's gastroscope: Eder, Metro-Tec, Cameron and A.C.M.I.[24]. Some modifications of the flexible portion of the gastroscope were made by Hermon Taylor, an English surgeon, and by Chamberlin in the United States[27] *(Figs. 35, 36)*.

Hermon Taylor's gastroscope was made in England. Its distal end could be moved but this required the passage of cables for orientation, and resulted in an increase in the diameter of the instrument which made some manoeuvers more difficult[43, 44].

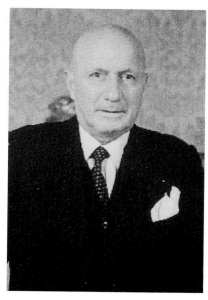

Fig. 32. Paolo Alessandrini, a leading gastroenterologist and director of the Institute for Digestive Diseases of the Rome Hospitals, one of the main advocates of Schindler's gastroscope in Italy. (courtesy of Dr. Sandro Alessandrini).

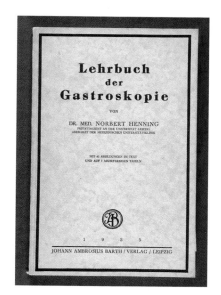

Fig. 33. A monograph on gastroscopy by Norbert Henning (1935). It described his rubber ball modification of the tip of Schindler's gastroscope and various devices for gastric photography.

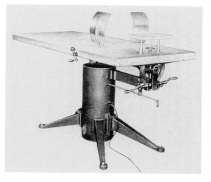

Fig. 34. Henning's examining table for endoscopy, particularly used for laparoscopy. (taken from his book).

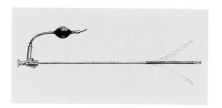

Fig. 35. The Hermon-Taylor gastroscope features a flexible tip but it was difficult to manipulate.

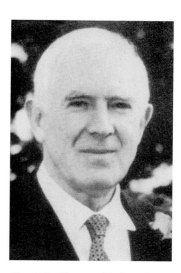

Fig. 36. Hermon-Taylor, distinguished British surgeon also known for his medical treatment of perforated gastric ulcers. (Fiftieth Anniversary, British Society of Gastroenterology).

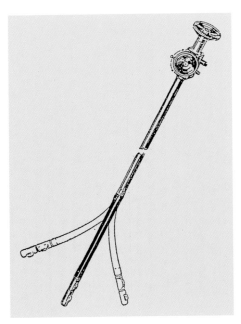

Fig. 37. *The Eder-Chamberlin gastroscope displaying the flexible movable tip (courtesy of Eder).*

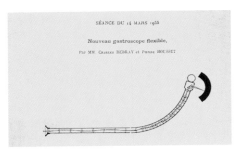

Fig. 38. *The O.P.L. gastroscope designed by Charles Debray in Paris (1955).*

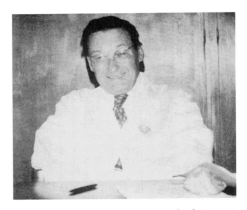

Fig. 39. *Charles Debray, a pupil of François Moutier, a renowned clinician and endoscopist, professor of gastroenterology at Hôpital Bichat in Paris. (author's collection).*

Chamberlin, an American endoscopist, ordered a similar instrument from the firm Cameron from Chicago[4]. His gastroscope was 51 cm long in its rigid portion and only 15 cm in its flexible part. The diameter of the rigid portion was 9.5 mm while that of the flexible tube was 11 mm.. The distal objective measured 4 cm. and a mirror which could be tilted, replaced the prism and provided a larger visual field. The angle of vision was 40 degrees and the tip could be moved about 30 degrees. Chamberlin believed that his gastroscope was easier to introduce than Hermon Taylor's instrument, but Schindler, who used it several times, thought that it had no real advantage over his own model *(Fig. 37)*.

Later, Streifeneder, an engineer from the Cameron factory, established his own firm under the name Eder. Following the suggestions of Eddy Palmer, one of the pioneers of gastroscopy in the United States, he succeeded in manufacturing an instrument only 9 mm in diameter in its wider portion which could be introduced through an oesophagoscope. A specific indication for this new gastroscope was the emergency examination of patients with gastrointestinal haemorrhage. This was done by Palmer and others[24, 30].

The O.P.L. gastroscope of Debray and Housset

In 1949, Charles Debray from Paris began to examine the possibility of manufacturing a French version of Schindler's gastroscope. In 1955, he presented the "Gastroflex" designed by Debray and Housset and made by the firm O.P.L.[7, 8] *(Figs. 38, 39)*.

The instrument had several advantages. The total length was 75.5 cm. The flexible portion was 37.5 cm in length and its diameter 11 mm. The diameter of the rigid portion was 8.5 mm. The total weight of the gastroscope was 310 grams. Like Schindler's gastroscope, it contained 52 optical elements with 34 lenses in the flexible portion. The images provided by the instrument were much better than those of the Schindler-Wolf gastroscope and pictures of considerable brightness could be taken. The angle of vision was wider and the flexibility of the instrument was greater. This model was used extensively in France. Debray succeeded in having O.P.L. design a thinner gastroscope only 10 mm in diameter, by eliminating the insufflation channel. However, the stomach had to be insufflated before the examination by means of a Camus tube.

The Storz semiflexible gastroscope *(Fig. 40)*

The Storz gastroscope, which was described and praised by Schindler in 1966, appeared several years later. The great advantage of the instrument, which was based on the classical model by Wolf-Schindler, was the incorporation of two lighting systems at the distal tip of the endoscope, provided by an external source of light transmitted by optical fibers. This resulted in a greatly improved illumination over other instruments. The addition of optical bundles increased the diameter of the instrument to 11 cm but with the advantage of eliminating the distal lamp, resulting in a shorter distal rigid tip. It was used extensively by Henning and his associates.

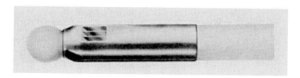

Fig. 40. Distal extremity of the semiflexible gastroscope designed by N. Henning and manufactured by Storz in Germany, featuring the distal rubber ball, an optical window and fiberoptic illumination. The last of the gastroscopes including a multiple lens system.

GASTROSCOPIC ACCIDENTS WITH SEMI-FLEXIBLE INSTRUMENTS.

Schindler[37] made a survey of 22,531 examinations, in which eight stomach perforations were reported, including three instances by Schindler himself, but with only one death. Another case of oesophageal perforation was reported somewhat later by Schiff[33]. The advent of fiberscopy did not avoid these accidents[9].

In 1951, Avery Jones and his associates[19] published a review on the risks of gastroscopy in Great Britain that was based on an analysis of 49,000 examinations made by 40 endoscopists. There were 75 accidents with 32 deaths, most of them due to oesophageal or gastric perforation. The majority of perforations occurred with gastroscopes fitted with a sponge tip which we have already described. Oesophageal perforations occurred mostly in the crico-pharyngeal region (with a mortality over 40 per cent). Most accidents were due to the use of the Hermon Taylor instrument which was more rigid and bulkier than the usual Schindler model. In 1964, Eddy Palmer published another survey of accidents due to gastroscopy, including 25,055 examinations with 0.108 per cent of perforations and 0.032 percent of deaths. Again, the Hermon Taylor gastroscope was responsible for more mishaps than the other instruments[29]. In 1957, Palmer made a wider inquiry addressed to the members of the American Society of Gastrointestinal Endoscopy which included 267,175 gastroscopies. There were 163 perforations with 25 deaths and 20 accidents due to anaesthesia[41]. It must be noted that in 20 of the 25 perforations the introduction of the endoscope was thought to have been easy[30]. Endoscopic biopsy which required the use of gastroscopes with wider diameters, was also a major cause of accidents[32, 40, 45].

To end this chapter we have a quote by Schindler which is still valid in part today, "Gastroscopic examination permits a differential diagnosis which is not possible by other means, and interpretation of pictures of disease conditions which formerly could not be diagnosed at all. The different forms of chronic gastritis and ventricular polyposis especially belong to this class".

Twenty years later, fiberscopy would bring about a revolution and open a new era of endoscopy.

REFERENCES

1 Benedict E.B. An operating gastroscope. Gastroenterology 1948;11: 281-295.
2 Berry L.H. Gastrointestinal pan-endoscopy. Springfield, (Ill), Ch.Thomas, 1974.
3 Boros E. Esophagoscopy by means of a flexible instrument. A new esophago-gastroscope. Gastroenterology 1947; 8: 724-728.
4 Chamberlin D.T. Description of a new gastroscope. Gastroenterology 1949; 12: 209-212.
5 Dagradi A.E., Stempien S.J. Rudolf Schindler. In memoriam. Gastrointest Endosc 1968; 15: 121-122.
6 Davis A.B. Rudolf Schindler's role in the development of gastroscopy Bull Hist Med. 1972; 46: 150-170.
7 Debray Ch., Housset P. Nouveau gastroscope flexible. Arch Mal Appar Dig. 1955; 44: 561-563.
8 Debray Ch., Housset P. Présentation d'un nouveau gastroscope biopsique. Ann Oto-Laryngol 1960; 77: 162-165.
9 Deutsch E. Hazard of perforation from passing fiberscope. Gastroenterology 1962; 43: 617-619.
10 Fischer I. Biographisches Lexicon der hervorragenden Ärzte der letzten fünfzig Jahre. Berlin, Urban & Schwarzenberg, 1932.
11 Franquela E. Valor diagnóstico de la gastroscopia Arch Med Cir y Espec. 1933: 36: 802-804.
12 Graulich R. Endoscopie en gastro-entérologie. Bruxelles Med. 1934; 14: 506-509.
13 Gurlt E. Biographisches Lexicon der hervorragender Ärzte aller Zeiten und Völker. V.C. Berlin, Wien, 1934.
14 Gutzeit K., Teitge H. Die Gastroskopie. Lehrbuch und Atlas. München, Urban & Schwartzenberg, 1937.
15 Hardt L.L. The flexi-rigid gastroscope. 1944; 3: 508-511.
16 Hellwig A. Die Entwicklung der Gastroskopie im Spiegel der deutschen Reichspatente (1877-1945) Meilensteine der Endoskopie. 2 Symposium der Internationale Nitze-Leiter Forschungsgesellschaft für Endoskopie. Wien, Literas Universitätsverlag, 2000.
17 Henning N. Erfahrungen mit dem flexiblen Gastroskop nach Wolf-Schindler. Münch Med Wschr 1932; 32: 1269-1271.
18 Hoffmann M. Optische Instrumente mit beweglicher Achse und ihre Verwendung für die Gastroskopie. Münch Med Wschr. 1911; 58: 2446-2448.
19 Jones F.A., Doll R., Fletcher C.M., Rodgers H.W. Risks of gastroscopy; survey of 49.000 examinations. Lancet 1951; 1: 647-649.
20 Kelling G. Gegliedertes, winklig-streckbares Gastroskop mit rotierbarem Sehprisma. München med Wschr 1898; 45: 1556-1559.
21 Kelling G. Endoskopie für Speiseröhre und Magen. Münch med Wschr 1989; 50: 1591-1594.
22 Kuttner I. Über Gastroskopie: ein gegliedertes Gastroskop, das durch Rotation gestreckt werden kann. Berlin klin Wschr 1897; 34: 912-939.
23 Modlin I.M., Farhadi J. Rudolf Schindler – a man for all seasons. J Clin Gastroenterol 2000; 31: 95-102.

[24] Monaghan J.F., Nast P.R. Gastroscopy. in Gastroenterology, H.L.Bockus (ed.) 2nd edition. vol 1, Philadelphia, Saunders, 1963: 318-328.

[25] Morales Noriega L. Sobre una nueva era de la gastrología. (el nuevo gastroscopio de Schindler) Arch Med Cir Espec. 1933; 36: 648-651.

[26] Moutier F. Traité de Gastroscopie et de Pathologie Endoscopique de l'Estomac, Paris, Masson, 1935.

[27] Neumann H.A., Hellwig A. Vom Schwertschlucker zur Glasfiberoptik. Die Geschichte der Gastroskopie. München, Urban & Vogel, 2001.

[28] Niwa H. History of Digestive Endoscopy, Tokyo, Nihon Medical Center, 1997.

[29] Palmer E.D. Risks of peroral endoscopy. US Armed Forces Med J 1954; 5: 974-994.

[30] Palmer E.D., Wirts C.W. Survey of gastroscopic and esophagoscopic accidents. Report of Committee on Accidents of American Gastroscopic Society. J.A.M.A. 1957; 164: 2012-2015.

[31] Rodriguez Olleros A., De La Viesca J.M. La gastroscopia, resultados de algunas observaciones. Medicina Latina 1933; 6: 238-251.

[32] Shallenberger P.L., DeWan C.H., Weed C.B., Reganis J.C. Biopsy through the flexible operating gastroscope. Gastroenterology 1950; 16: 327- 328.

[33] Schiff L., Shapiro N. Perforation of the stomach with the flexible gastroscope Am J Dig Dis 1941; 8: 260-261.

[34] Schindler R. Die diagnostiche Bedeutung der Gastroskopie. München med Wschr 1922; 69: 535-537.

[35] Schindler R. Ein völlig ungefährliches, flexibles Gastroskop. Münch Med Wschr 1932; 32: 1268-1269.

[36] Schindler R. Georg Wolf. Am J Dig Dis 1939; 5: 817-818.

[37] Schindler R. Results of a questionnaire on fatalities in gastroscopy. Am J Dig Dis 1940; 7:293-295.

[38] Schindler R. The rubber finger tip of the gastroscope. A warning. Gastroenterology 1949;13:473-473

[39] Schindler R. Gastroscopy. The endoscopic study of gastric pathology. Second edition. New York, Hafner, 1966.

[40] Shiner M. Gastric biopsy under direct visual control with the Hermon-Taylor gastroscope. Lancet 1956; 2271:178-179.

[41] Stempien S.J., Greene W.W. Gastroscopy under penthotal-curare anesthesia. Gastroenterology 1948;10: 978-981.

[42] Sussmann M. Ein biegsames Gastroskop. Therap d Gegenw. 1911; 52: 433-441.

[43] Taylor, Hermon. A new gastroscope with controllable flexibility. Lancet 1941; 2: 276-277.

[44] Taylor, Hermon. Difficulties and dangers of gastroscopy. Gastroenterology 1958; 35: 79-91.

[45] Tomenius J. An instrument for gastrobiopsies. Gastroenterology 1950; 15: 498-504.

[46] Walk L. The history of gastroscopy. Clio Med 1965; 1: 209-222.

[47] Wirts C.W., Carroll J.C., Wald D. Experience with operating gastroscope. Gastroenterology 1951; 19: 777-786.

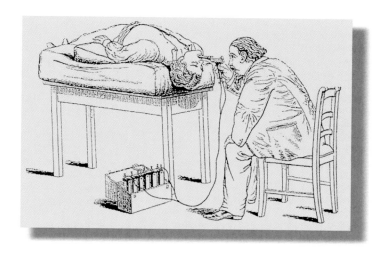

CHAPTER 5

Rigid
oesophagoscopy

THE FORERUNNERS

Since the classical antiquity, physicians have described blind efforts to retrieve foreign bodies impacted in the oesophagus using all kinds of pincers and clamps which we have already discussed in Chapter 1. The first attempts to inspect the entire gullet for diagnostic and therapeutic purposes started around 1870, as soon as laryngologists succeeded in visualising the pharynx and the upper oesophagus[19, 45, 52]. They were greatly helped by Karl Koller's discovery of local anaesthesia. Koller was a Viennese ophthalmologist to whom Freud suggested the use of cocaine as an anaesthetic in ophthalmology *(Fig. 1)*.

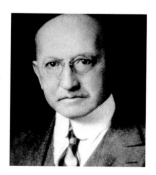

Fig. 1. Carl Koller (1857-1944), a Viennese ophthalmologist of Czech origin, was the first to use cocaine for local anaesthesia in ophthalmology following the suggestion of his friend Sigmund Freud. He later emigrated to the United States. He inaugurated the era of local anaesthesia, since then largely used in upper digestive endoscopy (courtesy of Revista Jano).

STOERK, SEMELEDER, BEVAN, DESORMEAUX

Around 1860 and prompted by the lighting system of García's laryngoscope, manufactured by Charrière, two Viennese physicians, Carl Stoerk (1832-1899)[65] and Friedrich Semeleder (1832-1901)[58], invented several instruments with which they could inspect the pharynx and the upper third of the oesophagus. These devices combined a frontal mirror with the reflecting system introduced by Czermak. Stoerk and Semmeleder examined the proximal oesophagus using a laryngeal mirror attached to a speculum shaped like a bivalve spoon, lit by a frontal mirror. Semeleder himself volunteered to be examined by Stoerck but the mucosal folds made vision difficult and no more than the first few centimeters of his oesophagus could be observed[4].

More successful attempts to proximal oesophagoscopy were made in 1868 by J. Alwin Bevan[1] at Guy's Hospital in London. His instrument was a rigid tube about 10 cm in length and 2 cm in diameter to which the endoscope was attached by means of a metal ring. The light source was a magnesium lighter made by a Mr. Mayer in Great Portland Street; the light ray was reflected onto a mirror at an angle of 45 degrees. According to Bevan, the magnesium light was sufficient to illuminate the entire oesophagus and even the stomach. Bevan replaced the tube by

ŒSOPHAGOSCOPE.

BY JOHN AYLWIN BEVAN, ESQ.

I BEG to draw the attention of the profession to a new means of diagnosis of the diseases of the throat and nose that I have discovered, by which, and with an ordinary candle, the precise position and nature of foreign bodies, strictures, morbid growths, &c., can be clearly seen ; obviating

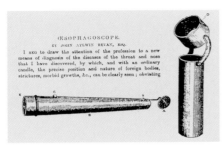

Fig. 2. Bevan's article published in The Lancet (1868) showing the devices which he invented for pharyngo-oesophagoscopy. The vertical instrument to the right was used for the extraction of foreign bodies.

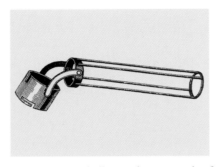

Fig. 3. Bevan's hollow endoscope made of thin metal rods, later criticised by Morrell Mackenzie (ref. 21).

another made of thin metal rods (rather similar to the "skeleton" tube designed years later by McKenzie). The endoscope was criticised by McKenzie who stated that "it had only theoretical value" and that Bevan did not seem to have any practical experience (some years later McKenzie's own instrument also became the subject of criticism by his contemporaries) *(Figs. 2, 3).*

Désormeaux also used his own "endoscope" for the examination of other cavities besides the urethra. He explored the uterine cervix and the rectum, and his assistant Labarraque, as we have already mentioned in chapter 2, was able to diagnose cases of oesophageal stricture due to the ingestion of lye; he also was able to discard the diagnosis of cancer of the oesophagus in a patient in whom oesophagoscopy had shown normal findings[4].

WALDENBURG, MACKENZIE, VOLTOLINI *(Figs. 4, 5)*

In 1868, Louis Waldenburg[70] began to use an instrument of his own design, and in 1870 he published its features in a Berlin weekly medical journal of which he himself was the editor. The endoscope consisted of a double telescopic tube whose outer part measured 7 cm in length and 1 cm in diameter; it was attached to a steel handle 14 cm in length. Both tubes were made of metal and the external one could be pushed down to 12 cm by means of a pin. If a mirror was introduced in the posterior wall of the pharynx, the upper oesophageal mucosa could be observed. In 1870, Waldenburg was able to diagnose a Zenker's diverticulum in a 40-year-old female.

KLINISCHE WOCHENSCHRIFT.

Organ für practische Aerzte.

Mit Berücksichtigung der preussischen Medicinalverwaltung und Medicinalgesetzgebung

nach amtlichen Mittheilungen.

Montag, den 28. November 1870. № 48. Siebenter Jahrgang.

III. Oesophagoskopie.

Eine neue Untersuchungsmethode.

von

L. Waldenburg.

Im Juni und Juli dieses Jahres behandelte ich einen in vieler Beziehung merkwürdigen Fall von Oesophagus-Erkrankung bei einer 40jährigen Frau. Das Leiden bestand seit 6 Monaten, und Pat. schrieb die Ursache desselben einem starken Drucke zu, der ihr an der linken Halsseite bei einem zu Thätlichkeiten

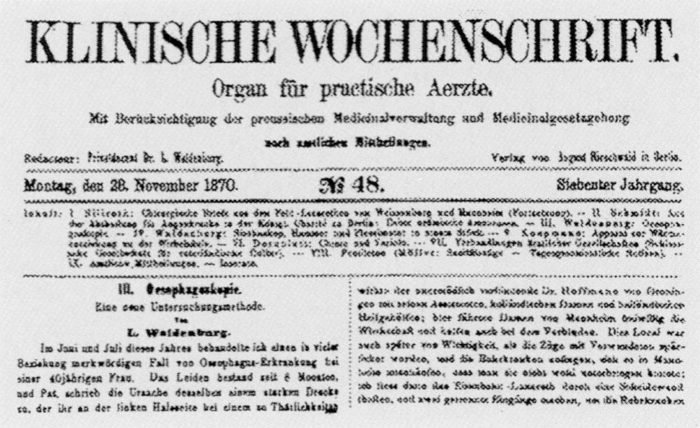

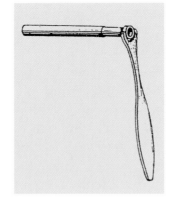

Fig. 4. Waldenburg was considered by many as the author of the first practical tool for performing oesophagoscopy. Heading of his article, published in 1870.

Fig. 5. Waldenburg's oesophagoscope. Original drawing from the author's article.

He was not unduly worried about illumination and almost exclusively used daylight, which he thought was sufficient,

but in winter and at dusk, he also used artificial light reflected on a concave mirror. He did not employ any lenses. Waldenburg also designed other instruments such as stethoscopes and pleximeters.

There followed more oesophagoscopic trials and in 1869 Stoerck[66] designed a flexible instrument resembling Waldenburgs' but consisting of metallic segments, anticipating the Nitze-Leiter's oesophago-gastroscope. It was 11 cm in length, and 20 mm in external diameter but the inside diameter was 11 mm. A rubber sheath covered Stoerck's tool to avoid mucosal lesions. It was coupled with a laryngeal mirror. Later on he convinced himself that rigid instruments were more advantageous for oesophagoscopy and he designed a 40 cm long rigid endoscope with a distal flexible portion made of eight metallic segments that could be straightened by means of a wire *(Figs. 6, 7)*.

A similar endoscope was designed by Voltolini, a Viennese otolaryngologist[69]; it consisted of a kind of long nasal bivalve speculum lit by means of a frontal lamp.

In 1880, Sir Morrell McKenzie (1837-1892), perhaps better-known as the main character of a notorious case of malpractice involving the Crown Heir Friedrich of Prussia, designed an instrument[47] which he named "skeleton-tube" as it was made of several thin metal rods. With this instrument, apparently for the first time, he extracted a foreign body (a splinter of bone) from the oesophagus. McKenzie's instrument was very light and was made of separate thin metal rods which resulted in a virtual tube. In 1880 he examined over 50 patients, but the endoscope had little acceptance among his colleagues[48] *(Figs. 8, 9)*.

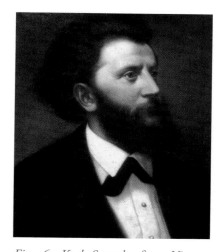

Fig. 6. Karl Stoerck, from Vienna, designed several instruments for the examination of the pharynx and the proximal oesophagus. (courtesy of the Institute for the History of Medicine, Vienna University, photograph taken around 1860).

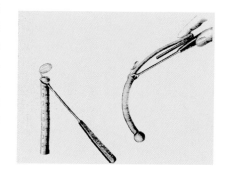

Fig. 7. Stoerck's articulated oesophagoscopes. Disappointed by his flexible instruments, he later recommended and used rigid oesophagoscopes (available for inspection at the Museum for the History of Endoscopy, Vienna University).

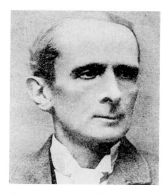

Fig. 8. Sir Morrell Mackenzie (1837-1892), distinguished British otolaryngologist (courtesy of Prof.Ramon Trias).

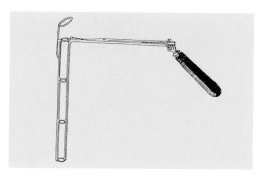

Fig. 9. Mackenzie's "skeleton" oesophagoscope (1871), partially patterned on Bevan's instrument, which was useful for foreign body extraction. However, it was also the subject of much criticism by his contemporaries (ref. 48).

In the United States, McKenzie's endoscope was soon displaced by Chevalier-Jackson's oesophagoscope[37, 38] which was also manufactured in Paris by Gentile, the successor of Charrière and Collin. The instrument consisted of a hollow tube adjusted to a handle at a right angle. This instrument is still used for the extraction of foreign bodies, a technique in which Chevalier-Jackson, his son and his successor, Gabriel Tucker, excelled. Chevalier-Jackson used a somewhat longer instrument to perform gastroscopies (see Chapter 3).

KUSSMAUL AGAIN

It was Kussmaul who again opened the way to progress. Because of the anatomical configuration of the oesophagus, he had a much greater success in his oesophagoscopy endeavours than with his attempts at gastroscopy. He used Désormeaux' endoscope for the first time in 1868, after watching the prowess of a professional sword swallower who had been persuaded to attend his clinic and be oesophagoscoped. As already mentioned in Chapter 3, Kussmaul and his first assistant, Müller, carefully observed how the sword swallower extended his head and neck during his performance, and Kussmaul concluded that a rigid oesophagoscope could be swallowed in a similar fashion. He first introduced a flexible wire guide and then the rigid hollow tube, lit by Désormeaux's alcohol-turpentine lamp. After numerous experiments, Kussmaul and Müller were able to provide a reasonable illumination for their instrument and used it to examine several patients with oesophageal lesions. They also travelled to many university clinics, taking the sword swallower with them[42]. The principle that guided these and all successive attempts was that a normal individual could swallow a straight rigid tube up to 45-50 cm in length and 13 mm in width, without untoward effects. The use of a sword swallower spread to other institutions and Brown Kelly[4] wrote that at Professor Marchick's university clinic in Vienna where he had had his endoscopy training, several people made a living by letting postgraduate students introduce endoscopes on them. A very popular volunteer called Adolph charged five schillings for each endoscopy!

According to Killian, Kussmaul was the first to identify an oesophageal tumor at the level of the tracheal bifurcation.

NITZE-LEITER'S OESOPHAGOSCOPE (Fig. 10)

Designed by the famous urologist Nitze together with Leiter, the instrument-maker, this instrument was flexible, being made of metal segments similar to those designed by Stoerck[53]. It was provided with a mirror which allowed vision, although poor, beyond the right angle made by the instrument. The endoscope was introduced on a seated patient, but the technique itself was rather difficult. It had little success and was soon replaced by Mikulicz's straight oesophagoscope.

JOHANNES VON MIKULICZ (1850-1905) *(Figs. 11, 12, 13)*

Johann or Johannes von Mikulicz (the particle "von" does not always appear in his signature) was born in Czernovicz (Bukovina), which at the time was part of the Austro-Hungarian Empire. He studied medicine in Vienna and continued his training in the well-known hospital "Allgemeines Krankenhaus" under the supervision of the famous surgeon Theodor Billroth who had organised a department of outstanding scientific quality[26]. Besides designing the first useful gastroscope, Mikulicz's contribution to oesophagoscopy was also very important. According to Starck, Mikulicz had seen Stoerck's demonstrations and had realised that an external source of light was totally insufficient for the examination of the distal third of the oesophagus and that internal illumination was necessary. He also deemed the flexible instruments of Kelling and Nitze-Leiter as useless for he was convinced that only totally rigid endoscopes introduced "in the same manner as sword swallowers do" would be useful in practice.

Around 1880, together with Joseph Leiter, he presented an oesophagoscope provided with a distal light. Mikulicz[50] stated that his instrument was as simple as

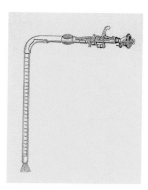

Fig. 10. The rectal angle flexible oesophagoscope designed by Nitze und Leiter included an optical system similar to that of their own cystoscope. It never became popular (ref. 19).

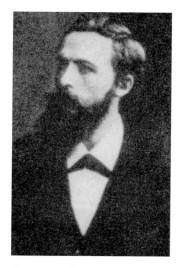

Fig. 11. Johann von Mikulicz, the distinguished surgeon, inventor of several prototypes of oesophagoscopes and gastroscopes.(courtesy Prof. M.Classen).

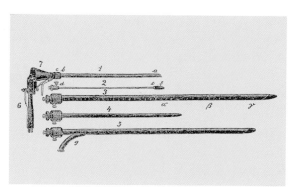

Fig. 12A. Mikulicz's oesophagoscope had a simple design and was manufactured in several lengths. Later it was coupled with Leiter's electroscope as a light source. Originally manufactured by Härtel in Breslau. (ref. 55).

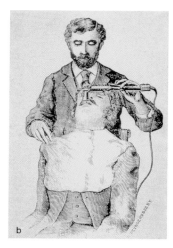

Fig. 12B. Oesophagoscopy with Mikulicz's instrument adapted to Leiter's electroscope. The patient is seated. (ref. 25)

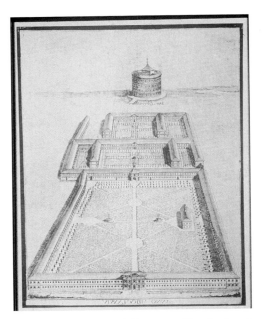

Fig. 13. The Vienna "Allgemeines Krankenhaus", the famous hospital where Mikulicz worked in Billroth's surgical clinic at the time of his first endoscopies. At the far end of the picture, the "Tower for the Mad" (Narrenturm), today a museum.

Leiter's urethroscope and that with an adequate technique the entire oesophagus could be examined; he used rigid tubes of different lengths depending on the level of the lesion to be examined. Each tube was 11-13 mm in diameter and was provided with a hard rubber tip guide to facilitate the introduction of the instrument; this was withdrawn before the examination. The endoscope included a thin tube containing a wire connected to a Bunsen battery at its proximal end and to a platinum filament lamp at its distal end. The incandescent platinum had to be cooled by means of a water stream that circulated through the tube. Later he used a miniature Edison lamp which did not require cooling; the illumination was provided by an external light source manufactured by Leiter under the name "electroscope"[51]. Mikulicz believed that his instrument was much more practical than Störck's "which often had mechanical troubles during withdrawal".

He soon realised that the examination was better tolerated when the patient was sedated; for this purpose, as for gastroscopy, he used morphine injections while other clinicians used local anaesthesia with cocaine, apparently much liked by the "professional" patients who agreed to be endoscoped many times. However, local cocaine was insufficient to prevent pain during the introduction of the tubes. Following Mikulicz, most endoscopists used morphine together with scopolamine for its anticholinergic properties.

In 1882, at the Berlin Congress of the German Society of Surgery, Mikulicz presented his findings in nearly 60 patients who he had examined oesophagoscopically. He was the first to observe that the proximal oesophagus was normally collapsed, a finding which greatly hindered the examination; from the thoracic oesophagus downwards, the lumen was open, a phenomenon which Mikulicz attributed to the negative intrathoracic pressure. He described foreign bodies, carcinoma of the oesophagus and secondary compressions due to aneurisms, in detail. He also gave an account of oesophageal peristalsis, while Kelling as well as Starck observed what appeared to be antiperistaltic contractions in the distal oesophagus.

Following Kussmaul's steps, Mikulicz also employed the services of an elderly lady who "swallowed" oesophagoscopes with great ease and helped Mikulicz and his assistants to develop new prototypes of instruments. Unfortunately for the immediate future of endoscopy, Mikulicz left Billroth's service to accept a chair first in Krakow and later in Breslau; with each change of residence his contacts with the endoscope manufacturers became more distant. Mikulicz was highly esteemed among his colleagues; according to Modlin[52], his name remains associated as an eponym to 18 diseases, syndromes, operations or instruments. Perhaps the best known of them is "Mikulicz syndrome" (hyperplasia of salivary and lacrymal glands).

It was a great pity that neither Kussmaul nor Désormeaux, Störck or Mikulicz published much on rigid oesophagoscopy, as in many hospitals the technique remained limited to the use of modified laryngoscopes for the examination of the upper oesophagus.

However, according to Kelling, Mikulicz's oesophagoscope was used extensively by Viktor von Hacker (1852-1933), a well-known Viennese surgeon who did "hundreds of examinations" with an improved version of the instrument[27, 28, 29]. Von Hacker was also one of Billroth's assistants and he had helped his teacher in doing the first gastrectomy with a gastrojejunal anastomosis, the so-called Billroth II gastrectomy. Von Hacker worked at the Sophien Spital in Vienna where he was Privatdozent (probably equivalent to assistant professor) and in 1888 he was appointed chief of the Department of Surgery at Graz University where he mainly worked on the treatment of oesophageal disease and in particular, on corrosive oesophagitis[30, 31]. In 1914 he invented an operation for replacing the oesophagus with a segment of transverse colon. Von Hacker published his surgical and endoscopic results extensively. He ended his days as "Rektor" of Graz University.

KELLING AND HIS ARTICULATED OESOPHAGOSCOPE *(Fig.14)*

In 1897, Kelling invented a flexible articulated oesophagoscope[41]. The instrument, 13 mm in external diameter, was made of several articulated metal segments, 1.45 cm in length. The segments were united by rivets and covered by a double rubber sheath. The instrument could be straightened by means of a metal wire placed along the shaft and pulled through an external handle shaped like a dented plier. The instrument was introduced with a mandrel ending in a sponge tip. For proximal illumination, Kelling used Caspers' lamp or Leiter's panendoscope. The distal light was provided by a platinum filament lamp encased on a metal rod and refrigerated by a mechanism similar to that of a urethroscope. It was used only for examinations with long tubes (45 cm). In the majority of cases, shorter tubes (30 cm) with a proximal light source were sufficient. The examination was done under morphine sedation (1 or 2 centigrams given subcutaneously). With his instrument, Kelling was able to extract foreign bodies and to dilate oesophageal strictures. He even suggested the tamponading of bleeding gastric lesions through the oesophagoscope! (see Chapter 9).

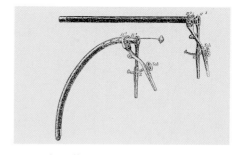

Fig. 14. Kelling's articulated oesophagoscope ("lobster tail") covered with a flexible rubber sheath. It was introduced curved and was straightened in the oesophagus thanks to a wire mechanism. (ref.41).

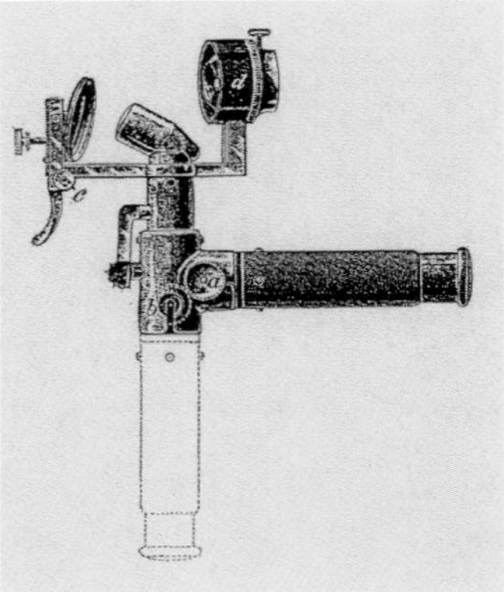

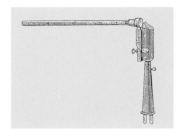

Fig. 15. Leiter's panelectroscope, the first of its kind. It could be adapted to a variety of endoscopes: oesophagoscopes, gastroscopes and cystoscopes (ref. 62).

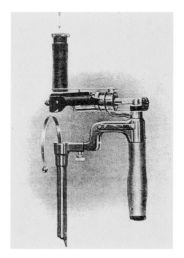

Fig. 16. Casper's panelectroscope which could be fitted to several kinds of instruments (ref. 49).

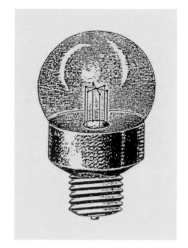

Fig. 17. Brünings' panelectroscope adapted to an oesophagoscope with its obturator. A complex instrument, it was handled with difficulty. (ref. 19).

THE EMERGENCE OF "PAN-ELECTROSCOPES"
(Figs. 15, 16, 17)

In 1879, Edison's discovery of the incandescent vacuum lamp helped to solve the problem of achieving acceptable illumination for oesophagoscopy and gastroscopy[20]. In 1887, Nitze presented the first endoscope that included an incandescent lamp[45], the so-called "Mignon" lamp. In the same year, Leiter made his first electroscope. The light source was a battery which provided electricity to the vacuum lamp placed at the handle of the instrument. The reflected light was a satisfactory source of illumination for the shaft of the endoscope. The "electroscope" could be adapted to various kinds of tubes for inspection of the urethra and the bladder, as well as the rectum and the oesophagus.

Other electroscopes which could be adapted as a light source to different kinds of endoscopes appeared on the market[25]. One of the most popular was that designed by Casper (1891). Leopold Casper was born in 1859 in Berlin, he was a pupil of Virchow and was appointed professor in 1922. His foremost activity was urologic endoscopy, and he was one of the first to catheterise urethers. In 1941 Casper emigrated to the United States and settled in New York where he acquired a great reputation as a urologist. He died there in 1959 when he was one hundred years old. Another electroscope, designed by Brünings[5], included a three filament lamp which was a feature of several oesophagoscopy and rectoscopy prototypes *(Figs. 18, 19, 20)*. All electroscopes were similar in that they were adapted to the proximal end of the endoscope and featured electrical lamps to avoid overheating of the shaft of the instrument *(Fig. 21)*.

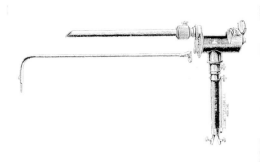

Fig. 18. Triple filament lamp, used with Brünings' electroscope (ref. 62).

Fig. 19. Von Hacker's oesophagoscope with its bevel distal end, fitted with Leiter's electroscope. The electrical part was manufactured by the firm Schwetter and Radl from Vienna in collaboration with Joseph Leiter (ref.62).

Thanks to the new illumination systems which replaced the cumbersome distal light sources and the platinum filaments which required water refrigeration, many endoscopists, like Mikulicz, von Hacker, Kelling and Rosenheim, could now work efficiently. However, other endoscopists such as Chevalier Jackson and Guisez, preferred to work with a hollow tube and a simple electrical lamp.

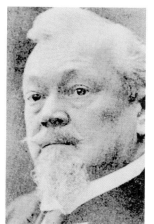

Fig. 20. Viktor von Hacker (1852-1933), Billroth's assistant who did a large number of oesophagoscopies in Vienna before being appointed professor of surgery and head of the surgical clinic at Graz University, of which he later became Rektor. (courtesy of Prof. Gunther Krejs, Graz University).

ROSENHEIM, KILLIAN AND BRÜNINGS
(Figs. 22, 23)

Until 1912, most oesophagoscopes featured a distal angle[4, 42] and some of them were telescopic, such as Lewisohn's, but the first to design a totally straight oesophagoscope was the Berlinese clinician Rosenheim. Based on Mikulicz's ideas, Rosenheim acquired considerable experience with his own oesophagoscope, which was manufactured by Hirschmann in 1895. The endoscope consisted of a straight tube adapted to a handle that made a right angle with the shaft of the endoscope. The instrument was inserted by means of a guide which was withdrawn at the beginning of the examination. Each set of instruments included tubes of several lengths and diameters, varying between 11.5 and 13 cm. Illumination was provided by means of an incandescent lamp attached to the handle of the endoscope, reflecting the

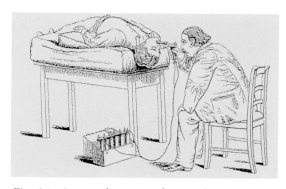

Fig. 21. An oesophagoscopy done with von Hacker's endoscope. The electroscope and an external battery are clearly seen (the endoscopist might have been von Hacker himself). (ref. 53).

parallel light rays into the tube by way of a small flat mirror[21]. However, the light source interfered with vision, and other clinicians recommended the use of a frontal Kirstein-type lamp[44] to ease manipulations through the endoscope (such as to extract foreign bodies or to introduce biopsy forceps).

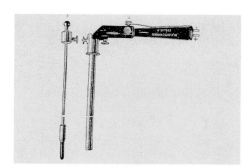

Fig. 22. Rosenheim's oesophagoscope, manufactured by W. Hirschmann in Berlin with an attached electroscope and the guide for its introduction. (ref. 19).

Fig. 23. Killian's oesophagoscope featuring a Casper type lighting system included in the handle. (ref. 19).

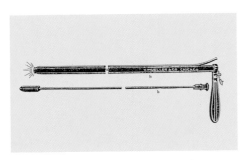

Fig. 24. *Chevalier Jackson's oesophagoscope, provided with a distal light but which could also be used with a frontal lamp. Originally manufactured by V. Mueller in Chicago, it was also made in Paris by the firm Gentile. (from the Gentile's catalogue, courtesy of Dr. J.Danón, Fundación Uriach).*

Some years later, Brünings[6] designed an improved instrument. The main innovation of his oesophagoscope was the use of two telescopic tubes, one external and the other a thin inner tube featuring lateral windows; this was pushed into the lumen of the first with the aid of a mandrel-guide.

CHEVALIER JACKSON, JEAN GUISEZ *(Fig. 24, 25)*

Chevalier Jackson made oesophagoscopy popular in the United States[37, 38]

His design was a simple hollow tube with distal illumination and manufactured in different lengths. Some of the tubes were long enough to enter the stomach and each one included a distal lamp with its own laryngoscope. This was used both as a handle and as an electroscope in a fashion similar to that of Rosenheim's and Brünings' endoscopes. This model of oesophagoscope was still in use in many centres around 1970[4]. In 1907, Jackson published his first book on oesophagoscopy and in 1911, Guisez published his own well-known treatise in Paris[22] *(Figs. 26, 27, 28).*

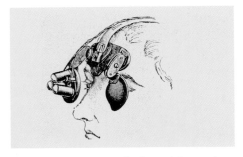

Fig. 25. *Guisez's triple frontal lamp, later replaced by a single more powerful lamp. (ref. 22).*

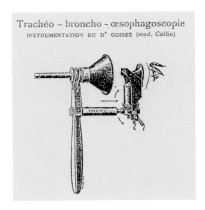

Trachéo – broncho – œsophagoscopie
INSTRUMENTATION DU Dᵀ GUISEZ (mod. Collin)

Fig. 27. *Guisez's oesophagoscope coupled with an electroscope. It could also be used with a frontal lamp which gave a larger field of vision. (Collin's catalogue, 1904, courtesy of Dr. J.Danón, Fundación Uriach).*

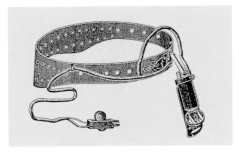

Fig. 26. *Kirstein's frontal lamp for oesophagoscopy, extensively used in Germany (ref. 62).*

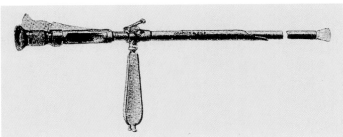

Fig. 28. *Bensaude's oesophagoscope, made by the firm Drapier in Paris (ref.22).*

Jean Guisez was the pioneer of oesophagoscopy in France. He used an instrument similar to that of Chevalier-Jackson; it was manufactured by Collin but had proximal rather than distal illumination. The light source was a 12 volt lamp with crossed filaments; an adjustable focus for monocular vision was attached to the handle at a right angle. The graduated endoscopic tube was provided with a metal guide with a flexible rubber terminal portion. In 1914, Collin made oesophagoscopes which varied in length from 22 to 40 cm and diameters between 9 and 13 mm. Another popular instrument was that of Bensaude, manufactured by the firm Drapier *(Fig. 29).*

SONDERDRUCK AUS

KLINISCHE WOCHENSCHRIFT

ORGAN DER GESELLSCHAFT DEUTSCHER NATURFORSCHER UND ÄRZTE

VERLAG VON JULIUS SPRINGER, BERLIN, UND J. F. BERGMANN, MÜNCHEN

JAHRG. 11 — 1. OKTOBER 1932 — Nr. 40, S. 1673/1675

ÜBER EIN NEUES OESOPHAGOSKOP FÜR DEN GEBRAUCH DER INNEREN KLINIK.

Von

Privatdozent Dr. NORBERT HENNING.

Aus der Medizinischen Universitätsklinik Leipzig (Direktor: Prof. Dr. MORAWITZ).

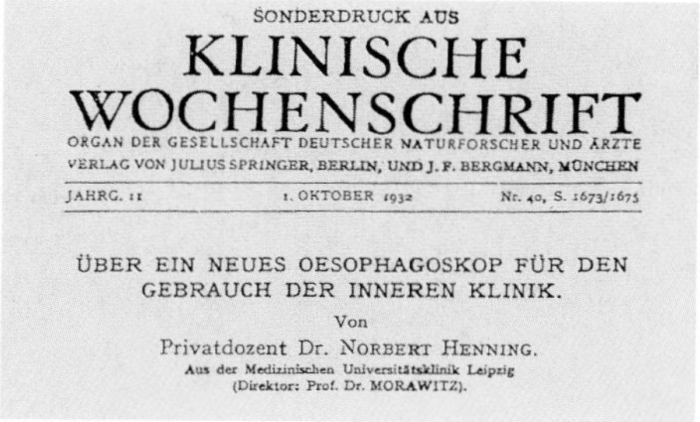

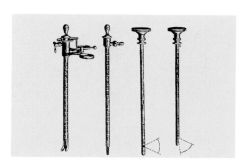

Fig. 29. Heading of Henning's article on his new oesophagoscope (1932).

BOROS' OESOPHAGOSCOPE

In 1947 Edwin Boros[2] from New York described an instrument in the journal "Gastroenterology". It consisted of a hollow tube, with a distal end made of a flexible metal coil, provided with a channel for illumination and another for the introduction of a rigid wire which could straighten the instrument and allow adequate frontal vision of the oesophageal surface. The instrument was easy to introduce thanks to its flexible extremity, but apparently it was never widely used. (The manufacturer's name does not appear in the article).

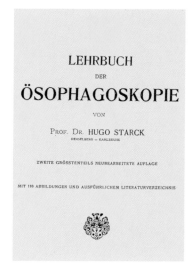

Fig. 30. Henning's optical oesophagoscope, possibly the last to be manufactured with an optical lens system. It was provided with a guide tipped with a rubber ball, and a channel for insufflation. Like Ringleb's cystoscope, the instrument could be used with two separate optical systems, one for oblique vision and the other for lateral inspection. The endoscope was manufactured in Berlin by Georg Wolf in 1932.

HENNING'S OPTICAL OESOPHAGOSCOPE *(Fig. 30, 31)*

In 1932, Henning[34] presented an instrument which may have been the last prototype of the optical oesophagoscopy era. Manufactured by Georg Wolf, this endoscope was 42 cm in length and 7.4 mm in diameter; it was comprised of a catheter as well as a wire guide with a rubber tip. The instrument coupled two optical systems; one prograde for frontal vision and the other for lateral vision by means of a prism. Both magnified the image twofold. In broad terms, if was inspired by Ringleb's cystoscope. Henning also used this endoscope to examine the trachea.

THE TECHNIQUE OF OESOPHAGOSCOPY
(Figs. 32, 33, 34, 35, 36)

Up until Mikulicz's time, oesophagoscopies were performed with the patient in a standing or a sitting position. Both were most uncomfortable for the patient and difficulties were encountered on attempts to spit saliva and mucous secretions during the examination.

LEHRBUCH

DER

ÖSOPHAGOSKOPIE

VON

PROF. DR. HUGO STARCK

HEIDELBERG – KARLSRUHE

ZWEITE GRÖSSTENTEILS NEUBEARBEITETE AUFLAGE

MIT 110 ABBILDUNGEN UND AUSFÜHRLICHEM LITERATURVERZEICHNIS

Fig. 31. Title page of Starck's famous handbook on oesophagoscopy (1914).

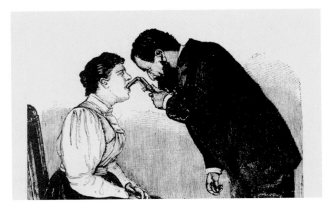

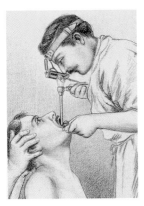

Fig. 32. Larygo-oesophagoscopy performed on a seated patient. (ref.49)

Fig. 33. Oesophagoscopy on a patient first seated and then recumbent (ref.49).

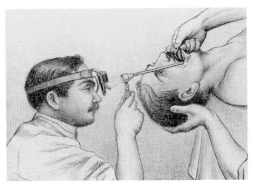

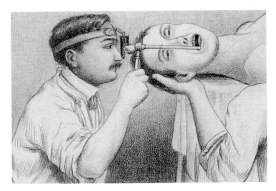

Fig. 34. Oesophagoscopy on a patient lying supine, the position preferred by Mikulicz and Rachet (ref. 49).

Fig. 35. Oesophagoscopy on a patient in the right lateral position (ref.49).

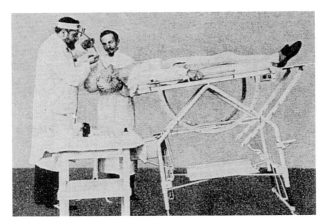

Fig. 36. Starck performing an oesophagoscopy on a patient lying supine (Starck, 1918).

Mikulicz's patients lay supine with their head bent back over the edge of examining table. Rosenheim recommended introducing the endoscope in this position after swabbing the pharynx with 10 per cent cocaine with the help of a laryngeal mirror. Other authors inserted Rosenheim's endoscope first on a seated patient while an assistant held his head firmly, and then had the patient lie down once the instrument had been inserted[25, 55]. In France, Guisez and Sencert used the sitting as well as the supine and lateral recumbent positions[24, 49].

In his book on oesophagoscopy[62], Starck mentions that the Barcelona laryngologist Botey used a mandrel made of transparent glass which he inserted in the metal oesophagoscope to be able to introduce the instrument in the upper part of the oesophagus under direct vision. Starck, Kölliker and Guisez preferred elastic guides, while Gottstein, a pupil of Mikulicz's, designed an instrument which had a soft metal tip instead of the rubber cap used by his mentor and which he believed was easier to disinfect[19].

EARLY THERAPEUTIC OESOPHAGOSCOPY

Foreign body extraction

Foreign body extraction from the oesophagus may well be the oldest therapeutic technique in gastroenterology. As we have already discussed, the first withdrawal attempts date back to the Stone Age and a myriad of devices and instruments have since been invented to extract objects from the upper digestive tract[4]. (see Chapter 1). The advent of the illuminated hollow endoscope greatly improved the manner in which these emergencies could be treated *(Figs. 37, 38)*.

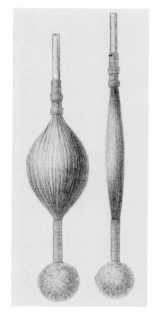

Fig. 37. Ferguson's "umbrella" used for the blind withdrawal of foreign bodies from the oesophagus (ref. 49).

The discovery of Roentgen rays helped a great deal in determining the exact location of foreign bodies in the oesophagus[4].This may be why optical oesophagoscopes lost ground as any manoeuvre through the solid instrument was difficult. The main difficulty was the extraction of foreign bodies, a technique in which both Chevalier Jackson in the United States and Guisez in France were indisputed masters. This was the beginning of therapeutic endoscopy. Around 1950, I had the chance to admire part of the amazing collection of objects extracted from the oesophagus by the Jacksons and Gabriel Tucker and associates which adorned the walls of the Chevalier Jackson Clinic at the Graduate Hospital of the University of Pennsylvania (nowadays at the Mutter Museum of the Philadelphia College of Physicians).

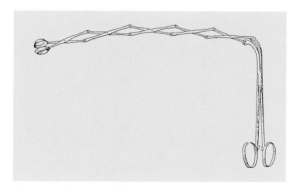

Fig. 38. Mathieu's folding clamp (ref. 49).

Jean Guisez at the Hôtel-Dieu and Albert Mathieu's associates at Hospital Saint-Antoine in Paris as well as L. Sencert in Nancy, also exhibited their extraordinary skill[24, 59]. All of them primarily used the oesophagoscope for the diagnosis and treatment of foreign bodies. They advised against blindly pushing the alien material into the stomach as had been done by Ambroise Paré, among others (1510-1590). The pushing manoeuvres usually ended in disaster, as shown by statistics compiled by Sencert in which he reported 8 deaths in 22 attempts![59]. The spontaneous propulsion of a foreign body through the oesophagoscope into the stomach was reported by von Hacker, Gottstein and Sencert, but none of them recommended forced blind pushing with rods or wires[19, 31, 59] (*Figs. 39, 40, 41, 42*).

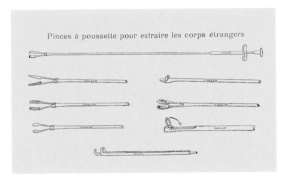

Fig. 39. Various devices for the extraction of foreign bodies (Collin's catalogue, 1907, courtesy of Dr. J Danón, Fundación Uriach).

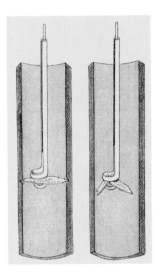

Fig. 41. Guisez's technique for fragmenting a bone (ref. 24).

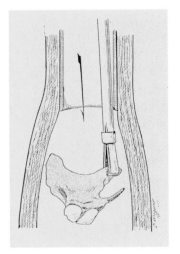

Fig. 40. Technique for the withdrawal of a denture using a "version" manoeuvre (ref. 24).

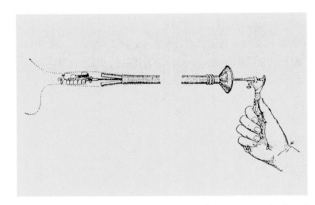

Fig. 42. Guisez's device for foreign body extraction (ref. 22)

However, the blind extraction of objects in the cervical oesophagus was done by means of several types of pincers, among them, the flexible articulated clamp used by Sencert. In the thoracic oesophagus blind extraction could be done with a De Graefe or a Froehlich basket, particularly useful to extract coins in children. However, in most cases extraction was attempted under endoscopic vision, using all kinds of hooks, pincers and clamps. In perusing the catalogues of instrument makers from the beginnings of the 20th century, the number of devices used for this purpose is awe inspiring. To extract dentures which were stuck horizontally in the oesophagus, Guisez succeeded in making true "versions". In other instances, other endoscopists such as Mikulicz, Killian or also Guisez, would use pincers similar to those used for urological lithotripsy, so as first to fragment large or hard objects such as metal pieces or bones.

In 1900, Gottstein reviewed 24 successful instances of treatment of oesophageal foreign bodies, among them 11 dentures[19]. In 1904 in Vienna, von Hacker published 27 of his own cases of extraction, 26 of which were successful. Reports rapidly accumulated. In 1905 Starck published 78 cases in which he attempted to remove a foreign body, with 70 successes[62]. In 1907, Sencert's assistant, Driout, compiled 88 cases with 80 good results, 26 in children[59]. The first Spanish contributions to therapeutic oesophagoscopy were made by Garcia Tapia[17] and by Botey in 1907[3] *(Figs. 43, 44, 45, 46).*

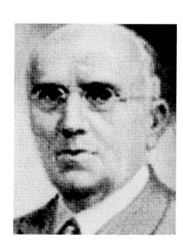

Fig. 45. Ricardo Botey (1855-1927). Otolaryngologist with vast experience in the extraction of foreign bodies with Killian's oesophagoscope. According to Starck, he used a mandrel made of transparent glass to introduce the endoscope under direct vision.(courtesy of Prof. M. Diaz Rubio).

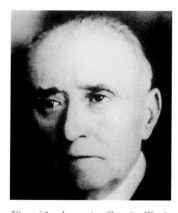

Fig. 43. Antonio García Tapia (1875-1950). In 1907 he published the first case of foreign body endoscopic extraction from the oesophagus in the Spanish literature. (courtesy of Prof. M. Diaz Rubio).

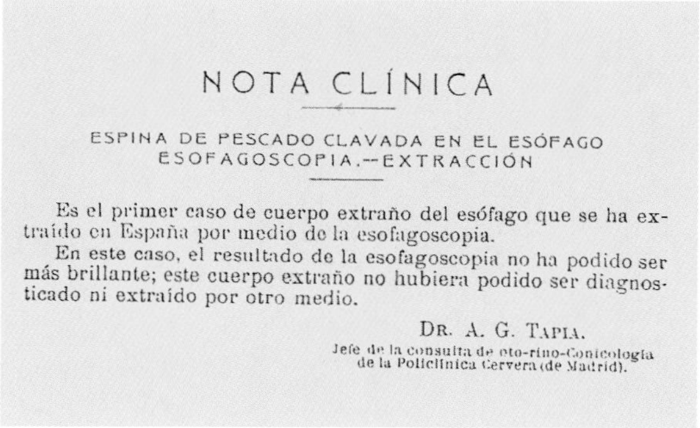

NOTA CLÍNICA

ESPINA DE PESCADO CLAVADA EN EL ESÓFAGO
ESOFAGOSCOPIA.—EXTRACCIÓN

Es el primer caso de cuerpo extraño del esófago que se ha extraído en España por medio de la esofagoscopia.
En este caso, el resultado de la esofagoscopia no ha podido ser más brillante; este cuerpo extraño no hubiera podido ser diagnosticado ni extraído por otro medio.

DR. A. G. TAPIA.
Jefe de la consulta de oto-rino-Conicología
de la Policlínica Cervera (de Madrid).

Fig. 44. Heading of the first paper published in Spain by A.Garcia-Tapia on the successful endoscopic extraction of a foreign body from the oesophagus(1907).

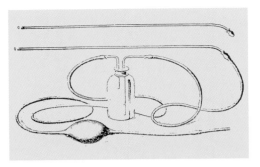

Fig. 46. Aspirator designed by Killian for oesophageal suction during oesophagoscopy. (ref. 3).

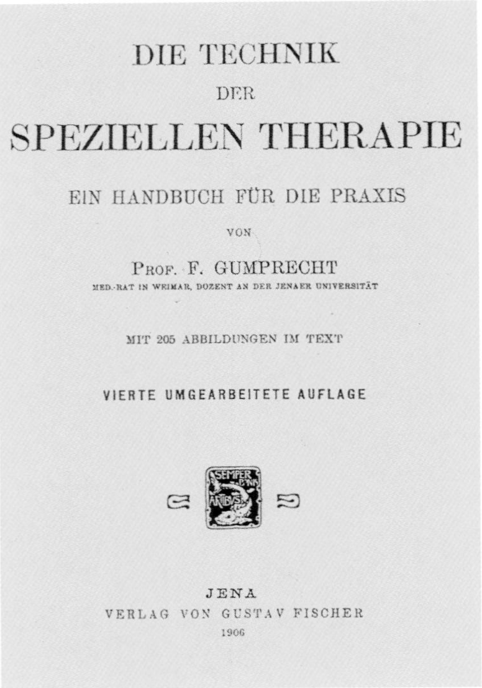

DIE TECHNIK
DER
SPEZIELLEN THERAPIE

EIN HANDBUCH FÜR DIE PRAXIS

VON

PROF. F. GUMPRECHT
MED.-RAT IN WEIMAR, DOZENT AN DER JENAER UNIVERSITÄT

MIT 205 ABBILDUNGEN IM TEXT

VIERTE UMGEARBEITETE AUFLAGE

JENA
VERLAG VON GUSTAV FISCHER
1906

Fig. 47. Title page of Gumprechts' book "Die Technik der Speziellen Therapie".

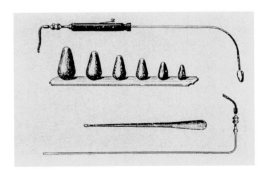

Fig. 48. Guisez's probes featuring distal metal olives for oesophageal dilation (Collin's catalogue, 1904, courtesy Dr. J.Danón, Fundación Uriach).

TREATMENT OF ORGANIC OESOPHAGEAL STRICTURES

Oesophageal stenoses, whether due to corrosive agents or to gastric reflux, are the other great issue in therapeutic endoscopy. In 1742, Manchard[49] had already recommended dilations. Procedures for blind dilation by means of dangerous devices such as metal rods were slowly replaced by dilating rubber probes of increasing diameters, provided either with a distal olive of various shapes or with a tip filled with lead pellets to ease the passage into the stomach. All these procedures are minutiously described by Gumprecht[25] (Figs. 47, 48).

Many experts considered dilation through the oesophagoscope to be the safest technique. Using the endoscope designed by his mentor, Désormeaux's assistant Labarraque, was the first to identify an oesophageal stricture. Once the diagnosis of stenosis was made, Sencert[59] recommended the instillation of novocaine to relax the muscular spasm which was usually present above the lesion. He then introduced a series of probes of progressive diameters. After a number of sessions, an acceptable luminal diameter was usually obtained and simple blind dilations could be done thereafter (Figs. 49, 50).

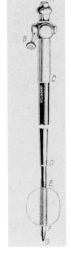

Fig. 49. Schreiber' probe for dilation of the oesophagus.

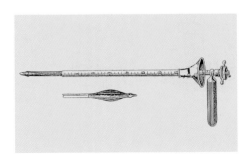

Fig. 50. Abrand's probe featuring a balloon and several metal wires for dilation (ref. 14).

Other endoscopists, such as von Hacker[31] and Starck[62], recommended prolonged dilations by means of a rubber probe introduced through the oesophagoscope and left in place for at least one hour. This method was successfully used by Starck, Rosenheim, Guisez and Sencert. The main danger was obviously the possibility of perforation, either above the stricture, a relatively common accident during blind dilation, or inside the stenotic area, an occurrence which even under oesophagoscopic visual control cannot be entirely avoided.

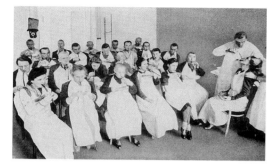

Fig. 51. Starck in his clinic performing oesophageal dilations on several patients with oesophageal strictures (courtesy of Prof. M.Classen).

Some physicians used linear or circular electrolysis by passing a straight or a circular knife plugged into an electrical current blindly or under visual control. The shape of the knife was adapted to dilating olives of various sizes. According to MacKenzie, all attempts at internal oesophagotomy fell into disrepute as the mortality was very high[48].

THE TREATMENT OF ACHALASIA (Figs. 51, 52, 53)

In the 19th century, the diagnosis of achalasia was made with difficulty and to correctly identify the disease as a functional disorder was a slow process. Oesophagoscopy proved that in many cases of megaoesophagus, a term invented by von Hacker, there was no organic stricture that could hinder the passage of the instrument through the cardia. Mikulicz coined the term "cardiospasm" for this disorder. Achalasia was treated by simple progressive dilations with rubber probes filled with lead pellets until a French 50 to 55 tube could be passed. However, it had already been observed that improvement was temporary and that after oesophagoscopy, forceful dilation using balloons was a better procedure. The most popular dilators were those designed by Gottstein and by Schreiber[19, 57]. Some authors recommended the use of manometers to control the dilation pressure which, according to Strauss, could safely reach 250 mm of mercury[56].

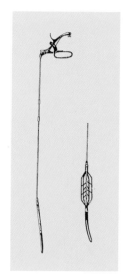

Fig. 52. Starck's mechanical dilator for the forceful dilation of the cardia. His dilator was used at the Hospital de Sant Pau until 1950.

Some devices made of a bundle of thin metal rods that could be opened like an umbrella became rather popular. They included dilators designed by Jacobi and by Starck. The latter's instrument was used extensively in Barcelona at the Hospital de Sant Pau until 1950. Starck's dilator was passed under fluoroscopic control on a seated patient; oesophagoscopic supervision was not required[63]. The technique consisted of bruskly opening an instrument which could be likened to a double umbrella and tearing the muscular fibres at the cardia. The procedure was not exempt of

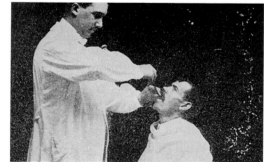

Fig. 53. Physician probing the oesophagus before performing a blind oesophageal dilation. (around 1920). (ref. 14).

danger and accidents such as haemorrhages and perforations were reported[68]. In 1929, Starck read a report on "Cardiospasm" at a meeting of the German Society for Digestive Diseases ("Deutsche Gesellschaft für Verdauungskrankheiten") in Berlin. He presented data on 219 patients with no cases of mortality[63, 64]. He did not observe haemorrhage after forceful dilation, although at oesophagoscopy after the procedure, the oesophageal mucosa appeared soiled with blood[54].

Starck's report was discussed by many, including Georg Kelling who favoured Heller's operation, and by Rudolf Schindler who had performed dilations with the Starck instrument on 11 patients; nine of them were clinically cured, another had an unsuccesssful course and troubles were encountered in the last patient, although fortunately, the intervention ended uneventfully. Although very rare, occasionally the "umbrella", once opened, could not be closed again because folds of oesophageal mucosa became herniated among the rods. Years later Starck himself publicly confessed that he had abandoned his instrument in favour of surgical myotomy!

Since that time, the development of oesophagoscopic instruments was practically always the domain of otolaryngologists or surgeons. The emergence of fibre lights substantially improved the vision of rigid oesophagoscopes but it was the appearance of the fibrescope and the possibility of examining oesophagus, stomach and duodenum with the same instrument that gradually shifted oesophagoscopy into the realm of the gastroenterologist. However, as recently as the late 1970s, a well-known book on the oesophagus was published in Switzerland[56]; it consisted of two parts, one on rigid oesophagoscopy written by Marcel Savary, an otolaryngologist, and a second on fibrescopy of the oesophagus, authored by a gastroenterologist, Gaudenz Miller (Fig. 54).

The indications for rigid oesophagoscopy were mainly limited to therapeutic procedures: the extraction of foreign bodies and alimentary particles, the haemosthasia of bleeding lesions and the sclerosis of varices. Rigid oesophagoscopy was employed also in some rare cases in which the fibrescope had been unable to provide a diagnosis. Savary and Miller mentioned the advantages of the fibrescope in patients in whom the cardia could not be examined adequately with rigid instruments, because of the existence of kyphosis, scoliosis or vertebral rigidity. Fibreoptics have advanced so greatly, especially since the invention of videoendoscopy, that the use of rigid instruments is rarely, if ever, justified today.

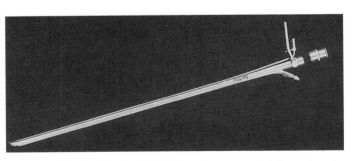

Fig. 54. The first "modern" rigid oesophagoscope: Hollinger's endoscope (1967) provided with fiberoptic cold light. (manufactured by G.Pilling, USA).

RISKS OF RIGID OESOPHAGOSCOPY

Many reports show that in about 2 per cent of cases it was not possible to introduce a rigid instrument[56]. In most centres, even with the most perfected endoscopes, rigid oesophagoscopy had always resulted in an unduly high morbidity and mortality. In a review made by Hafter and presented at the 10th International Congress of Gastroenterology (Budapest 1976), the risk of perforation, the most dreaded complication, varied between 0.2 and 1.9 per cent. A compilation of oesophagoscopies carried out between 1956 and 1972 in various countries showed that in 102,109 examinations with rigid instruments the percentage of perforations was 0.17, with a global mortality of 0.02 per cent[32]. Figures from one of the most reliable centres, the University O.R.L. Clinic in Lausanne, reported 4 perforations in 6,944 consecutive oesophagoscopies (0.06 per cent)[60].

The majority of data reviewed came from centres where at least one thousand examinations had been made and it is quite possible that in smaller unpublished series the incidence of complications was even greater. As expected, the majority of perforations occurred in the posterior wall of the pharynx and less often in the area of the cardia. Many accidents were probably due to inexperience of the examiner. Chevalier Jackson's popular advice "*look for the lumen of the oesophagus and follow it*" is still valid today, even if the new frontal vision fibrescopes have considerably changed the technique[46].

It may be interesting to read the conclusions made by Starck[60] in 1904 in a communication on oesophagoscopy which he read in Madrid during the International Congress of Medicine. Many are still valid today *(Fig. 55)*:

1. Oesophagoscopy can be performed in the majority of patients.
2. The most practical instruments are the rigid, not the flexible devices.
3. Oesophagoscopy is the best method to recognise and to localize foreign bodies.
4. Early diagnosis of cancer can only be done by oesophagoscopy.
5. Oesophagoscopy is the surest method for the diagnosis of mucosal lesions of the oesophagus (ulcers, inflammation, scars, stenosis).
6. In many cases the differential diagnosis between functional and organic strictures of the oesophagus is only possible by means of endoscopic examination.
7. Oesophagoscopy combined with intubation is the best method for examining the oesophagus.

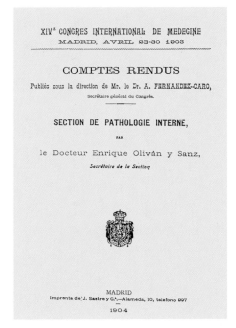

Fig. 55. Title page of the Proceedings of the International Congress of Medicine (Madrid 1904) in which Starck presented his conclusions on the value of oesophagoscopy (see text). (courtesy of Dr. J. Danón, Fundación Uriach).

REFERENCES

1 Bevan J.A. Oesophagoscope. Lancet 1868; 1: 470-471.

2 Boros E. Esophagoscopy by means of a flexible instrument. A new esophago-gastroscope. Gastroenterology 1947; 8: 724-728.

3 Botey R. La esofagoscopia directa en los cuerpos extraños del esófago. Anals de Medecina 1907; 1 (4) (25 April): 288-299.

4 Brown Kelly H.D. Origins of oesophagology. Proc Roy Soc Med 1969; 62: 781-786.

5 Brünings W. Die Technik der Bronchoskopie und Oesophagoskopie, Wiesbaden, J.F. Bergmann, 1908.

6 Brünings W. Die direkte Laryngoskopie, Bronchoskopie und Oesophagoskopie. Ein Handbuch für die Technik der direkten okularen Methoden. Wiesbaden, J.F. Bergmann, 1910.

7 Collin. (Maison Charrière) Fabricant d'Instruments de Chirurgie. Catalogue, Paris, Chez Collin, 1900.

8 Czermak J.N. Über den Kehlkopfspiegel. Wien med Wschr 1858; 8: 196-198.

9 Czermak J.N. Der Kehlkopfspiegel und seine Verwerthung für Physiologie und Medizin. (2ª edition) Leipzig, Wilhelm Engelmann 1863.

10 Edmonson J.M. History of the instruments for gastrointestinal endoscopy. Gastrointest Endosc 1991; 37: S27-S55.

11 Einhorn M. The inspection of the oesophagus and the cardia. New York Med J 1897; 66: 797-799.

12 Einhorn M. Report of a case of idiopathic dilatation of the oesophagus with cure and description of a new cardia dilator. New York Med J 1909; 89: 1077-1078.

13 Enciclopedia Universal Ilustrada Espasa: García, Manuel Vicente. 1924; vol. 25, p.765.

14 Fernández Martinez F. Tratado de exploración del aparato digestivo. Madrid, Javier Morata editor, 1930.

15 Fischer I Biographisches Lexicon der hervorzagenden Ärtze der letzten fünfzig Jahre. Berlin, Urban & Schwarzenberg, 1932.

16 García M. Physiological observations on the human voice. Proceedings of the Royal Society of London. 1855; 7: 399-410.

17 Garcia Tapia A. Espina de pescado clavada en el esófago. Esofagoscopia. Extracción. Clínica Moderna 1907; 61: 151-152.

18 Gentile. (ancienne Maison Collin). Catalogue Illustré, Paris 1934. (courtesy of Dr. J.Danón, Fundación Uriach).

19 Gottstein G. Technik und Klinik der Oesophagoskopie. Jena, Fischer, 1901.

20 Gröger H. Das Problem der Beleuchtung in der Endoskopie und seine Bewältigung. Das Wiener Endosckopie Museum. Eröffnungssymposium 1996, Wien, Literas Universitätsverlag 1997: 58-66.

21 Grünfeld J. Zur Geschichte der Endoskopie und der endoskopischen Apparate. Medizinische Jahrbüch Wien 1879: 237-291.

22 Guisez J. Traité des Maladies de l'Oesophage. Paris, J.B. Baillière 1911.

23 Guisez J. Les spasmes à forme grave de l'oesophage. Gazette Hôp Paris 1910; 83: 223-226.

24 Guisez J. Faits de l'oesophagoscopie. Considérations sur nos derniers cas d'extraction de corps étrangers de forme irrégulière par l'oesophagoscopie. Rev Hebdo Laryngol. 1908; 2: 548-556.

25 Gumprecht F. Die Technik der speziellen Therapie. Vierte umgearbeitete Aufgabe. Jena, Gustav Fischer, 1906.

26 Gurlt E. biographisches Lexicon der hervorragender Ärzte aller Zeiten und Völker. Berlin-Wien, VC. 1934.

27 Hacker von, V. Chirurgische Beiträge aus dem Erzherzogin Sophien Spital in Wien. Wien, Hölder, 1892.

28 Hacker von, V. Erfahrungen über die Endoskopie der Speiseröhre mit besonderer Berücksichtigung der Entfernung from Fremdenkörpern. Wien med Wschr 1894; 44: 2018-2019.

[29] Hacker von, V. Über die Technik der Ösophagoskopie. Wien klin Wschr 1896; 9; 91-112.

[30] Hacker von, V. Die Oesophagoskopie und ihre klinische Bedeutung. Beiträge zu klinischen Chirurgie. 1898; 20: 141-166.

[31] Hacker von V. Zur Statistik und Prognose der Verätzungen des Oesophagus und der im Gefolge derselben entstehenden Strikturen. Beitr z Chir Festschr Theodor Billroth Stuttgart, 1892: 123-137.

[32] Hafter E. The risk of oesophagoscopy and gastroscopy. in Ethical problems in the management of gastroenterological patients. F.Vilardell (ed.) Scand j Gastroenterol. 1977 (Suppl 47) 12:12-14.

[33] Heller E. Extramuköse Cardioplastik beim chronischen Cardiospasmus mit Dilatation des Oesophagus. Mitteil. Grenzgebiete Med Chir. 1913; 27: 141-149.

[34] Henning N. Über ein neues Oesophagoskop für den Gebrauch der inneren Klinik. Klin Wschr. 1932; 11:1673-1675.

[35] Housset P, Simoens A, Debray Ch. Esophagoscopy. in Vantrappen G, Hellemans J. (eds). Diseases of the Esophagus, Berlin - Heidelberg, Springer Verlag. 1974.

[36] Huizenga E. On esophagoscopy and sword swallowing. An Otol 1969; 78: 32-39.

[37] Jackson Ch. Tracheo-broncoscopy, Esophagoscopy, Gastroscopy. (St Louis), Laryngoscope, 1907

[38] Jackson Ch., Jackson Ch.L. Broncho-esophagology, Philadelphia, W.B. Saunders, 1930.

[39] Jackson, Ch., Jackson C.L. Diseases of the air and food passages of foreign body origin. Philadelphia, W.B. Saunders, 1936.

[40] Janeway H.H., Green N. Esophagoscopy and gastroscopy. Surg Gynec Obstet 1911; 13:245-253.

[41] Kelling G. Endoskopie für Speiseröhre und Magen. Gegliedertes oesophagosckop, welches durch Zug und Drehung streckbar ist. Münch Med Wschr. 1897; 34: 934-937.

[42] Killian G. Zur Geschichte der 0esophago- und Gastroskopie. Deutsch Zeitschr fur Chirurgie 1901; 58: 499-512.

[43] Kirstein A. Über Oesophagoskopie. Berlin Klin Wschr 1898; 27: 394-395.

[44] Kirstein A. Eine neue elektrische Stirn Hand und Stativ Lampe für Hals, Nose und Phr. Deutsch Med Wschr 1895;21: 462-466.

[45] Lauridsen L. Laterna magica in corpore humano. Steno Museum, Arhus, Svendborg, Isager Bogtryk, 1998.

[46] Lo Presti P.A. Clinical experience with a new foroblique fiber esophagoscope. Am J Dig Dis 1964: 9: 690-697.

[47] Mackenzie M. Diseases of the throat, London, Vincent Brooks, Day and Son, 1887.

[48] Mackenzie M. The use of the laryngoscope in diseases of the throat. 3rd edition, London, R.Hardwicke, 1871.

[49] Mathieu A, Sencert L., Tuffier TH. Maladies de l'estomac et de l'oesophage. Paris, Masson, 1913.

[50] Mikulicz, von. J. Über Gastroskopie und Ösophagoskopie. Centralbl. f. Chir. 1881; 43: 673-676.

[51] Mikulicz von J. Über Gastroskopie und Ösophagoskopie am Lebenden. Verhandlung Berlin, Dstch Gesell f. Chir 1882; 11: 30-38

[52] Modlin I. A brief history of endoscopy.Milano, Multi-Med, 2000.

[53] Newell O.K. The endoscopic instruments of Joseph Leiter of Vienna and the present development of endoscopy. Boston Med and Surg Journal 1887; 117: 530-537.

[54] Plummer H.S. Diffuse dilatation of the esophagus without anatomic stenosis. J.A.M.A. 1912; 58: 2013-2015

[55] Sahli H. Métodos de exploración clínica, Salvat, Barcelona, 1903.

[56] Savary M., Miller G. The Esophagus. Handbook and Atlas of Endoscopy. Solothurn (Switzerland), Verlag Gassmann 1978.

[57] Schreiber J. Die Dilatationssonde. Sammlung Klinische Vorträge, Leipzig, Breitkopf u. Härtel 1893: 703-724.

[58] Semeleder F. Uber oesophagoskopie. Wien. Medicinal Halle 1862; 3: 319.

[59] Sencert L. Corps étrangers de l'oesophage in Mathieu A, Sencert L, Tuffier Th. Maladies de l'estomac et de l'oesophage. Paris, Masson, 1913: 80-125.

60 Starck H. L'oesophagoscopie et sa valeur diagnostique. Comptes Rendus, XIV Congrès International de Médecine. Madrid, 1904: 300-305.

61 Starck H. Die direkte Besichtigung der Speiseröhre. Oesophagoskopie. Würzburg, Stuber, 1905.

62 Starck H. Lehrbuch der Ösophagoskopie. Würzburg, Kurt Kabitzsch, 1914.

63 Starck H. Die Behandlung der spasmogenen Speiseröhrenerweiterung. Münch med Wschr 1924; 71: 334-336.

64 Starck H. Kardiospasmus. Kardiotonisches Speiseröhrenerweiterung. Verhandl Gesell Verdauu Stoffwechelskr. Leipzig, G.Thieme, 1930:166-197.

65 Stoerk J. Die Untersuchung des Ösophagus mit dem Kehlkopfspiegel. Wien Med Wschr 1881; 9: 620-623.

66 Stoerk J. Ein neues Oesophagoskop. Wien med Wschr 1887; 37:1117-1119.

67 Stoerk J. Die Oesophagoskopie. Wien klin Wschr. 1896; 9: 625-631.

68 Vantrappen G., Hellemans J. Diseases of the Oesophagus. Berlin, Heidelberg, Springer Verlag, 1974.

69 Voltolini F.E. Über die Durchleuchtung des Kehlkopfes und andere Höhlen des menschlichen Körpers. Allgm Wien med Zeitung 1888; 33: 561, 581, 594.

70 Waldenburg M.L. Oesophagoskopie. Eine neue Untersuchungsmethode. Berlin Klin Wochenschr 1870; 48; 578-580.

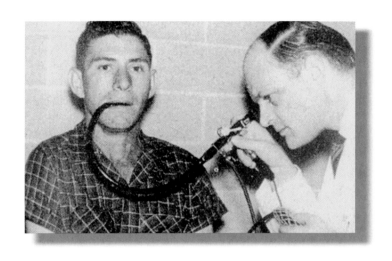

CHAPTER 6

The emergence of
optical fibre
fibrescopy

INVESTIGATING LIGHT TRANSMISSION

IN AN INQUIRY MADE IN THE UNITED STATES A FEW YEARS AGO, gastroenterologists were asked what they considered to be the most significant advances in gastroenterology over the last fifty years. The majority placed fibreendoscopy in first or second place in alternation with the discovery of the pathogenic role of Helicobacter pylori.

Taking into account how greatly endoscopy has contributed to the diagnosis of oesophago-gastric diseases and to the identification and documentation of intestinal and biliary disorders, while at the same time considering the wide variety of modalities of therapeutic endoscopy, I sincerely believe that fibrescopy should unquestionably have taken first place always. Its tremendous utility in clinical medicine is incomparable and from a social point of view, it has probably contributed to saving more lives than any other medical procedure, technique or discovery in our speciality[33].

Research into the history of fibrescopy is no easy task. It has evolved as the result of contributions from investigators working in many disciplines within the world of physics, optics, and medicine. For the interested endoscopist, the outstanding book by Jeff Hecht, "City of Light", is essential reading. In a pleasant yet detailed manner, the author relates the history of optical fibres, their development and their application in various scientific fields, including of course, medicine. This chapter owes much to his patient and exhaustive research[14] *(Fig. 1).*

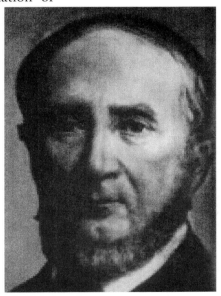

Fig. 1. Jean Daniel Colladon (1802-1893). Swiss engineer, professor of physics in Geneva. He studied the transmission of sound in the water of Lake Leman. He was the first to observe the transmission of light by total refraction from one end to the other of a water stream, a discovery which was used in various theatre productions in Paris (www.droits humains, org/Refug GE).

Possibly the first to demonstrate that light rays did not necessarily follow a straight path, but could travel through curved and bent forms, was Jean Daniel Colladon, a Swiss physicist from Geneva (1802-1893), who was interested in the illumination of public fountains. Colladon succeeded in directing a light ray through the

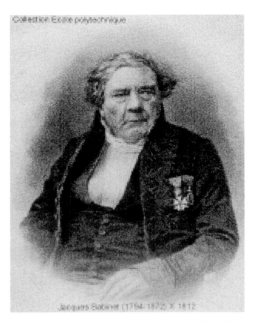

Jacques Babinet (1794-1872) X 1872

Fig. 2. Jacques Babinet (1794-1872). Professor of physics and astronomy in Paris. He was the first to study the transmission of light through solid materials such as glass fibres, putting into use Colladon's discovery of the total refraction of light inside a water stream. (courtesy of Bibliothèque Polytechnique, Académie des Sciences, Paris).

water flow of a cascade, and in 1841 he showed that light remained trapped in the water by the effect of total refraction. He also observed that if a thin stream of water met with an obstacle, the dispersed water droplets equally transmitted light. Colladon made displays of numerous light and water effects which were used at the Paris Opera House and at the Universal Exhibition of Paris in 1889. He also studied the transmission of sound under the water of Lake Leman, winning a prize from the Paris Académie des Sciences for this research, and invented an audiphone and contributed to the installation of electrical generators in Geneva, using the water of the Rhone river.

Colladon's ideas were developed by the Parisian professor of optical physics, Jacques Babinet (1794-1872); Babinet was born in Luzignan in 1794 and he died in Paris in 1872[3] *(Fig. 2).*

He was a very productive investigator and he invented a hygrometer, a polariscope, an air pump and a goniometer for measuring the refraction index of light. He was a professor at the Collège de France, the highest teaching institution in his country. In 1840 he was elected senior member of the Paris "Académie des Sciences".

Babinet became interested in Colladon's experiments and studied not only the illumination of water but also the transmission of light through glass plates curved in different shapes and positions. In his work "La polarisation de la lumière" (1845) Babinet suggested that this phenomenon might be used to manufacture "an instrument which could provide light to examine the inside of the mouth". He succeeded also in transmitting light rays through thin glass rods, thus anticipating fiberoptics. Babinet's goniometer for the measurement of light refraction is still employed by optical firms[14].

Thanks to Colladon, illuminated fountains proliferated in many European cities, starting in Paris which was named "La Ville Lumière", the City of Light, as a result of the illuminations made for the Universal Exhibition in 1889. The term, which is still used, inspired the title for Hecht's book. The illumination of fountains using water streams with different coloured sequences of varied shape and volume, reached its peak with the designs of the Spanish engineer Carlos Buigas, who created a magnificent coloured fountain in 1929 for the Universal Exhibition in Barcelona. Today it continues to draw crowds, impressed by the great variety of effects created with water and light. It was reproduced to a smaller scale in other fountains, such as the one he designed for the Paris "Exposition Universelle" in 1937[6] *(Figs. 3, 4).*

On the other hand, Babinet's observations that glass fibres could, like water, transmit light by total refraction of the light ray, stimulated numerous research projects. These led to the current development in fibre optics. The central idea of fibre optics is that the light which enters one extremity of a filament or tube made of transparent material will be totally reflected inside the wall of the tube or filament and transmitted to the opposite end. This will occur even if the fibres are bent or curved in any direction; glass as well as plastic materials of diameters varying between 5 and 100 microns have the same properties of transmitting light and are used today for very different purposes.

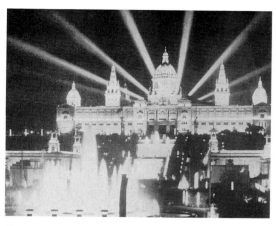

Fig. 3. Carlos Buigas, Spanish engineer from Barcelona, used Colladon's and Babinet's observations in his coloured fountains, such as that at Montjuich (Barcelona), built for the World Exhibition of 1929.

THE HISTORY OF GLASS FIBRES. BOYS, BAIRD AND HANSELL

The earliest manufacture of glass fibres dates back to the most remote antiquity and the Egyptians were already using glass beads and fibres as ornaments. In the 18th century, René Ferchauld de Réaumur, also known for his studies on digestion, succeeded in making glass fibres by rotating a wheel immersed in a cauldron filled with melted glass and extracting threads and fibres which remained stuck to the wheel. In the 19th century, several manufacturers were able to make thinner and more uniform fibres by immersing a hot glass tube in the melted glass. Once cooled, the tube was rotated on a wheel. Wigs, and ornaments for dresses were made with glass filaments. These became less fragile at the same time as they became longer and longer; some were 3 meters long, the maximum length that the diameter of the wheels would allow[14].

The brilliant English physicist Sir Charles Vernon Boys (1855-1944), well known for his investigations on the torsion of quartz fibres in the measurement of minute forces, succeeded in making several types of elastic glass fibres as resistant as steel, but apparently he was not interested in studying the possibility of transmitting light through his fibres. Boys, known also for his studies on the Newtonian constant of gravitation, was a professor at the Royal College and president of the London Academy of Sciences. He invented a radiomicrometer for measuring radiant heat[5].

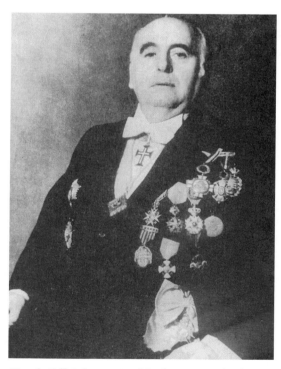

Fig. 4. Official portrait of Carlos Buigas, the designer of several coloured fountains at International Exhibitions in Barcelona, Paris and Los Angeles (courtesy of the Buigas family).

A few years later, around 1920, several factories produced very thin glass fibres which were resistant and very flexible and could be used for making fabric – the so-called "glass wool" still used today as an insulator *(Figs. 5, 6)*.

Other important forerunners were the innovations of the Scottish physicist John Logie Baird (1888-1946). Baird's main interest was television: as early as 1924 he had produced televised images of objects and in 1925 he transmitted recognisable images of people at the Royal Institution in London[1, 2]. Baird also studied optical fibres which he thought could be related to his work on television and in 1926 he patented the manufacturing of bundles of rigid glass or quartz tubes 0.3 mm in diameter and 50 mm in length, superimposed in parallel rows. In a transversal section they resembled the layout of a bee-hive. The fibres disposed in this way could transmit light from one end of the tube to the other without lenses or mirrors.

Baird never mentioned any specific application for his invention and apparently never pursued any further research along these lines but he got a patent for them in 1926 (British patent spec No. 020969/27). He then exclusively turned his attention to television, where he was a pioneer, particularly with colour television which he presented for the first time in 1928. Shortly before his death he had perfected a procedure for stereoscopic television[32] *(Fig. 7)*.

In 1926, an American, Clarence Hansell (1899-1967), applied both in the United States and the United Kingdom for a patent based on the transmission of light by cable through photoelectric cells which could transform light into optical signals and return them by means of other photoelectric cells. The design of the cables was not unlike Baird's: the filaments were made of quartz and were insulated from each other to avoid the loss of refraction, although he did not specify the method for insulating them. He mentioned that to be able to transmit light they should be congruent, that is, that both ends of the filaments should coincide. Hansell suggested his invention could be useful for surgical explorations. He was awarded a patent in 1930 which was negotiated with Marconi's firm for its development in Europe. As we shall see, further attempts to advance in this field –by physicists such as Van Heel and Hopkins– were hampered by this patent which apparently had no practical application[32].

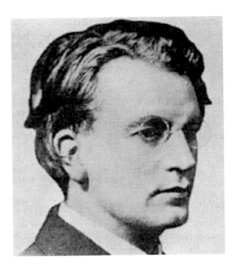

Fig. 5. John Logie Baird, one of the inventors of television, who also studied optical fibres and patented fibre bundles (ref. 2)

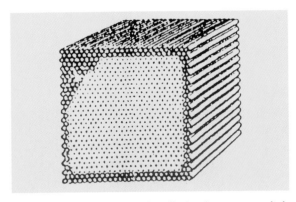

Fig. 6. Drawing of a fibre bundle for the patent on light transmission awarded to John Logie Baird (courtesy of the late L. Lauridsen).

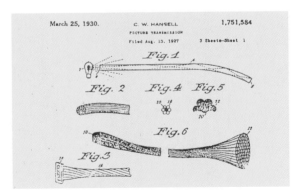

Fig. 7. Drawings from the patent awarded to Clarence Hansell 1926-1930. The light ray originated by the lamplight travelling through the fibre glass tube is clearly seen together with the fibre bundles (courtesy of the late L. Lauridsen).

PROPERTIES OF OPTICAL FIBRES *(Fig. 8)*

Optical fibres have many applications: glass or plastic filaments with diameters between 5 and 100 microns can be packaged into bundles containing thousands of fibres. Fibres 50 cm long can be manufactured as thin tubes, strings or cables which preserve the flexibility of individual fibres and may be twisted without losing the property to transmit light or images[23]. To protect them and to avoid light dispersion, the fibres must be coated with some material of lesser refraction. The figure shows a light ray entering a segment of a filament and reflected inside it. Optimal transmission requires the radius of the curvature of the light ray to be at least twenty times that of the radius of an individual fibre. The two ends of the fibre must be polished to allow transmission of images from one area to another. Depending on the diameter of the fibres, image resolution may be as great as 100 lines per millimetre[14].

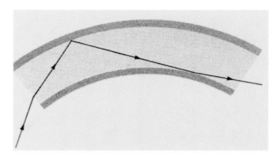

Fig. 8. The principle of fibre optics: total refraction of a light ray inside a tube protected by an insulating coating.

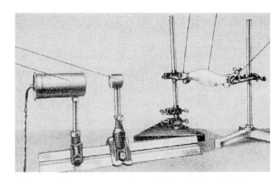

Fig. 9. Instruments devised by Heinrich Lamm (1930) to transmit images: to the left of the picture: an incandescent lamp of 25 volts as a light source. Towards the right: objective lens on a small stand. At the right end of the picture, the terminal portion of the fibre bundle directed to the ocular. (ref.29).

THE BIRTH OF FIBRE OPTICS. HEINRICH LAMM *(Figs. 9, 10, 11)*

Historians of fibreoptics agree that we owe the idea of applying the extraordinary innovation of optical fibres to medicine to Heinrich Lamm, a 20-year-old third-year medical student in Munich (Cand. Med) (erroneously cited as a gynaecologist by some authors). In a technical journal, Lamm published a paper in which he showed that a bundle of bent glass filaments of several microns in diameter could transmit light rays from one end to the other in spite of the bends[29]. Lamm (1908-1973) had attended gastroscopy sessions in Rudolf Schindler's clinic in Munich and had noticed how unpleasant it was for a patient to swallow a rather rigid instrument[14]. Lamm was probably aware of the experiments of light transmission through glass fibres that were taking place in several physics laboratories. Like Hansell, Lamm thought that fibres could transmit images as well as light provided that the two ends of each fibre were properly aligned and congruent.

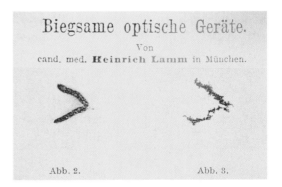

Fig. 10. The V shaped image of the filament of an incandescent lamp that Lamm succeeded in transmitting through glass fibres in his device (ref.29).

The young student invented a device by means of which he could show that glass fibres 40 microns in diameter could transmit the V image produced by the filament of an incandescent bulb and he published his findings in 1930.

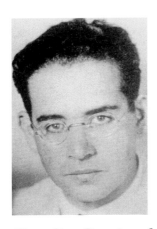

Fig. 11. Portrait of Heinrich Lamm in 1930 when he was a medical student in Munich. (courtesy of his son, Michael Lamm).

Lamm wrote in essence that "if one projects an image in the proximal surface of the fibre bundle (in his case, the filament of a light bulb), the image will be transmitted point by point to the surface of the other end of the fibres, where it can be observed by means of a lens which will used as an ocular. Even though the fibres are twisted or bent, the transmission of the image remains unaltered".

Although his research gave no practical results as the transmitted image was far from satisfactory (see *fig. 10),* Lamm ended his paper thanking Dr. Heurung from the Munich optical firm Rodenstock, Dr Schindler and Gerlach, a physics professor, for their advice. He wrote prophetically, "I hope that some optical instrument firm with more means and experience than I have, will succeed, thanks to my work, in making a clinically useful flexible gastroscope". Lamm tried to interest Schindler in his experiments but unfortunately, the latter was too busy with his own gastroscope designs to get deeply involved in the subject. However, in his remarks to Hirschowitz thirty years later when he presented his first fibrescope, Schindler recalled Lamm's efforts.

Lamm had applied for a patent for his discovery but he found that Clarence Hansell had already done so from a strictly theoretical point of view and had given up his European patent rights to the firm Marconi. The patent, which was never put to use by Marconi's group, later played an important role by obstructing the practical applications devised by Van Heel and Hopkins and their efforts to apply for patents. Lamm was of Jewish origin and emigrated to the United States where apparently he had no opportunity to pursue his work on fibre optics. However, his son Michael, has been kind enough to let me know that his father's medical career gave him much satisfaction and that he ended his days in 1974 as a respected surgeon in Texas[30].

PROGRESS: MÖLLER-HANSEN, O'BRIEN, VAN HEEL

Lamm's ideas and their possible application to the manufacture of endoscopes continued to develop, though slowly, thanks to a group of researchers in the field of optics. Among them in the first place I would like to mention Holger Möller-Hansen from Copenhagen whose goal was the same; to design a flexible gastroscope which could transmit images by means of fibre bundles[31] *(Figs. 12 y 13)*

Möller-Hansen, who had studied engineering, applied for a patent similar to Lamm's. The Danish physicist had been struck by the segmental vision system of flies consisting of individual superimposed sensitive neural fibres which resemble the sagittal drawings of the fibres included in Baird's patent. Möller-Hansen tried to coat the fibres with different substances of low refraction; he tried oils and even margarine. Both substances provided an almost transparent coating which would impede the external diffusion of light, and thus facilitate the total refraction of the light rays and their transmission. Unfortunately, the Danish patent office did not accept his application because of the earlier patent awarded to Hansell. His efforts were unfruitful and Möller-Hansen abandoned his work on glass fibres for other subjects; among other inventions, he managed to patent plastic bubble-lined envelopes[14].

Meanwhile, other physicists remained interested in the transmission of light and images through glass and quartz fibres (Figs. 14, 15).

Two scientists became leaders in the field: the Dutch physicist Abram Van Heel (1899-1966), professor of optics at Delft University[38], and the American Brian O'Brien[14]. Both studied ways to avoid the loss of total refraction of transmitted light due to friction among tightly bound glass fibres. O'Brien, an electro-optical engineer, worked in research at Rochester University and he was later appointed director of research at the American Optical Corporation, where among other activities, he put his energy into the design of giant screens for cinema and video. At the suggestion of his friend O'Brien, Van Heel developed the

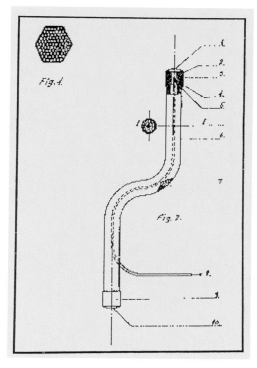

Fig. 12. Drawings made by Möller-Hansen to demonstrate the transmission of light through fibre bundles for a patent which was denied. (courtesy of the late L.Lauridsen).

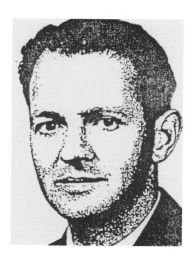

Fig. 13. Holger Möller-Hansen early in his career. (courtesy of Professor H.J.Reuter).

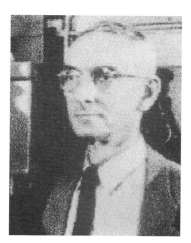

Fig. 14. Brian O'Brien, professor of optics at the University of Rochester (N.Y.) and adviser to Abram Van Heel, who became famous by designing photographic cameras for giant screens (courtesy Philips DP70).

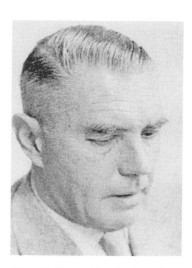

Fig. 15. Abram Van Heel, professor of optics at Leiden University, possibly the first to show the viability of image transmission through optical fibres. (www.optica.tn.delft.nl/history.htm)

idea of protecting the glass fibres by immersing them in liquids of low refraction index, as Möller-Hansen had previously done. He chose a metallic coating, but he found that it was not useful. Unfortunately, in 1951 transatlantic communications were poor and the collaboration between Delft and Rochester, which was giving such good results, could not proceed in practice. However, in 1952 Van Heel had made substantial progress and had been able to transmit images through bundles made of 400 fibres about 50 cm in length. They were congruent and coated with dark varnish. In July 1953, the Dutch scientific journal, "De Ingenieur" published a long article by Van Heel in which he described his method for the transmission of images through plastic fibre bundles 20 cm in length and 0.1 to 0.13 mm in diameter. Van Heel suggested the possible usefulness of his invention in medicine. It seems that the Dutch scientist was aware neither of Lamm's paper from 1930 nor of Möller-Hansen's research, which apparently was never given publicity[32].

Abram Van Heel had studied at Leiden University and he obtained his doctorate in 1925. He worked for one year in the Optics Institute of Paris University where he took part in the first tests with electronic computers. He continued his scientific career in the department of applied physics at Delft University where he was appointed professor in 1947. He was one of the founders of the I.C.O. (International Commission of Optics) of which he became President in 1950. In 1956 he edited the journal Optica Acta. He died suddenly, greatly respected, in 1966[38].

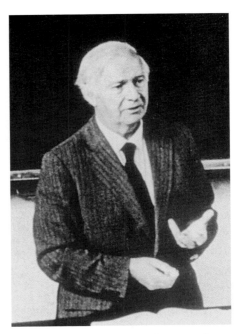

Fig. 16. Harold Hopkins during a lecture (courtesy of the late L.Lauridsen).

PRIORITIES AND CONTROVERSIES: HAROLD HOPKINS AND NARINDER KAPANY

After sending his paper to the "De Ingenieur", Van Heel apparently tried to establish his priority in the field by submitting a brief note to the prestigious journal "Nature". It had a much larger diffusion than the Dutch publication but his article was not published until January 1954[38], simultaneously with a longer paper by Harold Hopkins (1918-1994), a distinguished British physicist. Hopkins was born in Leicester in 1918 from parents of modest means. He graduated in physics in 1938 and was soon appointed assistant professor at London's Imperial College. He won acclaim in 1948 when he invented, with the help of the B.B.C., the first "zoom" lens. It is said that Hopkins's interest in fibrescopy began after a casual conversation with a London physician, Hugh Gainsborough, who complained about the poor acceptance of Schindler's semiflexible gastroscope among patients and prodded him to investigate the possibility of using some kind of flexible optical system to replace it[24] *(Fig. 16)*.

Hopkins, who was probably unaware of the early work on fibreoptics, started like others by transmitting light through a fine bundle of fibres 20 micron in diameter and over 1 meter in length. In 1952, Hopkins managed to get a grant from the Paul Instrument Fund of the Royal Society and this enabled him to take on a young research assistant of Indian origin, Narinder Kapany, a graduate from Agra University. The two worked with very thin fibres (25 microns in diameter) of the kind used to manufacture textiles. They were able to bundle together between 10,000 and 20,000 fibres and after cutting their ends into segments, made them coincide so that they would transmit light and images.

Hopkins and Kapany sent a letter to "Nature" *(Fig. 17)*. It was rapidly published in the same issue as Van Heel's[22]. Neither Hopkins' nor Van Heel's communication quoted the other, which clearly suggests that both authors had reached similar results, unaware of the work of the competitor. However, the delay of several months in publishing Van Heel's letter made some people suspicious that Hopkins had in some way influenced the editors to delay its publication until his own work had been completed. Nevertheless, it is obvious that in the future, the title of Hopkins letter which included "a flexible fibrescope" would attract the attention of gastroenterologists much more than the title of Van Heel's paper which limited itself to a description of the "transport of images". Hopkins was the first to employ the term "fibrescope"and his letter explicitly mentions its usefulness as a substitute for conventional endoscopes using lens systems[21]. His name is certainly much more familiar to endoscopists than that of Van Heel, although this is due also to other optical discoveries that Hopkins made some time later.

Retrospectively, it is clear that the two works complemented each other; Hopkins used a much greater number of very thin fibres without any kind of coating, while Van Heel used fewer and larger fibres but coated to avoid loss of light and image, as O'Brien had recommended earlier to him. Unfortunately, Van Heel did not acknowledge O'Brien's contribution in his letter to "Nature" and this caused serious animosity between the two scientists.

We have already described the late years of Heinrich Lamm in the United States; Van Heel, a respected university professor, like Möller-Hansen, turned his research to other areas; Kapany, Hopkins' coauthor, got a degree in optics at the Imperial College and the University of London.

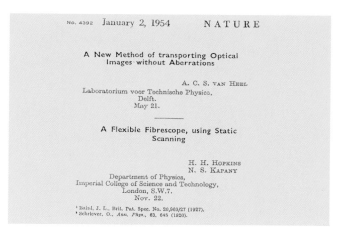

Fig. 17. The simultaneous publication in "Nature" of Van Heel's and Hopkins' letters on the transmission of images through optical fibres.

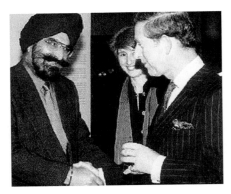

Fig. 18. Narinder Singh Kapany greeting Prince Charles of England. (source: the Narinder S. Kapany Foundation).

He then fell out with Hopkins and emigrated to the United States. In spite of rumours appearing in some publications that Kapany had to abandon his scientific activities and had to work as a restaurateur, the entire truth seems to be rather different[25] *(Fig. 18)*.

Kapany was appointed a professor at Rochester University and in 1960 he moved to California where he established the firm "Optics Technology" and later the firms "Kaptron" and "K2 Optics". He also got an appointment as Regents Professor at the University of California at Berkeley and another as a Consultant at Stanford University. He was awarded about one hundred patents for his research on optics, lasers, solar energy, monitorisation of pollution, etc. All these activities allowed him to become the leader of the Sikh Foundation which edits books and organises scientific programmes, art exhibitions and academic lectures. Kapany's curriculum (which can be easily perused on Internet) seems to belie the last assessment made by Hopkins on Kapany's work, "Kapany contributed nothing to the ideas of the project, he was only a pair of hands"[14].

A long and unpleasant fight for the patent of optical fibres followed. In spite of the probable priority of Van Heel for his paper in "De Ingenieur", O'Brien was awarded a patent for his idea of coating glass fibres with low refraction substances, while Hopkins' application was denied because of the previous patents of Hansell-Marconi and Baird. Neither did he succeed in obtaining more funds for his project and from then on, the development of fibre optics took place in the United States.

However, Hopkins continued his brilliant career[11] and he will be remembered for his pioneering work on fibre optics as well as for his invention of "cold light", that is, the use of optical fibres as an external source of light, and its transmission to the tip of an endoscope without generating heat. This major advance provided the basis of the lighting systems of all modern diagnostic and therapeutic endoscopes for which Hopkins was awarded a patent in 1960 (British patent spec 3257906; 1960). The patent was developed mainly by the German firm Karl Storz and it will be discussed in detail in the chapter on laparoscopy. Rather surprisingly, according to his admirers[11], Hopkins' great achievements were not adequately recognised by the British Government and his name never appeared in the Honours List annually awarded by the Crown.

This was the beginning of a long saga which started in Europe, went further in the United States and seems to have reached its final destiny in Japan with the current endoscopes in which image transmitting optical fibres have been superseded by the new video television technologies.

FIBRE OPTICS AND THE CLINICIAN:
BASIL HIRSCHOWITZ

Basil Hirschowitz was born in South Africa. He studied medicine at the University of Witswatersrand where, according to his own recollections, he witnessed his first gastroscopies with Schindler's instrument. He continued his studies in England where he was accepted as a registrar by Sir Francis Avery-Jones at the Central Middlesex Hospital. Avery-Jones had organised a gastroenterology unit there which soon acquired international recognition. Here Hirschowitz performed his first endoscopies[20]. His main interest at that time, however, was the study of gastric secretion and particularly that of pepsinogen. He moved to the United States where he worked under H. Marvin Pollard, a professor of gastroenterology at the University of Michigan at Ann Arbor. There he conducted several randomised clinical studies which had been promoted in the United Kingdom by Richard Doll and Leslie Witts, but which took longer to be recognised for their value in the United States.

Never failing to pursue his inquiries into the field of endoscopy, Hirschowitz made several attempts to televise an endoscopic examination. These were unsuccessful because of the poor technology at the time. In 1954, according to Keith Henley[15] who had also been a fellow with Sheila Sherlock in London and who had become a close associate of Pollard at Ann Arbor, he told Hirschowitz about Hopkins and Van Heels' letters which had just been published in "Nature". Henley was aware of these thanks to a registrar of Sheila Sherlock's, Tim Counihan[16]. Regaining interest in endoscopy[17] during a summer holiday, Hirschowitz visited Hopkins and Kapany in London. The team had succeeded in transmitting images through a fibre bundle, but according to Hirschowitz the lighting was poor and the image had a greenish tinge. When he returned to Ann Arbor, he began work in the Optics Institute of the University of Michigan thanks to a grant which Pollard had been able to obtain for him.

Unfortunately, he could not work with Kapany as he had moved to the United States to work for the optical firm "Bausch and Lomb". However, the physicist Wilbur Peters, from Michigan University, had become interested in the project and he recommended young Larry Curtiss, a physics student with a brilliant curriculum, as a substitute *(Fig. 19 y 20)*.

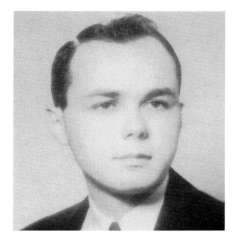

Fig. 19. Lawrence ("Larry") Curtiss, then an optics student at the University of Michigan, who had the remarkable idea of coating optical fibres with glass to avoid the dispersion of light and images, (courtesy of Mr. Lawrence Curtiss).

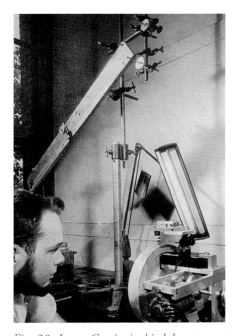

Fig. 20. Larry Curtiss in his laboratory at the University of Michigan with the equipment he used to insulate a glass tube with optical fibres of high refraction power, a technique which was essential to enable vision through a fibrescope. (courtesy of Ms Kathy Marquis, Bentley Historical Library, University of Michigan, in the collection: University of Michigan News and Information Services).

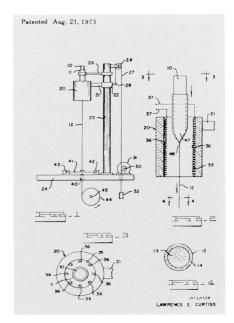

Fig. 21. Drawings presented by Lawrence Curtiss together with Basil Hirschowitz for their patent application in 1973 (U.S. Patent 3,753,672) (courtesy of Mr. Lawrence Curtiss).

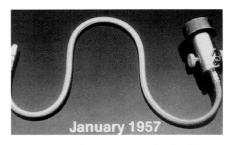

Fig. 22. The first prototype of a flexible gastroscope (courtesy of Prof. Basil Hirschowitz).

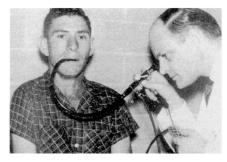

Fig. 23. Basil Hirschowitz using his gastroscope to examine a patient (the patient's name is unknown) (courtesy of Prof. Basil Hirschowitz).

Working together, Hirschowitz and Curtiss succeeded in making glass fibres with the help of the multinational firm, "Corning Glass", but they had to face the same problems as their forerunners: the loss of image due to the diffusion of light towards neighbouring fibres preventing the total refraction of light. After many trials that lasted several months using different coating substances such as lacquer, Curtiss[14] finally solved the problem with the ingenious idea of introducing an optical fibre of high refraction power inside a fine but wider glass tube of low refraction power and fusing both elements together in an oven constructed specially for the purpose. The result was a composite fibre consisting of a central zone of high refraction power, which transmitted the light, and an insulating external glass coat which prevented its external diffusion. According to Le Fanu[33], in Hirschowitz's own words, "When Curtiss first advanced the idea of fusing an optical glass fibre inside a tube of less refraction power, all the experts at the department laughed at him". But Curtiss and Hirschowitz were not discouraged. They continued their work, even including the manual tasks of putting the fibres together[15]. They finally managed to make 10 metre long fibres which were able to transmit light and could be rolled into balls.

These events occurred in December 1956 and at the end of the month, Hirschowitz, together with Peters and Curtiss, applied for a patent which covered the use of fibres for gastroscopy. In May 1957, Curtiss applied for a patent for his method for insulating light transmitting fibres by coating them with glass (US Patent 3,236,710). The same year, Hirschowitz presented his endoscope to his colleagues at the university. According to Keith Henley, the instrument "resembled an enormous worm fed an excess of growth hormone"[15]. Hirschowitz had the courage to swallow his thick "gastroscope" and confessed afterwards that it had not been a pleasant experience. A few days later, he performed an endoscopy on a lady with a peptic ulcer. The first clinical publication on fibregastroscopy appeared in the journal "Gastroenterology" in 1958[18]. It included Hirschowitz, the opticians Peters and Curtiss, and H. Marvin Pollard, Hirschowitz's chief, who had provided the economic aid necessary for the project *(Fig. 21)*.

In 1973, Curtiss perfected and patented his procedure for coating optical fibres (US Patent 3,753,672) while Hirschowitz had patented his first fibrescope (US Patent 3,010,357) in 1961. The granted patents bear the names of both Hirschowitz and Curtiss, together with Peters *(Figs. 22 y 23)*.

In spite of various attempts by Hirschowitz to convince manufacturers such as the American Optical Company, the G.U. of London and Eder in Chicago of the importance of fibrescopy, only the American Cystoscope Makers (A.C.M.I.) which had been founded by Reinhold Wappler in New York *(Fig. 24)* listened to him. The first prototype was made in 1960, and in 1961, the first commercial instrument appeared on the market, the ACM 4990. Little by little, fibrescopy began to be adopted by gastroenterologists and it became an accepted technique even by the most recalcitrant supporters of the semi-flexible Schindler-Wolf gastroscope. As Hirschowitz recently mentioned at a lecture during the World Congress of Gastroenterology (Bangkok 2002), the first fibregastroscope he used is now deposited at the Smithsonian Institution in Washington. In spite of their early refusal, the Eder company, as we shall see, later made colonoscopy and gastroscopy prototypes *(Fig. 25)*.

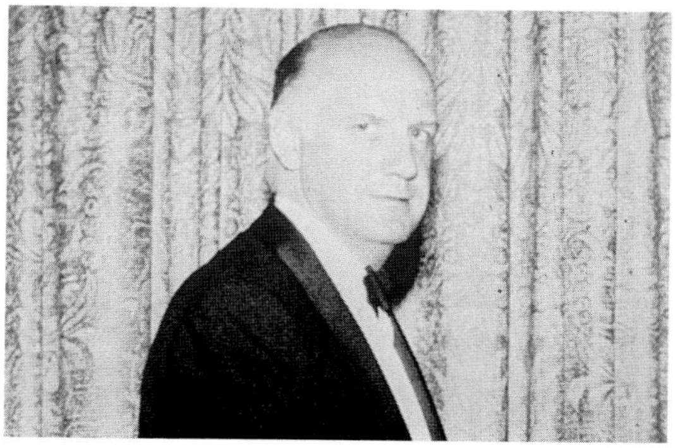

Hirschowitz, who had not abandoned his studies on gastric secretion, moved to the University of Alabama in Birmingham where he continued his brilliant research and where he is still active as professor of medicine. It was there in October 1960, where he started his first clinical programmes on gastroscopy.

Larry Curtiss[7], meantime, pursued a successful career in the medical industry as director of research and vice-president of A.C.M.I., and later, as a consultant to the firm Welch-Allyn, which was developing video-endoscopy. During his research activities, Curtiss was granted 11 patents, including the coating of glass fibres, diathermic snares, resectoscopes, spectrometers and spectroscopes. In 1973, he wrote an important review on high frequency currents and their use in digestive endoscopy[8].

Fig. 24. Reinhold Wappler Jr. He succeeded his father as head of A.C.M.I. and actively participated in the design and diffusion of the fibrescope. (courtesy of Mr. Reinhold Wappler Jr.)

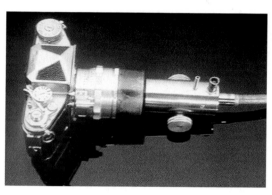

Fig. 25. The 35 mm Reflex Exacta camera used by Basil Hirschowitz for his first photographs (courtesy of Prof. Basil Hirschowitz).

THE FIRST FIBRESCOPE PROTOTYPES

Mark I, as the first prototype was named, was followed by Mark II, III, IV and finally by Mark V, the so- called "Hirschowitz gastro-duodenal fiberscope ACM 4990". With subsequent modifications, it was in use in various countries until the mid-1960s. The instrument's distal end had an incandescent lamp, a prism and an objective lens similar to that of a semi-flexible gastroscope. The deviation angle was 90 degrees but the vision was somewhat more reduced than that of the semi-flexible instruments: 45 degrees instead of the

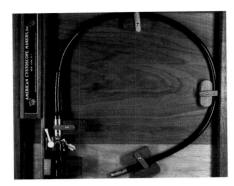

Figs. 26. First A.C.M.I. fibrescope employed in Barcelona around 1966 (F.O.5000)

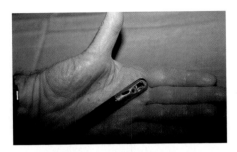

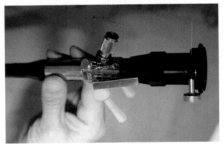

Fig. 27. and 28.- Head and terminal portion of the Hirschowitz fibrescope.

55 degrees in the latest Cameron gastroscopes and much less than the German Storz gastroscopes which had an angle of vision of 90 degrees *(Figs. 26, 27, 28)*.

The large diameter ocular piece allowed much light to enter, entailing, however, a reduction in the depth of the focus. This obliged the operator to constantly focus the image by means of a knob. The first instruments contained some 260,000 fibres, 24 microns in thickness, and the total diameter of the bundle was 12 mm. The first instruments, like the semi-flexible devices, only provided lateral vision and illumination was provided by an incandescent bulb which excessively heated the distal end of the first gastroscopes and sometimes caused mucosal burns. Some years later, "cold light", transmitted by optical fibres connected to an external light source replaced the lamp[10].

As was to be expected, Schindler[37], always belligerent, made several objections to the new fibrescopes. In his opinion, the proximal segment of the instrument should have been rigid to allow its proper orientation inside the stomach, recalling that he had had problems of this sort with the totally flexible lens gastroscope that Wolf had made for him (See Chapter 4) as the tip did not follow the rotations made with the ocular eyepiece. Other criticisms were the need to constantly focus the instrument because of the short focal distance and the narrow angle of vision, especially when compared to the latest semiflexible instrument made by Storz. The image of the first endoscopes was somewhat fuzzy and granular due to the imperfect coherence of the fibres. However, these problems were progressively solved, and even Schindler had to admit how easy it was for people with little experience to handle the instrument and to take photographs as well as films. Another inconvenience, which was solved by introducing a protective mouth piece, was that patients would frequently bite on the instrument, thus breaking fibres. The delicate fibres would also break after repeated use, adding to the black spots on the image.

Furthermore, like others, in our early experience at the Hospital de Sant Pau in Barcelona, we had many problems cleaning the instrument. As it was not completely waterproof the objective continually misted over and became soiled; the need for repairs was common. The gastroscopes had an excessively short life, particularly taking into account their high cost. In spite of these difficulties, all those who used the first ACMI endoscopes agreed that the future lay with optical fibres and that the manufacturing of an ideal device was just a matter of time.

In 1961, Hirschowitz received international recognition through a paper he wrote for The Lancet which was published together with colour photographs[19]. A few years later, several other firms, mainly Japanese, entered the field and contributed significant technical innovations. According to Kawai[28] (Figs. 29, 30, 31, 32), the first ACMI gastroscope employed in Japan was bought by Professor Kondo with his own funds. The first attempts to manufacture Japanese gastroscopes were made by the engineers of the Machida Corporation who succeeded in making fibres of very high quality, and in 1963 they presented their first commercial model which included a bundle of 50,000 fibres, the FGS type A[28]. In 1964, Takagi made the first gastroscopic biopsies in Japan, attaching a vinyl tube to the sheath of an ACMI gastroscope. In 1966, the firm Machida developed the prototype FGS-B which included a channel for biopsy as well as a mechanism for bending the tip of the instrument, used by Takemoto, among others. They later developed models FGS-K and C for cytology as well as the FES oesophagoscope, extensively employed by Kasugai in cases of gastric cancer[26, 27]. In 1967, this model was provided with cold light instead of an incandescent lamp, making photography and cinematography possible[28].

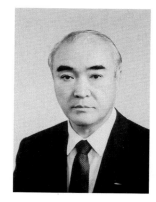

Fig. 29. Ichizo Kawahara, Doctor in Engineering, who designed numerous endoscopes for the firm Olympus. (courtesy of Olympus Inc).

In 1967, according to a survey made by John Morrissey[34], the endoscopy market included 14 different models of semi-flexible gastroscopes equipped with lens systems, 22 types of fibrescopes and 13 different gastrocameras.

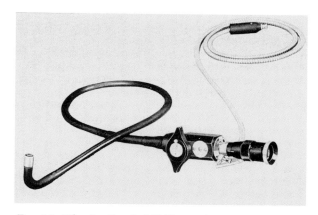

Fig. 30. The Lo Presti ACMI oesophagogastroscope with frontal vision and movable tip. (courtesy of A.C.M.I.).

As years went by, Machida left the field to the Olympus Company. Internationally known for their photographic cameras, they had developed the gastrocamera which, since 1965, included a gastrocamera-fibrescope for direct vision of the photographic field. Their model GFT was followed by the GFT-A which had a distal tip that could be bent. It became very popular in Japan[35]. Olympus also manufactured the GFB model with lateral vision, especially adapted for biopsy and cytology examinations, as well as the EF oesophagoscope with frontal vision (Figs. 33, 34, 35).

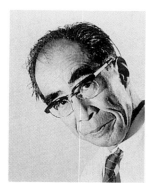

Fig. 31. Professor Taikoro Kondo, pioneer of fibregastroscopy in Japan (courtesy of Olympus Inc.)

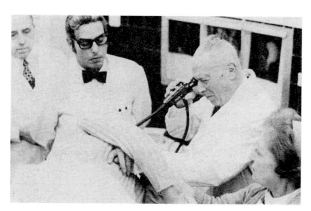

Fig. 32. Dr. E. Vidal-Colomer performing a gastroscopy with one of the first A.C.M.I. instruments at the Hospital de Sant Pau (Barcelona).

119

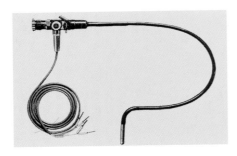

Fig. 33. The Machida FGS gastroscope, extensively used by Takemoto and his associates. It included a biopsy channel and a mechanism for bending the tip. (from a Machida leaflet).

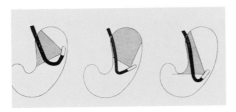

Fig. 34. Inversion manoeuvre with the Machida FGS-B gastroscope (courtesy of Dr. R. Ottenjann).

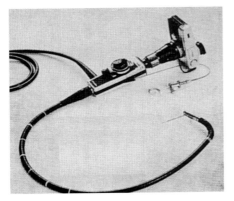

Fig. 35. The Olympus GFB-K gastroscope provideed with "cold light" illumination (1972). (courtesy of Olympus Inc.)

Olympus engineers and particularly Mr.Ichizo Kawahara[28] developed another instrument with lateral vision and a channel for biopsy which was also very useful for photography. A.C.M.I. made an oesophagogastroscope with frontal vision, the Lo Presti Mark 87 and 89 models. The latter had better manual control and a suction channel as well as a movable tip. The Eder company, which in 1969 had marketed a fibrescope, the model Eder-Villa, and the firm Bausch and Lomb where Kapany had been working, lost ground and were left out of the race (Fig. 36).

In 1963, Hirschowitz introduced an oesophagoscope in which "cold light" from glass fibres replaced the incandescent lamps[21]. A longer instrument, providing frontal vision, replaced those featuring lateral vision for the routine examination of the upper digestive tract. These instruments differed from the original gastroscopes in several ways, particularly in the advantage of the frontal vision design which would be applied later to all endoscopes used to examine tubular structures in the body, such as the colon, the bronchi, the small bowel, the urethra and even the biliary tree. An additional channel allowed the optical system to be washed during the examination, as well as the introduction of tubes, brushes and biopsy forceps. Another improvement, mentioned previously, was the introduction of cold light illumination, which eliminated the need for a distal lamp. Soon, the orientation of the instrument was perfected by means of wires that allowed the flexible distal tip of the gastroscope to be bent and the possibility to perform retrovision manoeuvres for

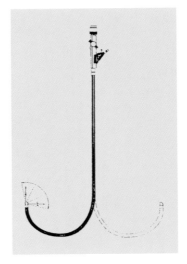

Fig. 36. A gastroscope designed by Dr. F. Villa for the Eder Company of Chicago (around 1973, source: Eder Co. advertisement).

the gastric fundus and the cardia. According to Haubrich[13], the first instrument that became really popular in the United States was the frontal vision endoscope which was 75 cm long. A few years later, instruments of 110 cm in length were made. These permitted adequate examination of the duodenum, essential progress at a time when duodenal ulcer disease was the most important problem facing the gastroenterologist. An excellent review of the first accomplishments of fibrescopy has been written by J. F. Morrissey[34] *(Fig. 37)*.

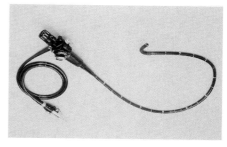

Fig. 37. The Olympus GIF-K2 gastroscope which around 1973 was replacing other instruments as it was easier to handle and provided better vision of the duodenum. (courtesy of Olympus Inc.).

The Japanese firm Machida as well as the American Eder Company developed instruments which combined frontal and lateral vision. Since then, other endoscopes with lateral vision and greater length have been used for cannulation of the Ampulla of Vater and the radiographic examination of the bilio-pancreatic tract which will be discussed in Chapter 12. Endoscopy prototypes appeared soon afterwards and around 1971 Olympus marketed several GIF models (GIF P, GIF D2) which had great versatility and excellent vision. They rapidly replaced outdated instruments[35].

Fibrescopes were the basic instruments of modern endoscopy for many years until they were progressively replaced by the videoendoscopes. Fibrescopy has also been successfully used in veterinary medicine[36].

INITIAL RISKS OF FIBRE OESOPHAGO-GASTROSCOPY

An evaluation of the risks of the first fibrescopic examinations seems necessary at this point. As with any new technique, the initial period was not entirely accident-free: perforations at the zone of the cardia and during attempts to visualise the duodenal bulb occurred on occasion. Schindler, always contentious, reportedly considered the fiberscope more dangerous that his own semi-flexible instrument[37]. In the United States in 1969, Davis published a case of oesophageal perforation with a gastrocamera fibrescope. During the 10th International Congress of Gastroenterology in Budapest in 1976, a symposium took place in which several multicentric reports on the risks of endoscopy and other diagnostic procedures were presented[12]. After 1966, statistics on oesophago-gastric perforations during fibrescopy began to appear. In Table 1, the great diversity of the data, varying between 0.11 and 0.007 per cent, can be appreciated. The statistics included 395,162 gastro-oesophageal examinations with a global percentage of perforations of 0.033 per cent. There were more oesophageal than gastric perforations, particularly among elderly people. Approximately one in eight perforations had a fatal outcome. Other injuries included bronchial aspiration (rare) and cardiovascular accidents demonstrated by electrocardiography. Haemorrhage following a mucosal biopsy was an infrequent event. Hafter assessed the risk of complications after gastroscopy at around 1/1000.

TABLE 1. PERFORATIONS IN OESOPHAGO-GASTRIC FIBRESCOPY

Author	Year	N. Examinations	%Perforations
Ariga	1966	70,400	0.03
Katz	1969	35,448	0.02
Maruyama	1972	45,246	0.007
Schiller (BSGE)	1972	23,563	0.11
Stadelmann	1973	99,426	0.029
Silvis	1974	111,415	0.011

REFERENCES

[1] Baird, John Logie. (article on vision) Enciclopedia Espasa, Appendix n. 10, Barcelona, Espasa Calpe SA 1933: 1156.

[2] Baird M.H.I. John Logie Baird and Television. Eye of the World. arts.Waterloo.ca/FINE/juhde/baird962.

[3] Babinet Jacques. Encyclopédie Larousse L3. vol 1. Paris, 1966.

[4] Berci G, Forde K.A. History of endoscopy. What lessons have we learned from the past? Surg Endosc 2000; 14: 5-15.

[5] Boys Ch.V. Encyclopaedia Britannica, vol 2, Chicago, 1987.

[6] Buigas Carlos. Creador de las fuentes de Montjuich y tantas cosas más.WWW weblandia.com/cerdanyola/buigas.htm.

[7] Curtiss L.E. Personal letter to the author, 2002.

[8] Curtiss L.E. High frequency currents in endoscopy: a review of principles and precautions. Gastrointest Endosc 1973; 20: 9-12.

[9] Davis J.S. Esophageal perforation by the gastrocamera gastroscope. Gastrointest Endosc 1969;15: 201-203.

[10] Elewaut A., Cremer M. The history of gastrointestinal endoscopy –the European perspective. in Classen M., Tytgat, G., Lightdale Ch. Gastroenterological Endoscopy. Stuttgart, Thieme, 2002: 7-30.

[11] Gow, J.G. Hopkins' contribution to Medicine. Das Wiener Endoskopie Museum. Eröffnungssymposium, 1976. Wien, Literas Universitäts Verlag, 1997: 67-72.

[12] Hafter E. The risk of oesophagoscopy and gastroscopy in Ethical problems in the management of gastrointestinal patients. (F.Vilardell (ed.) Scand J Gastroenterol 1977 (Suppl 47) 12:12-14.

[13] Haubrich W.S., Edmonson J.H. History of endoscopy. in Gastroenterologic Endoscopy (M.Sivak ed.) 2 nd edition. Vol 1, Philadelphia, WB Saunders Co. 2000: 2-15.

[14] Hecht J. City of Light. The story of fiberoptics. New York, Oxford. Oxford University Press, 1999.

[15] Henley K.S. Personal letter to the author, 2002.

[16] Henley K.S. History of fiberoptic endoscopy. (letter) Gastroenterology 1980; 78: 1123.

[17] Hirschowitz B.I. History of fiberoptic endoscopy (reply) Gastroenterology 1980; 78: 1123.

[18] Hirschowitz B.I., Curtiss L.E., Peters C.W., Pollard H.M. Demonstration of a new gastroscope the "fiberscope". Gastroenterology 1958; 35: 50-53.

[19] Hirschowitz B.I. Endoscopic examination of the stomach and the duodenal cap with the Fiberscope. Lancet 1961; 1: 1074-1078.

[20] Hirschowitz B.I. A personal history of the fiberscope. Gastroenterology 1970; 76: 864-869.

[21] Hirschowitz B.I. The fibreoptic era in endoscopy —beginnings and perspectives. Ital J Gastroenterol 1989; 21: 247-250.

[22] Hopkins H. H., Kapany N. A flexible fiberscope, using static scanning. Nature 1954; 173: 39-41.

[23] Hopkins H.H. The physics of the fiberoptics endoscope. in Endoscopy. G.Berci (ed.) New York, Appleton Century Crofts, 1976: 27-63.

[24] Jennings CR. Harold Hopkins (Letter to the editor) Arch Otolaryngol, Head & Neck Surg. 1998; 124: 1-2.

[25] Kapany, Narinder Singh ji. Curriculum Vitae. www. Sikh Foundation. Org.

[26] Kasugai T. Gastric biopsy unde direct vision by the fiberscope. Gastrointest Endosc 1968; 14:126.

[27] Kasugai T. Endoscopy in Japan with special reference to detection of gastric cancer. Gastrointest Endosc 1969; 15: 204-205.

[28] Kawai K., Niwa H., Fujita R. The History of endoscopy. The Japanese point of view. in Classen M., Tytgat, G., Lightdale Ch. Gastroenterological Endoscopy. Stuttgart, Thieme, 2002: 32-41.

[29] Lamm H. Biegsame optische Geräte. Zeit. Instrumentenk 1930; 50: 579-581.

[30] Lamm M. Personal letter to the author, 2002.

[31] Lauritsen L. Die Priorität zur Einführung des Fiberlichtes. Das Wiener Endoskopie Museum. Eröffnungssymposium, 1996. Wien, Literas Universitäts Verlag, 1997: 88-100.

[32] Lauritsen L. Laterna Magica in Corpore Humano. Svenburg, Isager Bogtryk, 1998.

[33] Le Fanu, J. The Rise and Fall of Modern Medicine. New York, Carroll & Graf, 1999: 195-196.

[34] Morrissey J.F., Tanaka Y., Thorsen W.B. Gastroscopy. A review of English and Japanese literature. Gastroenterology 1967; 53: 456-476.

[35] Morrissey J.F., Tanaka Y., Thorsen W.B.. The relative value of the Olympus model of CT-5 gastrocamera and Olympus model GT-F gastrocamera fiberscope. Gastrointest Endosc 1968; 14: 197-200.

[36] Riedelberger K. Gastroskopie beim Pferd. Meilensteine der Endoskopie. Wien, Literas Universitätsverlag. 2000: 255-260.

[37] Schindler R. Gastroscopy. The endoscopic study of gastric pathology. 2nd edition. New York, Hafner, 1966: Introduction, p.XXXIV.

[38] Van Heel A.C.S. A new method of transporting optical images without aberrations. Nature 1954; 173: 39.

[39] Van Heel A.C.S. www. optica.tn.tudelft.nl/history.htm 2001.

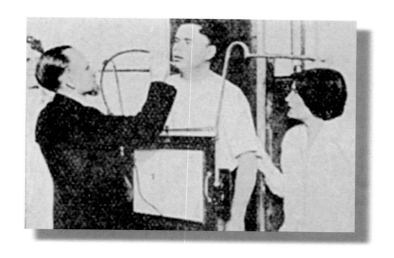

CHAPTER 7

....

The history
of endoscopic
documentation

PAINTINGS, WATERCOLOURS AND DRAWINGS

SINCE THE EMERGENCE OF ENDOSCOPY, PHYSICIANS HAVE TRIED TO document the images seen through their instruments. The famous Désormeaux treatise on endoscopic urology[15] contains excellent colour drawings of vesical calculi. Many articles published by the first endoscopists are illustrated in black and white, but Elsner's book on gastroscopy[17], published in 1911, includes several plates of coloured drawings of gastric lesions. In Schindler's atlas of 1922[51] as well as in Henning's book of 1935[28], there are several coloured pictures of stomach diseases. Henning's monograph features watercolours as well as coloured pictures of the original black and white photographs. Of even better quality are the watercolours painted by Mrs. Claire Escoube in the splendid book by Moutier (1935)[39]. Other illustrations, perhaps not quite as brilliant, are those drawn in 1966 by Gladys McHugh and Eve Vermonde for the second American edition of Schindler's "Gastroscopy"[52]. *(Figs.1, 2, 3, 4).*

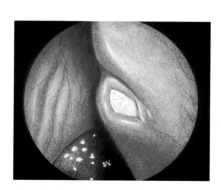

Fig. 1. Gastric ulcer. Watercolour from Elsner's book "Die Gastroskopie"(1911).

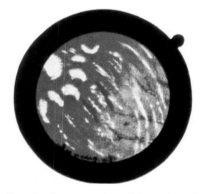

Fig. 2. Acute gastritis. Watercolour by Gladys McHugh for Schindler's "Gastroscopy" (1966).

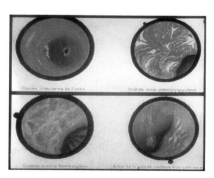

Fig. 3. Original watercolours by Ms Claire Escoube for F. Moutier's book "Traité de Gastroscopie" (1935). (courtesy of Prof. Michel Cremer).

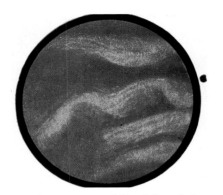

Fig. 4. Large gastric folds. Coloured photograph from the book "Die Gastroskopie" by Norbert Henning (1935).

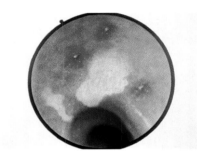

Fig. 5. Erosive gastritis. Watercolour by R. Alemany at Hospital de Sant Pau, Barcelona (around 1940).

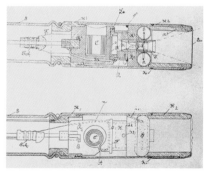

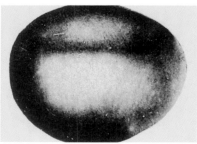

Fig. 6. A) Two drawings of the distal end of Kelling's gastrocamera, showing the lens and the film roll. B) photograph of large folds at the cardia taken by Kelling (1897).

However, in my opinion, nobody has surpassed Mr.R. Alemany from Barcelona. His drawings and watercolours of endoscopic images were so magnificent that Dr. Henry Bockus, on visiting Hospital de Sant Pau to negotiate the Spanish translation of his famous "Gastroenterology", offered him a permanent contract with the publishing firm W. B. Saunders in Philadelphia; Alemany accepted and remained with the company for the rest of his professional life *(Fig. 5)*.

INTRAGASTRIC PHOTOGRAPHY: KELLING, LANGE AND MELTZING

The development of photography gave further impetus to the attempts to document images. As we have already mentioned, several endoscopists hired artists who were present in the examining room and produced drawings, paintings and watercolours. Nevertheless, most clinicians believed that photography, once perfected, would provide much more objective images of their observations.

As in other fields of digestive endoscopy, Georg Kelling was again the first to publish photographs of gastric lesions using a small camera attached to a rubber tube. He apparently took advantage of a patent which had been awarded to a Mr. Oelbermann in 1890[44] and described the instrument in a report published in the German Archives for Digestive Diseases in 1897[34]. It consisted of a tube protected by a flexible sheath, inside which thin wires were coupled to a small photographic camera whose shutter could be released from outside.

A lens and the roll of film, which was protected by a small lid, were placed near the objective of the camera between two incandescent lamps *(Fig. 6)*.

An inflatable balloon pushed the camera forward, opened the lid and at the same time lit the lamps. The distal tip of the tube which contained the camera was 5 cm in length and the diameter of the instrument was 16 mm. The roll of film was 7 mm in width and 15 cm in length, allowing for twelve exposures. According to the photographic plates that accompanied the article, Kelling took pictures of normal gastric mucosa, a carcinoma and enlarged folds at the cardia (see figure 6). Even though the results were initially promising, they were not clinically valid, as later recognised by Kelling himself.

One year later, in 1898, Lange and Meltzing[35] published a paper in which they presented their instrument, an authentic forerunner of the Japanese gastrocameras which would be introduced fifty years later. Judging from the very few months elapsed between this and Kelling's article, they were obviously unaware of the former. One of the authors, Fritz Lange, was born in Dessau[24] and he studied medicine in Jena, Leipzig and Munich. In 1896 he was a surgical assistant in Rostock where he probably met C.A.Meltzing who in 1893, while still a medical student (Med. Cand.), had written a thesis on diaphanoscopy of the stomach at the University Polyclinic in the same town. Lange later became assistant professor in orthopaedic surgery in Munich, and went on to become a full professor. He died in Bad Tolz in 1952. Little is known of Meltzing other than the fact that he pursued his career as a medical practitioner in Duisburg (Rhineland) *(Figs. 7, 8, 9, 10)*.

The two apparently started to design their gastrocamera independently – Meltzing in Rostock and Lange in Munich. It was a most ingenious instrument. Like Kelling's device, it consisted of a miniature photographic camera fitted at the tip of a gastric tube; an incandescent lamp was located close to the objective. Near the tip was a metal cylinder containing the rolled photographic film, which was 50 cm in length and 5 mm in width. The instrument was covered with a rubber sheath and the outside diameter was 11 mm, much smaller than that of Kelling's gastrocamera (16 mm.). By means of a system of wires, the film could be unwound and some 50 pictures could be taken. Another wire opened the shutter of the objective and lit the lamp. Air could be insufflated through a distal opening in the sheath.

Preparation of the patient was very simple: a clear liquid diet was prescribed the night before the examination and the following day, sparkling mineral water was administered to cleanse the stomach. The examination lasted some 15 minutes and the film was previously loaded in a dark room. At the time of their article, Lange and Meltzing had examined 15 patients. They succeeded in visualising the vessels of the gastric mucosa in two instances and in another case they diagnosed a gastric cancer. Nevertheless, the authors had to admit that they had many failures and the method was soon abandoned.

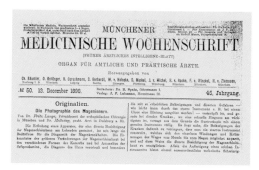

Fig. 7. The Lange and Meltzing gastrocamera. Title page of their original article (1898).

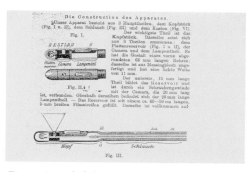

Fig. 8. Detailed drawing of the gastrocamera. At the distal end the lamp is clearly seen, as well as the microfilm and the window of the photographic camera.

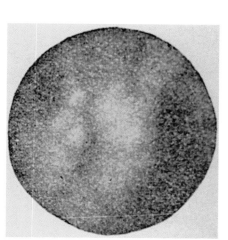

Fig. 9. Enlarged photograph from Lange and Meltzing's paper. The quality of the images was rather poor.

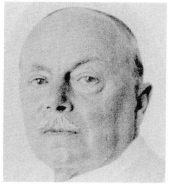

Figs. 10. Fritz Lange, one of the inventors of the gastrocamera. He became a respected professor of orthopaedic surgery at Munich University (copyright unknown).

THE "GASTROPHOTOR": HEILPERN, PORGES AND BACK

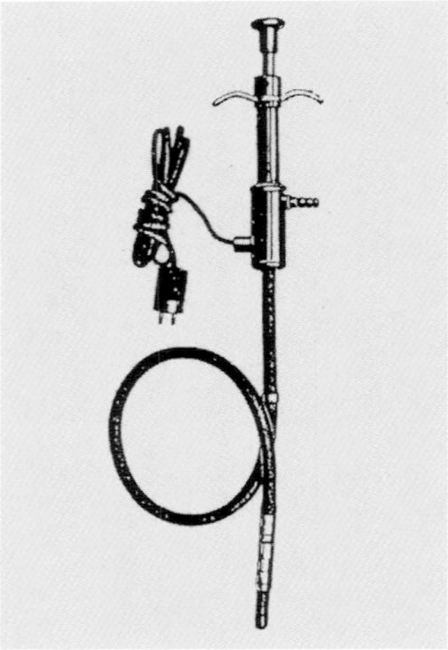

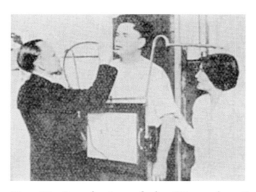

Fig. 11. A general view of Heilpern, Porges and Back's gastrocamera which they named "Gastrophotor".

The endeavours of Lange, Meltzing and Kelling had no immediate followers. A patent for a gastrocamera was apparently awarded to a Dr. Von Schrijver, but according to comments made later by Heilpern, this device was neither used nor written about. Thirty years later, two Viennese physicians, Professor Otto Porges and his associate Heilpern, helped by an engineer, Mr. G. Back, presented their gastrocamera model at the meeting of the German Society for Digestive Diseases ("Deutsche Gesellschaft für Verdauungskrankheiten") in Berlin (18 October 1929). The next year they published a detailed account of their experiences[25] *(Figs. 11, 12, 13, 14)*.

The instrument they designed essentially consisted of a small metal tube, 12.5 mm in diameter and 8 cm in length, fitted at the end of a soft tube. The cylinder contained two square cameras, one on top of the other. Each one was 4.75 cm long and was provided with 16 miniature windows distributed in two superimposed rows with shutters instead of lenses. The openings were paired to provide stereoscopic vision and oriented in all directions, with a clearance angle of 90 degrees. Thus the operator could obtain four pictures simultaneously with each take, or two stereoscopic pictures. Illumination between the two cameras was provided by a tungsten lamp protected by a thick glass window. The instrument could take 16 pictures (8 stereoscopic views).

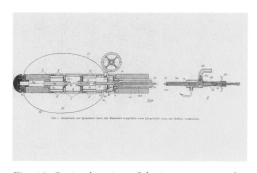

Fig. 12. Introduction of the "Gastrophotor" under fluoroscopic control (collection of Dr. J. Vilardell).

The camera was introduced on a seated patient and the stomach was previously emptied with an Ewald tube. The operator handled the wires which opened the shutters of the windows and a

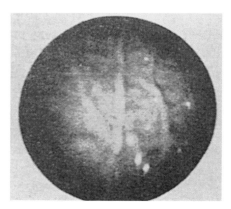

Fig. 13. Sagittal section of the instrument, rather similar to the original Lange and Meltzing's gastrocamera

Fig. 14. Enlarged black and white photograph of the gastric mucosa taken with the "Gastrophotor". Prominent gastric folds are well seen (ref. 26).

balloon provided enough air to distend a fine rubber sheath which protected the instrument and allowed space to take the pictures on a distended stomach. Endeavours were made to introduce the tip of the instrument near the pylorus under fluoroscopic control. A transformer was used to increase the voltage and to provide the necessary power for illumination. On pushing a button, the tungsten filament of the lamp fused each time, providing a very brilliant light (equivalent to 15000 bougies) for 1/100 second.

The black and white photographs had stereoscopic relief and once developed, they were enlarged and read. The gastrocamera achieved some degree of popularity but was abandonded when the Schindler-Wolf gastroscope appeared on the market. Heilpern and Porges[26] published an atlas of stomach photographs in 1936. The gastrocamera was also used in France by C. Garin and P. Bernay from Lyon[7, 21, 22] who published several pictures, most of which the authors themselves considered to be of poor quality. Not withstanding, Garin presented a report on the gastrocamera diagnosis of stomach cancer at the 2nd International Congress of Gastroenterology (Paris 1937) (see Chapter 14).

Like Henning[28], Schindler also used the "Gastrophotor", and compared the gastrocamera pictures with the images seen with his gastroscope, concluding that the "gastrophotor" was of little use. In his book on gastroscopy, he[52] reports that he took hundreds of photographs of his housemaid's stomach and saw many falsely abnormal images. Henning also employed the gastrocamera and although he considered the pictures were technically acceptable, he believed the problem was that "one took pictures of something that one had not seen, and that therefore one had to interpret images of something which one had not been able to visualise", resulting in what he called "mythical interpretations"[28].

Around 1940 there was renewed interest in this instrument as Back, the engineer who had originally designed the instrument, had emigrated to the United States and together with a New York firm, was able to market the camera. However, in his 1929 presentation, Porges stated that his instrument had been copied in America from an earlier imperfect prototype and that the name "Gastrophotor" had been used against his will!

Schindler[47] recognised that some American gastroenterologists, such as H. Rafsky[47], successfully used the gastrocamera to document images previously seen by gastroscopy. Using the same instrument, P. W. Ashner and M. M. Berck[1], likewise published photographs of various gastric lesions (peptic ulcers and carcinomas).

However, other endoscopists like Charles Debray[13] later made unfavourable comments on the "gastrophotor", raising criticisms which were to be equally valid for the Japanese gastrocameras —mainly that the instruments could not examine the entire stomach and that the blind examination, taking into account

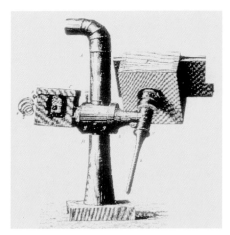

Fig. 15. Theodor Stein's photourethroscope (1874). The "Photoendoskop" was the first attempt to manufacture an instrument for photography under visual control. (courtesy of Prof. H.J.Reuter).

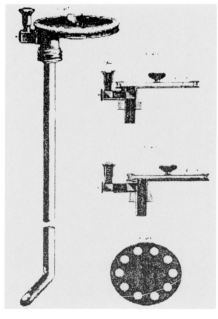

Fig. 16. Nitze's photographic cystoscope made by Hartwig in Berlin (1874). The "Photographierkystoskop" consisted of a glass disk provided with ten round openings which were successively rotated through the objective of the photographic camera. By means of the light provided by an incandescent lamp at the tip of the cystoscope, 10 pictures could be taken on glass and enlarged 10-12 times. Exposure times were around 3/10ths of a second. However, the pictures had to be taken blindly. (courtesy of Prof. H.J.Reuter).

the speed of the exposures, could possibly miss lesions hidden beyond folds of the mucosa, especially if air insufflation had been inadequate. Moreover, developing and enlarging these small photographs required advanced technology which could not be found everywhere.

HENNING'S GASTROCAMERA

In 1931, the firm Georg Wolf made a prototype consisting of four miniature photographic cameras fitted with lenses. Light was provided by two lamps. The instrument was shown to Henning who worked with it for a while but later dismissed it for the same reasons invoked by Debray, that is, his conviction that "one should take pictures only of things that one can see"[44].

PHOTOGRAPHY THROUGH THE ENDOSCOPE

As in other fields related to endoscopy, urologists and otolaryngologists were the first to take pictures through their instruments. In 1858, Czermak from Prague[12] tried for the first time to photograph his own larynx by means of a frontal mirror and a laryngoscope similar to that of Manuel García (see Chapter 5). He succeeded in taking pictures using a lens and a camera with four objectives which could make four snapshots. Coupled in pairs, they could produce a stereoscopic effect.

In 1874, Theodor Stein, a urologist, designed a photo-urethroscope which he called "Photo-endoskop", consisting of a bellow camera screwed to a modified Désormeaux endoscope. He first used gas light and later magnesium light which allowed him to take pictures of the urethra with an automatic camera given the name "Heliopiktor"[55].

In 1874, Nitze[45] also attempted to take pictures. He designed a "Photographierkystoskop" for Hartwig, an instrument maker with whom he was associated. It consisted of a camera and a glass disk and ten pictures 2.8 mm in diameter could be taken and enlarged 10-12 times. The light provided by an incandescent lamp located at the tip of the cystoscope lasted 3/10ths of a second. Joseph Leiter, who had quarrelled with Nitze, soon followed suit with a similar photocystoscope (Figs. 15, 16).

Successive attempts helped in perfecting the photographic techniques. Some time later, in 1929, Karl Otto Ringleb (1875-1946), a pupil of Nitze's who became professor of urology in Berlin, published a magnificent atlas of black and white cystoscopic pictures; several photographs of the bladder mucosa show veins and arteries in great detail *(Figs. 17, 18).*

PHOTOGRAPHY WITH RIGID GASTROSCOPES

Turning to gastroenterology, in 1926, Elsner tried to take pictures through his rigid gastroscope with little success owing to the poor illumination resulting from the absorption of light by the lens system of the instrument[18].

Henning was more successful, and in 1931 he adapted a reflex camera to the rigid Elsner's gastroscope as modified by Schindler[27]. His camera was able to take six pictures without having to load more film. In his 1935 book on gastroscopy, Henning published a series of black and white photographs of the stomach, some of which provided more than acceptable views of the mucosa. Just before World War Two, in 1938, Henning was able to take photographs in colour with exposure times of 1/2 to 1 second[29] *(Figs. 19, 20, 21, 22, 23).*

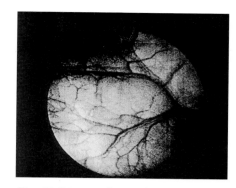

Fig. 17. Picture taken with Ringleb's photo-cystoscope. In 1913, Ringleb and Fromme published an atlas of cystoscopy with detailed black and white pictures of the bladder mucosa (ref.19).

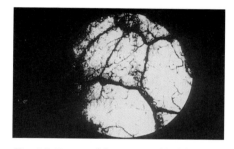

Fig. 18. Image of the urinary bladder taken by Fromme and Ringleb in 1913 with Ringleb's instrument. The blood supply of the mucosa is clearly seen (ref.19).

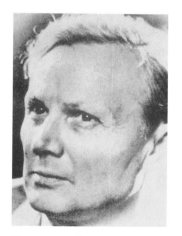

Fig. 19. Norbert Henning, one of the most creative gastroenterologists of his time. He contributed enormously, first in Leipzig and later in Erlangen, to the progress of digestive endoscopy (collection of Dr. J.Vilardell).

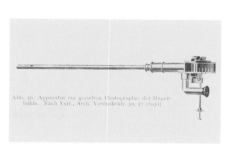

Fig. 20. Henning's photographic instrument adapted to a modified Elsner's rigid gastroscope, (1931). (ref.28).

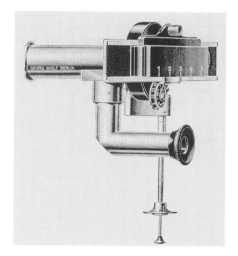

Fig. 21. A detailed view of the photographic camera with the film roll introduced. (ref.28).

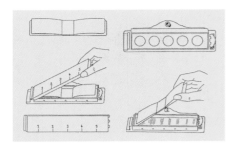

Fig. 22. Loading the film roll in Henning's photogastroscope (ref.28).

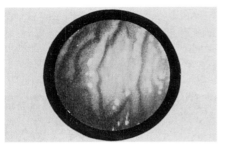

Fig. 23. Detail of a black and white picture taken by Henning showing several irregular longitudinal gastric folds. (ref.28).

PHOTOGRAPHY WITH SEMI-FLEXIBLE GASTROSCOPES

As Charles Debray had already pointed out, the advent of the Schindler-Wolf gastroscope, which included more than fifty lenses, made photography even more difficult. This was because the optical system absorbed so much light that sufficient exposure time was practically impossible even for black and white films. Henning tried to adapt his reflex camera to semiflexible gastroscopes, with poor results[27]. In 1937, Moutier in Paris also tried to take pictures with the Schindler instrument, using a camera designed by an engineering friend of his, a Mr. Kitroser[40]. He used black and white films with exposure times as long as 5 seconds. The best images were enlarged and then coloured, as Henning had done earlier, but again results were mediocre.

In a popular American science journal a few years later –in 1940– W. Hull[30] showed that good black and white pictures could be taken with the Schindler-Wolf gastroscope in conjunction with a Leica and the Carl Zeiss Micro-ibso adapter. The first colour pictures with this instrument were taken by Harry Segal and his associates[53]. Segal managed to increase the voltage of the light source by means of a 25 volt incandescent lamp which at the time of the exposure could reach a brightness of 80 volts. A synchronous mechanism provided both the increase in the voltage and the film exposure. Segal used 35 mm Kodachrome film for artificial light and exposure times of 1/2 second. The diameter of the pictures was 6 mm. His instrument consisted of a vertical periscope for the endoscopic examination, an adapter between the camera and the eyepiece of the endoscope, a solenoid for the diaphragm of the objective, a prism with its solenoid and a stand. Other endoscopists followed him[6] *(Figs. 24, 25, 26).*

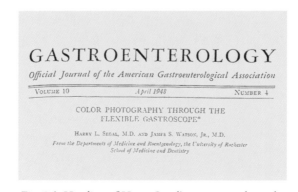

Fig. 24. Heading of Harry Segal's paper on colour photography through Schindler's semi-flexible gastroscope (1948).

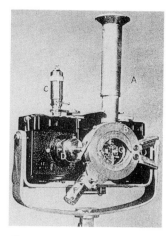

Fig. 25. Prototype of photographic camera used by Harry Segal (from ref.53). (by permission from the A.G.A. and Elsevier).

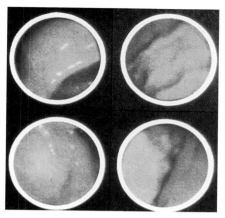

Fig. 26. Colour photographs taken with Segal's instrument. Kodachrome film for artificial light, exposures of 1/2 second. (by permission from the A.G.A. and Elsevier).

In Paris, Debray[13] used a photographic device similar to Segal's but he was not able to take pictures of the same quality. The problems were always the same: poor light and exposure times that were too long for photographing a mobile organ like the stomach. However, in 1955 Robert Nelson[42] was taking colour pictures of good quality and routinely documenting his findings. He used the Eder-Chamberlin gastroscope which had a shorter flexible segment and therefore fewer lenses. It also had a movable distal segment with which the focal distance between the objective and the gastric wall could be better ajusted, thus providing better focused pictures. The camera was a Leica, without an objective, that was screwed to a double prism periscope made by Leitz. But in contrast with Segal's instrument, its ocular piece was on the same plane as that of the gastroscope. A special 25 volt lamp which could reach 60 volts by manipulating a rheostat provided sufficient light. The film which Nelson used was mainly Ektachrome with exposure times of 1/2 second. Not only did Nelson get good pictures with this instrument but he was also able to follow and document the peristaltic movements of the gastric antrum through a series of black and white stills and movies with exposure times of 1/4 second[43] (Fig. 27).

GASTROPHOTOGRAPHY WITH AN ELECTRONIC FLASH

In 1956, Debray and Housset[13] presented a series of colour photographs made with an intragastric electronic flash set at the tip of the gastroscope. Following their directions, the instrument was designed by Grammont, an engineer, and manufactured by the firm O.P.L. (Optique Levallois-Perret) (Figs. 28, 29, 30).

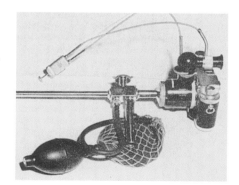

Fig. 27. Nelson's photographic camera (1955). A Leica camera is screwed on a double prism Leitz periscope. By means of a rheostat, the lamp could reach 60 volts. Exposure times were similar to those of Segal's (1/2 second). (from ref.42). (by permission from the A.G.A. and Elsevier).

135

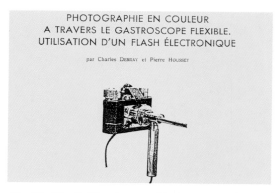

Fig. 28. The O.P.L. photographic instrument designed by Charles Debray and Pierre Housset for colour pictures using an electronic flash. (ref.13).

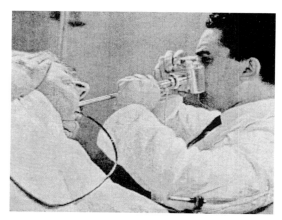

Fig. 29. Pierre Housset taking pictures with his gastroscope (author's collection).

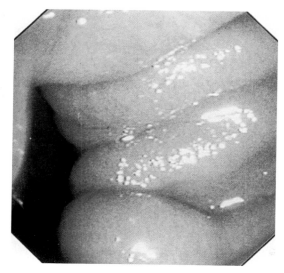

Fig. 30. Anastomotic gastritis. Coloured photograph taken with the O.P.L. electronic flash camera (author's collection).

The instrument consisted of three parts:

1) A "Gastroflex" gastroscope, which was an improved version of Schindler's instrument, of smaller diameter and more flexible. It had two protected wires, one for connecting the incandescent lamp used for observation, and the other coupled to a flash lamp. The distal lamp socket had two holes, one for the observation lamp and another one for the miniflash lamp. Both were covered with plexiglas.

2) A reflex camera screwed to the gastroscope which replaced the eyepiece. The small size allowed the use of commercial Kodachrome "daylight" films. The film roll advanced 20 mm each time and about 30 pictures 6.5 mm in diameter could be taken. These were later projected on a screen by means of a standard slide projector. The view-finder could be focused to suit the operator's vision. The flash light lasted 1/1000 second and was synchronised with the shutter opening by means of a rotating mirror.

3) An electrical source which provided a 180 volt current for the flash lamp during the exposure as well as 30 volts for the observation lamp.

This sketchy description should suffice to realise the technical complexity of the instrument and the possible dangers of its use. In its day, the O.P.L. photogastroscope represented an important advance in endoscopic technology and provided images which were often of great quality. A similar flash model was employed by Fourès and Caroli for their laparoscope (see Chapter 13.).

THE JAPANESE GASTROCAMERA

Around 1950, blind intragastric photography acquired a new perspective thanks to the ingenuity of a Japanese team comprising Drs Uji and Hayashida[37] and the Olympus engineers, M. Fukami and M. Sugiura[33]. They developed a new gastrocamera which consisted of a miniature camera attached to a flexible tube and connected to a control unit. The distal camera had a wide angle lens, a flash lamp, a film roll and openings for air insufflation to keep the gastric walls distended and away from the camera objective. Under the camera but above the lens of the objective, there was a powerful lamp. A cleaning spray used before the examination prevented soiling of the lens. The tube was made of a flexible metal coil covered with a vinyl sheath which contained a wire for handling the camera and advancing the roll of film. The camera allowed 32 pictures to be taken and the film was 5 mm in diameter *(Figs. 31, 32, 33, 34, 35)*.

The technique was quite simple, not very different from that employed earlier with the "gastrophotor"; after air insufflation, the fasted patient was examined by introducing the tube as near to the pylorus as possible. As in diaphanoscopy, the position of the camera could be assessed in a darkened room by the glow of the lamp inside the abdomen (see Chapter 1). Once

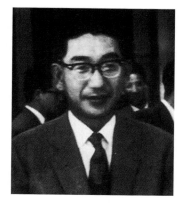

Fig. 31. Dr. T. Uji of the Surgical Department of Tokyo University Branch Hospital. He designed the first gastrocamera together with engineers from Olympus (courtesy of Olympus Inc.).

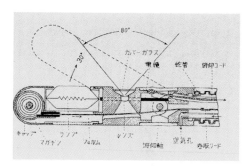

Fig. 32. First gastrocamera prototype, Olympus GT-I (courtesy of Olympus Inc.).

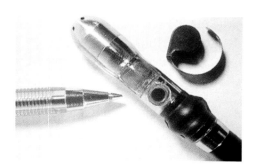

Fig. 33. The distal end of the gastrocamera (alongside a pencil to compare sizes). (courtesy of Olympus Inc.)

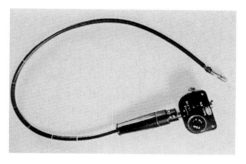

Fig. 34. Outline of the gastrocamera according to one of its pioneers, Prof. Sadataka Tasaka (1st World Congress of Endoscopy, Tokyo, 1966).

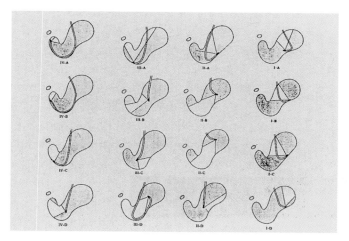

Fig. 35. Visual field of the gastrocamera in various positions (composite picture made from several separate drawings from the Atlas of Drs Ashizawa and Kidokoro (1970).

the camera was judged to be as far down as possible, the operator started taking photographs. The camera was then slowly withdrawn and by bending the distal tip and rotating the instrument, an almost complete view of the gastric walls was obtained.

Around 1956, new prototypes of gastrocameras were marketed such as the type III. This included a tip which could be moved in opposite directions as well as an improved flash mechanism. The cooperation of Olympus engineers, in particular M. Fukami, played an essential role in the ensuing progress. In 1960, another model (GTV) was manufactured. This one was thinner (8.5 mm in diameter) and more flexible[33, 57]. Magnificent pictures were taken with the GTV instrument[2]. Another gastrocamera especially adapted to ultraviolet light became fairly popular in Japan, as U.V. light allowed a more detailed inspection of the gastric mucosa[31].

The gastrocamera was an immediate success in Japan where large campaigns for the early detection of gastric cancer had been organised. In 1959, a gastrocamera club had 500 members[20]. In the United States, where it was divulged by John Morrissey at the University of Wisconsin[38], the gastrocamera was used fairly frequently. It also had its fans in Europe, especially in Germany. The greatest problem was the developing of the colour films which until 1966 had to be processed in Japan. When a workshop and a photography laboratory opened a short time later in Hamburg, films could be developed and Olympus gastroscopes repaired. In 1966, Morrissey[38] reckoned that there were some 10,000 gastrocameras in use in Japan, with the capacity of annually examining more than half a million people. More than 3,000 hospitals were using the gastrocamera[57]. The technique was practically devoid of risk and Oshima[46], one of its leading champions, published the results of a survey based on the examination of 81,731 patients, with only 8 accidents (0.009 percent) —none of which were fatal.

Gastrocamera examinations were included in large Japanese programmes for the detection of gastric cancer; they were performed by nurses but the pictures were analyzed by physicians[33]. In Europe, during the years when the gastrocamera examination reached its peak (1970-1971), about 20,000 photography cartridges were developed each year in Hamburg[29]. In Barcelona, our own experience with the gastrocamera was rather unsatisfactory as the films sent off to be

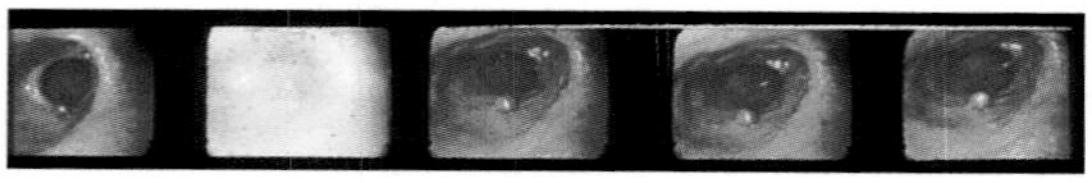

Fig. 36. Gastrocamera photographs taken by Dr. J. Segura at Hospital de Sant Pau in Barcelona around 1968. A small benign-looking polyp in the gastric antrum is readily identified.

developed in Hamburg were often returned 5-6 days later, by which time a clinical decision had already been made by other means, particularly through fibrescopy which was progressing very quickly at that moment *(Figs. 36)*.

The major objection to the gastrocamera had been stated by Schindler and Henning many years earlier concerning the

138

"gastrophotor" –that is, the lack of visual control. In spite of the development in 1964 of a gastrocamera attached to a fibrescope, the Olympus model GTF A, the progress of conventional photography with the standard fibrescopes prevented its diffusion outside Japan. After 1975, the use of the gastrocamera began to decline, and in 1983 Olympus ceased manufacturing the instrument[33] *(Figs. 37, 38)*.

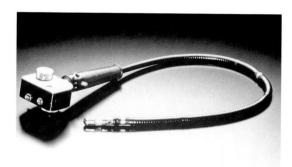

Fig. 37. Gastrocamera with fibrescope designed by Olympus in 1964 (courtesy of Olympus Inc.).

The gastrocamera provided enormous help in mass surveys for the early detection of gastric cancer in asymptomatic individuals in Japan. Its usefulness for making a diagnosis in patients with gastric symptoms was seldom appreciated in the West because of the progress of the biopsy and cytology techniques that were already available.

CINEGASTROSCOPY

Henry Colcher[9], a Belgian physician who had to flee the German occupation of his country, and who worked at New York's Columbia University in the gastroenterology service run by Dr. Charles Flood, designed a device for endoscopic cinematography using an external cold light transmitted to the tip of the gastroscope *(Figs. 39, 40)*.

The films were loaded in a 8 mm. reflex camera (Camex) providing 8 exposures per second. The system could be adapted to Schindler's semi-flexible gastroscope as well as to the fibrescope and for the first time provided films of the stomach in movement which were of excellent quality.

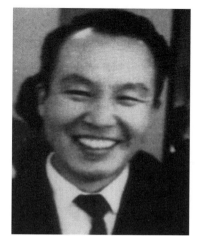

Fig. 38. M. Fukami, an Olympus engineer, who decisively contributed to the development of the gastrocamera (courtesy Olympus Inc.).

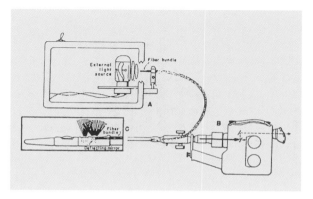

Fig. 40. Benedict's gastroscope used by Henry Colcher for cinegastroscopy (courtesy of the late Henry Colcher)

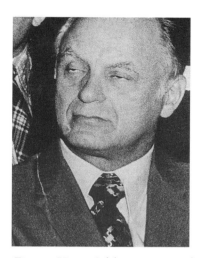

Fig. 39. Henry Colcher, promoter of cinegastroscopy in the United States (authors' collection).

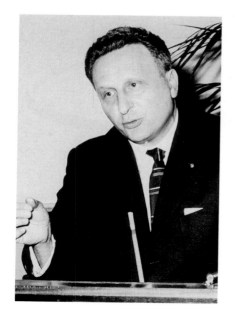

Fig. 41. Sacha Segal from Reims, pioneer of endoscopic cinematography with the gastroscope as well as with the laparoscope (courtesy of Dr. Alain Segal).

Colcher had made his first attempts to cinegastroscopy in 1959, using Benedict's semi-flexible gastroscope, introducing a fibre bundle 2 mm in diameter into the biopsy channel of the instrument to carry the light provided by an 750 Watt outside lamp. A similar arrangement was adopted by the firm Storz for lighting its gastroscope[10]. Colcher also used a potent internal lamp which was switched off intermittently to avoid overheating. His favourite cameras were the 8 mm and the 16 mm French Beaulieu, particularly the Beaulieu super 8, and the preferred film was Ektachrome[11].

Sacha Segal, a Frenchman from Reims[14, 54], was also a pioneer of cinegastroscopy. He recommended holding the gastroscope firmly and rotating it along the axis of the camera to attain a focal distance of 50 mm whereby the entire 16 mm roll of film could be used. He also employed the Beaulieu camera whose advantage was that it included a diaphragm-mirror which allowed the transmission of light. By means of a screen with a scale of the same diameter as that of the endoscopic image as seen through a 50 mm lens, the endoscopic examination and the filming could be performed simultaneously. Once calibrated, a photoelectric cell, synchronised with the speed of the film, determined the amount of light the film would receive. Other attempts at cine-endoscopy were made in the United States by Belber using a fibreendoscope[4], and in Venezuela by Valencia-Parparcén and Beker[58] (Figs. 41, 42, 43, 44).

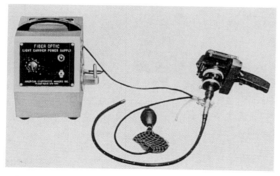

Fig. 42. The A.C.M.I. LoPresti oesophagoscope with an attached photographic camera (courtesy of A.C.M.I.)

Throughout the decade 1970-1980, Colcher, Segal and other gastroenterologists managed to present very good endoscopy films at many international meetings until the emergence of video-endoscopy put an end to these exhibitions.

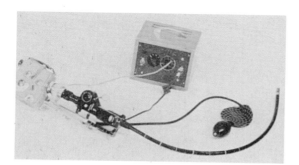

Fig. 43. Olympus GTF endoscope to which a Camex movie camera has been adapted.(courtesy of the late Henry Colcher).

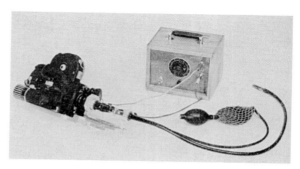

Fig. 44. A.C.M.I. endoscope to which an Arriflex camera for cinematography has been adapted (courtesy of the late Henry Colcher).

ENDOSCOPY AND TELEVISION

In 1963, an exhibition of black and white televised endoscopy took place at a meeting of the American Society of Gastrointestinal Endoscopy[48]. There had been some previous examples: in 1960, Dubois de Montreynaud and Bruneau[16] had televised bronchoscopies and Debray and his associates had performed a laparoscopy on a dog which was televised in colour. Other endoscopists, such as Berci[5] in the United States, also performed televised gastroscopies. At the World Congress of Endoscopy (Tokyo 1966), Adolf Wiebenga from Amsterdam[59] presented his experience with televised colonoscopy. At the Second World Congress (Rome 1970), examples of television endoscopy were presented by the Americans Rider and Puletti[49] and by the Japanese Suzuki[56] *(Fig. 45)*.

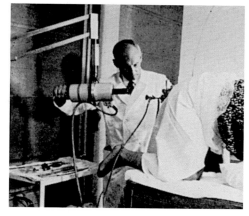

Fig. 45. First attempt to televise a colonoscopic examination by Adolf Wiebenga (Amsterdam 1966) (ref.59).

PHOTOGRAPHY THROUGH THE FIBRESCOPE *(Fig. 46)*

With the advent of fibrescopy, all the techniques which had been used with semi-flexible optical instruments were applicable to the fibre endoscopes[32]. Starting with his first examinations, Hirschowitz used a reflex photographic camera for a great many years (Chapter 6). At the First World Congress of Endoscopy (Tokyo 1966), several reports on photography through the fibrescope were presented. McCray and Winawer[36] from New York took pictures of the oesophagus with a Nikon F camera which allowed two exposures per second. They used high speed Ektachrome 125 ASA. In 1966, the Japanese firm Machida still manufactured telescopic rigid oesophagoscopes for the extraction of foreign bodies. These devices used cold light and photographs

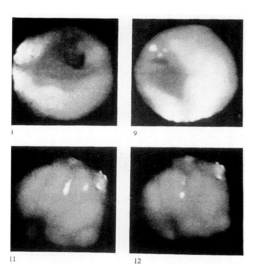

Fig. 46. First pictures of the stomach taken with a reflex camera by Basil Hirschowitz (courtesy of Prof. Basil Hirschowitz).

and films of good quality could be taken. On the other hand, Olympus had already marketed gastroscopes which included a camera and a distal opening for suction and insufflation. Henry Colcher[11] took pictures and did some cinegastroscopy using the Eder fibrescope and a Camex camera and also used an adapter with which he could screw the Camex apparatus to a gastrocamera. But in these early times, everybody agreed that the quality of the pictures was better with the semi-flexible instruments than with the fibrescopes[11]. At the previously-mentioned 1966 Tokyo Congress, several participants questioned whether cinematography was really necessary: against cinematography were the high costs involved, as stressed by the Japanese endoscopists during the discussion of Colcher's paper[10]. It goes without saying that videoendoscopy —which allows such easy storage of images— has made any such discussion quite irrelevant.

A NEW REVOLUTION: VIDEO-ENDOSCOPY

In 1983, during the combined annual meeting of the American Gastroenterological Association (A.G.A.) and the American Society of Gastrointestinal Endoscopy (A.S.G.E.) the firm Welch-Allyn, mostly known for manufacturing optical instruments in the fields of otology and ophthalmology, exhibited a new instrument which caused a tremendous impact: the video-endoscope. It looked rather like an ordinary fibrescope except for the objective lens which had been replaced by a small sensor. Only a few millimetres in diameter, this was able to transmit images of excellent definition onto a television screen. The instrument contained a bundle of optical fibres which carried light into the cavity to be examined, but the image was produced by a charge coupled device (CCD) which had been invented in 1966. The CCD, or "chip", revolutionised endoscopy and video instruments rapidly began to replace the usual fibreoptic endoscopes.

BASIC ELEMENTS OF VIDEOTRANSMISSION *(Fig. 47)*

The CCD was invented by Willard S. Boyle and George E. Smith, both engineers working for the Bell Research Laboratories and interested in a way to improve the video-telephone as well as in new types of memory for semiconductors for computers. According to information received through Bell Laboratories, on the 17th October 1969 in just one hour, the two researchers designed the basic structure of the CCD, established the basis for its function, listed its possible applications in the field of imaging and memorising, and invented the term "Charged Couple Device". As of 1981, the CCD began to be applied to fields as diverse as spatial telescopes for their high sensitivity to light, videocameras, high definition television, digital photographic cameras, fax and photocopying machines.

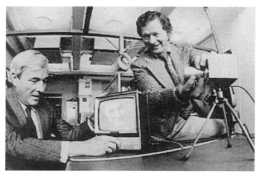

Fig. 47. George Smith and Willard Boyle from the Bell Research Laboratories were awarded the C & C prize for their invention of the CCD (source: the Bell Research Laboratories).

The CCD has immensely improved not only surgical endoscopy techniques[3] but also teaching opportunities, by allowing a great number of individuals to follow diagnostic examinations and operations *(Fig. 48)*.

The CCD can be broadly defined as an image sensor integrated in a circuit included in a small silicone plate. When a light particle (photon) collides with the CCD, a current is generated. Each photon originates an electron and an electronic "void" with a positive charge. The more photons impact on the CCD, the more charges are produced. The device is made in such a way that it includes a large number of photosensitive elements (pixels) which are arranged as a

142

reticulum in a very small area. When the image is focused over the reticulum by means of a lens, each pixel generates electrons in proportion to the number of photons it receives. The integration in the space of the pixels with different electrical charges turns into an electric representation of an image.The electrical charges of the pixels aligned into one row can be transferred to the next row in the CCD by changing the voltage. By moving the charges from one row of pixels to another inside the reticulum, it is possible to eliminate the charges of the chip, a process called coupling. The CCD of an endoscope may contain hundreds of thousands of pixels. To fill a screen with an image, the CCD must have an adequate number of rows and columns of pixels. The CCD measures the intensity of the light (photon) but the colour of the image depends on its wavelength. The CCDs that transmit colour contain three types of pixels (for red, blue and green). Their combination produces the other colours.

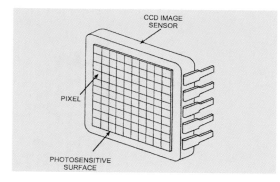

Fig. 48. Drawing of a CCD chip (Coupled Charge Device). On the right side of the chip, five connections for electrical contact. (courtesy of Olympus Inc.).

THE APPLICATION OF THE CCD TO ENDOSCOPY

Since the Welch Allyn presentation in 1983, there has been a continuous flow of innovations. The Japanese instrument makers, Olympus, Fuji and Pentax, soon introduced their own video-endoscopes. It is obvious that this new modality of endoscopy entails a great change in the way that the instruments are employed as they no longer require the direct observation through an eye piece, but only direct monitoring on a screen. This greatly facilitates endoscopic manoeuvres such as endoscopic therapy and the entire field of surgical endoscopy. Many physicians today are therefore familiar with endoscopic images that previously required the use of some kind of ocular teaching attachment. Further significant progress as the result of videoendoscopy has been its application in veterinary medicine[50]. One drawback to date however, has been the difficulty in transporting the entire set of equipment from one place to another, especially for emergency cases when endoscopy must be done "in situ" (Figs. 49, 50, 51).

Other advantages provided by videoendoscopy are the ease with which images can be stored in computers and on CDs, the digitalisation of images, the use of chips of great magnification and the use of spectroscopy. These exciting new openings are in no way restricted to the bounds of a book on history, but already have a firmly established role to play in the future.

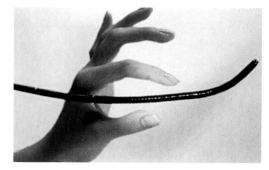

Fig. 49. Prototype of the Olympus CIF XP 160 endoscope, the diameter is only 5.6 mm, thanks to the terminal chip. (courtesy of Olympus Inc.).

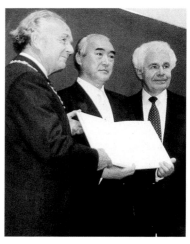

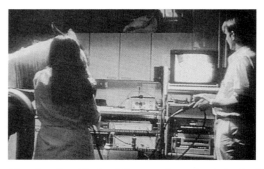

Fig. 51. Dr. K. Riedelberger, from the School of Veterinary Medicine at Vienna University, performing video gastroscopy on a horse (ref.50). (with permission).

Fig. 50. Ichizo Kawahara, Doctor in Engineering and Director of Olympus, receiving an Honorary Degree for his contributions to endoscopy from the Technical University in Munich. The award is given by Professors Meitlinger, President of the University and Dudel, Dean of the Medical Faculty. (OMGE News).

REFERENCES

[1] Aschner P.W., Berck M.M. Clinical experience with gastrophotography. Ann Surg 1930; 91: 875-879.

[2] Ashizawa S., Kidokoro T. Endoscopic color atlas of gastric diseases. Tokyo, Bunkodo Co, 1970.

[3] Barlow D.E. Flexible endoscope technology: the video image endoscope. en Sivak M. Gastroenterologic Endoscopy. Philadelphia, WB Saunders, 2000: 29-49.

[4] Belber J.P. Intraduodenal cinematography in normal and pathologic duodenal bulb. Gastrointest Endosc 1969;15: 160-161.

[5] Berci G. Endoscopy and television. Brit Med J 1962; i: 1610-1613.

[6] Bernstein B.M. Review of intragastric photography. Am J Dig Dis 1937; 4: 102-104.

[7] Bernay P. La gastrophotographie. Paris, Masson, 1931.

[8] Boyce W., Bishop D. Polaroid endophotography. Gastrointest Endosc 1968; 14:186-189.

[9] Colcher H., Katz G.M. External source of light for color cinematography through the gastroscope. Am J Gastroenterol 1961; 35: 518-521.

[10] Colcher H. Cinegastroscopy and still photography of the stomach. Proceedings 1st World Congress of Gastrointestinal Endoscopy. Tokyo 1966:109-114.

[11] Colcher H. Gastrophotography and cinegastroscopy. Progress in Gastroenterology. (GBJ Glass (ed.) Vol.1. New York, Grune & Stratton, 1968: 97-128.

[12] Czermak J.N. Der Kehlkopfspiegel und seine Verwerthung für Physiologie und Medizin, Leipzig, Engelmann, 1863.

[13] Debray Ch., Housset P. Photographie en couleur a travers le gastroscope flexible. Utilisation d'un flash eléctronique. Sem Hôp Paris 1956; 32 (30 juin): 2238-2243.

[14] Debray Ch., Housset P., Segal S., Paolaggi A., Pette F. La photographie et la cinematographie endoscopiques digestives. Etat actuel en France. Sem Hôp Paris 1961: 37: 963-969.

[15] Desormeaux A.J. De l'endoscope et de ses applications au diagnostic et au traitement des affections de l'urèthre et de la vessie, Paris, J.B.Baillière, 1865.

[16] Dubois de Montreynaud J.M.,Bruneau J., Jomain J., Traité pratique de photographie et cinematographie médicales, Vol I Paris, Paul Montel 1960.

[17] Elsner H. Die Gastroskopie. Leipzig, G.Thieme, 1911.

[18] Elsner H. Mein verbessertes Gastroskop. Dtsch Med Wschr 1923; 49: 253-255.

[19] Fromme F., Ringleb O. Lehrbuch der Kystophotographie, Wiesbaden, I.F.Bergmann, 1913.

[20] v.Gaisberg U. Gastrocamera im Kampf gegen das Magenkarzinom. Eröffnung Symposium, Wiener Endoskopie Museum, Wien, Literas Universitätsverlag, 1997: 124-136.

[21] Garin C., Bernay P. La gastrophotographie. Lyon Médical 1939; 151: 753-755.

[22] Garin C., Bernay P. La gastrophotographie. premiers résultats. Arch Mal Appar Digest 1931; 21: 558-562.

[23] Goyena J.R., Islengh J.P., Hofmamm H. Gastrophotography. General information concerning endogastric photography and its technique. Rev Gastroenterol 1936; 3: 158-175.

[24] Gurlt E. Biographisches Lexicon der hervorragender Ärzte aller Zeiten und Völker. Berlin - Wien, V.C. 1934.

[25] Heilpern M.J., Porges O. Über die Gastrophotographie, eine neue Untersuchungsmethode. Klin Wschr 1930; 9: 15- 17.

[26] Heilpern M.J., Porges O., Hofmann H. Atlas der Gastrophotographie. Leipzig und Wien, Franz Deuticke, 1936.

[27] Henning N. Eine neue Apparatur zur endoskopischen Photographie der Magenschleimhaut. Arch für Verdauungskrh. 1931; 50: 27-33.

[28] Henning N. Lehrbuch der Gastroskopie, Leipzig, Ambrosius Barth, 1935.

[29] Henning N., Keilhack H. Die gezielte Farbenphotographie in der Magenhöhle. Deutsche Med Wschr 1938, 64: 1392-1393.

[30] Hull W.M. Inside the body. Popular Science (May) 1940.

[31] Kaneko E., Utsumi Y., Yoshitoshi Y. On special photography of gastric mucosa. Proceedings 1st World Congress of Gastrointestinal Endoscopy, Tokyo 1966:191-193.

[32] Kawahara I., Ichikawa H. Flexible endoscope technology. in Sivak M. (ed.) Gastroenterologic Endoscopy. Philadelphia, W.B. Saunders, 2000:16-28.

[33] Kawai K., Niwa H., Fujita R., Shimizu S. The history of endoscopy: the Japanese perspective. en M. Classen, G.N.J, Tytgat, Ch.J. Lightdale. Gastroenterological Endoscopy, Stuttgart, Thieme, 2002.

[34] Kelling G. Sonde zum photographieren Speiseröhre Arch Verdauungskr. 1897; 3: 299-311.

[35] Lange F., Meltzing C.A. Die photographie des Mageninneren. Münch med Wschr 1898; 50: 1585-1588.

[36] McCray R.S., Winawer S.J. Successful still photography with the fiber esophagoscope. Proceedings 1st World Congress of Endoscopy, Tokyo, 1966:1-4.

[37] Modlin I. A brief History of Endoscopy, MultiMed, Milano, 2000.

[38] Morrissey J.F. Gastrointestinal endoscopy: Twenty years of progress. Gastrointest Endosc 1983; 29: 53-56.

[39] Moutier F. Traité de gastroscopie et de pathologie endoscopique de l'estomac. Paris, Masson, 1935.

[40] Moutier F. Presentation de photographies originales de la muqueuse de l'estomac, obtenues avec le gastroscope flexible. Arch Mal Appar Dig 1937; 27: 327.

[41] Nakayama K., Endo M., Kobayashi S., Suzuki S. Differential diagnoses by esophagoscopy on the picture of the esophageal mucus membrane. Proceedings 1st World Congress of Gastrointestinal Endoscopy, Tokyo 1966:12-17.

[42] Nelson R.S. Routine gastroscopic photography. Gastroenterology 1956; 30: 661-668.

[43] Nelson R.S. Movements of the gastric antrum. Gastroenterology 1956; 30: 669-675.

[44] Neumann H.A., Hellwig A. Vom Schwertschlucker zur Glasfiberoptik. Die Geschichte der Gastroskopie. München, Urban & Vogel, 2001.

[45] Nitze M. Zur Photographie der menschlichen Harnröhre. Berlin Med Wschr 1893; 31: 744-745.

[46] Oshima H. Neue Untersuchuingsmethode mit der Gastrokamera in der Magenhöhle. Med Klinik 1965; 60: 1807-1809.

[47] Rafsky H. Intragastric photographs in neutral colors. Rev Gastroenterol 1942; 9: 202-220.

[48] Rider J.A., Hirschowitz B. Clinical session. American Society for Gastrointestinal Endoscopy. San Francisco 29th May, 1963.

[49] Rider J.A., Puletti E.J, Colombini P.N. An evaluation of color television gastroscopy. Proceedings 2nd World Congress of Gastrointestinal Endoscopy, Padova, Piccin, 1972:149-153.

[50] Riedelberger K. Gastroskopie beim Pferd. Meilensteinen der Endoskopie, Wien, Literas Universitätsverlag, 2000: 255-260.

[51] Schindler R. Lehrbuch und Atlas der Gastroskopie. Munich, I.F. Lehmann, 1923.

[52] Schindler R. Gastroscopy. The endoscopic study of gastric pathology. New York, Hafner, 1966.

[53] Segal H.L., Watson J.S. Color photography through the flexible gastroscope. Gastroenterology 1948; 10: 575-584.

[54] Segal S. Filming technique in gastric endoscopy. Advances in gastrointestinal endoscopy. Proceedings 2nd World Congress of Gastrointestinal Endoscopy. Padova, Piccin, 1972: 167-168.

[55] Stein S.T. Das Photoendoskop Berl Klin Wschr 1874; 47: 31-33.

[56] Suzuki H., Joh S., Kusakari K., Watanabe Y. Multiple usage color TV endoscope. Proceedings 2nd World Congress of Gastrointestinal Endoscopy, Padova, Piccin, 1972: 155-156.

[57] Tasaka S. Progress of gastrocamera examination. Proceedings 1st World Congress of Gastrointestinal Endoscopy, Tokyo 1966: 70-77.

[58] Valencia-Parparcén J., Beker S. Fiberscope and endoscopic cine-photography. Proceedings 1st World Congress of Gastrointestinal Endoscopy. Tokyo, 1966: 78-81.

[59] Wiebenga A. Rectosigmoidoscopy: a comparison using colour photography, colour movie film and black and white television, including video-tape recording. Proceedings of the First World Congress of the International Society of Endoscopy, Tokyo, 1966: 387-393.

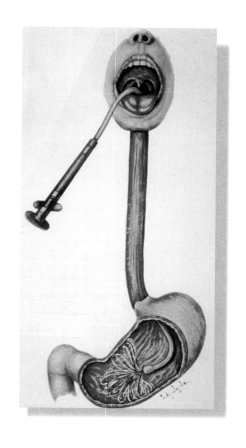

CHAPTER 8

The evolution of ancillary procedures: biopsy and cytology. Endoscopic ultrasonography

PART ONE: BIOPSY AND CYTOLOGY

THE EVOLUTION OF DIAGNOSTIC CYTOLOGY

THE FIRST PHYSICIAN TO MENTION THE POSSIBILITY OF USING A microscopic technique for the study of cells in the diagnosis of digestive cancer was probably Lionel Beale (1828-1906), a famous British pathologist[2]. At the end of the 19th century, several German physicians, among them Boas[4], Reineboth[40] and Rosenbach[41], published instances of cancer of the stomach diagnosed by the finding of small fragments of neoplastic tissue in the fluid of gastric washings. In 1909, Giovanni Marini[32] *(Figs. 1, 2),* who was working at the University Department of the famous internist Augusto Murri in Bologna, was the first to demonstrate isolated cancer cells by examining the gastric contents in patients with carcinoma. Marini used a Faucher tube to wash the stomach and observed the samples which he obtained directly under the microscope. There is no doubt that at least some of the drawings of the cells which illustrate his paper as well as those of a monograph which he later published, show features that are compatible with current cytologic criteria for malignancy. Marini found neoplastic cells in 32 of 37 patients with gastric cancer, he used a micrometric method to measure nucleus-nucleolus relationships and he described several abnormalities which were later confirmed by the criteria developed by Papanicolaou *(Fig. 3).*

In Paris, Loeper and Binet[31] perfected Marini's technique by using several stains. They were apparently able to identify malignant cells in seven instances of carcinoma. They used haematoxylin-eosin or toluidine blue for staining their slides. However, gastric cancer at that time was usually diagnosed by palpation of the tumour or by diaphanoscopy and the great majority of the diagnosed malignancies were large inoperable lesions, which explains the high diagnostic yield of cytology.

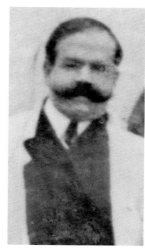

Fig. 1. Giovanni Marini, assistant physician at the University Clinic of Prof. Augusto Murri in Bologna (courtesy of Prof. E.Pisi, Bologna).

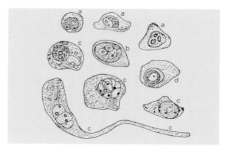

Fig. 2. Cells obtained by Marini, some of them exhibiting current criteria for malignancy (a "tadpole" cell, often present in squamous carcinomas, is clearly identified).

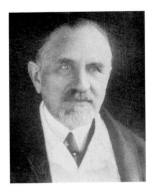

Fig. 3. Maurice Loeper, a gastroenterologist from Paris and one of the first to diagnose gastric cancer by cytological examinations (collection of Dr. Jacinto Vilardell).

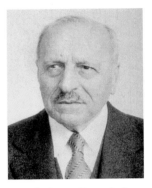

Fig. 4. George Papanicolaou, pioneer of gynaecologic cytodiagnosis. He established the current criteria for malignancy (personal collection).

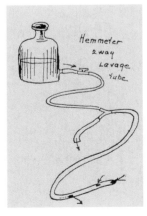

Fig. 5. Hemmeter's gastric tube. Drawing modified from Rehfuss treatise (ref. 39).

Reading these publications today, I found it surprising that in spite of the spectacular advances in radiology, a field of research that was apparently so promising, very little was explored. With endoscopy there has been a revival in cytologic techniques as samples can be easily obtained under direct vision.

From 1940 onwards, renewed interest was seen in cytological diagnosis thanks to the work of George Papanicolaou[38], a gynaecologist *(Fig. 4)* of Greek origin who was working in New York. In 1943 he published his famous monograph on the diagnosis of uterine cancer from cervical smears. Papanicoloau established solid criteria for malignancy which he had painstakingly discovered and which allowed him to find early cancers of the uterine cervix. Papanicolaou's criteria, with some modifications, are still used all over the world for the cytological diagnosis of gynaecological cancer as well as in malignancies of the gastrointestinal tract, the lungs and other organs.

Some American gastroenterologists, in particular Cyrus Rubin, then a research fellow at the University of Chicago under Drs Kirsner and Palmer, followed Papanicolaou's investigations and applied his staining techniques and his criteria for malignancy to the examination of cells obtained from the oesophagus and the stomach using various abrasive and washing techniques.

ABRASIVE CYTOLOGY TECHNIQUES

Hemmeter's tube

At the end of the 19th century, John C. Hemmeter from Baltimore[19], one of the first presidents of the American Gastroenterological Association *(Figs. 5, 6)*, invented a device which he particularly employed for the diagnosis of gastric carcinoma. The tube-like instrument was useful for several purposes: for the biochemical analysis of acid and pepsin in gastric juice which were often reduced or absent in cases of cancer, for the detection of lactic acid, often found in high amounts in advanced carcinoma, as well as for the microscopic examination of gastric contents in search of Oppler-Boas bacilli often present in advanced carcinoma.

Hemmeter's tube had both a distal and a lateral opening, fashioned with rough edges which

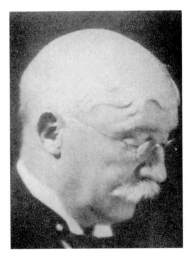

Fig. 6. John C. Hemmeter, one of the first American gastroenterologists. He made many studies on gastric secretion (courtesy of Dr. J. Kirsner, Chicago).

would abrade the gastric wall and collect small fragments of tissue and isolated cells. Hemmeter looked for cytological characteristics of malignancy such as "karyokinetic figures" and both typical and atypical mytotic figures. He used his abrasive method in 48 cases of cancer and although he did not publish detailed statistics, he stressed its diagnostic value, emphasising the minimal risk of his technique unless forced aspiration, which could provoke a haemorrhage, was performed.

Hemmeter also suggested performing radiographic examinations of the stomach, which had been started in 1895 by Roentgen in Germany. Hemmeter used lead acetate diluted in plastic bags which were swallowed by the patient, but the technique was unsuccessful and was rapidly replaced by bismuth suspensions and later by barium salts.

Henning's "Zelltupfsonde"

The first "modern" abrasive instrument was a tube devised by Norbert Henning[20], the so-called "Zelltupfsonde", which consisted of a flexible rubber tube provided with a wire guide, tipped with a small rubber sponge covered by a fine piece of cellophane. The instrument was introduced blindly and the wire was pushed so that the cellophane protection would break in the stomach, avoiding contamination by oesophageal cells. The protruding sponge was then rubbed against the gastric walls for a few minutes and reintroduced into the tube. Once the tube was withdrawn, the sponge was washed and the resulting fluid centrifuged and stained using Papanicolaou's or Giemsa's stains.

Panico's balloon

Also at the beginning of 1950, Panico and Papanicolaou[37] designed an abrasive balloon for oesophago-gastric cytology which had some acceptance in the United States. It consisted of a double-lumen rubber tube ending with a metal olive to which a small latex balloon was attached. The balloon was covered with a *(Fig. 7)* fine knotted silk mesh. Once the tube was introduced in the stomach and its contents aspirated, the balloon was inflated so that it could slowly progress towards the pylorus pushed by the stimulated peristaltic movements. On continuation, the balloon was deflated and the instrument was slowly withdrawn. The silk mesh, to which neoplastic cells would possibly adhere, was then washed in saline solution and the fluid centrifuged and stained according to Papanicolaou's method. Some modifications made by

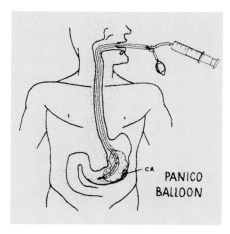

Fig. 7. Panico's Balloon (drawing modified from a brochure on the diagnosis of digestive cancer by the American Cancer Society, 1953).

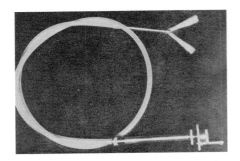

Fig. 8. Ayre's brush. The two brushes were rotated clockwise in the stomach. (Manufacturer's brochure).

Rubin[42] and by Japanese authors did not improve the expected results and the balloon, which was quite uncomfortable for the patient, was abandoned around 1953.

Ayre's and Nieburg's brushes *(Fig. 8)*

In 1953, Ayre[1] introduced another device, the so-called "gastric brush". It consisted of a polyethylene tube which was fitted at its distal end with a metal tip enclosing a double-winged brush. This was projected inside the gastric cavity by means of a tiny spring activated by pushing a wire plunger attached to the rotor handle of the instrument. Once the instrument was fully inserted, it was withdrawn about an inch. The brush was then forced out of the sleeve and gently rotated clockwise while slowly withdrawing the device. On continuation, the rotor handle was pulled into its original position and the tube was withdrawn. The bristles were then smeared onto glass slides. Two to four slides were usually prepared. The brush could also be washed with Ringer's solution and the lavage fluid centrifuged and processed according to the usual cytology techniques.

Herbert Nieburgs[35], a cytologist at New York's Mount Sinai Hospital, devised a similar instrument which was less rigid *(Fig. 9)* and consisted of a bundle of soft nylon threads which were pushed out of the flexible sleeve and inside the stomach by means of a wire to which they were attached. The nylon threads were then brushed blindly against the gastric walls. None of these devices became popular due to the same problem: the blind abrasion without any visual control.

Cabré-Fiol's "mandrel-sound" *(Figs. 10, 11, 12)*

A much more precise and useful instrument for the cytodiagnosis of oesophageal and gastric cancer was the so-called "mandrel-sound" invented by Vicente Cabré-Fiol[6], a gastroenterologist from Barcelona who, while working at the Hospital de Sant Pau in the early fifties, designed a semi-rigid double-lumen tube made of radiopaque plastic material. A metal wire which ended in a soft rubber cap to avoid trauma to the mucosa was introduced in one of the two channels of the tube. A bundle of nylon threads attached below the cap remained inside the tube during the insertion of the device. A second channel was used to aspirate the stomach contents and to wash the stomach after brushing.

The instrument was inserted into the stomach under fluoroscopic monitoring and was pushed as near as possible to the suspicious lesions. The

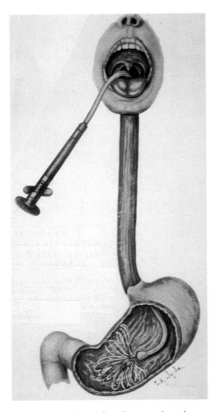

Fig. 9. Nieburgs' brush introduced into the stomach (courtesy of Dr. H. Nieburgs, New York).

wire was then gently pushed, the nylon threads were projected into the gastric lumen and the area was brushed repeatedly (between 10 and 12 times). The wire was pulled and the nylon threads were again encapsulated into the tube. Next, the stomach was washed through the second channel of the tube and the device was withdrawn. The nylon threads were then washed and centrifuged and processed together with the fluid obtained by gastric lavage according to Papanicolaou's technique. The great advantage of Cabré-Fiol's procedure was that abrasion was done under radiologic control, allowing a better sampling of the suspected lesion and the additional use of washings to collect more cytological samples.

Cabré-Fiol's method was extensively used in Barcelona[7, 8] until the advent of fibrescopy and was adopted by other Spanish centres.

Other abrasive systems, mainly used for oesophageal cytology, such as Hershenson's instrument made with a piano wire and a gauze fitted to a sponge[22], or Debray's "Cyto-rape"[11], met with little acceptance. A few years later, endoscopic brushes coupled with Japanese and American fibrescopes were universally used.

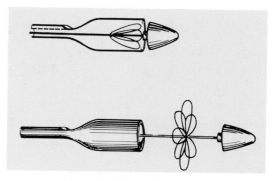

Fig. 10. Cabré-Fiol's "mandrel-sound". The nylon threads are attached to the mandrel which is provided with a distal rubber cap. The instrument was introduced with the nylon threads protected inside the cap at the end of the double lumen tube.

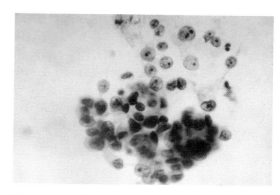

Fig. 11. Malignant cytologic smear obtained with Cabré-Fiol's instrument.

WASHING TECHNIQUES

Disappointed with the results that he obtained with Panico's balloon, Cyrus Rubin[42], then a research fellow at the Gastroenterology Service of Drs Palmer and Kirsner at the University of Chicago, devised a washing method using an isotonic solution injected under pressure to dislodge neoplastic cells from the gastric mucosa, taking advantage of their lesser adherence properties as compared to those of normal epithelial cells. For this purpose, he used a radiopaque tube between 16 and 18 F in size, and after checking its correct position under fluoroscopy, he injected Ringer's or normal physiologic solution, exerting pressure with a large 100 ml syringe. Moving the tube, he was able to sample practically the entire gastric mucosal surface. About 500 ml of fluid was injected. After rotating the patient in different positions, gastric contents were then aspirated *(Fig. 13)*.

For oesophageal diagnosis, lavage with a 50 ml syringe was sufficient and aspiration of the injected solution had to be rapid to avoid regurgitations or pain in instances of malignant strictures. Rubin's group achieved excellent

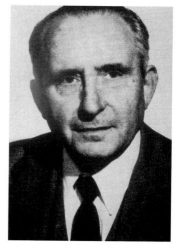

Fig. 12. Vicente Cabré Fiol, gastroenterologist of the Hospital de Sant Pau, a pioneer in abrasive digestive cytology in Spain.

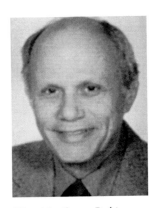

Fig. 13. Cyrus Rubin, one of the leaders of gastroenterologic cytodiagnosis in the United States (World Gastroenterology News).

results with this method which we used at the University of Pennsylvania in the late fifties, although the results were no better than with Cabré-Fiol's technique and were more time-consuming. Later modifications adding chymotrypsin to the washing fluid to increase cellular exfoliation did not bring significant advantages. The greatest problem with the method was the scant number of cells obtained in comparison to abrasion; it required the meticulous microscopic examination of at least six different smears by an expert cytologist. Sometimes many hours were required to obtain a diagnosis in a single case.

The results obtained with different cytologic techniques until the early sixties are presented in Table 1.

TABLE 1. ACCURACY OF NON-ENDOSCOPIC DIAGNOSTIC CYTOLOGY (adapted from reference n.7)

Author	N.Cases	Pos(%)	Method
Seybolt,Papanicolaou (1957)	114	66	abrasive balloon
Raskin et al. (1959)	131	95	washings
Reece et al. (1961)	115	84	washings
Seppala (1961)	151	80.5	washings
Henning et al. (1964)	227	73.5	abrasion (a)
Cabre-Fiol et al. (1968)	316	88.6	abrasion (b)

(a) "Zelltupfsonde"
(b) Mandrel-sound and washings

THE BEGINNINGS OF ENDOSCOPIC CYTOLOGY

Although some oesophagoscopists, such as Chevalier Jackson[23], had made smears of material retrieved during their examinations, we have not found any specific references to oesophageal cytologic diagnosis in the literature as most endoscopists were only taking biopsies.

Since the beginnings of fibrescopy, most instruments were provided with an additional channel for biopsy, through which a brush could be introduced or washings of the suspicious area done, always under visual control. Biopsy forceps were developed at that time and in the same fashion as in the case of non-endoscopic cytology, endoscopists employed lavage as well as abrasive techniques. After 1965, Japanese authors began to gather considerable experience with these methods[26, 30].

Among the authors who performed endoscopic cytology, particular mention should be made to Norbert Henning's followers in Erlangen, in particular

Siegfried Witte[50] who had been using the blind "Zelltupfsonde" (in 1970 he studied 16 patients with gastric cancer and found tumour cells in all of them), as well as the groups led by Cabré-Fiol in Barcelona and by Debray in Paris, both of whom had built up notable cytological experience[49]. (Table n.2).

TABLE 2. ENDOSCOPIC CYTOLOGY OF GASTRIC CANCER
(adapted from reference n.7)

Author and Method	N.Cases	Positive	False P.
Washings			
Kasugai (1974)	512	96.0	2.0
Ishioka (1976)	278	92.8	0.9
Brushings			
Witte (1974)	96	89.6	1.2
Kasugai (1974)	73	87.6	-
Perez Mota (1974)	59	89.8	1.4
Maass (1975)	194	68.0	4.7
Prolla (1977)	110	81.8	0.7
Pilotti (1977)	78	83.3	-
Cabre-Fiol (1978)	515	92.2	1.1

THE DEVELOPMENT OF ENDOSCOPIC GASTRIC BIOPSY

Blind gastric biopsy

By the end of the 19th century, Fenwick[17], Boas[4], Ewald[16] and Einhorn[14] had found small particles of gastric epithelium in the fluid recovered after stomach washings which appeared when forceful aspiration had lodged small pieces of mucosa into the holes of the gastric tube *(Fig. 14)*.

The Wood's and Tomenius instruments.

Around 1949-1950, a new technique for suction gastric biopsy was developed simultaneously in Australia and in Sweden, putting into practice the old observations that small fragments of gastric mucosa would be sucked into the hole of a hollow tube by the negative pressure produced by vigorous aspiration *(Figs. 15, 16, 17)*.

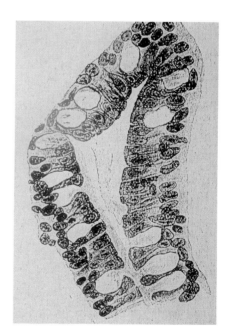

Fig. 14. Fragment of gastric mucosa aspirated with Ewald's tube, showing atrophic gastritis with intestinal metaplasia (from Boas, ref. n.4).

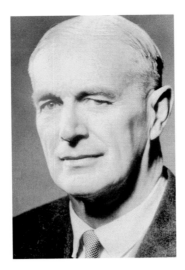

Fig. 15. Ian Wood from Australia, a pioneer of blind gastric biopsy (courtesy of Dr. J. Saint-John, Melbourne).

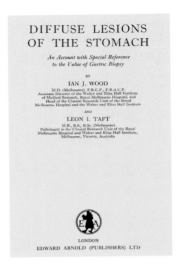

Fig. 16. Ian Wood's book on gastritis based on the study of stomach biopsies obtained with his instrument.

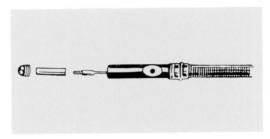

Fig. 17. Wood's biopsy tube. To the left of the picture, the cylindrical knife which is screwed to the mandrel. To the right, the capsule featuring a round lateral hole through which the mucosa is aspirated (ref. 47).

Both Ian Wood[51] and John Tomenius[45] had the idea of using a knife to excise these fragments of mucosa. For this purpose, they used sharp cylindrical blades which would cut the pieces of mucosa sucked into the lateral hole at the distal end of a tube. The diameter of the hole, the amount of negative pressure and the duration of aspiration were the prime factors required to obtain a biopsy large enough to allow histologic study.

The Wood biopsy instrument was 100 cm in length and had marks at 45, 55 and 65 cm. It was introduced down to the 65 mark and the mucosa was aspirated with the patient lying in the left lateral position. After aspiration, the biopsy was obtained by forcefully pulling the wire to which the knife was attached. The tube was rotated 180 degrees, withdrawn 2-4 cm., and the cutting was repeated to obtain a second biopsy. The instrument was then pulled out.

The proximal half of the instrument designed by Tomenius was rigid, while the distal portion was flexible, like Schindler's *(Figs. 18, 19)* gastroscope. The external diameter of the tube was 10 mm. The hole at the distal end could be 1, 1.5 or 2 mm in diameter, according to the size of the biopsy that was required. The circular knife had to be pushed forward to cut the mucosa. Tomenius mainly used the instrument with the 2 mm hole which allowed the aspiration of muscularis mucosae. The tip of the tube was protected by a rubber ball similar to those featured in Henning's gastroscopes. The size of the tube allowed as many as seven mucosal fragments to be taken in a single operation.

Cheli, Brandborg, Debray and Crosby's tubes.

Most prototypes inspired in Wood's and Tomenius' instruments had a similar arrangement: a semi-flexible plastic tube, a metal tip provided with a lateral hole and a circular knife blade attached to a wire or a mandrel which had to be pulled abruptly to allow the cutting blade to excise a piece of mucosa. The Brandborg and Rubin tube[5] used in the United States was provided with a hydraulic pump which allowed the successive withdrawal of several biopsy fragments. Rodolfo Cheli from Genova devised a tube[9] which was used in several Italian centres *(Figs. 20, 21)*.

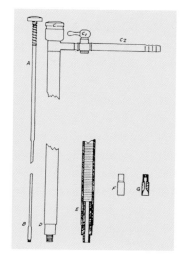

Fig. 18. The Tomenius instrument: A) head of the guide wire with spring. B) terminal end where the blade is attached. F and G; C) tap to control aspiration. D) and E) distal hollow part of the instrument which lodges the aspirated gastric mucosa (redrawn from ref. 45).

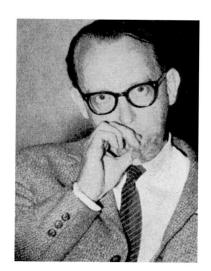

Fig. 19. John Tomenius, gastroenterologist at the Serafimer Hospital in Stockholm, a pioneer of blind gastric biopsy.

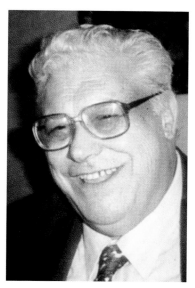

Fig. 20. Rodolfo Cheli, pioneer of blind gastric biopsy in Italy (author's collection).

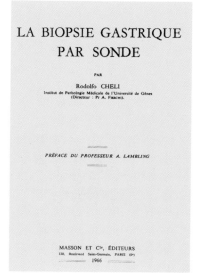

Fig. 21. "La biopsie gastrique par sonde", a book by Rodolfo Cheli which introduced blind gastric biopsy in the European Continent.

157

The Crosby capsule, which was mostly used to biopsy the small bowel, was also employed in the stomach when the obtention of large mucosal fragments was required as in the case of hypertrophic gastric folds[10].

The Henning-Heinkel biopsy tube

The best practical instrument for blind gastric biopsy was designed by Norbert Henning and Klaus Heinkel in Erlangen[21] and was extensively used by Heinkel[18] *(Figs. 22, 23, 24)*.

It consisted of a semi-rigid tube with a ball-shaped rubber tip similar to that of Henning's gastroscopes. At the proximal end, the biopsy knife was controlled by a handle shaped like scissors which activated a wire and a spring coil. This controlled the cutting. The suction pressure was monitored manometrically and usually reached 300 to 400 mg of mercury for 3-4 seconds. The instrument provided good quality specimens of the gastric walls of the gastric body. Heinkel developed a more flexible tube to biopsy the antrum, but the results were unsatisfactory as it was difficult to pull the wire when flexed inside the gastric cavity.

Blind gastric suction biopsy was used mostly for the study of diffuse gastric lesions, such as chronic gastritis which may affect large areas of the stomach mucosa and where great precision in the location of the samples was not needed. The accuracy of blind biopsy for the diagnosis of circumscribed lesions such as carcinoma was low unless the lesion was large.

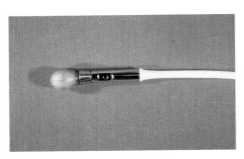

Fig. 22. The Henning-Heinkel gastric biopsy instrument, featuring a distal rubber ball like those employed in Henning's gastroscopes (Hospital de Sant Pau).

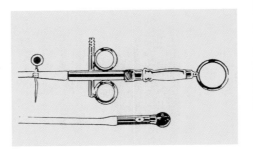

Fig. 23. A view of the handle and the scissor-like mechanism to control the depth of the biopsy (Hospital de Sant Pau).

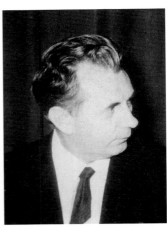

Fig. 24. Klaus Heinkel, an associate of Norbert Henning's, who introduced blind gastric biopsy and pioneered fibrescopy in Germany (author's collection).

Between 1950 and 1960, many studies on gastritis were carried out based on endoscopic appearances but mostly on histological diagnoses made by means of blind biopsy[15, 47, 52]. Gastritis was classified with some variations according to different authors, as superficial, atrophic or gastric atrophy. Only the emergence of fibrescopy, which allowed taking biopsies of the entire gastric surface, demonstrated that blind suction biopsy could provide reliable information on the morphology of the gastric body walls but not on that of the antral mucosa where gastritis was most often present. After 1967-1968, suction biopsy was definitely replaced by endoscopic biopsy under visual control.

ACCIDENTS OF BLIND GASTRIC BIOPSY

Table 3 lists some of the haemorrhagic complications of blind biopsies reviewed from the literature by Klaus Heinkel[18].

TABLE 3. INCIDENCE OF HAEMORRHAGE EN BLIND GASTRIC BIOPSY (adapted from reference n.18)

Author	N.Cases	N. Haemorrhage	percent
Debray et al (1953)	550	0	-
Rubin et al. (1955)	200	2	1.0
Joske et al. (1953)	623	10	1.6
Coghill, Williams (1955)	454	9	2.1
Heinkel, Henning (1965)	8036	2	0.025
Cheli (1966)	2800	4	0.14

ENDOSCOPIC GASTRIC BIOPSY

The pioneer of endoscopic gastric biopsy was undoubtedly Chevalier Jackson[23] who, using his rigid gastroscope, was able to obtain *(Fig. 25)* biopsies of stomach lesions aided by his incomparable technical skill[39]. In 1906, he performed his first endoscopic biopsies and later stated that "in malignant lesions one can obtain samples without any risk in vegetant lesions but in ulcerated suspicious flat lesions it is not justified to biopsy the edges of the lesion even when it looks easy because of the risk implied". In 1935, together with his son[24], he wrote, "to obtain tissue through the hollow gastroscope is easy and we have done it in hundreds of cases without any complications, thus showing that if adequate precautions are taken, there is no danger". Other pioneers were Swalm and Morrison[44] who compared endoscopic aspects with the histological findings obtained with Jackson's open gastroscope.

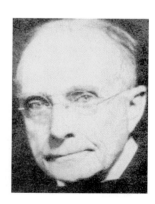

Fig. 25. Chevalier Jackson, the great American endoscopist (courtesy of Dr. Joseph B.Kirsner).

Other attempts to endoscopic gastric biopsy were made by Kenamore[28] and by Benedict[3] using semi-flexible gastroscopes and biopsy forceps inserted into an accessory channel. Results were mediocre. For the study of gastritis, Kenamore used forceps which could be adapted to Schindler's gastroscope and which were manufactured by the firm Phillips-Drucker of St Louis.

Benedict's gastroscope

The "Benedict operating gastroscope"[3], made in 1949 by the firm A.C.M.I., featured a channel through which a biopsy forceps could be inserted. The forceps were pushed outside the instrument by a mechanism similar to that used in cystoscopy to catheterise the urethers. This gastroscope was used mostly in the United States but it never became popular because of its size and its large diameter. It was mainly used only when there was the need to obtain biopsies[34] (Figs. 26, 27).

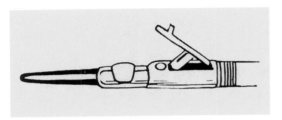

Fig. 26. Benedict's semi-flexible gastroscope, showing the mechanism for taking biopsies under visual control (ref. 47).

Monaghan, an experienced gastroscopist at the University of Pennsylvania who at first was enthusiastic about the instrument, gradually abandoned it feeling that it was too cumbersome and difficult to introduce, but mostly because of the patient's discomfort during the examination. Monaghan stated[34], "I have had the unfortunate experience, after demonstrating biopsy with this method, of losing follow-up patients whom I had used for teaching purposes for years. Others in whom gastroscopy would have been very important in following the progress of their inflammatory disease, have refused further instrumentation".

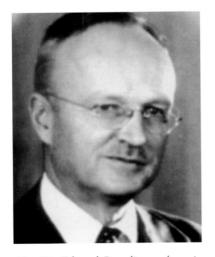

Fig. 27. Edward Benedict, endoscopist and surgeon from Boston (courtesy A.S.G.E.).

SUCTION GASTROSCOPIC BIOPSY

Debray and Housset[12] designed a gastroscope manufactured by O.P.L. in Paris with an additional channel for biopsy and provided with a mechanism not unlike that of the Benedict instrument (Fig. 28). It included a biopsy tube similar to Tomenius' for blind suction biopsy. Working with Avery Jones in London[43], Margot Shiner also adopted a similar tube to perform biopsies through the Hermon-Taylor gastroscope. Tomenius himself modified his biopsy tube so that it could be used with a semi-flexible gastroscope[46] (Fig. 29).

What is quite clear however, is that all these instruments had perforce an increased diameter and patients were reluctant to accept them. Schindler stated in his book that patients violently refused to be examined with Benedict's gastroscope.

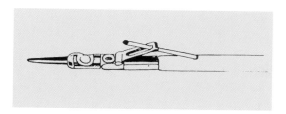

Fig. 28. Tip of the O.P.L. gastroscope used by Debray and Housset, provided with a lever that lifts the aspiration biopsy tube (courtesy of the late P.Housset).

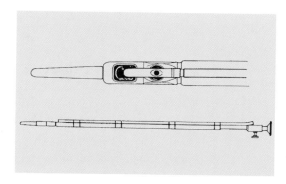

Fig. 29. Margot Shiner's endoscopic suction biopsy instrument fitted at the tip of Hermon-Taylor's gastroscope (courtesy of the late Margot Shiner).

One of the pioneers of biopsy with the semi-flexible gastroscope, Emmanuel Deutsch from Boston[13], performed biopsies under general anaesthesia, but results with these instruments were far from satisfactory. Positive diagnoses of cancer were made in 15 to 60 per cent of cases at the most, as it was difficult to accurately select the site of biopsy with available optical systems[48].

THE FIRST FIBRESCOPIC BIOPSIES

Japanese endoscopists rapidly led the field of endoscopic biopsy and cytology, as gastric cancer had a very high prevalence in Japan. Many endoscopists did biopsies and cytological examinations simultaneously. Among them, special mention should be made to the work of Tatsuzo Kasugai[25, 26, 27] at the Aichi Cancer Centre in Nagoya. In the mid-1960s, using both endoscopic biopsy and lavage cytology under visual control, he made a positive diagnosis in 494 of 512 instances of proven gastric cancer – an impressive result *(Figs. 30, 31)*. From 1970 onwards, the cytological and biopsy diagnosis of gastric malignancies has been greatly developed in all countries[29, 33, 36] (Table n. 4).

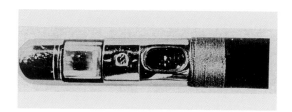

Fig. 30. Tip of the Olympus gastroscope for cytology washings and biopsies (courtesy of Olympus Inc.).

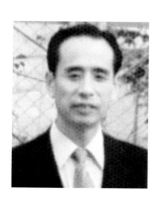

Fig. 31. Tatsuzo Kasugai (courtesy of Dr. Gabriel Nagy, Sydney).

TABLE 4. ACCURACY OF GASTROSCOPIC BIOPSY IN EUROPE
(Survey made in 1970)

Author	Instrument	N.Biopsies	Positive
Mirelli	ACMI	629	55.0
Heinkel	Machida	400	70.0
Banche	Storz	228	65.0
Debray, Housset	Olympus GFB	145	60.0
Sala, Vilardell	Olympus GFB	145	60.0
Schmid	Olympus GFB	450	73.0 (V)
			41.0 (U)
Demling, Ottenjann	Olympus GFB	1200	80.0

(V) proliferating lesions.
(U) ulcerated lesions.

REFERENCES

1 Ayre J.E., Oren B.G. A new rapid method for stomach cancer diagnosis; the gastric brush. Cancer 1953; 6:1177-1181.

2 Beale L.S. The Microscope in Medicine. 2 ed. London, J.A.Churchill, 1858.

3 Benedict E.B. An operating gastroscope. Gastroenterology 1948; 11: 281-283.

4 Boas I. Diagnostik und Therapie der Magenkrankheiten, Leipzig, Georg Thieme, 1896.

5 Brandborg L., Rubin C.E., Quinton W.E.. A multipurpose instrument for suction biopsy of the esophagus, stomach, small bowel and colon. Gastroenterology 1959; 37: 1-16.

6 Cabré-Fiol V. Procedimiento para la obtención de muestras para citología endogástrica. Rev Esp. Enferm Apar Dig. 1953; 12: 186-189.

7 Cabré-Fiol V., Vilardell F. Cytological diagnosis of digestive cancer. Quadriennal Reviews. VI World Congress of Gastroenterology. Madrid 1978, Rev Esp Enferm Apar Dig. (Suppl) 1978: 23-44.

8 Cabré-Fiol V., Oló García R., Vilardell F. Five years of cytologic diagnosis of gastric cancer by "exfoliative biopsy" Proceedings 1st World Congress Gastroenterol, Washington 1958. Baltimore, Williams & Wilkins, 1958:1006-1007.

9 Cheli R. La biopsie gastrique par sonde, Paris, Masson et Cie, 1966.

10 Crosby W.H., Kugler H.W. Intraluminal biopsy of the small intestine. The intestinal biopsy capsule. Am J Dig Dis 1957; 2: 236-241.

11 Debray Ch., Housset P., Martin E., Marche Cl., Garat J.P. Un nouveau procedé de cyto et d'histodiagnostic. L'aspiration par sonde râpe où cyto-râpe. Arch Mal Appar Dig 1967; 56: 988-989.

12 Debray Ch., Housset P., Papchin A, Verdier A. Our experience of the diagnosis of cancer of the stomach by controlled gastrobiopsy under fiberscope. in Advances in Gastrointestinal Endoscopy. Proceedings 3nd. World Congress of Gastrointestinal Endoscopy, Padua, Piccin 1971: 355-354.

13 Deutsch E. Gastroscopy. New Engl J Med 1954; 250: 468-471.

14 Einhorn M. Clinical observations on erosions of the stomach and their treatment. Med Record N.Y. 1894; 45: 780-785.

15 Elster K., Rösch W., Ottenjann R. Evaluation of the expansion of chronic gastritis by endoscopic "stufenbiopsie". in Advances in Gastrointestinal Endoscopy. Proceedings 3nd. World Congress of Gastrointestinal Endoscopy, Padua, Piccin 1971: 787-793.

[16] Ewald C.A. Klinik der Verdauungskrankheiten. Berlin, August Hirshwald, 1893.

[17] Fenwick S. On atrophy of the stomach and the nervous affections of the digestive organs. London, J & A Churchill, 1880.

[18] Heinkel K. Gastric suction biopsy. in Gastroenterology, H.L. Bockus (ed) 3rd edition, vol. I. Philadelphia, W.B. Saunders, 1974:573-578.

[19] Hemmeter J.C. The early diagnosis of cancer of the stomach. Med Rec NY 1899; 56: 577-583.

[20] Henning N., Witte S. Eine neue Methode zur Zytodiagnostik der Magenkrankheiten. Deutsch Med Wschr 1952; 77: 1-4.

[21] Henning N., Heinkel K. Die Saugbiopsie als Untersuchungsmethode in der Magendiagnostik. Münch med Wschr 1955; 97: 832-837.

[22] Hershenson L.M., Lerch V, Hershenson M.A. Esophageal cytology by a gauze sponge smear technique.JAMA 1958; 168: 1871-1875.

[23] Jackson Ch. Gastroscopy. Med Record 1907; 71: 549-555.

[24] Jackson Ch., Jackson C.E. Peroral gastroscopy, including examination of supradiaphragmatic stomach. JAMA 1935; 124: 269-271.

[25] Kasugai T., Kato Yagi M., Yamoka Y. Endoscopic and biopsy diagnosis of gastric sarcoma. in Advances in Gastrointestinal Endoscopy. Proceedings 3rd. World Congress of Gastrointestinal Endoscopy, Padua, Piccin 1971: 239-241.

[26] Kasugai T. Gastric biopsy and cytology under direct vision in the diagnosis of malignant gastric tumor. in Advances in Gastrointestinal Endoscopy. Proceedings 3nd. World Congress of Gastrointestinal Endoscopy, Padua, Piccin 1971: 753-766.

[27] Kasugai T. Gastric biopsy under direct vision by the fibergastroscope. Gastrointest Endosc 1968; 15: 33-39.

[28] Kenamore B. Biopsy forceps for flexible gastroscope. Am J Dig Dis 1940; 7: 539-540.

[29] Kidokoro T., Takezoe K., Soma S. Clinical application of a biopsy fibergastroscope. in Advances in Gastrointestinal Endoscopy. Proceedings 3nd. World Congress of Gastrointestinal Endoscopy, Padua, Piccin 1971: 773-776.

[30] Kobayashi S., Kasugai T., Yamaoka Y., Yoshii Y., Naito Y. Improved technique for gastric cytology utilizing simultaneous lavage and fibergastroscopy. Gastrointest Endosc 1969; 15: 198-200.

[31] Loeper M., Binet E. Cytodiagnostic des affections de l'estomac. Bull Mem Soc Med Hôp Paris 1911; 31: 563-568.

[32] Marini G. Über die Diagnose des Magenkarzinoms auf Grund der cytologischen Untersuchungen des Spühlwassers. Arch Verdauungskrankh 1909; 15: 251-259.

[33] Mekel R.C.P., Van Reinsburg S. Optic fibre oesophagoscopy combined with biopsy for the diagnosis of oesophageal cancer. in Advances in Gastrointestinal Endoscopy. Proceedings 3nd. World Congress of Gastrointestinal Endoscopy, Padua, Piccin 1971: 387-392.

[34] Monaghan J.F., Nast P.R. Gastroscopy. in Gastroenterology H.L.Bockus (ed). 2nd edition. Vol. I. Philadelphia, W.B.Saunders, 1963: 318-328.

[35] Nieburgs H.F. Cytologic procedures. A.M.A. Scientific Exhibits p.259, New York, Grune & Stratton 1955.

[36] Okuda S., Morii T., Inui H., Senda N., Hosoi S. Biopsy and water-jet cytology by color television fiberscope for diagnosis of early gastric cancer. in Advances in Gastrointestinal Endoscopy. Proceedings 2nd. World Congress of Gastrointestinal Endoscopy, Padua, Piccin 1971: 793-800.

[37] Panico F.G., Papanicolaou G.N. Cooper W.A. Abrasive balloon for exfoliation of gastric cancer cells. JAMA 1950; 143:1308-1309.

[38] Papanicolaou G.N. Atlas of Exfoliative Cytology. Cambridge (Mass) Harvard University Press, 1954.

[39] Rehfuss M. The diagnosis and treatment of diseases of the stomach. Philadelphia, W.B. Saunders, 1927.

[40] Reineboth H. Die Diagnose des Magenkarzinoms aus Spühlwasser und Erbrochenen. Deutsch Arch Klin Med 1896; 58: 63-69.

41 Rosenbach O. Über die Anwesenheit von Geschwulst Partikeln in dem durch die Magenpumpe entleertes Mageninhalte bei Karzinoma Ventriculi. Deutsch Med Wschr 1882; 33: 452-454.

42 Rubin C.E., Massey B.W., Kirsner J.B., Palmer W.L. Stonecypher D.D. The clinical value of gastrointestinal cytologic diagnosis. Gastroenterology 1953; 25: 119-138.

43 Shiner M. Duodenal biopsy. Lancet 1956; 1: 17-19.

44 Swalm W.A., Morrison L.M. Gastroscopic and histologic studies of the stomach with gastric and extra-gastric disease during life and at autopsy. Am J Dig Dis 1941; 8: 391-397.

45 Tomenius J. An instrument for gastrobiopsies. Gastroenterology 1950; 15: 498-504.

46 Tomenius J. A new instrument for gastric biopsies under visual control. Gastroenterology 1952; 21: 544-549.

47 Vilardell F. Enfermedades difusas del estómago. Barcelona, ed. Científico-Médica, 1962.

48 Vilardell F. Gastrobiopsy and cytology. Results of a European survey. in Advances in Gastrointestinal Endoscopy. Proceedings 3rd. World Congress of Gastrointestinal Endoscopy, Padua, Piccin 1971: 767-772.

49 Vilardell F. Problems of gastric exfoliative cytology. Digestion 1969; 2: 61-63.

50 Witte S. Endoscopic cytology of the digestive system in Advances in Gastrointestinal Endoscopy. Proceedings 3nd. World Congress of Gastrointestinal Endoscopy, Padua, Piccin 1971: 239-241.

51 Wood I.J., Doig R.K., Motteram R., Hughes A. Gastric biopsy, report of fifty-five biopsies using a new flexible gastric biopsy tube. Lancet 1949; 1: 18-19.

52 Wood I.J., Taft L.I. Diffuse lesions of the stomach. London, Edward Arnold, 1958.

PART TWO:
ENDOSCOPIC ULTRASONOGRAPHY

THE ADVENT OF ENDOSCOPIC ULTRASONOGRAPHY

The emergence of sonography

According to "Dorland's Medical Dictionary", ultrasonography is defined as the visualisation of deep structures of the body by recording the reflections or (echoes of) pulses of ultrasonic waves directed into the tissues. Diagnostic ultrasonography utilises a frequency range of 1 million to 20 million Hertz (cycles per second) or 1 to 20 MHz. Such waves are transmissible only in liquids and solids. Ultrasonography is also called sonography or echography.

Diagnostic ultrasound developed from the Sonar, a system to detect the presence of objects under water by acoustic echo. Interest in this method arose from the danger of icebergs in navigation; it rendered great services in the detection of submarines during World War Two[19].

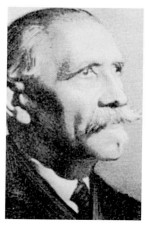

The development of the Sonar owes a great deal to a French physicist, Paul Langevin, who played a leading role in this research. Langevin, also known at that time for his intimate relationship with Marie Curie, had invented the "Hydrophone". This instrument could detect sounds under the water and had proved its usefulness during the First World War for tracking down the noise made by the engines of German submarines. Langevin was later one of the discoverers of ultrasound, which he used to analyse sounds reflected by dense bodies immersed in water. He was soon joined by British and American physicists who, during World War Two, greatly perfected the detecting devices, and the Sonar (Sound Navigation and Ranging:SONAR) was born. Sound waves emitted or reflected by an object are detected by the sonar apparatus and analysed for the information they contain[19] *(Fig. 32)*.

Fig. 32. Paul Langevin (1878-1946), inventor of the "hydrophone", one of the discoverers of ultrasound and pioneer of its use in the detection of solid masses in water (SONAR) (source: Académie des Sciences, Paris).

Ultrasonics in medicine. The early experiences.

In a review on ultrasonics and its scientific application published in Great Britain in 1939, L.Bergmann[1] suggested the possibility of using echograms in the diagnosis of human disease. However, it was only in 1950 that a British surgeon and former military officer, John J. Wild, who had emigrated to the United States, published an epoch-making paper, "The use of ultrasonic pulses for the measurement of biologic tissues and the detection of tissue density changes"[22]. Wild stated that his experiments "demonstrated that it should be possible to detect tumours of the accessible portions of the gastrointestinal tract both by density changes and also, in all probability, by failure of tumour tissue to contract and relax". In 1956, he had produced "echograms" of tissues and presented promising results in the diagnosis of cancer of the breast[23]. With the help of John Reid, an electrical engineer, he had examined 117 cases of breast pathology with his linear real-time B-mode instrument but hinted also at the diagnosis of tumours of the lower large bowel. He then produced a rectal scanner, with a transducer that was inserted rectally, and which could gauge the thickness of the rectal wall and detect prostatic enlargements *(Figs. 33, 34)*.

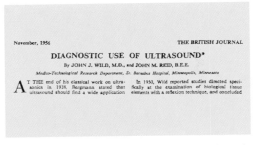

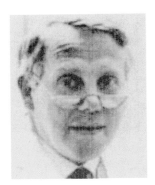

Fig. 33. Heading of Wild's paper in 1956 on the diagnostic use of ultrasound.

Fig. 34. John Julian Wild, pioneer of the use of ultrasound for diagnostic purposes (from ref. 21, copyright unknown).

John Julian Wild[21] was born in England in 1914 and he studied medicine at Cambridge. During World War Two he was staff surgeon in several hospitals in London and in 1944 he joined the Royal Army Medical Corps. He then left for the United States and worked as a fellow in the surgical department of the University of Minnesota where he became interested in measuring bowel wall thickness. For this purpose he conceived the idea of using pulse echo ultrasound generated by a discarded machine employed during the war to train flyers to read radar maps. He coined the term "echography" for the ultrasound examination.

However, he was not the only one to be interested in ultrasonics and the paternity of abdominal ultrasound examinations has also been attributed to Douglass Howry from Denver who, according to a paper that he published in 1952, had been able to obtain images of a gallbladder filled with calculi in 1948[12]. In 1963, his colleague and coworker, Joseph Holmes from Denver, described their early experiences with abdominal sonography[11]. Primitive transducers and water-bath coupling were certainly limiting conditions for the procedure which was very uncomfortable for many patients[12]. Holmes' long-time associate, Howry, has provided an interesting account of their early experiences with ultrasound[13]. The first paper dealing with ultrasonography of the pancreas was published in 1970 by Freimanis of Ohio State University[8].

Ultrasonography took some time before it was readily accepted by clinicians for the diagnosis of abdominal masses. In 1958, Ian Donald, a professor of gynaecology at Glasgow University, using first a Mark IV Kelvin Hughes flaw detector and later a B-type scope, compared the results of ultrasound examination with findings at surgery and concluded that the sonographic technique was still very crude and that although fluid masses (cysts) were readily diagnosed, other lesions were identified with difficulty. He said, "Our clinical judgement should not be influenced by ultrasonic changes"[6].

Nevertheless, slowly but steadily, ultrasonography improved in performance. Patients who had to be immersed in water to facilitate ultrasound transmission by the early instruments were no longer required to do so, and the advent of real-time ultrasound greatly improved matters[7]. Yet in 1984, a prospective study of 500 patients performed in England[3] concluded that for the detection of gallstones both ultrasound and oral cholecystography were equally effective, and suggested that both techniques should be used for a complete gallbladder assessment. However, the advent of grey scale images that were far superior to the early B-mode images and real-time imaging further enhanced the accuracy and possibilities of ultrasound. Four years later, in 1988, a position paper by the American College of Physicians[9] stated that real-time ultrasound was the diagnostic technique of choice for gallbladder disease, although "the oral cholecystogram still had a role in the evaluation of the gallbladder".

Intraluminal ultrasonography

Soon investigators tried to improve the accuracy of ultrasound scanners by placing the instruments as close as possible to the suspicious lesions. Fiberscopes would be the ideal tools to achieve this. However, real-time sector scanning and recording were developed mainly by cardiologists for the assessment of the dynamic activity of the heart. In 1978, a scanning system using a single transducer introduced into the oesophagus was developed at Nagoya University by Hisanaga and co-workers[10]. This team used a small instrument (13mm x 5mm x 21mm in size and a 2.25 to 3.5MHz generator) which provided images of high quality. The safety of the introduction of an US probe into the oesophagus opened the way to the adaptation of similar devices for the study of lesions of the upper digestive tract. In the late 1970s, small diameter probes introduced either singly or coupled to an endoscope, began to be tested in several gastroenterology centres.

Transgastroscopic ultrasonography *(Fig. 35)*

In 1976, transgastroscopic ultrasonography was first attempted by Lutz and Rösch[15] at Erlangen University. The 3 mm diameter probe was manufactured

Transgastroscopic Ultrasonography

H. Lutz, W. Rösch

Department of Internal Medicine, University of Erlangen-Nuremberg

Fig. 35. Heading of the paper on echography through the endoscope by Lutz and Rösch from Erlangen.(1976).

by the Siemens company and could be advanced through the operative channel of a TGF Olympus endoscope. However, the fully flexible probe which operated with an ultrasonic frequency of 4 MHz., provided only an A sonogram and images no better than those already produced in the sixties. The probe allowed the detection of cystic and solid masses and the authors suggested its usefulness for puncturing pancreatic pseudocysts.

Real-time endoscopic ultrasonography

Real-time scanning in endoscopic gastroenterology had to wait until 1980, when it started nearly at the same time in the USA and in Germany. A team from the Mayo Clinic, led by Eugene DiMagno, presented an ultrasonic endoscope[4]: an ACMI side-viewing gastroduodenoscope (model FX-5) was modified by attaching a probe to the end of the instrument so that both optics and ultrasound were oriented on the same side. The resulting rigid tip of the instrument was 13 mm in diameter and 80 mm long. The real-time image was generated by a 10 MHz 64-element linear array. The field of view was 3 cm wide and 4 cm deep. A digital-scan converter provided NTSC standard television format which enabled videotaping. The instrument included an adjustable gray scale. They first tried the instrument in dogs; by 1982, they had examined 22 human subjects[5] *(Figs. 36, 37, 38)*.

Similar attempts were also made in 1980 in Frankfurt by Meinhard Classen and his co-workers[20]. They used an ultrasonic probe incorporated to a side-viewing

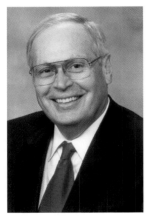

Fig. 36. Eugene DiMagno from the Mayo Clinic, pioneer of ultrasound endoscopy (courtesy Dr.E. DiMagno).

Methods and Devices

ULTRASONIC ENDOSCOPE

EUGENE P. DIMAGNO   JAMES L. BUXTON
PATRICK T. REGAN   ROBERT R. HATTERY
DAVID A. WILSON   JOSE R. SUAREZ
PHILLIP S. GREEN

Gastroenterology Unit and Department of Radiology, Mayo Clinic and Mayo Foundation, Rochester, Minnesota 55901; and Bioengineering Research Center, SRI International, Menlo Park, California 94025

Fig. 37. Heading of the first paper published by DiMagno and associates on ultrasound endoscopy (1980).

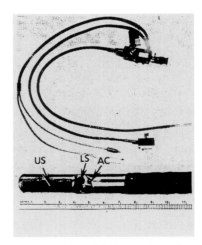

Fig. 38. The modified ACMI FX ultrasound endoscope (1980) (courtesy of Dr. DiMagno).

168

Olympus GFB 3 gastroscope. The 5 MHz frequency allowed for good resolution and the ultrasonic probe was covered by a balloon containing olive-oil as a transmitting medium. Eighteen patients with different biliary and pancreatic conditions were examined. Their investigations were presented at the 11th ASNEMGE Congress of Gastroenterology that took place in Hamburg in 1980[17]. Since then, EUS has been used increasingly and extensively in the staging of gastrointestinal tumours, in laparoscopy, in conjunction with colour Doppler analysis, for the puncture of pancreatic pseudocysts and the detection of choledochal stones and for diagnosis and selected therapy interventions using fine needle punctures[2, 14, 16, 18] *(Figs. 39, 40)*.

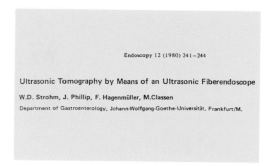

Fig. 39. Heading of the paper published by Meinhard Classen's team on ultrasonic endoscopy using an Olympus instrument (1980).

REFERENCES

[1] Bergmann L. Ultrasonics and their scientific application. London, Bell, 1938.

[2] Chack A, Hawes R.H., Cooper G.S., Hoffman, B.,Catalano M.F., Wong R.C.K. Prospective assessment of the utility of EUS in the evaluation of gallstone pancreatitis. Gastrointest Endosc 1999; 49: 599-604.

[3] De Lacey G., Gaijar B., Twonby B., Levi J., Cox A.G. Should cholecystography or ultrasound be the primary investigation for gallbladder disease? Lancet 1984; 1: 205-207.

[4] DiMagno E.P., Buxton J.L., Regan P.T.,Hattery R.R., Wilson D.A.,Suarez J.T., Green P.S. The ultrasonic endoscope. Lancet 1980; i: 629-631.

[5] DiMagno E.P., Regan P.T., Clain J.E., James E.M., Buxton J.L. Human endoscopic ultrasonography. Gastroenterology 1982; 83: 824-829.

[6] Donald I., MacVicar J., Brown T.G. Investigation of abdominal masses by pulsed ultrasound. Lancet 1958; i: 1188-1195.

[7] Ferrucci J.T. Body ultrasonography. (second of two parts)New Engl J Med 1979; 300: 590-602.

[8] Freimanis A.K., Asher W.M. Development of diagnostic criteria in echographic study of abdominal lesions. Am.J.Roentgenol Radium Ther Nucl Med. 1970; 108: 747-755.

[9] Health and Policy Committee, American College of Physicians. to study the gallbladder. Position paper. Ann Intern Med 1988; 109: 752-754.

[10] Hisanaga K., Hisanaga A. A new real-time scanning system of ultra-wide angle and real-time recording of entire adult cardiac images. Ultrasound Med 1978; 4: 391-402.

[11] Holmes J.H., Howry D.H. Ultrasonic diagnosis of abdominal disease. Am. J.Dig. Dis. 1963; 8: 12-31.

[12] Howry D.H., Bliss W.R. Ultrasonic visualization of soft tissue structures of the body. J Lab & Clin Med 1952; 40: 579-592.

[13] Howry D.H. Brief atlas of diagnostic ultrasound radiologic results. Radiol Clin North Am. 1965; 3: 433-452.

[14] Liu C.L., Lo, C.M., Chan J. K.F., Poon R. T.P. Lam C.M.,Fan S.T. Detection of choledocolithiasis by EUS in acute pancreatitis: a prospective evaluation in 100 consecutive patients. Gastrointest Endosc 2001; 54: 325-330.

[15] Lutz H., Rösch W. Transgastroscopic ultrasonography. Endoscopy 1976; 8: 203-205.

[16] Menzel J., Domschke W Gastrointestinal miniprobe sonography: the current status. Am J Gastroenterol 2000; 95: 605-616.

[17] Rösch T., Classen M. Gastroenterologic endosonography. New York, Thieme, 1992.

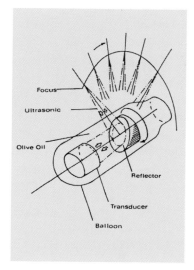

Fig. 40. Drawing of the ultrasound probe used by Classen's group in Frankfurt (courtesy Prof. Meinhard Classen).

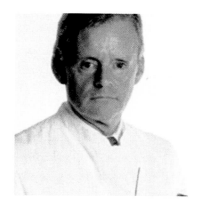

Fig. 41. Prof. Meinhard Classen and his team introduced ultrasonic endoscopy independently, in 1980.

[18] Rösch T., Kassem A.M. Endoscopic ultrasonography in Gastroenterological Endoscopy. M.Classen, G.N.J. Tytgat, Ch.J. Ligthdale (eds) Stuttgart-New York, Thieme, 2002: 199-220.

[19] Seibert J.A. One-hundred years of medical diagnostic imaging technology Health Phys 1995; 69: 695-720.

[20] Strohm W.D., Phillip J., Hagenmüller F., Classen M. Ultrasonic tomography by means of an ultrasonic fiberendoscope. Endoscopy 1980; 12: 241-244.

[21] Ultrasound.net/jjwildbio.html

[22] Wild J.J. The use of ultrasonic pulses for the measurement of biologic tissues and the detection of tissue density changes. Surgery 1950; 27: 183-188.

[23] Wild J.J., Reid J.M. Diagnostic use of ultrasound. Brit J Phys Med. 1956; 19: 248-257.

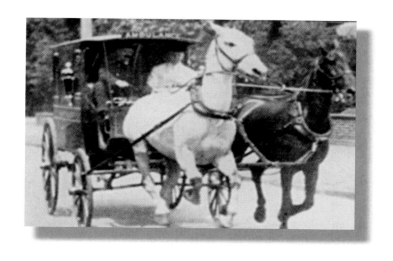

CHAPTER 9

· ·

Endoscopic control of upper gastrointestinal haemorrhage

THE EVOLUTION OF UPPER DIGESTIVE HAEMORRHAGE OVER THE YEARS

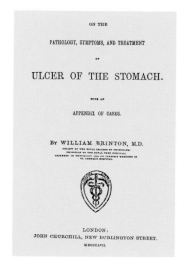

Fig. 1. Front page of the book by William Brinton (1823-1867) on "Ulcer of the Stomach" published in London in 1857.

DIAGNOSIS, PROGNOSIS AND TREATMENT OF UPPER DIGESTIVE bleeding is as worrying a problem for the clinician in the 21st century as it was at the end of the 19th century. In spite of the progress made in diagnosis as well as in therapy, massive haemorrhage is still a cause of high mortality and apparently has not decreased over the years.

As early as 1857, William Brinton considered that haemorrhage was a severe complication of gastric ulcer[5] on the basis of 200 personal cases observed at Saint-Thomas Hospital in London as well as of experiences from other centres. He distinguished between mild bleeding due to "congestion" of the mucosa around the ulcer and severe haemorrhage due to penetration of the ulcer into an artery. The latter was less frequent —only one third of his cases. He assessed the mortality of ulcer haemorrhage as being one death in twenty cases, and found it was four times more frequent in men than in women. The mean age of the patients whom he had treated was 43 years *(Fig. 1)*.

Around 1930, Rivers[73] published a series of 668 patients admitted to the Mayo Clinic for haematemesis; the diagnosis of intrinsic gastric lesion was made in 90 percent of cases. As far back as these days, he called attention to the relationship between haemorrhage and erosive gastritis or duodenitis, entities which were only rarely identified by the surgeon[74].

Another study made at that time by Ernest Bulmer[7] on 526 patients admitted to the Birmingham General Hospital for haematemesis between 1902 and 1926, revealed that bleeding was due to acute ulcers in 218 instances and due to to chronic ulcers in 249; twenty-five patients had oesophageal varices and 7 bled from a gastric cancer. Male predominance was almost twice the number of female patients. Between 1926 and 1931, when the study ended, the ratio had barely changed *(Fig. 2)*.

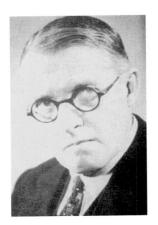

Fig. 2. Ernest Bulmer (1900-1967), Chief of the Medical Service at Birmingham General Hospital and one of the pioneers of gastroscopy in the U.K. Author of a meticulous longitudinal study on the evolution and mortality of upper gastrointestinal haemorrhage in England (courtesy of the British Society of Gastroenterology).

In the first edition of his well-known treatise (1946), Henry L. Bockus[3] recorded a mortality of 10 per cent in massive haemorrhage. F. Avery Jones[37, 38] reviewed 1,764 patients with peptic ulcer and published a global mortality of 7.7 per cent in patients who had had a haemorrhage. Around that time, clinicians began to realise that perhaps 75 per cent of patients suffered only from mild bleeding that required little more than expectant observation[71], a figure not very different from that quoted by Brinton one hundred years earlier! In 1954, Atik[1] recorded a mortality of 42 percent in a series of 296 patients with massive haemorrhage treated either medically or surgically.

Literature reviews show that urgent endoscopy could have made an etiological diagnosis in the great majority of instances of bleeding. However, even with the routine use of endoscopy, little progress was made in reducing the mortality of bleeding patients until the advent of therapeutic endoscopy. Even now mortality due to massive haemorrhage has decreased only slightly as the age of patients admitted to hospital is constantly increasing, and this obviously has an unfavourable effect on the global prognosis[2].

The large discrepancies in the published figures concerning gastrointestinal bleeding mortality illustrate the difficulties in comparing old statistics. Systems used to compile the observations and the methodology for selecting patients admitted to the wards vary greatly. It is obvious that before the emergence of efficient means of transportation many patients with massive haemorrhage died before arrival at the hospital and admissions were merely a reflection of the large numbers of patients who recovered from mild or moderate bleeding. This may explain why Ewald[18], a man with tremendous clinical experience, could state that he had never seen a patient die due to upper gastrointestinal haemorrhage! and that according to Leube[49], mortality due to haemorrhage was only 1.1 per cent. Nevertheless, in 1900 Fenwick recorded the more realistic figure of 3.4 per cent for mortality in massive haemorrhage[20] *(Figs. 3, 4)*.

A review[83] of 1,000 gastroduodenal ulcers treated in our service at Hospital de Sant Pau in 1966 showed that 15.4 percent of patients had a previous history of gastrointestinal bleeding. This figure was not unlike that reported in Paris by Lambling and Bonfils[46] with the same proportion of bleeding gastric ulcers (22 percent). At that time it was stated that the origin of digestive bleeding could be ascertained in only 42 percent of cases and that the clinical course of a bleeding ulcer was unpredictable[29]. Gastroscopy was not mentioned in these reports.

After 1970, the mortality rates for gastric and duodenal ulcer began to decrease in young patients, while they continued to rise in elderly female patients according to data from several Western countries such as Germany,

Great Britain and the United States[9, 39, 40, 58, 59]. Admissions for ulcer haemorrhage have clearly diminished in the last decades at our centre, Hospital de Sant Pau, as in other European centres. Nowadays, upper gastrointestinal endoscopy can provide a diagnosis in the great majority of cases. Rather surprisingly, practically no gastroenterology textbook published prior to 1950 refers to gastroscopy as a diagnostic tool in case of haemorrhage. Although some authors such as Eusterman[17] in 1935, mentioned endoscopy as a technique which might be useful in selected cases, neither Bockus[3] nor Rehfuss[72] considered gastroscopy to be useful and instead employed Einhorn's string test to determine the origin of bleeding, especially when only melaena was detected.

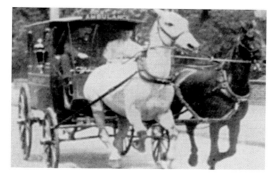

Fig. 3. Ambulance employed at the end of the 19th century in Philadelphia for transportation of patients (original picture at the University of Pennsylvania archives, copyright unknown).

NON-ENDOSCOPIC DIAGNOSIS OF THE ORIGIN OF BLEEDING

In the early 20th century, very few clinicians dared to introduce a tube into the stomach of a bleeding patient in search of blood in the gastric contents[18]. Most physicians thought that intubation was dangerous and preferred to wait.

In his investigations at the Hamburg-Eppendorf hospital[47], Hermann Lenhartz (1854-1910)[21] found a mortality of only 2.1 percent in a series of 146 patients admitted for haemorrhage and treated with gastric lavage and early feeds. Starting in 1935 at Bispebjerg Hospital in Copenhagen, Einar Meulengracht[55] treated 251 bleeding ulcer patients with early feedings and encountered only 3 deaths, showing that the procedure had clear advantages. Other clinicians followed suit. Intubations and gastric lavage became more popular and allowed early feedings; they also opened the way to attempts to introduce endoscopes into the stomach during the bleeding episode. But it was a still a long time before endoscopy was used in patients with haemorrhage without waiting for many days for the bleeding to subside. In any case, gastroenterologists preferred radiological examinations which they considered devoid of danger and which they often performed themselves *(Figs. 5, 6)*.

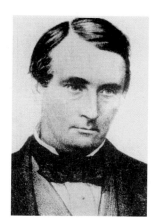

Fig. 4. Samuel Fenwick (1821-1902), consultant physician at the London Hospital, who wrote the first clinical and pathological description of gastric atrophy and related it to pernicious anaemia, and also several studies on gastric ulcer (courtesy of Astra Inc.).

EINHORN'S STRING TEST

Einhorn's string test, which consisted of having the patient swallow a thin silk string about 85 cm in length graded in centimetres and featuring a small weight at its distal end, was mainly used in Philadelphia by Bockus[3] and Rehfuss[72] to

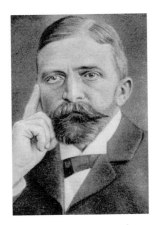

Fig. 5. Hermann Lenhartz (1854-1910). Professor of Medicine and Chief of Medicine at the Hamburg-Eppendorf Hospital, the first to use gastric lavage followed by early feedings in bleeding ulcer patients (collection Dr.Jacinto Vilardell).

localise the site of bleeding in patients with maelena. The string was withdrawn the following day and studied for blood stains and their location. If the blood was found between the 44 and 54 cm marks, it was thought to be caused by a gastric ulcer on the lesser curve of the stomach and when stains were found below 56 cm, the source of the bleeding was considered the duodenum[72]. Einhorn devised this test to diagnose ulcers that were not visible on the x-ray examination as he thought that the ulcer would often leave a trace of blood on the string. The test proved to be unreliable, although it was used at the Graduate Hospital of the University of Pennsylvania at least until 1955 when I saw it performed. It was used in conjunction with radiology amd later replaced by the endoscopic examination *(Fig. 7).*

The intravenous injection of fluorescein, which allowed the blood stain on the string to become fluorescent when there was active bleeding, did not meet the expectations it created[70]. Other techniques based on the same principle, such as the intravenous injection of a radioactive isotope and the subsequent determination of radioactivity in the aspirated gastrointestinal contents or by means of an ingested miniature Geiger counter, also failed in their task[54, 67]. With its many advantages, fibrescopy replaced these sophisticated but unreliable procedures.

GASTROSCOPIC DIAGNOSIS OF ACUTE HAEMORRHAGE.

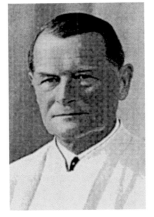

Fig. 6. Einaar Meulengracht (1887-1976). Professor of medicine in Copenhagen, he favoured early feedings in bleeding ulcer patients instead of keeping them on an empty stomach, opening the way to the introduction of tubes and endoscopes in the stomach of these patients (copyright unknown).

Rovsing, Kraft, Herrick: According to Haubrich[28], the first to use an endoscope to determine the cause of a gastric haemorrhage was the Cleveland surgeon F.C.Herrick[32]. In 1911 he suggested introducing a cystoscope he designed himself into the stomach to attempt visualisation of a bleeding lesion through a small gastrotomy performed during surgery. He used a 20 cm long, 18 mm x 12.5 mm wide instrument, provided with a distal lamp, an obturator and a thin adjacent hollow tube for insufflation. With this tool, he succeeded in diagnos-

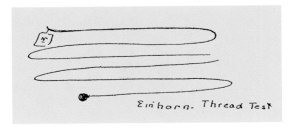

Fig. 7. The Einhorn string, often used by Rehfuss and by Bockus (adapted from ref.72).

ing a small pyloric ulcer in a 22-year-old female who had bled. Recovery was uneventful. However, in an addendum to his paper, Herrick recognised that in a more thorough review of the literature he had found that a similar technique had already been used in Europe. As a matter of fact, three years earlier, Thorkild Rovsing[75], professor of surgery in Copenhagen, had introduced a cystoscope in the stomach of a 50-year-old patient and after insufflation through the drainage channel of the instrument he had been able to visualise the entire gastric cavity, although he did not find any suspicious lesion. Through the German firm Louis and H. Loewenstein, he ordered an "operative gastroscope" with which he and his first assistant Ludwig Kraft examined 24 patients with various gastric lesions. Some time later, Kraft[45] employed this method to examine patients with massive gastric haemorrhage. He published a report on five patients, one of whom died as a result of gastric wall necrosis following burns due to overheating of the endoscope lamp. Both Rovsing and Kraft made a small incision in the stomach wall, previously freed from adhesions, and protected it with a tobacco pouch-type suture. They then proceeded to ligate the bleeding vessel *(Fig. 8: A, B, C) (Fig. 9).*

These attempts to control haemorrhage had no followers until fifty years later when Youmans and his group[89] introduced a cystoscope in the stomach of a patient with a malignant bleeding gastric ulcer and in another with acute multiple ulcers and were able to stop the haemorrhage using monopolar electrocoagulation.

However, most endoscopists remained reluctant to use these instruments in instances of haemorrhage. In a 1950 textbook on peptic ulcer –considered at the time as the definitive treatise on the subject– the authors[35] warn that gastroscopy may induce gastric bleeding. Even later, in 1964, a well-known Hungarian surgeon[43] wrote that in a patient with a debilitating massive haemorrhage " gastroscopy never gives a positive result and is therefore contraindicated". And he certainly was not the only one to think in this way.

Schindler himself[78] wrote that in the immediate period after a haemorrhage "gastroscopy is contraindicated, but it may be useful when the bleeding has been controlled....if the surgeon insists on operating, it will be useful to perform gastroscopy before the intervention to determine the origin of the bleeding and help in the surgical strategy". Around the same epoch, Avery Jones[38] stated that gastroscopy should not be

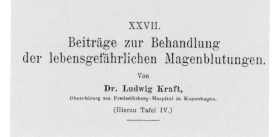

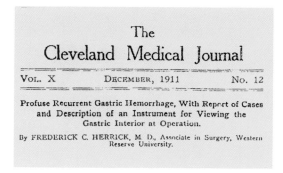

Fig. 8. A: Heading of Rovsing's paper (1908) on pre-operative endoscopy in digestive haemorrhage. B. Heading of Kraft's paper, on the same subject (1910). C. Title of Herrick's paper on surgical endoscopy in gastric haemorrhage, published in 1911.

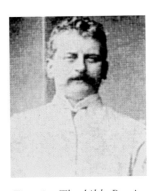

Fig. 9. Thorkild Rovsing (1862-1927), Professor of Surgery in Copenhagen, the first to introduce a cystoscope in the stomach through a gastrotomy to visualise the gastric mucosa. Mostly known for his publications on acute appendicitis (Rovsing's sign) (courtesy of Dr. Aksel Cruse, Aarhus).

considered an alternative to the radiological examination and that if judged necessary, it could be performed before operation in the anaesthesia room. Avery Jones thought at that time that gastroscopy was of little use in massive haemorrhage and that it involved risks. It took him many years to change his opinion. In 1957, Marvin H. Pollard[71], another well-known clinician from Ann Arbor University, also wrote that gastroscopy was of little use in massive bleeding and that it involved a substantial risk. Obviously, all these authors were using the semi-flexible Schindler-type endoscope.

However, in 1937, Norbert Henning[31], a talented endoscopist with enormous experience working in Leipzig, mentioned that on only one single occasion did he induce bleeding in a patient with obstructive jaundice using the rigid gastroscope. Henning insisted that gastroscopy was an important diagnostic tool in massive haemorrhage produced by erosions in which there were often no clinical symptoms.

After 1930, gastroscopy gradually began to be used to examine patients who had experienced a gastrointestinal haemorrhage. Following Felix Hoffman's synthesis of acetyl-salicylic acid and its widespread use, some clinicians started to associate the sudden appearance of bleeding with the ingestion of salicylates. Direct examination of the gastric mucosa with the gastroscope was able to produce the definitive proof of the association *(Figs. 10, 11)*.

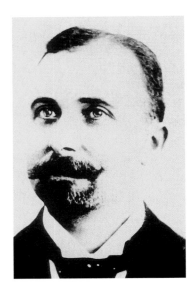

Fig. 10. Felix Hoffman (1868-1946), a German chemist, who was the first to synthesise acetyl-salicilic acid; he took part in the early clinical tests with the drug (courtesy of Bayer Inc.).

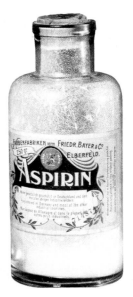

Fig. 11. Aspirin was first marketed in Germany. Nobody could then imagine the important role that the drug would play in the aetiology of gastric bleeding (courtesy of Bayer Inc.).

British clinicians were the first to endoscopically demonstrate the presence of erosions and ulcerations in the stomach of patients who had been taking aspirin. In 1938, Arthur Douthwaite[15] published an experimental study in which he showed the presence of hyperaemia and submucosal haemorrhages in the stomachs of several volunteers who had been administered aspirin (*Fig. 12*).

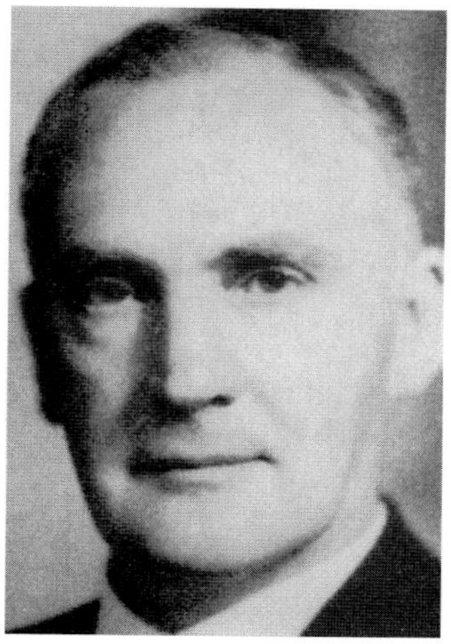

The following example on the value of early gastroscopy in a case of haemorrhage of uncertain origin was published by Sir Arthur Hurst[34]. He described a patient who since the age of 18 was taking aspirin regularly for recurrent headaches. On admission to Guy's Hospital in London after a massive haematemesis, a radiological examination showed no lesions. Once the haemorrhage had subsided, Hurst decided to perform a gastroscopy after having the patient ingest two fragmented tablets of aspirin. Endoscopy showed aspirin particles adhering to the gastric mucosa surrounded by echymotic areas and blood extravasation. According to Hurst, this was the first observation in which gastroscopy conclusively demonstrated that a gastric haemorrhage could be induced by the ingestion of aspirin (*Fig. 13*).

In 1950, Olsen and Moersch[60] from the Mayo Clinic performed rigid gastroscopy on several patients admitted with haemorrhage of unknown origin and succeeded in diagnosing the cause of the bleeding.

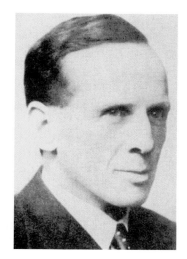

Fig. 12. Arthur Douthwaite (1896-1974), British pharmacologist and gastroenterologist. The first to employ a gastroscope to demonstrate the lesions in the gastric mucosa produced by acetyl-salicilic acid (courtesy of the British Society of Gastroenterology).

EDDY PALMER AND THE "VIGOROUS" DIAGNOSIS OF GASTROINTESTINAL HAEMORRHAGE

Starting in 1945, Eddy Palmer, a gastroenterologist in the American Army, began to use emergency endoscopy and radiology for the diagnosis of acute digestive bleeding. Between 1945 and 1960 Palmer treated 862 adult patients admitted for bleeding using both diagnostic methods simultaneously. In 1951, he published a monograph entitled "Diagnosis of Upper Gastrointestinal Hemorrhage" which is now a classic[61]. In his book, Palmer analysed his technique and his results in detail. Palmer's opinion, which was not shared by many, was that it was imperative to establish the origin of a haemorrhage as soon as possible, and that both the presumptive clinical diagnosis and the physical examination were very often erroneous. He also believed that radiology was less useful than endoscopy in the diagnosis of bleeding erosions and in gastric ulcers located in the fundic region of the stomach which were missed by the radiologist. In Palmer's experience, the longer one waited to perform endoscopy, the greater the likelihood of missing the diagnosis as many acute erosions would disappear in a few days (*Figs. 14, 15, 16*).

Fig. 13. Sir Arthur Hurst (1879-1944), famous British physician, author of a well-known text-book on "Gastric and Duodenal Ulcer" and founder of the British Society of Gastroenterology (collection of Dr. Jacinto Vilardell).

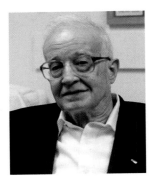

Fig. 14. Eddy Palmer in a recent photograph, a pioneer in the early aggressive diagnosis of gastrointestinal haemorrhage (courtesy of Dr. Eddy Palmer).

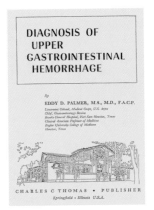

Fig. 15. Title page of Eddy Palmer's monograph on the early diagnosis of upper gastrointestinal bleeding, published in 1951.

Palmer describes his technique in the following way: "after admission, patients received gastric lavage with ice water by means of a large bore (30F) tube in order to empty the stomach as well as to stop bleeding". This procedure had already been carried out by some older clinicians in German-speaking countries. Lavage was continued until the aspirated fluid no longer showed visible traces of blood. Immediately after lavage and a previous injection of atropine and phenobarbital, Palmer performed oesophagoscopy with the Eder-Hufford endoscope. This was followed by gastroscopy with the thin Eder gastroscope which could be inserted through the hollow oesophagoscope. Taking the relatively narrow visual field into account, he used a telescopic lens which provided a magnification of 4 times to examine the mucosa. Palmer agreed that instruments other than the Eder-Hufford endoscope, used separately, could be equally useful (Fig. 17).

It was obviously very important to perform the examination as rapidly as possible. After endoscopy, patients had a barium radiological examination. Palmer stated that with his method he had reached 87.1 percent of correct diagnoses, especially because of the ease with which erosions and gastric ulcers were diagnosed. He also stressed the important number of lesions such as duodenal deformities and oesophageal varices identified by the radiologist, which were not causing any bleeding. In spite of these excellent results, most gastroenterologists were still reluctant to employ aggressive diagnostic methods on the bleeding patient.

In 1969, Palmer published his results in 23 years of experience based on 1,400 patients[62]. He was probably the first to report that erosive oesophagitis caused a greater percentage of haemorrhages (7 per cent) than previously thought. Global mortality in his series was 7.9 percent and he had only one severe accident (perforation of a Zenker's diverticulum).

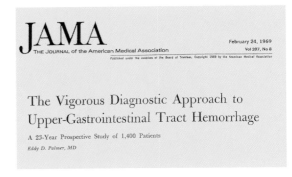

Fig. 16. Heading of Eddy Palmer's paper from 1969, describing in detail his experience with 1,400 bleeding patients in whom emergency endoscopy had been performed.

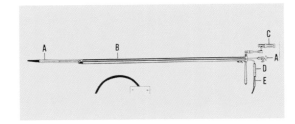

Fig. 17. The Eder-Hufford oesophago-gastroscope, used by Eddy Palmer, Benjamin Sullivan and other American endoscopists for the early diagnosis of gastrointestinal bleeding, (courtesy of Eder Inc.).

OTHER ADVOCATES OF EARLY ENDOSCOPY

Sir Francis Avery Jones: With the passage of time, Avery Jones changed his mind and became a strong believer in early investigations to ascertain the cause of bleeding in upper gastrointestinal haemorrhage[39]. In his service at the Central Middlesex Hospital in London, gastroscopies were performed without accidents in patients who had had recent haemorrhage. Using the Hermon-Taylor gastroscope (see Chapter 4), his team examined 116 of a series of 217 patients in whom neither the clinical examination nor radiology had provided a diagnosis, and found 86 lesions – 65 of which were gastric ulcers. In 1960, they published their results with the early gastroscopic examination followed by a barium swallow using a portable x-ray machine. Obviously neither the Hermon Taylor endoscope nor the Schindler-Wolf which they used in elderly patients could visualise the duodenum, and therefore all diagnoses of duodenal ulcer were only made by the radiologist. However, endoscopy proved its worth in the diagnosis of gastric ulcer (more than 80 percent correct diagnoses) and also its harmlessness[8, 9] *(Fig. 18).*

J.J. Desneux, Ch. Debray, P. Housset, D. Katz: In Brussels, Jean Jacques Desneux[14], who died prematurely, performed urgent endoscopy which he documented with excellent photographs. Emergency endoscopy was also done in Paris at Hospital Bichat in Charles Debray's service[13], especially by Pierre Housset[33], who organized an ambulant service for the performance of urgent endoscopy in several hospitals of the city. In Jerzy Glass' service at New York Medical College *(Figs. 19, 20, 21),* David Katz[41] began to perform emergency endoscopies around 1960. Like Eddy Palmer, he noted the high percentage of acute erosions which were causing massive bleeding (28 percent of his patients). These lesions would probably have gone undiagnosed if endoscopy had been done late or if only radiology had been utilized.

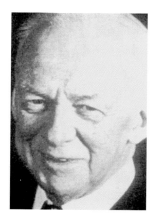

Fig. 18. Sir Francis Avery Jones (1910-1998), gastroenterologist at the Central Middlesex Hospital in London, one of the first to endorse early diagnostic investigations in patients with upper gastrointestinal haemorrhage (courtesy of the late Sir Francis Avery Jones).

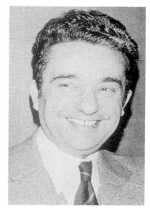

Fig. 21. Pierre Housset, an associate of Charles Debray who designed the O.P.L. semi-flexible gastroscope which he extensively employed in the urgent diagnosis of digestive haemorrhage in Paris (authors' collection).

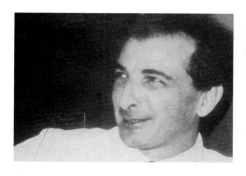

Fig. 19. Jean-Jacques Desneux, a distinguished Belgian gastroenterologist, one of the first in 1950 to introduce the emergency endoscopic examination in the management of haemorrhage (courtesy of Prof. Michel Cremer).

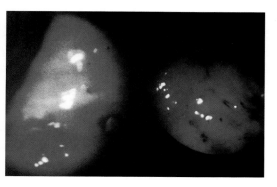

Fig. 20. Colour photograph obtained by J.J. Desneux with the O.P.L. gastroscope in a patient with haemorrhagic gastritis (courtesy of Prof. Michel Cremer).

However, in spite of the high accuracy of the endoscopic diagnosis, clearly confirmed in a review commissioned by the A.S.G.E.[25], there were many doubts about the practical value of the early examinations and their impact on therapy, at least until the development of endoscopic techniques for local haemostasia[41, 59, 80]. In the last twenty-five years, the prognostic value of the finding of a visible vessel at the base of an ulcer or the presence of a clot, has allowed satisfactory identification of patients at risk of rebleeding[22].

THE DEVELOPMENT OF THERAPEUTIC ENDOSCOPY

The control of variceal bleeding

Variceal haemorrhage is always a fearful complication with mortality no less than 50 percent[6] and a risk of recurrence after initial control of the bleeding episode around 70 per cent[26].

Tamponade of bleeding varices

Kelling, a forerunner of so many procedures of digestive endoscopy, wrote the following sentence, reproduced by Neumann[58], "I don't want to leave unmentioned that in the rare cases in which a fatal haemorrhage from oesophageal varices may occur, I try to tampon the oesophagus with gauzes at least one metre long". Other surgeons, such as Crafoord[12], sporadically employed variceal tamponade. In 1930, Karl Westphal (1887-1952), professor of medicine at Hannover, employed for the first time Gottstein's dilating balloon distended with water and placed inside the oesophagus to control a variceal haemorrhage in two patients with alcoholic cirrhosis[88]. In both instances, the balloon remained in place for 24 hours and massive bleeding was stopped. Westphal, a prominent figure in German gastroenterology and friend of the famous laparoscopist Heinz Kalk (who was to write his obituary), recommended that a Gottstein balloon (see chapter 5) should be available in all hospital emergency departments for that purpose. Nevertheless, it took twenty years for variceal tamponade with balloons to become an accepted procedure *(Figs. 22, 23)*.

In 1947, Rowntree[76] employed a latex balloon attached to a Miller-Abbott tube to treat a patient with liver cirrhosis who was bleeding profusely to the point that sclerosing injections through the oesophagoscope were impossible. The procedure was successful and Rowntree tried to interest the firm Georg Pilling in its production, apparently without success. However, Sengstaken and Blakemore were more fortunate and a balloon that they designed for this purpose became popular in many hospitals all over the world.

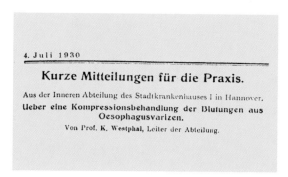

4. Juli 1930

Kurze Mitteilungen für die Praxis.

Aus der Inneren Abteilung des Stadtkrankenhauses I in Hannover.
Ueber eine Kompressionsbehandlung der Blutungen aus Oesophagusvarizen.
Von Prof. K. Westphal, Leiter der Abteilung.

Fig. 22. In 1930 Karl Westphal (1887-1952) employed a balloon for the first time to apply pressure on bleeding oesophageal varices. (obituary written by Heinz Kalk, Deutsch med Wschr 25 Jan.1952).

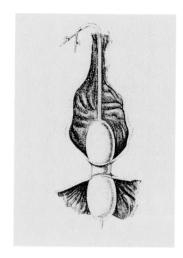

Fig. 23. Gottstein's dilating balloon used by Westphal to tamponade a variceal haemorrhage in two patients with cirrhosis of the liver (from Mathieu A. et al. Maladies de l'Estomac et de l'Oesophage, 1913).

The Sengstaken-Blakemore balloon.

On the seventh of December 1949, at a meeting of the Southern Surgical Association, Robert Sengstaken (1923-2000) (who would later make a brilliant career in neurosurgery) and Arthur Blakemore (1897-1970), a distinguished vascular surgeon, presented a balloon for the tamponade of bleeding oesophageal varices. They published their favourable experience in 30 patients the following year *(Figs. 24, 25)*.

The device[79], still in use on occasions, consists of a tube with four channels fitted with a balloon at the distal end. This is inflated to compress the oesophageal walls, and another small balloon is used to apply pressure on the gastric fundus. Both balloons are connected to an independent tube. A third channel serves for gastric suction. The tube, which is used for insufflation of the oesophageal balloon, is connected to a manometer to monitor pressure in the oesophagus. Continuous traction of the balloons is necessary and this

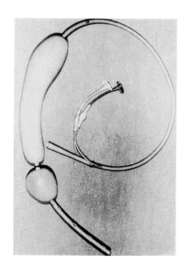

Fig. 25. Sengstaken-Blakemore balloon first employed around 1950 and still occasionally used at Hospital de Sant Pau (Davol Rubber Co. Providence, R.I.).

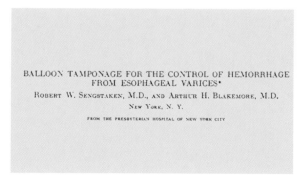

BALLOON TAMPONAGE FOR THE CONTROL OF HEMORRHAGE
FROM ESOPHAGEAL VARICES*
ROBERT W. SENGSTAKEN, M.D., AND ARTHUR H. BLAKEMORE, M.D.
NEW YORK, N. Y.
FROM THE PRESBYTERIAN HOSPITAL OF NEW YORK CITY

Fig. 24. Heading of the original paper by Sengstaken and Blakemore on tamponade of oesophageal varices.

requires careful monitoring. Although the technical procedure may vary somewhat from one centre to another, the compression of the oesophageal balloon is maintained for 24 hours with permanent patient vigilance. The gastric balloon is usually kept distended for another 24 hours. In spite of the numerous accidents and ill effects reported[11], in experienced hands the Sengstaken balloon has saved many lives, at least temporarily[68, 69, 86].

Other balloons, such as the Linton-Nachlas device (1966) which was specifically employed for the control of gastric varices,[50] were designed in the ensuing years. The Linton instrument consisted of a tube ending in a balloon which could be distended with air up to 800 ml and two channels for simultaneous suction of the oesophagus and the stomach. The large size of the intragastric balloon allowed compression of gastric varices and oesophageal varices at their origin with somewhat more efficacy than the Sensgtaken instrument. It avoided direct compression of the oesophagus, thus preventing erosions on an already fragile oesophageal mucosa. Several authors pointed out the drawbacks and the dangers of balloon tamponade[11, 82] and balloons were gradually replaced by pharmacological therapies (parenteral pituitrine and its analogues) and by endoscopic methods which had little acceptance until the advent of the simpler and less dangerous fibrescopes. Nowadays, Sengstaken and Linton balloons are very seldom employed (two or three times per year at Hospital de Sant Pau).

Sclerosing oesophageal varices

Attempts to introduce a "cure" for oesophageal varices began with the initiative of the famous Swedish thoracic surgeon, Clarence Crafoord. In his article published in 1939, Crafoord[12] mentioned that treatment of oesophageal bleeding from varices had always been conservative, based on transfusions, rest and sedatives. Like others, he had occasionally performed tamponade of varices and had tried surgical ligation of the varices in desperate cases either by the transpleural or the transabdominal routes. Crafoord had the idea of using the same technique that was employed in his clinic to obliterate haemorrhoids, that is, the local injection of a sclerosing agent; in his case, quinine clorhydrate. His assistant Frencker, an endoscopist, designed a needle which could be introduced through a rigid oesophagoscope. The first patient treated was a 17-year-old girl with splenomegaly and oesophageal varices who had had splenectomy without success. The radiological examination showed oesophageal varices and an oesophagoscopy performed by Frenckner confirmed the presence of varices from below the upper oesophageal sphincter appearing as a bunch of grapes *(Fig 26, 27, 28)*. He injected the sclerosing solution (2 ml quinine solution) into the three more prominent varices without untoward effects. The injection was repeated every second day, each time more distally, into the remaining varices.

One month later, the varices had disappeared and three years later the patient was well although some residual varices were detected by the radiological examination. Unfortunately, Crafoord's paper includes no references and as it was published in an O.R.L. journal it received scarce attention from gastroenterologists.

Nevertheless, after 1940, otolaryngologists such as Herman Moersch from the Mayo Clinic[56, 57], who was a very experienced oesophagoscopist, used a similar technique with reasonably good results, but again no impact was made on gastroenterologists. Moersch gave an injection of 1 ml 2.5 per cent sodium morrhuate in each quadrant and at different levels. He treated a heterogeneous group of patients, usually under general anaesthesia, and by 1941 he had treated 11 patients.

Moersch[57] attributed the idea of sclerosing varices to the well-known surgeon from the Mayo Clinic, Waltmann Walters, who had suggested the technique in 1933 during the discussion of a paper presented at the Staff Meetings of the Clinic[85]. Walters had said, "An additional method of reducing the amount of venous blood in the esophageal varices might be injection of periesophageal or para-oesophageal plexus of veins with some non-irritating yet sclerosing solution, a method similar to that employed for obliterating varicous veins in the legs. The solution should be injected with a very small needle so as to prevent undue bleeding from the needle puncture in the vein. Should bleeding occur, ligation of the vein at the site of the needle puncture could be carried out".

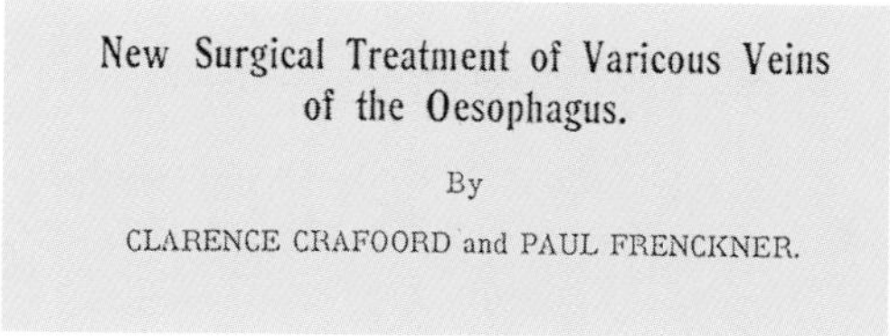

Moersch then tried to produce oesophageal varices in dogs, without success. Douglas McGill, a gastroenterologist at the Mayo Clinic, has told me that many years later, Moersch, long retired, was invited to a clinical presentation on sclerotherapy of bleeding varices through the fibrescope and commented that although the instruments had been much improved, the technique was the same that he had used fifty years earlier! (Fig. 29).

Cecil Patterson, a gastroenterologist, was another pioneer of the sclerosing treatment of varices in the United States; he started treating patients in 1946 and in 1947 he published his results in 24 patients submitted to several sclerosing sessions. Six patients died but among the 18 others who survived, only 8 episodes of

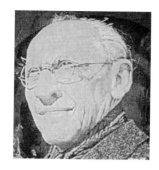

Fig. 26. Clarence Crafoord, born in 1899 and retired in 1966, famous Swedish thoracic surgeon, who for the first time treated oesophageal varices by injecting sclerosing agents through the oesophagoscope (source: Karolinska Institute).

New Surgical Treatment of Varicous Veins of the Oesophagus.

By

CLARENCE CRAFOORD and PAUL FRENCKNER.

Fig. 27. Heading of Crafoord and Fraencker's 1939 paper. It passed almost unnoticed by gastroenterologists, possibly because it was published in an O.R.L. journal.

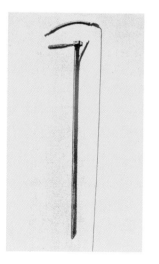

Fig. 28. Needle designed by Fraencker and Crafoord for endoscopic sclerosis of varices (adapted from ref. 12).

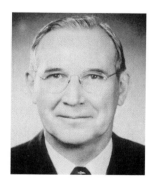

Fig. 29. Herman Moersch, otolaryngologist and oesophagoscopist at the Mayo Clinic (Rochester, Minn) who, following Crafoord, employed a technique for sclerosing oesophageal varices in 1940 (courtesy Dr. Douglas McGill).

bleeding were detected during follow-up. Patterson was so enthusiastic that he even said, "To the best of my knowledge, no other method is able to protect these patients with oesophageal varices so efficiently from a recurrence of haematemesis"[65, 66].

Besides Crafoord and Frencker, another pioneer in Europe was Macbeth[52] (identified as Mac Beth in some articles), an otolaryngologist from Oxford. In 1949, he performed sclerosing injections by means of a needle which he himself had designed, on 30 patients, 14 of whom had cirrhosis and the rest portal hypertension due to other causes. He and Kempe[44], a Swedish otolaryngologist, employed sodium morrhuate instead of quinine. In 1958, Johnston[36] began to perform sclerotherapy in Belfast using rigid oesophagoscopes and injections of ethanolamine (Varistab). In 1973, he published his experience of 15 years which consisted of 115 patients who, after control of the haemorrhage by means of a Sengstaken balloon, received sclerosing injections. Haemorrhage was controlled in 93 percent of cases, with a single sclerosing session.

With the fibrescope, the tool the gastroenterologists had started to use, they became more interested in this kind of therapy and in 1976, Loren Pitcher[69] was apparently the first to use sclerosing needles through a fibrescope in patients with bleeding varices.

Treatment of haemorrhage of gastric origin

According to Neumann[58], Kelling –always inventive– wrote in regard to the management of bleeding peptic ulcer, "In the case of a life-threatening gastric haemorrhage, are we authorised in some way to tamponade the bleeding through the oesophagoscope? That question can only be answered through experiments in animals".

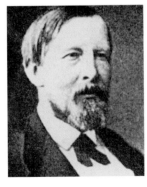

Fig. 30. Adolf Kussmaul (1822-1902), who employed lavage and aspiration of the stomach for the treatment of gastric haemorrhage (see Chapter 1) (courtesy of the Falk Foundation).

In cases of gastric haemorrhage, many early 20th century authors[16, 19, 53] recommended absolute rest, nothing by mouth and an ice bag over the stomach region. However, some clinicians such as Ewald and Kussmaul, who had designed a suction tube to treat gastric dilatation (see Chapter 1), dared to introduce a tube into the stomach to perform gastric lavage with iced water, or even to introduce a solution of ferric perchloride, although others considered that any manipulation of the patient could be dangerous[72] *(Fig. 30)*.

Possibly the first to use gastric lavage in the United States in regard to the management of bleeding peptic ulcer was Kaufmann from New York[42]. He had seen it performed in Kussmaul's clinic 25 years beforehand. Kaufmann repeatedly injected 300 ml of water which was emptied by simple postural drainage.

In cases of recurrent haemorrhage, Mathieu[53] from Paris emptied the stomach and then used a solution of ferric perchloride, injecting and aspirating the fluid repeatedly, following the recommendations of Louis Bourget (1856-1913), a professor of medicine in Lausanne[4]. In 1913 Mathieu wrote, "For the past 10 years I have been washing the stomach of bleeding patients who have gastric retention, without difficulties in inserting the tube or encountering adverse effects"[53]. Bourget's procedure was also mentioned by Knud Faber[19] from Copenhagen and by René Gutmann[27] from Paris. Others believed that ferric perchloride was useless and that it could induce nausea and vomiting in some patients[42]. On the other hand, Elsner thought that ice water lavage or ferric per-chloride administration should be undertaken only as last resort therapeutic measures[16] *(Fig. 31)*.

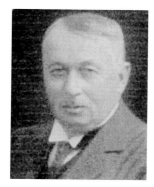

Fig. 31. Louis Bourget (1856-1913). Born in Yverdon (Switzerland), he studied medicine in Geneva and became professor of medicine in Lausanne. He recommended gastric lavage with ferric perchloride for the treatment of gastric bleeding. Author of various papers on the biochemical and clinical aspects of gas-troenterology. (Collection Dr. Jacinto Vilardell).

In the early 1930s, Horace Soper from Saint-Louis[81] was a firm supporter of gas-tric lavage to eliminate blood clots. He left a catheter "in situ", through which he injected a thrombin solution, watched for a recurrence and initiated early feedings. Other authors quoted by Ivy[35] added calcium chloride or an epineph-rin solution as a vasoconstrictor in the water used for lavage, but the data avail-able are sparse and inconsistent.

Many surgeons were in favour of an immediate surgical intervention as the clin-ical course of the patients was unpredictable and mortality of early surgery was much less than that of a delayed operation[27]. Other surgeons favoured simple gastric tamponade, although Rovsing considered it useless[75], or diathermo-coag-ulation following gastrotomy[27].

Wangensteen and gastric freezing

In the late fifties, Owen Wangensteen[87], a surgeon from the University of Minnesota, began to employ an ingenious device to freeze the stomach and to control bleeding in this unorthodox way. After pharyngeal anaesthesia, a double lumen tube ending in a balloon was introduced into the stomach. A mixture of water and alcohol (equal parts) was washed through the channels of the tube. It had previously been cooled in a refrigerator at temperatures between –15 and–20 centigrades for 45 to 60 minutes. About 600-800 ml of fluid were injected and circulated. In 1962 Wangensteen published satisfactory results using this technique, which he attributed to the inhibitory effect of freezing on gastric acid secretion. Wangensteen's device was marketed and employed in several centres, including Hospital de Sant Pau. However, accidents were reported (aspirations, rupture of the balloon, pneumonias, etc.) and at the same time, the promising early results were not confirmed in adequate controlled studies[77]. In our experi-ence, recurrent haemorrhage was not uncommon after the procedure and it was abandoned a few months later *(Figs. 32, 33)*.

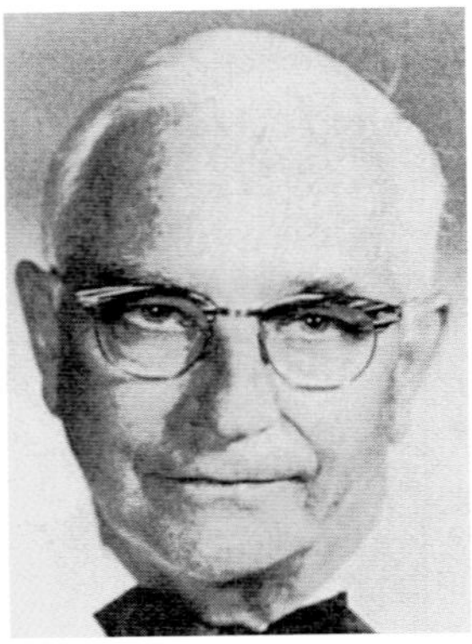

Endoscopic therapies *(Figs. 34, 35, 36)*

Local endoscopic therapies for bleeding gastric lesions, especially of peptic ulcers, began roughly 25 years ago and are not therefore open to discussion in a historical monograph such as this[10]. One great step forward has been the development of specific units for the care of gastrointestinal emergencies where the patient is treated by specialised personnel and endoscopy or other measures can be performed without undue delay[30, 48, 84], especially in instances of massive haemorrhage.

Sclerosing therapies

However, it may be relevant to mention the first cases of bleeding ulcer treated by direct injection of the lesion with various agents such as adrenaline, polydocanol, thrombin and so on. More than twenty-five years have elapsed since Nib Soehendra[80] published his first results at the Hamburg-Eppendorf Hospital –of such tradition in the field of gastroenterology– using local endoscopic therapy. He was rapidly followed by other endoscopists, mainly European *(Fig. 37)*.

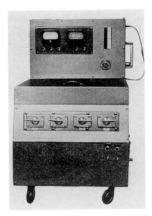

Fig. 32. Owen Wangensteen (1899-1981), Professor of surgery at the University of Minnesota in Minneapolis. In 1963 he invented a machine to freeze the stomach and thus control gastric bleeding. The procedure was not successful (courtesy of Dr. J.Puig-Lacalle).

Fig. 33. A Japanese version (Juntendo University) of Wangensteen's device for gastric freezing, presented at the First World Congress of Digestive Endoscopy (Koike et al., Tokyo 1966).

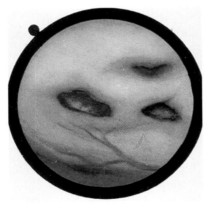

Fig. 34. Acute bleeding gastric ulcers (François Moutier, 1935).

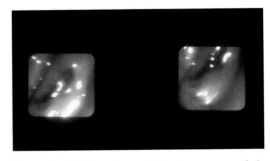

Fig. 35. Bleeding ulcer of the lesser curve of the stomach (Collection of the Digestive Endoscopy Unit, Hospital de Sant Pau).

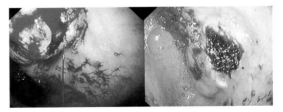

Fig. 36. Jet bleeding from an acute ulcer, before and after endoscopic therapy with Argon beam (courtesy of Dr. J.R.Armengol-Miró).

Electrocoagulation therapy

For many years, surgeons had treated patients with inoperable bleeding gastric cancer by means of a gastrotomy followed by a palliative procedure, usually electrocoagulation[17, 27]. As already discussed, Yeomans treated two bleeding lesions through a cystoscope[89]. Fibrescopes have allowed the use of electrocoagulation, particularly in the United States, following reports by Papp in 1974. In 1976, Papp had successfully treated 40 bleeding lesions without untoward results[63, 64].

Laser treatments which have been useful in other fields were also tried in attempts to stop ulcer bleeding, especially in Erlangen[23, 51], but it was soon realised that sclerosing therapies had similar results at a much lower cost; laser therapy for bleeding is no longer used. Argon coagulation is likely to enjoy success but the technique is still in the early stages[10] *(Fig. 38)*.

The favourable effect of early endoscopy and haemostatic therapy was not clearly demonstrated until 1990 when a study from Scotland was published[24].

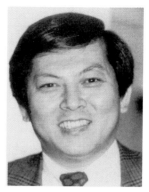

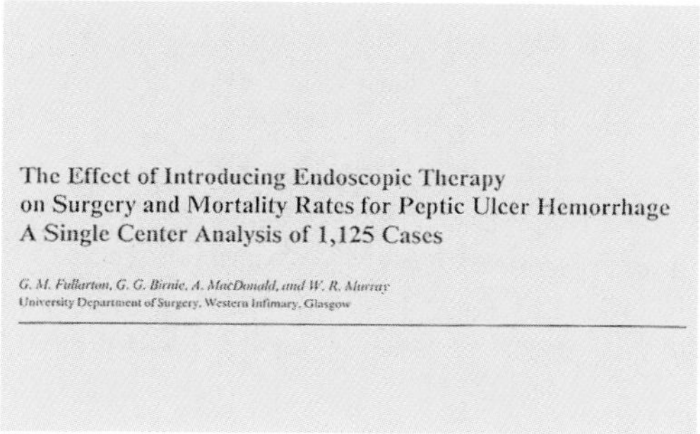

Fig. 37. Nib Soehendra, professor of endoscopy, Hamburg University and Head of the Endoscopy Centre, Hamburg-Eppendorf Hospital. The first to use sclerosing injections directly on a bleeding gastric ulcer (courtesy of Prof. H. Niwa).

The Effect of Introducing Endoscopic Therapy
on Surgery and Mortality Rates for Peptic Ulcer Hemorrhage
A Single Center Analysis of 1,125 Cases

G. M. Fullarton, G. G. Birnie, A. MacDonald, and W. R. Murray
University Department of Surgery, Western Infirmary, Glasgow

Fig. 38. Heading of Fullerton's paper showing for the first time the positive impact of endoscopic treatment on the outcome of upper gastrointestinal haemorrhage (1990).

REFERENCES

[1] Atik M., Simeone F.A. Massive gastrointestinal bleeding; study of two hundred-ninety-six patients at City Hospital of Cleveland. A.M.A. Arch Surg 1954; 69: 355-365.

[2] Bloom B.S., Fendrick A.M., Ramsey S.D.. Changes in peptic ulcer and gastritis/duodenitis in Great Britain. J Clin Gastroenterol 1990; 12: 100-108.

[3] Bockus H.L. Peptic Ulcer Disease. en Gastroenterology vol I, Philadelphia, W.B.Saunders, 1946.

[4] Bourget L. Les Maladies de l'Estomac et leur Traitement. Paris, Baillière, 1912.

[5] Brinton W. On the Pathology, Symptoms and Treatment of Ulcer of the Stomach. London, John Churchill, 1857.

[6] Burroughs A.K., Heygere F., McIntyre N. Pitfalls in studies of prophylactic therapy for variceal bleeding. Hepatology 1986; 6: 1407-1413.

7 Bulmer E. Mortality from haematemesis. Lancet 1932; 2: 720-722.

8 Chandler G.N., Watkinson G. The early diagnosis of the causes of haematemesis. Quart J Med 1959; 28: 371-395.

9 Chandler G.N., Cameron A.D., Nunn A.M., Street D.F. Early investigations of haematemesis Gut 1960; 1: 6-13.

10 Classen M (editor) Section on Therapeutic Procedures. en M.Classen, G.N. Tytgat, C.J.Lightdale: Gastroenterological Endoscopy, Stuttgart, G.Thieme, 2002: 262-301.

11 Conn H.O., Simpson J.H. Excessive mortality associated with the balloon tamponade of bleeding varices J.A.M.A. 1967; 202: 585-591.

12 Craafoord C., Frenckner P. New surgical treatment of varicous veins of the oesophagus. Acta Oto-laryngologica 1939; 27: 422-429.

13 Debray Ch., Housset P. Emergency oeso-gastroscopy in haemorrhages of the upper-digestive tract —Its significance (150 examinations). in Advances in Gastrointestinal Endoscopy. Proceedings of the 2nd World Congress of Gastrointestinal Endoscopy (1970), Padova, Piccin Medical Books, 1972: 259-262.

14 Desneux J.J. La gastroscopie d'urgence dans les hémorragies digestives aigües. Acta Chir Belgica 1952; 51: 747-760.

15 Douthwaite A.H., Lintott G.A.M. Gastroscopic observations of the effect of Aspirin and certain other substances on the stomach. Lancet 1938; 2: 1222-1223.

16 Elsner H. Lehrbuch der Magenkrankheiten für Ärzte und Studierende. Berlin, Karger, 1909.

17 Eusterman G.B., Balfour D.C. The Stomach and Duodenum, Philadelphia, W.B. Saunders, 1935: 763-769.

18 Ewald C.A. Klinik der Verdauungskrankheiten, Berlin, August Hirschwald, 1893.

19 Faber K. Magen und Darmkrankheiten, Berlin, Springer, 1923.

20 Fenwick S., Fenwick W.S. Ulcer of the Stomach and Duodenum and its Consequences. London, J. and A. Churchill, 1900.

21 Fischer I. Biographisches Lexicon der hervorzagenden Ärzte der letzten fünfzig Jahre. Berlin, Urban & Schwarzenberg, 1932.

22 Foster D.N., Miloszewski K.J.A.,Losowski M.S. Stigmata of recent haemorrhage in diagnosis and prognosis of upper gastrointestinal bleeding. Brit Med J 1978: 1: 1173-1177.

23 Frühmorgen P., Bodem F., Reidenbach H.F., Kaduk B., Demling L. Endoscopic laser coagulation of bleeding gastrointestinal lesions with report of the first therapeutic application in man. Gastrointest Endosc 1976; 23: 73-75.

24 Fullarton G.M., Birnie G.G., MacDonald A., Murray W.R. The effect of intoducing endoscopic therapy on surgery and mortality rates from peptic ulcer hemorrhage. A single center analysis of 1,125 cases. Endoscopy 1990; 22: 110-113.

25 Gilbert D.A., Silverstein F.E., Tedesco F.J. Symposium: the National A.S.G.E. Survey on gastrointestinal bleeding.III Endoscopy in upper gastrointestinal bleeding. Gastrointest Endosc 1981; 27: 94-99.

26 Graham D., Smith. H The course of patients with variceal hemorrhage. Gastroenterology 1981; 80: 800-809.

27 Gutmann R.A. Les Syndrômes Douloureux de la Région Épigastrique. Paris, G.Doin, vol.I. 1947.

28 Haubrich W.S. Edmonson J.M. History of Endoscopy. in Gastroenterologic Endoscopy. M.Sivak (ed) vol.1, Philadelphia, W.B. Saunders, 2000: 2-15.

29 Hawkins C.F. Diseases of the Alimentary Tract. London, William Heinemann, 1963.

30 Hellers G., Ihre T. Impact of change to early diagnosis and surgery in major upper gastrointestinal bleeding. Lancet 1975; 2: 1250-1251.

31 Henning N. Lehrbuch der Gastroskopie. Leipzig, Johann Ambrosius Barth, 1935.

32 Herrick F.C. Profuse recurrent gastric hemorrhage, with report of cases and description of an instrument for viewing the gastric interior at operation. Cleveland Med Journal 1911; 10: 969-976.

33 Housset P. (personal communication).

34 Hurst A. Aspirin as a Cause of Haematemesis. en Selected Writings of sir Arthur Hurst (1879-1944) edited by T. Hunt. London, British Society of Gastroenterology, 1970: 90-91.

35 Ivy A.C., Grossman M.I., Bachrach W.H. Peptic Ulcer, Philadelphia, Blakiston Co, 1950: 832-833.

36 Johnston G.W., Rodgers H.W.. A review of 15 years experience in the use of sclerotherapy in the control of acute haemorrhage from oesophageal varices Br J Surg 1973; 60: 797-800.

37 Jones F.A., Haematemesis and melaena. Brit med J 1943; 1: 689-691.

38 Jones F.A. Haematemesis and melaena. en F.Avery Jones (ed.) Modern Trends in Gastroenterology. London, Butterworth, 1952: 432-443.

39 Jones F.A. Hematemesis and melena with special reference to causation and to the factors influencing the mortality from bleeding peptic ulcers. Gastroenterology 1956; 30: 166-190.

40 Katschinslki B.D., Zachewitz H., Goebell H. Non-steroidal antinflammatory drugs and mortality from peptic ulceration in West Germany, 1952-1989. Dig Dis Sci 1992; 37: 385-390.

41 Katz D., Douvres P., Weisberg H., McKinnon W., Glass G.B.J. Early endoscopic diagnosis of acute gastrointestinal hemorrhage: Demonstration of the relatively high incidence of erosions as a source of bleeding. J.A.M.A. 1964: 188: 405-408.

42 Kaufmann J. The treatment of hemorrhage from gastric ulcer with special reference to gastric lavage. Am J Med Sci 1910; 139: 790-800.

43 Kelemen E. Physical diagnosis of acute abdominal diseases and injuries. Budapest, Akadémiai Kiadó, 1964.

44 Kempe S.G., Koch H. Injection of sclerosing solutions in the treatment of the esophageal varices. Acta Oto-Laryng (Stockholm) (Suppl) 1954; 118: 120-129.

45 Kraft L. Beiträge zur Behandlung der lebensgefärlichen Magen Blütungen. Arch f. Klin Chirurgie. 1910; 93: 557-580.

46 Lambling A., Bonfils S., Baratgin B. les hémorragies del ulcères gastro-duodénaux. Étude de 254 observations. Arch Mal Appar Dig. 1957; 46: 73-79.

47 Lenhartz H. Eine neue Behandlung des Ulcus Ventriculi. Deutsch Med Wschr 1904; 30: 412-415.

48 Lepore M.J., Grace W.J. Role of the intensive care unit in gastroenterology. Am.J.Gastroenterol 1969; 51: 493-497.

49 Leube v. W.O. Beiträge zur Diagnostik der Magenkrankheiten. Deutsch Arch f. Klin Medicin. 1883; 33: 1-21.

50 Linton R.R. The treatment of esophageal varices. Surg Clin North Am 1966; 49: 485-495.

51 Loizou L.A. Endoscopic laser treatment for peptic ulcer and variceal haemorrhage. in Lasers in Gastroenterology, Krasner N. (ed). London, Chapman & Hall, 1991: 75-108.

52 Macbeth R. Treatment of oesophageal varices in portal hypertension by means of sclerosing injections. Brit Med J 1955; 2: 877-880.

53 Mathieu A., Sencert L., Tuffier Th. Traité Médico-Chirurgical des Maladies de l'Estomac et de l'Oesophage. Paris, Masson editeurs, 1913.

54 McKibbin B., Watson B.W. Localization of intestinal bleeding using a miniature Geiger counter. Gut 1953; 4: 82-87.

55 Meulengracht E. Treatment of haematemesis and melaena with food. Lancet 1935; 2: 1220-1222.

56 Moersch H.J. Treatment of esophageal varices by injection. Proc Staff Meet Mayo Clin 1940; 15: 177-178.

57 Moersch H.J. Further studies on the treatment of esophageal varices by injection of a sclerosing solution. Ann Otol Rhinol Laryngol 1941; 50:1233-1244.

58 Neumann H.A., Hellwig A. Vom Schwertschlucker zur Glasfiberoptik. Die Geschichte der Gastroskopie. München, Urban & Vogel, 2001: 49.

59 Nord H.J. Diagnosis and management of acute upper gastrointestinal bleeding. in H.J.Nord and P.G. Brady (eds). Critical Care Gastroenterology, New York, Churchill & Livingstone, 1982: 59-78.

60 Olsen A.M., Moersch H.J. The role of gastroscopy in the diagnosis of upper gastrointestinal hemorrhage of obscure origin. Gastroenterology 1950; 14: 292-299.

61 Palmer E.D. Diagnosis of Upper Gastrointestinal Hemorrhage. Springfield,Ill. Ch. Thomas, 1951.

62 Palmer E.D. The vigorous diagnostic approach to upper-gastrointestinal tract hemorrhage. A 23 year prospective study of 1400 patients. J.A.M.A. 1969; 207: 1477-1480.

63 Papp J. Endoscopic electrocoagulation in upper gastrointestinal hemorrhage. A preliminary report. J.A.M.A. 1974; 230: 1172-1173.

64 Papp J. Endoscopic elecrocoagulation of upper gastrointestinal hemorrhage J.A.M.A. 1976; 236: 2076-2079.

65 Patterson C.O.,Rouse M.O. Injection treatment of esophageal varices. J.A.M.A. 1946; 130: 384-386.

66 Patterson C.O. the sclerosing therapy of esophagel varices. Gastroenterology 1947; 34: 391-395.

67 Pillow R.P., Hill L.D., Ragen F.,Siemsen J.S., Wallace I.A. Newer methods for localization of obscure small bowel bleeding. J.A.M.A. 1962; 179: 23-26.

68 Pitcher J.L. Safety and effectiveness of the modified Sengstaken-Blakemore tube: a prospective study. Gastroenterology 1971; 61: 291-298.

69 Pitcher J.L. Medical management of bleeding esophagogastric varices. Gastrointestinal Emergencies, Oxford, Pergamon Press, 1976: 261-268.

70 Pittman F.E. the fluorescein string test. An analysis of its use and relationship to barium studies of the upper gastrointestinal tract in 122 cases of gastrointestinal tract hemorrhage. Ann Intern Med 1964; 60: 418-429.

71 Pollard M.H. Upper gastrointestinal hemorrhage. in Gastroenterologic Medicine, M.Paulson (ed) Philadelphia, Lea & Febiger, 1969: 571-582.

72 Rehfuss M.E. Diagnosis and Treatment of Diseases of the Stomach. Philadelphia, W.B. Saunders, 1927.

73 Rivers A.B., Wilbur D.L. The diagnostic significance of hematemesis. JAMA 1932; 98: 1629-1631.

74 Rivers A.B. A clinical study of duodenitis, gastritis and gastrojejunitis. Ann Intern Med 1931; 4: 1265-1281.

75 Rovsing T. Gastroduodenoskopie und Diaphanoskopie. Arch. f. klin Chirurgie. 1908; 86: 575-588.

76 Rowntree L.G., Zimmerman E.F., Todd M.H., Ajar J. Intraesophageal venous tamponade. Its use in a case of variceal hemorrhage from the esophagus. J.A.M.A. 1947; 135: 630-631.

77 Ruffin J.M., Grizzle J.E., Hightower N.C. et al. A cooperative double-blind evaluation of gastric "freezing" in the treatment of duodenal ulcer. New Engl J Med 1969; 281: 16-19.

78 Schindler R. Gastroscopy, Chicago, University of Chicago Press, 1937.

79 Sengstaken R.W., Blakemore A.H. Balloon tamponage in the control of hemorrhage from esophageal varices. Ann Surg 1950; 131: 781-789.

80 Soehendra N., Werner B. New techniques for endoscopic treatment of bleeding gastric ulcer. Endoscopy 1976: 8; 85-87.

81 Soper H.W. The treatment of hematemesis by retention catheter. J.A.M.A. 1931; 97: 771-775.

82 Spellberg M. Emergency upper G.I. endoscopies. in Ethical Problems in the Management of Gastroenterological Patients. F.Vilardell (ed) Scand J Gastroenterol 1977;12 (suppl 47) 19-20.

83 Vilardell F. Les hémorragies et les perforations des ulcères gastroduodénaux et leurs traitements. Rev de Med (Paris) 1966; 7: 851-867.

84 Villanueva C., Balanzó C. A practical guide to the management of bleeding ulcers. Drugs 1997;53: 389-403.

85 Walters W. Discussion. Proc. Staff Meet Mayo Clin. 1933; 8: 163-165.

86 Watkinson G. Use of Sengstaken balloons. in Ethical Problems in the Management of Gastroenterological Patients. F.Vilardell (ed) Scand J Gastroenterol 1977; 12 (suppl 47) 39-41.

[87] Wangensteen O.H., Orahood R.C., Vorhees A.B. y cols. Intragastric cooling in the management of hemorrhage from the upper gastrointestinal tract. Amer J Surg 1963.; 105: 401-412.

[88] Westphal K. Über die Kompressions Behandlung der Blutungen aus Esophagus Varizen. Deutsch Med Wschr. 1930; 56: 1135-1136.

[89] Youmans C.R. Jr., Patterson M., McDonald D.F., Derrick J.R. Cystoscopic control of gastric hemorrhage. Arch Surg 1970; 100: 721-723.

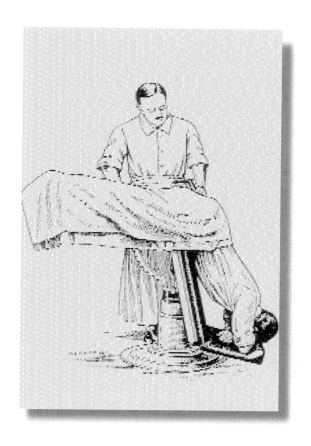

CHAPTER 10

The evolution of rigid rectosigmoidoscopy

INTRODUCTION

RECTOSCOPY WAS THE FIRST INSTRUMENTAL EXAMINATION EVER employed in gastroenterology due to the ease of insertion of instruments through the anal orifice and also because of the high incidence of anorectal disease. According to some historians, the introduction of specula in the rectum should be attributed to Egyptian physicians[29]. In many medieval Arab manuscripts and in Western sculptures such as capitals from Romanesque cloisters, scenes depicting physicians exploring the anorectal region of patients are often found.

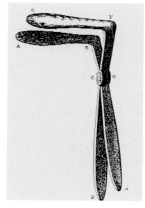

Fig. 1. Bronze anoscope from Roman times, found in Pompei (courtesy of the late Dr. J. Arán).

Schreiber[47] wrote that Hippocrates had employed some type of speculum to make anoscopies, and among objects found in the ruins of Pompei, there were instruments made of bronze, a very resistant metal, very similar to the bivalve specula of the 19th century *(Figs. 1, 2)*.

In texts from Arab medicine, various types of cannulae and specula are described and surgery of haemorrhoids was a relatively common practice at least since the 15th century[48]. At the end of the 19th century, the anus and the rectum were explored by means of specula and rigid tubes, simply using daylight or some kind of external illumination. However, the examination of the higher rectum and the sigmoid required longer and more complex tools. In German treatises of the 19th century, rectal endoscopy was named romanoscopy or recto-romanoscopy, from the name of the first rectal fold, the so-called "plica rectoromana"[16]. In other countries, physicians, gynaecologists, urologists and surgeons used the terms anuscopy and rectoscopy[29, 44].

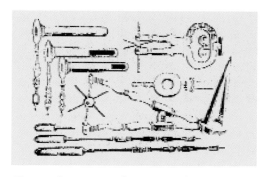

Fig. 2. Instruments for ano-rectal examinations apparently employed by Fabrizio d'Acquapendente. (courtesy of the late Dr. J. Arán).

According to Georg Gottstein (1857-1918), professor of medicine first in Breslau (today Wroclaw, Poland) and later in Berlin and the author of a comprehensive review of rectosigmoidoscopy published in the early years of the 20th century, but which unfortunately includes no bibliographic references[16], the American William Otis was the first to perform rectoscopy. However, Raoul Bensaude[5], a pioneer of proctology in France, stated that Howard Kelly, another American, was the first to show –in 1895– that a totally straight tube could be introduced as far as the rectosigmoidal junction.

After Bozzini, who invented an instrument with enough light to examine part of the urethra and the lower rectum, his successors also tried to visualise body cavities with their own devices. Thus the Frenchman, Pierre Salomon Segalas probably examined the rectum as Désormeaux and Sir Francis Cruise later did with their endoscopes (see Chapter 2). The main difficulty was to obtain sufficient light, although illumination of the rectum was easier than that of the narrow urethra to which urologists had dedicated so much effort. In Vienna we were able to see an "enteroscope", designed by Josef Leiter, the maker of the Mikulicz' gastroscope which is depicted in figure 18. It consisted of a hollow metal tube of small diameter and a thin rod to which a small recipient containing a platinum filament was distally attached. However, illumination was still too feeble to examine anything other than the rectal ampulla.

ANOSCOPES

The anoscope was the oldest instrument invented to examine the anorectal area; small metal tubes, with or without an obturator, bivalve specula and separating clamps may be found in many drawings from the most remote antiquity.

Current rigid endoscopes are more preferable for the examination of the anorectal region than fibrescopes. A few years ago, S.M. Kelly and associates[26] demonstrated that an anoscope may detect internal haemorrhoids, fissures and condilomas better than flexible sigmoidoscopes even when a good retrovision manouevre can be accomplished. Hypertrophy of anal papillae, a relatively frequent cause of bleeding, may also elude fibrescopic observation, which according to Kelly, may miss up to 20 percent of lesions in this area.

Anoscopes by Kelly and Bensaude: The first "modern" anoscopes were designed by Kelly[25] and Bensaude[5]. They were very similar: a short metal tube with a funnel-like distal end cut more or less obliquely. The instrument was provided with a handle and a round metal obturator to help in the painless introduction through the anal canal. External illumination was usually provided by a frontal lamp. Kelly's "sphincteroscope", made by Arnold in Baltimore[25], was conical in shape and 4 cm long (see figure).The diameter of the distal part attached to the funnel was 2.5 cm while the diameter of the funnel was 5 cm *(Figs. 3, 4)*. Bensaude's anoscope[11] was very similar and was made by Collin in Paris *(Figs. 5, 6)*.

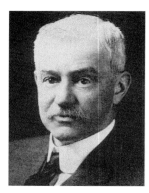

Fig. 3. Howard Atwood Kelly (1858-1943). Gynaecologist and proctologist, professor at Johns Hopkins University in Baltimore, a pioneer of rectoscopy (copyright unknown).

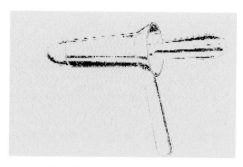

Fig. 4. The "Sphincteroscope", an anoscope by Kelly (1890), conical in shape and ending in a funnel (manufactured by Arnold in Baltimore)(ref.25).

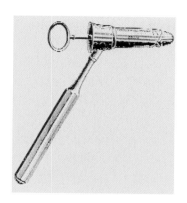

Fig. 5. Bensaude's anoscope made by the firm Collin, similar to Kelly's instrument. (Catalogue Collin, Maison Charrière, Paris 1903) (courtesy of Dr. J.Danón, Fundación Uriach).

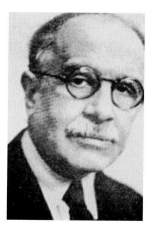

Fig. 6. Raoul Bensaude, the father of French proctology. (collection Dr. Jacinto Vilardell).

The technique of anoscopy was (and continues to be) very simple, such as Kelly described it in 1895: "the instrument is used by pushing it into the rectal ampulla and then slowly withdrawn until the sphincter circle closes well over it; by withdrawing it slowly and pushing it back a little, the whole sphincter area is brought beautifully into view".

Glass anoscopes: The anoscopes designed by two Americans, Hill and Roberts, were more sophisticated. Both were made of glass: Hill's anoscope[22] consisted of a straight glass tube with an oval window on one side. The distal end was round with another small window, which allowed insufflation. A similar instrument, also made of glass and including a side opening for therapeutic applications or probing suspected fistulae, was described by Roberts[45]. The advantage of these instruments was the large visual field provided by the transparent glass, avoiding mucosal prolapse which might occur in specula with blades (Figs. 7, 8).

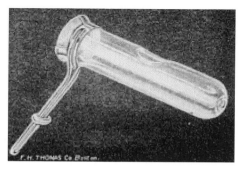

Fig. 7. T.C.Hill's glass anoscope (1906), featuring a lateral oval window. The blunted end had an orifice which allowed air insufflation (ref. 41).

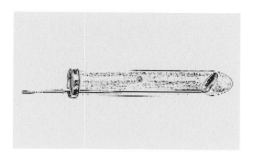

Fig. 8. Glass anoscope by Dudley Roberts (1910). A modification of Hill's anoscope, it included a rotating mirror which allowed complete examination of the rectal ampulla (ref.45).

ANAL DILATORS *(Figs. 9, 10)*

Other instruments that deserve mention are anal dilators, which allowed rectal examination in case of sphincter stenosis. Probably the first instrument of this kind on record was the paediatric speculum described by Bodenhammer.

These instruments were made of two blades and a double handle fitted with a dented wheel, a spring or a screw that would keep the blades opened. The most popular specula in the European continent were those of André Cain, recommended by Bensaude, and the dilators designed by Trelat, Noel Hallé and Nicaise, all made in 1900 in Paris by Collin, the successor of Charrière[11]. Kelly also designed a conical sphincter dilator featuring a scale graded in millimetres, from 20 mm at the distal end to 50 mm in its wider part, thus allowing to gauge the diameter of the dilation[25].

A more complex dilator was designed in Paris by Savignac[11]. The Spaniard Fermin Martinez[35] also described a light anal dilator featuring ondulated blades which made expulsion of the instrument difficult in case of rectal contractions due to intolerance to the examination *(Figs. 11, 12)*.

THE RECTOSCOPE

A rectosigmoidoscope is basically a hollow tube of a calibre appropriate for the width of the bowel. The first instruments were all made of metal, often chromated in their interior to favour the internal diffusion of light and with a scale in centimetres on the outside wall. The use of a magnifying lens was described by Gottstein as early as the early 20th century.

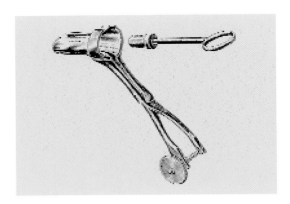

Fig. 9. Anal dilator designed by André Cain, recommended by Bensaude. (Catalogue Collin, Maison Charrière. Paris 1903) (courtesy of Dr. J.Danón, Fundación Uriach).

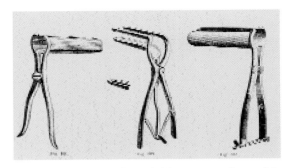

Fig. 10. Two types of rectal dilators manufactured by Collin in Paris. Trelat's dilator (left) and Nicaise dilator (right). (Catalogue Collin, Maison Charrière, Paris 1903) (courtesy of Dr. J.Danón, Fundación Uriach).

Soon after World War 1, rectoscopes made from plastics –especially bakelite– began to appear, particularly in the United States, and more recent developments include disposable plastic instruments[28]. Most rectosigmoidoscopes measure 25 cm in length and their external diameter varies between 1.5 and 1.9 cm[41].

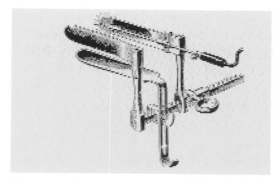

Fig. 11. Dilating anoscope designed by Savignac in Paris (Catalogue Collin, Maison Charrière, Paris 1903) (courtesy of Dr. J.Danón, Fundación Uriach).

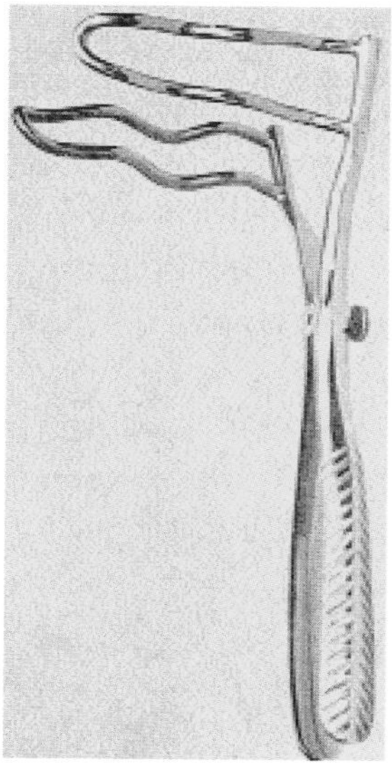

Fig. 12. Rectal speculum by Fermin Martinez (1918) (ref.35).

The first rectoscopes

The early French[5] and German[16] proctologists recognised that the rectoscope originated in the United States. Like the anoscope, the rectoscope, a longer version of the same instrument, consisted of a hollow metal tube, an obturator and an external source of light. Most instruments featured a scale graded in centimetres on the outside and their length was usually 25 cm. In many cases, light provided by a frontal mirror was reflected inside the tube in the same way as a laryngoscope or an oesophagoscope. In general, further progress was inhibited by the flexures above the rectum.

The presence of faeces in the bowel, the painful nature of the examination when anal pathology was present and also the uncomfortable kneeling position, which many patients (especially of the female sex) considered physically and psychologically degrading, were factors that impeded a rapid development of the technique.

Problems were also caused by the difficulty in achieving an adequate cleansing of the bowel in spite of the previous administration of enemata. Technical problems differed little from those encountered during oesophagoscopy, although the larger caliber of the rectum allowed the use of wider and better lit instruments without the difficulties involved in introduction through the pharynx.

Bodenhamer's rectoscope

William Bodenhamer (1808-1905), the leading proctologist in the United States in the 19th century[27], was born in Pennsylvania and he studied medicine at the Worthington Medical College of Ohio where he graduated in 1839. After working in several American institutions he soon specialised in proctology and finally established his practice in New York. He published several scientific books in which he criticised the procedures employed by his colleagues for the treatment of fissures, fistulae and haemorrhoids, and also wrote other popular works for the layman. As early as that time (in the mid-19th century), he recommended fibre-rich foods such as wholemeal bread and bran, as well as oranges, figs and prunes for the treatment of constipation, recommendations no different from those made one century and a half later. Bodenhamer designed various types of instruments, among them a long bivalve ano-rectoscope[8], a paediatric speculum for use in congenital anal stenoses[7] and the so-called "recto-colonic endoscope" (1863) which we will describe later as the first example of a semi-flexible rectoscope *(Figs. 13, 14, 15)*.

Among his publications, special mention should be made of his treatise on congenital malformations of the ano-rectal area, although his best known work was one on the physical examination of the rectum, with an appendix on haemorrhoid ligation[7]. His last publication on rectal atony appeared the year he died, 1905.

William K.Otis

Otis[53] was the son of the famous urologist Fessenden Otis and better known for his design of an optical system for cystoscopes which he designed together with Reinhold Wappler, the A.C.M.I. instrument maker[38]. He became interested in rectoscopy and also invented his own instruments for this purpose although his main interest was always urology[39].

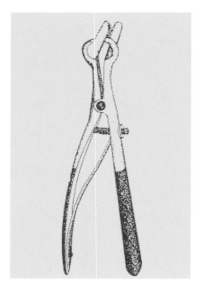

Fig. 13. Paediatric speculum-dilator designed by Bodenhamer (1879) (ref. 7).

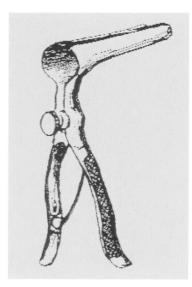

Fig. 14. Speculum-rectoscope by Bodenhamer (ref. 7).

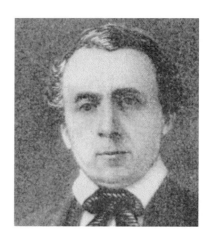

Fig. 15. William Bodenhamer (1808-1905), possibly the best known American proctologist in his time (from Pennington, ref. 41).

Kelly's rectoscope

As in many other instances, priority in the design of a rectoscope for clinical use was also given to another physician, Howard Kelly[24]. Kelly, was a gynaecologist but he was interested in digestive disease. He was a professor of gynaecology at Johns Hopkins Medical School in Baltimore and in 1905, among other publications, he wrote a book on appendicitis with beautiful colour illustrations. His first prototype (1895) consisted simply of a hollow metal tube provided with a handle and a blunt obturator[25]. Kelly's entire set consisted of: 1) a short rectoscope, 14 cm in length and 22 mm in diameter, 2) a long rectoscope (20 cm long and 22 mm in diameter) and 3) a 35 cm long sigmoidoscope, also 22 mm in diameter. All his instruments were provided with the same type of blunt obturator and a stout handle (*Figs. 16, 17*).

Kelly used sunlight as the means of illumination, but later preferred lighting from an external electric lamp placed near the sacrum. The light was directed into the rectum from the frontal mirror worn by the operator. A 42 cm rod fitted with a spoon served to eliminate faecal material, and another copper rod enveloped with cotton wool was used for cleansing the visual field.

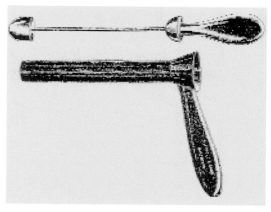

Fig. 16. Rectoscope by Howard A.Kelly (1895) (ref.25).

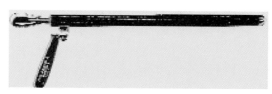

Fig. 17. Sigmoidoscope by Howard A. Kelly (1895). (ref.25)

INSTRUMENTS FEATURING INTERNAL ELECTRICAL LIGHT

A few years later, in the same way as in oesophagoscopy, frontal mirrors and external lights were replaced by internal lamps, placed either proximally or distally. Many clinicians and instrument makers devised "polyscopes" or "electroscopes" supplied with electrical light and to which several types of endoscopic tubes of many shapes and diameters could be fitted to examine either the larynx, the bladder or the rectum. The most popular were the electroscopes made by Joseph Leiter in Vienna, Gustave Trouvé in Paris or the panelectroscopes designed by Brünings, Schreiber and Levi, which are modifications of an original electroscope invented by Leopold Casper, a Viennese urologist who emigrated to the United States. A "light concentrator" ("Lichtkonzentrator") designed by Gottstein and provided with a prism placed beyond the window of the endoscope was used by some proctologists[16] (*Fig. 18*).

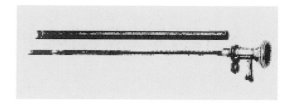

Fig. 18. "Enteroscope" designed by Joseph Leiter in Vienna. The light source was a platinum filament. (1880) (courtesy of the Institute for the History of Medicine, Vienna University).

Kelly's rectoscope, which was coupled to Casper's electroscope by Herzstein (Kelly-Herzstein rectoscope), became popular in Germany until Strauss presented his own instrument provided with a distal lamp.

Electrical anoscopes

Several instrument makers adapted a lighting system to their anoscopes. All models were similar in that they included either a distal lamp or a proximal illumination fitted to the handle of the instrument, generally a low voltage lamp such as a "Mignon" lamp. In the United States, the most widely used of these endoscopes was that designed by Hirschman[41] and modified by Pennington. It was lit by a lamp fitted on a rod which could be introduced through the anoscope. In France, the most popular anoscope was that designed by Hartmann[21] and manufactured by the firm Gentile (successor of Charrière-Collin); the lamp was screwed at the handle of the instrument *(Fig. 19, 20, 21)*.

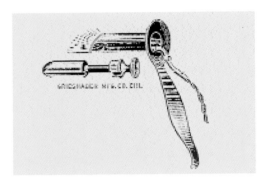

Fig. 19. Anoscope provided with electrical illumination designed by Hirschman and modified by Pennington (ref. 41).

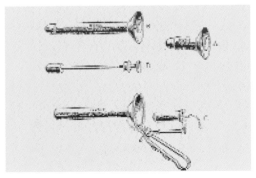

Fig. 20. Ano-rectoscope by Hartmann featuring distal illumination (1908). (Catalogue Collin, Maison Charrière, Paris 1903). (courtesy of Dr. J.Danón, Fundación Uriach).

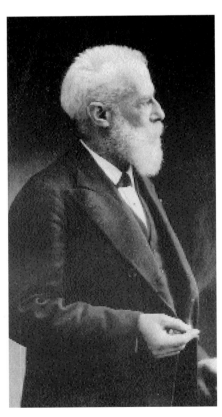

Fig. 21. Henri Hartmann, famous Parisien surgeon, specialised in rectal surgery, author of the rectal exclusion operation after colectomy (Hartmann's operation). (collection Dr. Jacinto Vilardell).

Electrical rectoscopes

Remarkably, the design of the rectosigmoidoscope has changed very little since the late 19th century, except for the fact that lamps have now been replaced by "cold light". This is provided by optical fibres following Hopkins' principles, widely used in laparoscopy (see Chapter 6). Current endoscopes are lit by optical fibre rods placed distally and controlled by a simple transformer. Cold light rectoscopes were introduced in Germany before the fibrescopes by the firm Richard Wolf. According to Waye[55], some metal models are practically indestructible, but they have recently been replaced by disposable plastic tubes. However, little by little they are also being superseded by fibresigmoidoscopes (see Chapter 11).

Trouvé's rectoscope: Among the instruments that the ingenious Trouvé manufactured, his rectoscope deserves a special place[16]. It was provided with a distal lamp (1903) *(Fig. 22)*.

Leone Levi's microendoscope: Among the numerous attempts to explore body cavities with electric light, Leone Levi's polyscope should be mentioned. He presented his instrument in 1904 in Madrid at the 14th International Congress of Medicine[31]. Leone Levi was born in 1861 in Genoa, Italy. He had multiple interests in medicine: he was professor of dermatology, but also specialised in venereal disease and otolaryngology. In 1890 he invented a technique for suturing the larynx *(Figs. 23, 24)*.

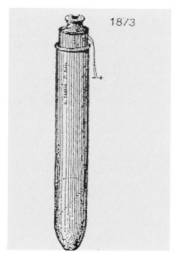

Fig. 22 Rectoscope designed by Gustave Trouvé featuring electrical lighting (1873) (from Trouvé's Manuel d'Electrologie Médicale, Paris, 1893).

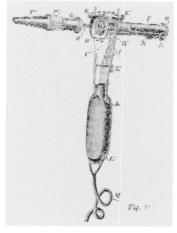

Fig. 23. "Microendoscope" designed by Leone Levi from Genoa (1903) which could be adapted to various types of endoscope, similar to the panelectroscopes by Casper and Brünings (ref.31).

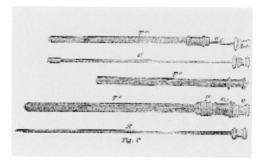

Fig. 24. Endoscopy tubes employed by Levi presented at the 19th International Congress of Medicine, Madrid, 1904 (ref.31).

His instrument was derived from Casper's electroscope and consisted of: 1) a metal piece which included two electrical lamps fed by the current provided by low weight accumulators controlled by a rheostat. A switch allowed the lights to be turned on and off; 2) a system of movable lenses which could be adapted to several focal distances; 3) an adapter fitted to the metal piece to which several tubes could be screwed according to the cavity to be examined.

The instrument was provided with a stout handle in which the electrical wires were fitted. The light source was external and magnifying lenses were also included in the instrument set.

Rectoscopes with distal light systems

Rectoscopes by Beach, Tuttle and Pennington: Again the matter of priority arises in regard to electric rectoscopes. In his well-known treatise on "Rectum, Anus and the Pelvic Colon", Pennington states that in 1899 he had shown a proctoscope provided with a small portable lamp which could be introduced in the distal end of the tube and that in 1901 Beach had published a rectoscope featuring a handle and an independent rod fitted with a distal electrical lamp which could light the visual field through a glass window to avoid soiling. However both the American and the European literature usually attribute the invention of the first practical sigmoidoscope with distal lighting to J.P.Tuttle[52] in 1902 *(Figs. 25, 26)*.

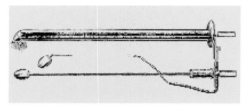

Fig. 25. Rectoscope by J.P.Tuttle (1902). Generally regarded as the first rectoscope with electrical lighting (ref.16)

Tuttle's rectoscope consisted of a metal tube provided with an obturator ending in a metal olive. The distal end of the rod of the obturator was flexible and could be bent to pass through the rectosigmoid junction. A channel which contained the electrical wires was attached to the outer surface of the endoscope. According to Pennington, Tuttle's instrument was quite similar to the one designed by Beach one year earlier. Therefore Tuttle's priority is quite dubious and can probably be better attributed either to Beach or to Pennington himself *(Figs. 27, 28)*.

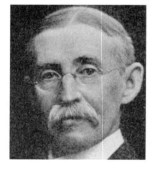

Fig. 26. J.P.Tuttle, well-known American surgeon and proctologist (ref. 41).

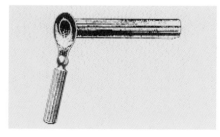

Fig. 27. The Beach rectoscope which according to Pennington, antedated that of Tuttle (1901) (ref. 16).

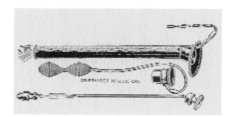

Fig. 28. Pennington's rectoscope, repeatedly modified since the first prototype from 1899. The instrument shown here probably dates from 1918 (see text for details).

Most instruments resembled each other: for rectoscopy, 12 cm tubes were used, while the longer ones (30-35 cm) served to examine the sigmoid colon. Most tubes featured a graded scale on their outer surface. Beach designed a glass covering to protect the lamp and to make sterilisation possible[4].

Pennington's rectoscope, which went through several improvements, consisted of a metal tube including in its wall an auxiliary channel which contained the light carrier. The instrument was provided with a perpendicular handle. The proximal end of both the endoscope and the obturator were bent one inch at an angle sufficient to permit the auxiliary tube to emerge outside the line of vision, which Pennington thought to be an advantage. It was made by the firm Grieshaber from Chicago.

Brünings rectoscope: As well as an electroscope and an oesophagoscope which became very popular, Brünings also designed a rectoscope. This was made in several lengths but featured a single long obturator which could be employed with all the different rectoscopes. Once the obturator was withdrawn, a glass window was screwed onto the proximal end to permit insufflation. The light source was his own electroscope[16] *(Fig 29, 30).*

The Strauss rectosigmoidoscope: Widely employed in Germany after 1903, it was the prototype on which the majority of instruments used in Europe were based[50]. It consisted of a graded hollow tube fitted with an insufflation balloon, a handle and an obturator ending in a metal olive, as well as a light carrier with a distal lamp. A glass window could be screwed on at its proximal end to avoid loss of insufflated air. The control switches for both the insufflation and the lighting systems were located at the head of the instrument. As opposed to Tuttle's endoscope where it was attached to the external surface, the light carrier was placed inside the tube. This arrangement was repeated in all rectoscopes from then on. The lamp was placed 2 cm inside the end of the rectoscope to avoid obstruction of vision by the faeces. A rheostat allowed control of the intensity of the light; Strauss insisted that his "cold light" never produced excessive heat, although the term "cold light" has today a very different meaning! The diameter of the tube was 2 cm for the sigmoidoscope and 2.5 cm for the rectoscope. Strauss also designed an eyepiece with a magnifying lens as well as another prototype featuring a prism which could transmit images to two tubes disposed as a V. This allowed simultaneous observation by two physicians and was very useful for teaching purposes[51] *(Figs. 31, 32).*

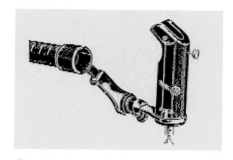

Fig. 29. Brünings' electroscope, employed by various endoscopists for rectoscopy as well as for other endoscopic examinations (ref. 16).

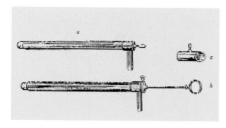

Fig. 30. Brünings' rectoscope could be easily fitted with the electroscope as a light source. It was manufactured in several lengths but with a single obturator (ref.16).

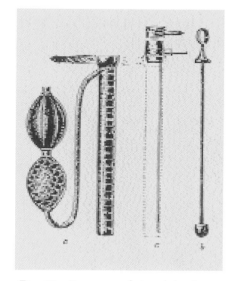

Fig. 31. Rectoscope designed by Strauss (1903), probably the most popular rigid instrument. It included distal lighting and a double balloon for insufflation (ref.50).

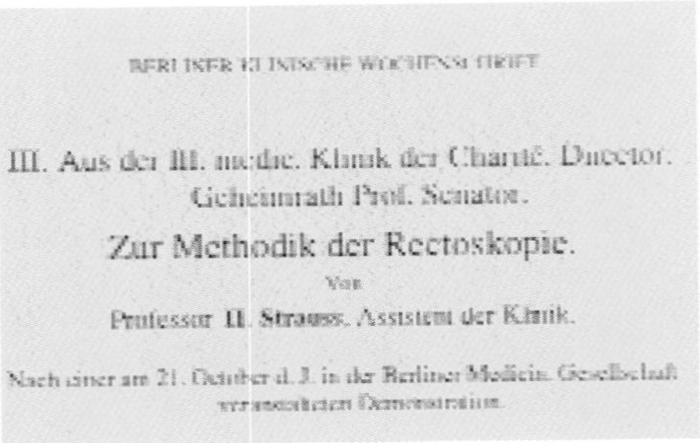

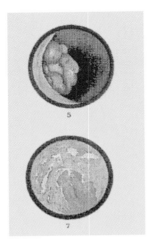

BERLINER KLINISCHE WOCHENSCHRIFT

III. Aus der III. medic. Klinik der Charité. Director.
Geheimrath Prof. Senator.

Zur Methodik der Rectoskopie.

Von

Professor H. Strauss, Assistent der Klinik.

Nach einer am 21. October d. J. in der Berliner Medicin. Gesellschaft
veranstalteten Demonstration.

Fig. 32. Heading of the main paper by Strauss on rectoscopy (1903).

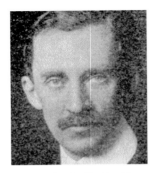

Fig. 33. Drawings published by Lockhart-Mummery using a modified Strauss rectoscope and presented at the London Clinical Society in 1905. Above, sigmoid carcinoma, below, ulcerative colitis (ref. 32).

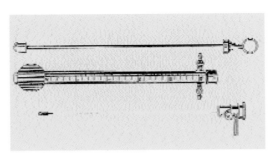

Fig. 34. J. P. Lockhart-Mummery, famous British proctologist and the first of a dynasty of specialists (ref. 41).

Hermann Strauss[18] was born in Heilbronn in 1868. He studied in Berlin and worked as Oberartz for 10 years in the university clinic of the famous internist Hermann Senator (1843-1911) at "La Charité" in Berlin. In 1910, he was appointed chief of internal medicine at the Jewish Community Hospital in Berlin. His last known publication, before the advent of Nazism, is dated 1928. He died in the Theresienstadt concentration camp in 1944. His instruments were manufactured by the firm of Louis and Heinrich Loewenstein, both of whom also disappeared during the Nazi era.

Lockhart-Mummery's rectoscope: This instrument was described by P. Lockhart-Mummery on the 27 January 1905 at a session of the Clinical Society of London. The author acknowledged that it was a modification of the Strauss rectoscope. With his tube, Lockhart-Mummery could examine "every inch of the mucous membrane from the anus to the middle of the sigmoid flexure". He explored several patients in the Sims or knee-chest positions and succeeded in visualising cancerous lesions in the sigmoid colon. The instrument had a rounded edge to avoid damage to the mucosa during insertion. The presentation was illustrated by many projections[32, 33] *(Figs. 33, 34).*

Insufflation and "pneumatic" rectoscopes: Another important development was the routine use of insufflation to facilitate the progression of the instrument. According to Gottstein, the first to employ insufflation in endoscopy was the American gynaecologist J. Marion Sims who in 1848 had performed insufflation of the vagina to enlarge the visual field. There were heated discussions in regard to the safety of the technique and accidents such as perforations, were reported. However, in due time insufflation became an accepted procedure. It was done by means of a rubber balloon which allowed the entry of air. A transparent glass eye piece was screwed on to close the proximal end of the rectoscope, sometimes coupled to a magnifying lens. The rectoscopes featuring insufflation devices were called "pneumatic rectoscopes". An original variation of the standard pneumatic rectoscope was designed in the United States by Beer (1911). It consisted of a rubber bulb which was attached 1 cm from the end of the shaft of the tube. It could be insufflated after insertion of the rectoscope, not unlike an oesophageal dilator such as the Gottstein instrument (see Chapter 9). Beer's instrument, which apparently provided "controlled" insufflation, was not successful[41] *(Fig. 35).*

Fig. 35. The Beer rectoscope (1911) provided with an inflatable rubber sleeve attached to its distal end. The light source was a distal lamp on a light carrier, manufactured by William Wood & Co. (ref.16).

The Schreiber and Friedel rectoscopes: The rectoscope devised by Julius Schreiber[47] was similar in some ways to Strauss' instrument: it was 40 cm long and included an obturator with a conical tip featuring several grooves, as well as a graded scale with multiple perforations. The instrument was marketed in France by Collin under the name of Friedel's rectoscope[11] *(Fig. 36)*.

In addition to Tuttle's treatise of 1902[52], Schreiber's book, "Die Rekto-romanoskopie" (1903), describes the procedures followed in Germany in detail and is particularly valuable[47]. Julius Schreiber (1848-1932) was no doubt unaware of the achievements of American proctologists; he worked as an assistant in Naunyn's clinic[14] and spent most of his later life as professor of clinical medicine in Koenigsberg, where besides his recto-sigmoidoscope, he designed one of the first oesophagoscopes and a dilator for the treatment of achalasia (see Chapter 5).

Luys' rectoscope: This instrument was designed by the distinguished French urologist Georges Luys (1870-1953). It was derived from his own cystoscope. Luys was well-known as he had invented a "urine segregator" to separate urine from the two urethers during cystoscopy. His instruments were manufactured by Collin early in the 20th century. The entire set consisted of a graded metal tube 30 cm long provided with a metal obturator, a shorter instrument 18 cm in length, a 2 volt distal lamp on a metal rod carrier, a handle to which the tubes could be screwed, a glass eyepiece and two magnifying lenses[34] *(Figs. 37, 38)*.

Rectoscopy instruments were not cheap and the full Luys set as described in the Collin catalogue (Paris 1908) was priced at 185 FF, a respectable sum.

Montague's rectoscope: Another ingenious instrument was devised twenty years later by the American proctologist Montague (1926). It consisted of a hollow metal tube inside which another tube – which served as an obturator– carried the distal lamp fitted on a rod attached to the obturator. The inside of the tube was painted black to avoid the reflection of light. A lateral slit on the outside tube made therapeutic manoeuvres easier[36] *(Fig. 39)*.

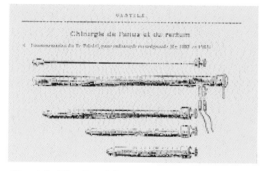

Fig. 36. The Friedel rectoscope manufactured in Paris by the firm Gentile (successors of Charrière), a French version of Schreiber's rectoscope (ref.11).

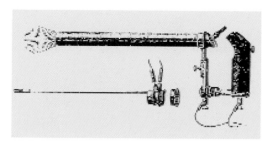

Fig. 37. Rectoscope by Bensaude with Brünings electroscope fitted in its handle (ref. 5).

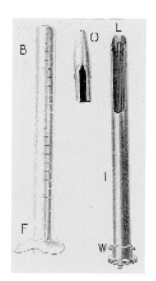

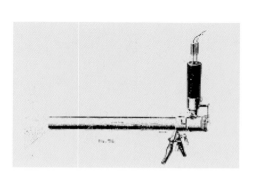

Fig. 38. Rectoscope with distal lighting designed by G. Luys and marketed in Paris by the firm Collin (1911).

Fig. 39. Montague 's rectoscope. From the left: the external tube, the tip of the obturator and the inner tube carrying the distal illumination (ref. 36).

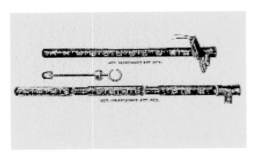

Fig. 40. "Telescopic" rectoscope designed by von Aldor, a gastroenterologist in Karlsbad (nowadays Karlovy Vary) (ref. 16).

"Telescopic" endoscopes

Another curious instrument which seems to be inspired by the early oesophagoscopes designed by Turck and by Waldenburg (see Chapter 5) was the Rubsamen instrument, manufactured by Heynemann in Leipzig. It consisted of a short rectoscope, 10 cm in length, for inspection of the rectal ampulla. A 30 cm thinner sigmoidoscope could be introduced into this. Heynemann also made a more complex endoscope, the "Stoeckle-Heynemann rectoscope", which included tubes of various lengths and diameters. Another rectoscope invented by Von Aldor, an internist from Karlsbad (now Karlovy Vary, Czech Republic), consisted of three different segments which could be fitted onto each other. The shorter instrument was introduced first, guided by an obturator, and the other segments were added successively as necessary to examine more distal portions of the bowel[1] *(Fig. 40)*.

Around 1911, a rectoscope provided with distal illumination was designed by Heinrich Stern and manufactured by Wappler[54]. It included a telescopic lighting system that could slide inside the tube. The distal end of the rectoscope was cut at an oblique angle, so that the lamp protruded from the lumen and provided better illumination.

Bensaude's rectoscope

According to Bensaude[5], three surgeons, Quénu, Duval and Hartmann were the first to employ a rectoscope in France. Raoul Bensaude, the most famous of French proctologists, published his first paper in 1907. He designed endoscopes 20 to 30 cm long with their lumen painted black. He also devised paediatric rectoscopes and some thin (10 mm in diameter) instruments for use in case of anal stenosis. He mainly used a rectoscope 25 cm long and 2 cm in diameter. He used two sorts of light sources: an external 12 volt lamp, coupled to Brünings' electroscope (see figure 37), or an internal lighting system consisting of a 3 volt lamp on top of a metal rod similar to the instrument used by Tuttle. Bensaude always controlled the intensity of the lighting by means of a rheostat. He usually examined patients in the knee-chest position *(Fig. 41)*.

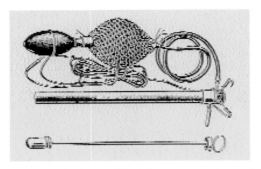

Fig. 41. The last model of the rectoscope designed by Bensaude in 1920, made by the firm Drapier in Paris, and provided with two coupled balloons, the larger one serving to control the rate of insufflation (from the Drapier & Cie catalogue).

First rectoscopy attempts with semi-flexible instruments

Bodenhamer semi-flexible rectoscope: Just like the oesophagoscopists who attempted to design semi-flexible instruments to pass the cricopharyngeal area, proctologists faced a similar challenge with the rectosigmoid flexure. Bodenhamer's instrument was 14 inches in length (35 cm) and its distal end was made up of flexible segments rather similar to the first "lobster-tail" oesophagoscopes devised by Störck in Vienna (see Chapter 5). A whale-bone obturator served to introduce a straight instrument, but after its withdrawal the distal flexible end could be bent and introduced further. A laryngeal mirror reflected the external light and allowed visualisation of the mucosa above the rectal plicae. The lighting system consisted of an external lamp and a lens, probably inspired by the early laryngoscopes[7] *(Fig. 42)*.

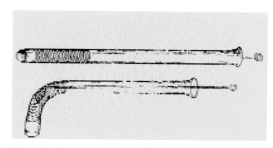

Fig. 42. Rectoscope by Bodenhamer with a flexible distal segment, featuring an internal mirror and external illumination (ref. 16).

Eduard Rehn's semi-flexible rectoscope: In 1921, the German surgeon Eduard Rehn designed a rectoscope featuring a typical "lobster-tail" flexible distal portion[42]. Rehn was the son of the famous surgeon Ludwig Rehn and father of another well-known surgeon, Jorg Rehn. Eduard Rehn was born in 1880 and retired in 1952[43]. He was appointed professor of surgery in Freiburg and became known mainly for his prophylactic treatment of postoperative venous thromboses with anticoagulants. His instrument was 40 cm in length and was lit by Brünings' panelectroscope. The flexible segments were longer than those designed by Bodenhamer *(Figs. 43, 44)*.

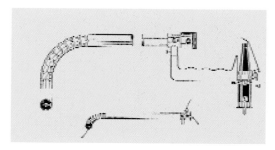

Fig. 43. Semiflexible rectosigmoidoscope designed around 1920, by Eduard Rehn (see text for details) (ref. 42).

Rehn led the way to flexible sigmoidoscopy[40] and to total colonoscopy as his technique for introducing the 40 cm instrument required the patient to swallow a silk thread which ended in a little glass bead before the examination. Rehn administered a laxative to the patient and usually 48 hours later the bead would appear through the anus. He would then attach the bead and the thread to his endoscope and in this way help its progression inside the bowel, as Italian gastroenterologists would do 50 years later when they attempted the first total colonoscopies (see Chapter 11). Rehn's instrument was used in France by Bensaude[5] but he thought that its use should be limited to patients who had a wide mesocolon which would not hinder the passage of the instrument.

Instruments featuring proximal illumination

Starting from 1920, rectoscopes featuring proximal illumination were more and more employed especially in the United States; their main advantages were the avoidance of the distal lamp, which easily became soiled, and the fact that if light

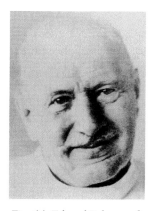

Fig. 44. Eduard Rehn, professor of surgery in Freiburg (Germany). Photograph taken towards the end of this life (courtesy Prof. J. Rehn).

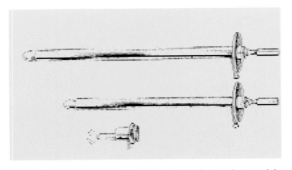

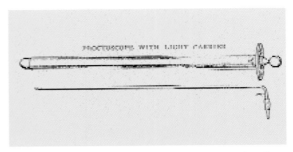

Fig. 45. Rectoscope with proximal lighting designed by Lyon-Bartle around 1925. Widely used at Dr. H.L.Bockus' clinic at the University of Pennsylvania Graduate Hospital (author's collection).

Fig. 46 Rectoscope made by the firm Wappler (later A.C.M.I.) with distal lighting to which proximal illumination could be adapted by means of Squier's electroscope (price of the set: $ 12.50 (Wappler Catalogue, 1918).

was powerful, the generated heat transmitted to the metal tube of the endoscope made the patient uncomfortable. Among these instruments one of the most popular was the Lyon-Bartle rectoscope[6] manufactured in two sizes, 25 and 30 cm, with a diameter of 1.5 cm. An instrument measuring 45 cm was also available to be used in patients with megacolon. This rectoscope was extensively used in Dr. H. L. Bockus' service at the Graduate Hospital of the University of Pennsylvania. It also included a simple eyepiece with a glass window and a lamp with a lens which was screwed onto the tube once the obturator had been withdrawn. The rectoscope was sturdy and easy to clean, and very useful for training endoscopists *(Figs. 45, 46, 47)*.

The so-called "Wappler set", marketed by A.C.M.I., consisted of a cystoscope, an urethroscope, an oesophagoscope and a rectosigmoidoscope, as well as a speculum for the examination of the ear[54]. All instruments shared the same lighting system provided by a proximal lamp, the "Squier light carrier". Wappler also made the Yeomans proctoscope which included a proximal lamp, introduced by an obliquely placed rod, and a rectoscope with an external light carrier similar to Tuttle's instrument[54].

THE TECHNIQUE OF RECTOSCOPY

Cleansing the bowel

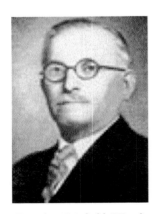

Fig. 47. Reinhold Wappler (1870-1933), born in Germany, founder of American Cystoscope Makers, he contributed decisively to the design and manufacture of all kinds of endoscopic instruments ("Wappler diagnostic set") (courtesy of A.C.M.I.- Zircon).

The prescription of clysters and enemata was known to the Egyptians, the Greeks and the Romans, and it is no wonder that early endoscopists tried to clean the rectum by means of enemata. Strauss recommended physiological saline solutions[5]. It has been shown that without an enema rectoscopy may fail in as many as 50 percent of cases[55] and also that the enema fluid will not modify the appearance of the mucosa[37].

Anaesthesia

The great majority of clinicians thought anaesthesia unnecessary, although in patients with painful anal lesions, Strauss recommended applications of 2 percent novocaine while other specialists favoured cocaine or eucaine. Gottstein thought that general anaesthesia and its accompanying risk should be used only in exceptional cases.

The position of the patient for rectoscopy

In his exhaustive review of rectoscopy, Gottstein commented that the first endoscopic examinations of the lower parts of the body were done for the diagnosis of urologic problems; no wonder that the first proctologic examinations were often made by urologists who positioned the patient as for a standard urologic examination.

The lithotomy position: Used by the first proctologists. The patient lay supine with the pelvis raised for anal inspection. However, introduction of any instrument longer than a simple anal speculum was difficult[16] *(Figs. 48, 49).*

The knee-elbow position: It is necessary to stress that this position, used by Kelly – chiefly a gynaecologist – was mainly used for inspection of the vaginal cavity. The patient was prone, resting on the knees and elbows as can be seen in many illustrations[25]. For many patients, especially the elderly, this position was rather uncomfortable. Nevertheless, French and German proctologists usually preferred this position, also popular in Spain and Italy. The greatest drawback was the difficulty in achieving a correct forward tilt of the pelvis which would allow the straightening of the rectosigmoid and thus the insertion of the tube beyond the sigmoid flexure. In addition to Kelly – who used to restrain the patient with leather straps – Schreiber and Strauss favoured the knee-elbow position.

The Sims position: The American gynaecologist James Marion Sims (1813-1883),who introduced endoscopic insufflation[3], generally employed the left lateral position, also preferred by Lockhart-Mummery and other British practitioners. This position is still used today, especially if the examination has to be performed on a hospital bed. The patient lies on his left side with the knees flexed and the buttocks well outside the edge of the bed (Bockus recommended

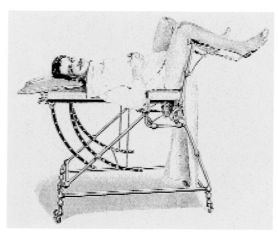

Fig. 48. The lithotomy position, the first to be employed by urologists for rectal examinations (ref. 16).

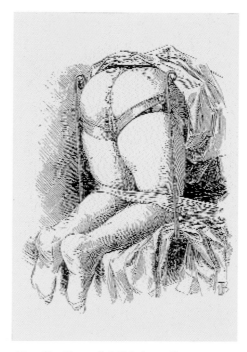

Fig. 49. Howard Kelly's knee-elbow position. The patient remains in place thanks to a strap fixed under her buttocks (ref.25).

a distance of 15 cm). This position was also often used in Germany by Gottstein *(Figs. 50, 51, 52).*

The Hanes "inverted" position: In his attempts to examine the large bowel beyond the recto-sigmoid junction, Hanes[20] found that the introduction of the sigmoidoscope was easier and better accepted by the patients if they were tilted forwards, to allow the descent and the straightening of the colon. The position was first used in 1906 by Hanes and his associate Mathews. Granville Hanes was a professor of ano-rectal disease at the University of Louisville (Kentucky). He designed a table that could be tilted and which became very popular in the United States. Other tables of this type allowed tilting of the patient to the point where the head almost touched the ground. Until the advent of fibrescopy, this table was used extensively in the United States and in particular at the University of Pennsylvania. The patient's position can be seen in fig. 53 (not all patients found it comfortable!) *(Fig. 53).*

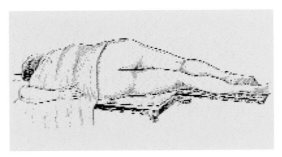

Fig. 50. The Sims lateral position used among others by Gottstein and by British proctologists (ref.16).

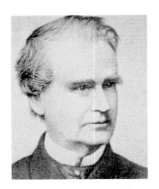

Fig. 51. Marion Sims (1813-1883), a distinguished American gynaecologist, the first to use vaginal insufflation, leading the way to rectal insufflation procedures (courtesy the late Dr. J.Arán).

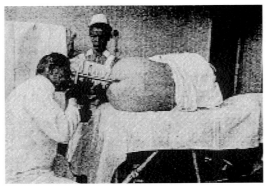

Fig. 52. Gottstein performing a rigid sigmoidoscopy in the lateral position (ref.16).

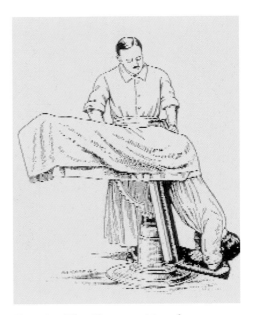

Fig. 53. The Hanes position for rectoscopy (1908), widely used in the United States. The patient kneels and is then tilted forwards. (ref.20).

Practitioners have been using rigid sigmoidoscopy less over the last 30 years as examination is often impossible beyond the rectosigmoid junction no matter which manoeuvres are attempted. Shatz and Freitas[49] showed that a 25 cm rectosigmoidoscope may be inserted as far as the sigmoid but no further. Flexible sigmoidoscopy is better tolerated, and in the majority of instances it may reach a distance between 45 and 60 cm. By means of clips left in the most distant area examined, Lehman[30] showed that if a distance of 60 cm is reached the entire sigmoid colon may be explored in 81 percent of cases. It is no wonder that in many institutions rigid sigmoidoscopy has been entirely replaced by fibrescopy except for the examination of the anorectal region.

Accessory devices

Pennington and Strauss used two coupled rubber balloons of the same size for insufflation, while Bensaude also employed two balloons although one was much larger than the other, apparently for better control of insufflation *(Fig. 54)*.

A rectoscopy set comprised several rods wrapped with cotton wool for cleansing, metal probes used for dilation, and several types of clamps and pincers to extract foreign bodies, such as hardened faecal material, or to take biopsies. Gottstein's biopsy clamp was widely used for oesophagoscopy as well as for sigmoidoscopy; another clamp covered by a rubber sheath was used for the extraction of foreign bodies.

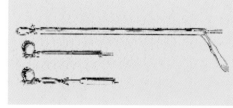

Fig. 54. Diathermy loop by Arthur Foges for the excision of polyps (1911) (ref. 15).

Polypectomies and the cauterization of tumours

Polypectomies were first carried out at the end of the 19th century, almost as soon as the first rectoscopes appeared on the market. Several types of clamps were used for biopsy as well as for the excision of small polyps[17]. Possibly Kelly was the first to employ dentated pincers, clamps and scissors to treat small lesions *(Figs. 54, 55)*. He also described galvano-cauterization with metal loops for the excision of pedunculated polyps. Similar devices were employed at the Mayo Clinic by Louis Buie[10], who used to leave in place a metal loop screwed to a clamp which remained "in situ" for 24 hours. The clamp was then unscrewed and the polyp usually fell off and was expelled two or three days later. Schreiber recommended using a thermocautery, Gottstein an electrocoagulation probe with high frequency current, and Foges, author of a well-known book on rectoscopy, a diathermal loop attached to a rectoscope. Foges' device was widely used in Germany[15, 16].

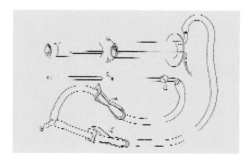

Fig. 55. Instruments for polyp fulguration employed by Louis Buie at the Mayo Clinic (ref. 41).

Photography through the rectoscope

According to Gottstein, photography of the rectum was first done around 1903 by Sabatschnikov and Fedorov in Russia. I have been unable to find any information about Sabatschnikov, but the Soviet Encyclopaedia describes Sergei Petrovich Fedorov (1869-1936) as a professor of surgery at the Medical Academy at St.Petersburg. He is mentioned as a consultant in some correspondence between Czar Nicholas II and the Empress that can be found on the Internet. Although his publications are mostly in Russian, in a paper that appeared in 1898 in the Proceedings of the German Society for Surgery, Fedorov (listed as von Fedorov) described his own rectoscopic technique and mentioned the usefulness of photography[13]. In Germany, Strauss used a photographic camera to document his findings. Much later, around 1930, Bensaude in France designed a photorectoscope manufactured by the firm S.F.O.M. Fifty years later the introduction of quartz rods and glass fibres as light carriers made photography an easily available procedure. The cameras made by the firm Wolf in Germany were widely employed in Germany. A rectoscope made by Fourès for Charles Debray in Paris with the Fourestier lighting system consisting of a very potent 150 volt lamp and quartz rods as light carriers, provided pictures of outstanding quality[12] (see Chapter 8). In 1966, coloured pictures taken with several prototypes of fibre rectosigmoidoscopes were presented[56] at the First World Congress of Digestive Endoscopy in Tokyo (Fig 56, 57, 58, 59).

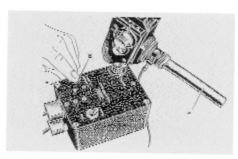

Fig. 56. Bensaude's photorectoscope made by S.F.O.M. (around 1950).

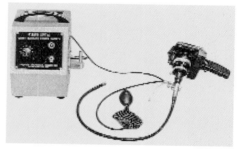

Fig. 57. Fibre optics rectoscope shown at the first World Congress of Endoscopy (Tokyo 1966).

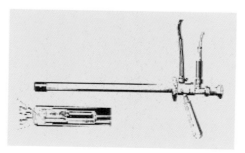

Fig. 58. Cold light photorectoscope (1969) manufactured by the firm Richard Wolf in 1969 (courtesy of the firm R.Wolf).

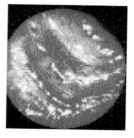

Fig. 59. Picture obtained with the cold light Fourestier-Fourès photorectoscope at the Hospital de Sant Pau.

RISKS AND ACCIDENTS

Risks of rectoscopy: As all rigid rectoscopes have very similar features and are used in the same way, the statistical data of most publications allow valid comparisons. In his writings, Foges stated that he had performed over 4,000 rectoscopies without accidents[15]. Gottstein insisted that accidents of rectosigmoidoscopy were few and that he had personally experienced no accidents in more than 1,000 such examinations. However, at that time (towards the end of the 19th century), cases of perforation were reported due to the insertion of the instrument with undue pressure, during therapeutic manoeuvres or because of excessive air insufflation. Lockart-Mummery, Strauss and others documented perforations due to the excessive penetration of the obturator or to uncontrolled insufflation. Schreiber reported a case of perforation after polypectomy.

According to the American Medical Association[2], rectosigmoidoscopy is a procedure with very little risk. Between 1925 and 1934, Louis Buie's team at the Mayo Clinic performed 41,475 rectoscopies. No significant problems occurred in 91 percent up to 25 cm. using a 1.5 cm diameter tube. By 1945, at the Graduate Hospital in Philadelphia, Dr.H.L. Bockus and associates had done more than 75,000 rectosigmoidoscopies without major mishaps[6].

In a series compiled years later, Bolt[9] described 5 cases of bowel perforation among 172,351 examinations, and in another series published by the Mayo Clinic, Jackman[24] reported 4 perforations in 350,000 examinations. In three of these cases, perforation occurred in areas of the sigmoid which had been previously resected and anastomosed.

In a review published in 1977, Hafter[19] assessed the risk of perforation by sigmoidoscopy as between 0.2 and 0.006 percent. According to Hafter, the incidence of perforations after polypectomy was around 0.3 percent.

In recent years, the frequency of perforation after rigid sigmoidoscopy has been calculated to be between 1/10,000 and 1/20,000 examinations, while that of flexible sigmoidoscopy is around 1/5,000[55].

REFERENCES

[1] Aldor L. von. Über die Aetiologie und die Behandlung der Hemorroidenblütung. Med Klinik 1914; 10: 637-641.

[2] A.M.A. Diagnostic and therapeutic technology assessment. Rigid and flexible sigmoidoscopies. J.A.M.A. 1990; 264: 89-92.

[3] Bailey, H., Bishop W.J. Notable Names in Medicine & Surgery. 2nd edition. London, H.K. Lewis, 1946.

4 Beach W.M. A new proctoscope and sigmoidoscope. J.A.M.A. 1901; 36: 1783-1784.

5 Bensaude R. Traité d'Endoscopie, Paris, Masson, 1926.

6 Bockus H.L. Proctosigmoidoscopy. in Gastroenterology. Vol II. Philaldelphia, W.B. Saunders, 1946.

7 Bodenhamer W. The physical exploration of the rectum. New York, William Wood & Co. 1870.

8 Bodenhamer W. A theoretical and practical treatise on the haemorrhoidal diseases. Giving their history, nature, cases, pathology, diagnosis and treatment. New York, William Wood, 1884.

9 Bolt R.J. Sigmoidoscopy in detection and diagnosis in the asymptomatic individual. Cancer 1971: 28: 121-126.

10 Buie L.A. Practical Proctology. Philadelphia, W.B. Saunders, 1926.

11 Collin. Maison Charrière, Catalogue des Instruments, Paris 1908.

12 Debray Ch., Segal S., Leymarios J. Rectosimoidian photography and cinematography in colour with cold light. Proc. 1st World Congress International Society of Endoscopy, Tokyo 1966: 394-397.

13 Fedorov S.P. (von) Über Rektoscopie und einige kleinen operative Angriffe im Rektum. Verhandlungen Deutsche Gesell f. Chirurgie. Berlin, 1898; XXVII, pr2: 438-441.

14 Fischer I. Biographisches Lexicon der hervorzagenden Ärtze der letzten fünfzig Jahre. Berlin, Urban & Schwarzenberg, 1932.

15 Foges A. Atlas der rectalen Endoskopie. Berlin, Urban & Schwartzenberg, 1910.

16 Gottstein G. Die Rectosigmoidoskopie in Abderhalden E. Handbuch der biologischen Arbeitsmethoden. Abt IV, Teil 6/I 1920: 864-906.

17 Gumprecht F. Die Technik der speziellen Therapie. 4ª edition, Jena, Gustav Fischer, 1908.

18 Gurlt E. Biographisches Lexicon der hervorragender Ärzte aller Zeiten und Völker. Berlin-Wien, V.C. 1934.

19 Hafter E. Risks of sigmoidoscopy and colonoscopy in Ethical Problems in the Management of Gastroenterological Patients. (F.Vilardell ed.) Scand J Gastroenterol 1977; 12 (Suppl 47) 21-22.

20 Hanes G.S. A new position for the diagnosis and treatment of diseases of the rectum and sigmoid flexure. J.A.M.A. 1908; 51: 1134-1136.

21 Hartmann H. Proctoscopie et sigmoidoscopie. Arch Mal Appar Dig 1908; 11: 257-258.

22 Hill T.C. A Manual of Proctology. Philadelphia, Lea & Febiger, 1923.

23 Hillemand P., Bensaude A., Loygue J. Les Maladies de l'Anus et du Canal Anal. Paris, Masson, 1955.

24 Jackman R.J. Rigid tube proctosigmoidoscopy. In Berry LH (ed) Gastrointestinal Panendoscopy. Springfield (Ill) Charles C. Thomas 1974: 439-460.

25 Kelly H.A. A new method of examination and treatment of diseases of the rectum and sigmoid flexure. Ann Surg 1895; 21: 468-478.

26 Kelly S.M., Sanowski R.A., Foutch P.G. et al. A prospective comparison of anoscopy and fiber endoscopy in detecting anal lesions. J Clin Gastroenterol 1986; 8: 658-660.

27 Kleiner S.B. William Bodenhamer –early American proctologist. Am J Dig Dis Nutr 1934; 1: 601-603.

28 Kravetz R.E. A look back. Proctoscope. Am J Gastroenterol 2001; 96: 1918.

29 Lauridsen L. Laterna Magica in Corpore Humano. Svendborg, Isager Bogtryk, 1998.

30 Lehman G.A., Buchner D.M., Lappas J.C. Anatomical extent of fiberoptic sigmoidoscopy. Gastroenterology 1983; 84: 803-808.

31 Levi, L. Le applicazioni del microendoscopio nel campo della clinica medica generale. Comptes Rendus, XIV Congrès International de Médecine. Madrid, 1904: 752-759.

32 Lockhart-Mummery P. An instrument for the examination of the rectum and sigmoid flexure. (The electric sigmoidoscope) Transactions Clin. Soc. London 1904-1905: 38: 212-214.

33 Lockhart-Mummery J.P. The Sigmoidoscope –a Clinical Handbook on the Examination of the Rectum and Pelvic Colon. London 1906.

[34] Luys G. La rectoscopie. Clinique Par. 1907; 2: 487-488.

[35] Martinez F. Nuevo dilatador de ano. Arch Esp Enferm Apar Dig 1918; 1:107-113.

[36] Montague J.F. The modern treatment of haemorrhoids. Philadelphia, J.B. Lippincott, 1926.

[37] Niv Y. Enema preparation for proctosigmoidoscopy does not cause mucosal changes. Endoscopy 1990; 22: 199-200.

[38] Otis F.N. A description of the instruments and apparatus of the author, with directions for their use in operations of the genito-urinary organs, New York, Putnam and Sons, 1875.

[39] Otis W.K. Concerning the new electro-cystoscope N.Y. Med J 1905; 85: 625-628.

[40] Overholt B. Clinical experience with the fibersigmoidoscope. Gastrointest Endosc 1968; 15: 27.

[41] Pennington J.R. A Treatise on the Diseases and Injuries of the Rectum, Anus and Pelvic Colon. Philadelphia, Blakiston, 1923.

[42] Rehn E. Fortschritte in der Rektoskopie u. Sigmoidoskopie. Zentrbl. f. Chir 1921; 48: 1598-1601.

[43] Rehn J. Erlebte Chirurgie. Landsberg/Lech, Ecomed, 1997.

[44] Robert B., Roig y Bofill E. Enfermedades del Aparato Digestivo, Madrid, Biblioteca de la Revista de Medicina y Cirugia Prácticas, 1889.

[45] Roberts D. A new anal speculum. JAMA. 1910; 54: 124-125.

[46] Rosenheim T. Über die praktische Bedeutung der Romanoskopie. Berl Klin Wschr. 1905; 13 (Fest.Num): 11-14.

[47] Schreiber J. Die Recto-Romanoskopie, Hirschwald, Berlin, 1903.

[48] Segal A., Segal S., Willemot J. Originalité de la medecine arabe dans l'endoscopie spéculaire du corps humain. Proceedings of the XXIX International Congress of the History of Medicine. Sections A & B, vol 1. Cairo,1986: 268-277.

[49] Shatz B.A., Freitas E.L. Area of colon visualized through the sigmoidoscope. J.A.M.A. 1954;156: 717-719.

[50] Strauss H. Zur Methodik der Rectoskopie. Berlin Klin Wschr. 1903; 48: 1100-1104.

[51] Strauss H. Erfahrungen über die Endoskopie der Flexura Sigmoidea. Berl Klin Woschr 1905; 13: 1137-1142.

[52] Tuttle J.P. A Treatise of Diseases of the Anus, Rectum and Pelvic Colon, London, Henry Kimpton, 1903.

[53] Valentine F.C. William Kelly Otis. Centralblatt Harn und Sex organe 1906; 17: 592.

[54] Wappler R. Catalogue of the Wappler Electric Manufacturing Co. No 2, 1918.

[55] Waye J.D. Colonoscopy and proctosigmoidoscopy. in Bockus Gastroenterology, 5th edition, W.S. Haubrich, F. Schaffner, J.E. Berk (eds) vol.1, Philadelphia, WB Saunders 1995: 316-330.

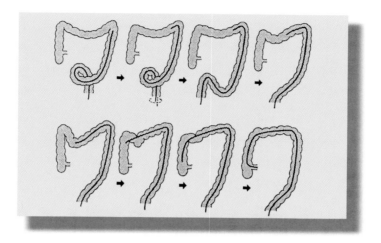

CHAPTER 11

The development
of fibrecolonoscopy

T̲HE GROWING ENTHUSIASM FOR FIBREOPTIC ENDOSCOPY AMONG gastroenterologists soon induced them to attempt examining the colon in the same fashion as the oesophagus and the stomach, especially after the appearance, of the first fibrescopes with frontal vision, such as that designed by Hirschowitz in 1963. The first colonoscopes were short and quite difficult to handle, but soon instrument makers in the United States (Eder, A.C.M.I.) and Japan (Machida, Olympus) began to manufacture prototypes of flexible sigmoidoscopes to replace the more dangerous and unpleasant rigid instruments that could seldom reach further than 30 cm (see Chapter 10).

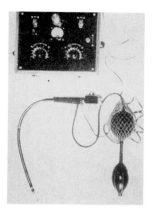

Fig.1 First sigmoidocamera designed by F. Matsunaga. Presented at the First World Congress of Gastroenterology (Washington 1958) (courtesy of Olympus Inc)

THE SIGMOIDOCAMERA, A COLONIC GASTROCAMERA

Stimulated by the success of the gastrocamera around 1950, the firm Olympus developed a similar model for photography of the colon. The main promoter of this new technique was Professor Fujio Matsunaga of Hirosaki University who presented the first prototype which was a modification of the type II gastrocamera in 1958[19]. The method consisted of inserting first a rigid sigmoidoscope and then introducing the "sigmoidocamera" into its lumen with the aim of taking pictures beyond the distal end of the metal tube (in his publications, Matsunaga uses also the term "cavocamera" for his device). The first models manufactured by Olympus were shown by Matsunaga during the First World Congress of Gastroenterology (Washington, 1958). They were 75 cm long and the films employed were Anscochrome-Tungsten *(Figs 1, 2)*.

The instrument could only be employed to take pictures of areas of the colon that could be seen through the rigid sigmoidoscope or a little beyond it. Some years later, between 1960-1970, other prototypes were manufactured. These were 1.5-2 m long and 5 mm in diameter. Although these instruments were considerably longer, Matsunaga succeeded in photographing the distal colon in only 22 percent of cases *(Figs. 3, 4, 5)*.

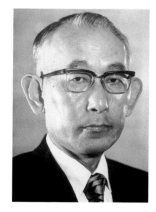

Fig. 2. Fujio Matsunaga, professor at Hirosaki University (Japan) (courtesy of Prof. Keiichi Kawai).

223

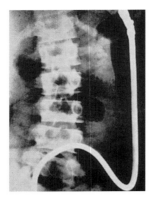

Fig. 3. Radiograph of Matsunaga's sigmoidocamera in the splenic angle of the colon (courtesy of Olympus Inc.).

Around 1960, Professor Hirohumi Niwa and associates[26] developed a new type of sigmoidocamera based on the gastrocamera type V. With this device they were able to take pictures up to the splenic flexure and for the first time, they suggested the possibility of reaching more proximal segments of the colon. Although the Niwa sigmoidocamera type II had greater manoeuverability, technology progressed rapidly and Olympus soon manufactured the sigmoidocamera type III. This model was introduced under fluoroscopic control and did not require insertion through a rigid endoscope. However, pictures were often of poor quality due to the presence of faecal material, the narrow lumen of the colon and the limited number of exposures available. After 1966, Niwa, as well as Matsunaga, abandoned the sigmoidocamera for the first fibrecolonoscopes which could be coupled to an external photographic camera[27] (Figs. 6, 7, 8).

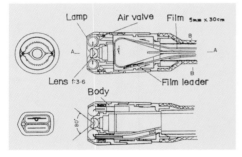

Fig. 4. Drawing of Matsunaga's sigmoidocamera, very similar to a gastrocamera. The lens, the two distal lamps and the film loader are well seen (1966) (courtesy of Olympus Inc.).

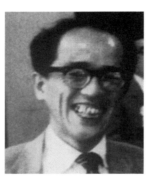

Fig. 5. M. Sugiura, engineer of the Olympus firm, one of the leaders in the manufacturing of the gastrocamera and the sigmoidocamera (courtesy of Olympus Inc.).

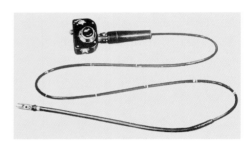

Fig. 6. Sigmoidocamera by Niwa (Olympus). Presented at the First World Congress of Endoscopy (Tokyo, 1966) (courtesy of Prof. H. Niwa).

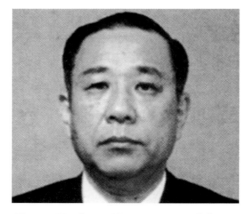

Fig. 7. Hiruhomi Niwa, pioneer of the sigmoidocamera and of colonoscopy in Japan (courtesy of Prof. H. Niwa).

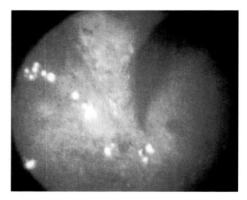

Fig. 8. Picture obtained with Niwa's coloncamera. Ulcerations and erosions in the sigmoid colon compatible with the diagnosis of ulcerative colitis (courtesy of Prof. H. Niwa).

THE FIRST ATTEMPTS AT COLONOSCOPY IN THE UNITED STATES

In 1963, Robert Turell, a well-known New York proctologist, designed several instruments for sigmoidoscopy including optical fibres. He first developed a standard rectoscope coated inside with rigid fibre bundles which transmitted a powerful light along the shaft of the instrument and provided excellent illumination of the bowel mucosa. He also designed a rectoscope with a proximal lighting system using external fibre bundles[38]. Finally, he adapted the A.C.M.I. oesophago-gastroscope to colonoscopy succeeding in some instances to inspect the bowel beyond the sigmoid flexure (Fig. 9).

Also in 1963, Suzanne Lemire and A.E. Cocco[18] were able to visualise the left colon using a frontal view gastroduodenoscope, which we surmise was "sacrificed" for that purpose.

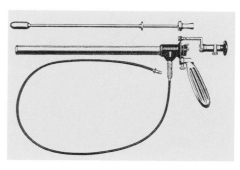

Fig. 9. Rigid sigmoidoscope designed by Turell, internally coated with optical fibres (courtesy A.C.M.I. - Zircon).

THE FIRST COLONOSCOPIES IN JAPAN

Other trials were made in Japan using standard oesophago-gastroscopes. In 1963, Oshiba and Watanabe tested the first colonoscope designed by the engineers of the Machida company. Meanwhile, using instruments designed by Olympus, Niwa[26] and Kazanawa[16] started collecting experience with other prototypes and presented their first findings in 1965. Unfortunately, none of these instruments or techniques reached the international recognition which they deserved as all the reports by these clinicians were published in Japanese.

In 1965, Niwa[26] developed the first prototype of colonoscope with the technical advice of the Olympus engineers. The visual angle of the lens was 35º and the tip of the endoscope was stiff and could not be bent. The instrument was quite rigid and insertion down to the descending colon was very difficult. Even in the sigmoid colon the distal end of the fibrescope remained stuck to the mucosa and vision was therefore often blurred. Moreover, when withdrawing the instrument, illumination was dimmed when the distance from the objective became too great[29].

The next prototype featured a prograde optical system which could be replaced at will by one with lateral vision, but the distal end of the endoscope had to be unscrewed each time that it was necessary to change the optical system. The instrument had little practical value and was never commercialised.

In 1966, the frontal optical system was replaced by a rotating prism with an oblique angle of deviation on the optical axis of 105 degrees and an angle of

225

vision of 40 degrees. A knob at the proximal end of the endoscope controlled the rotation of the lens. This allowed both a frontal and a lateral view without further manipulations. With this colonoscope, which was presented at the First World Congress of Digestive Endoscopy in Tokyo, Niwa's team achieved a satisfactory view of the sigmoid colon but the instrument was still rigid and difficult to introduce. Niwa then concluded that the colonoscope should be more flexible and that it should be provided with an oblique vision optical system. The result was a short colonoscope (1968), 67 cm long. It had a mechanism that allowed the tip to be flexed vertically and it was used to inspect the sigmoid colon[17]. Vision was slightly oblique (19 degrees) and the instrument was furnished with controls of the same kind as the oesophagoscope –already on the market. This colonoscope allowed a satisfactory and efficient view of the sigmoid colon, especially when considering that the majority of colonic tumours are located in this area[28].

The endoscope was later prolonged 25 cm. and the foroblique lens was replaced by a frontal one which was marketed as Olympus colonoscope SB. In the meantime, in 1968, Matsunaga designed another prototype with which he tried to visualise the right colon. This new instrument was 120 cm long and featured a tip that could be bent in all four directions (model CF-SB). It was tried, among others, by Dean in Edinburgh[8]. In 1970, a 200 cm long version of the instrument was manufactured. It was the predecessor of the LB colonoscope but introduction was still difficult and the right colon could be reached only in 10 percent of cases. In 1970, Yamagata designed another colonoscope which was produced by the Machida company. It was a modification of the duodenoscope made by this firm in 1967-1969 and the basis for the Machida colonoscope type VII which was 190 cm long and was marketed sometime later *(Figs. 10, 11)*.

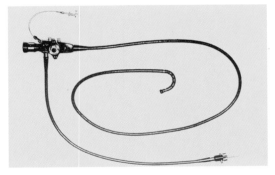

Fig. 10. Prototype of Matsunaga's colonoscope (1969) Presented at the Second World Congress of Digestive Endoscopy, Rome-Copenhagen, 1970 (ref. 20).

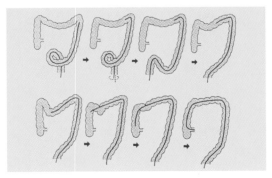

Fig. 11. Insertion of the colonoscope according to Matsunaga (1970) (ref. 20).

Matsunaga also designed another colonoscope for the firm Olympus[20]. Instruments improved gradually and in 1968-1969 models 2 and 3 of this colonoscope were introduced. The colonoscope was 2 m. in length and was provided at its distal end with a 2.5 cm pointed metal end, a mechanism for air insufflation and a canal for cleansing the distal lens with a water jet. The tip of the endoscope could be bent 120 degrees in four directions. The optics consisted of a fixed-focus system with a visual angle width of 60 degrees. The observation range was 5 to 70 mm. However, the passage of the instrument beyond the transverse colon was still very difficult and inspection of the ascending colon was possible in only 10 percent of instances. In 1974 the Olympus factory developed a colonoscope with a frontal optical system but a 30º oblique lens; the endoscope was of variable stiffness and greater flexibility in the distal segment.

This colonoscope was a great improvement over previous models, yet progress was much slower than in upper digestive endoscopy. This was mainly because of the peculiar anatomical structure of the large bowel with its plicae and flexures, and also because the greater diameter of the bowel lumen caused many difficulties in orientation and handling. Unfortunately, as the procedure was done blindly, the fibrescope could bent and twist over its own axis and even form a complete loop at its distal end making manipulation impossible. All these problems required much greater technical skill than that required for oesophago-gastroscopy.

It seemed obvious that colonoscopy required a meticulous anatomical and functional study of the colon in order to conform the instrumental technique to the special configuration of the bowel. This is what Bergein Overholt did.

THE SIGMOIDOSCOPES OF BERGEIN OVERHOLT

It is curious that the most significant contributions to the early history of fibrescopy, whether of the upper or the lower digestive tract, originated in the Department of Medicine at the University of Michigan at Ann Arbor. We have already discussed the role of Basil Hirschowitz[15], then a fellow in the Gastroenterology Service run by Marvin Pollard, in starting fibre oesophago-gastroscopy in collaboration with the Optics Institute of the University and the A.C.M.I. engineers. Similar circumstances developed in regard to colonoscopy. As Overholt himself explains in "The History of Colonoscopy"[31], four years after the first fibre gastroscopy performed there, in 1961, Bergein Overholt –a medical intern in the medical department –applied for a fellowship at the Public Health Service. He was interviewed by Dr. Howard Gowen who complained that that same morning he had undergone a very unpleasant and painful rigid sigmoidoscopy. Overholt was aware of the developments of fibrescopy and discussed with him the need to design a "flexible sigmoidoscope" using the same principles that guided the design of oesophago-gastroscopes *(Fig. 12)*.

The Public Health Service awarded a grant to the firm "Optics Technology" of California whose president was no other than Narinder Kapany, Hopkins' associate in the development of fibreoptics, who had emigrated to the United States (see Chapter 6). The initial attempts at instrument design and development were unsuccessful as more information on the anatomy and configuration of the colon was needed for the optical engineers to develop the mechanical devices essential for producing a practicable prototype.

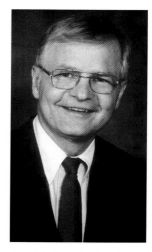

Fig. 12. Bergein Overholt, a pioneer of colonic fibrescopy in the United States (courtesy of Dr. B. Overholt).

Thanks to a research grant awarded to him by the firm Dow-Corning, Overholt was able to obtain the materials necessary to perform enemas of "silastic" foam, a mixture of silicones and a cathaliser which could be injected into the rectum like a barium enema. The foam gelled rapidly and resulted in a soft and spongy cast of the rectosigmoid. It was easily expelled through the rectum by the bowel contractions. This method had been used unsuccessfully for diagnostic purposes as a complement of the radiological examination[5]. Overholt then made a reverse hollow silastic mould of the expelled solid silicone material, thus obtaining a real anatomic model of the lumen of the bowel in which fibre instruments could be inserted and tested *(Figs. 13, 14)*.

Although many firms seemed to be interested in the colonoscope, the first prototypes of flexible fibre sigmoidoscopes were developed by the Illinois Institute of Technology Research and the Eder company, which had considerable experience in rigid and semiflexible oesophagoscopes and gastroscopes. A series of technically difficult animal experiments preceded clinical testing of the instruments.

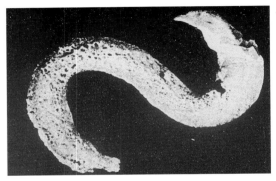

Fig. 13. Silicone foam cast of the sigmoid colon of the type used by B. Overholt to study the anatomy of the colon. From this a reverse silastic mould could be made in which endoscope prototypes could be tested.

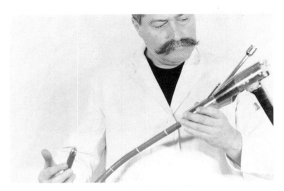

Fig. 14. Prototype of the flexible sigmoidoscope designed in 1963 at the Illinois Institute of Technology Research (courtesy of B. Overholt).

FEATURES OF THE OVERHOLT PROTOTYPE

The instrument designed by Overholt was 50 cm long. The external diameter was about 5/8 of an inch (16.5 mm). Fibre light bundles from an external light and an optical fibre bundle ran the length of the instrument. A 1 mm. diameter channel was used for insufflation or for washing and cleaning the distal lens. Another channel, 5 mm in diameter, permitted the introduction of tubes for aspiration as well as biopsy clamps made at the Illinois Institute of Technology Research. The sigmoidoscope was equipped with knobs at its proximal end to provide some control of the tip on the instrument *(Figs. 15, 16)*.

In February 1966, at the Veterans Hospital at Ann Arbor, Overholt was the first to use colonoscopy to confirm the presence of a sigmoid carcinoma previously suspected by radiological examination. Like others before him, Overholt employed a rigid sigmoidoscope as a guide for the introduction of the fibrescope beyond 25 cm. A comparative study with the rigid sigmoidoscope later revealed that this instrument reached the distance of 25 cm in only 45-50 per cent of cases, while the fibrescope reached 25 cm in 80 percent of the same patients and at least 30 cm

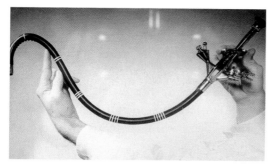

Fig. 15. Flexible fibresigmoidoscope (phase II) designed by B. Overholt and the engineers of the Eder company (1963) (courtesy of Dr. B.Overholt).

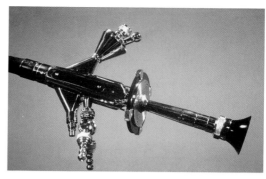

Fig. 16. Close view of the 1966 Eder sigmoidoscope (Phase II) (courtesy of Dr. B.Overholt).

of the colon could be inspected in 40 percent. In May 1967 the first series of patients studied with the flexible sigmoidoscope was presented at a meeting of the American Society for Gastrointestinal Endoscopy and published the following year in the Society's journal[30]. While there were many skeptical gastroenterologists with doubts about the value of the new instrument, there were at least as many enthusiasts. In the course of time the optimism of the latter was confirmed *(Fig. 17)*.

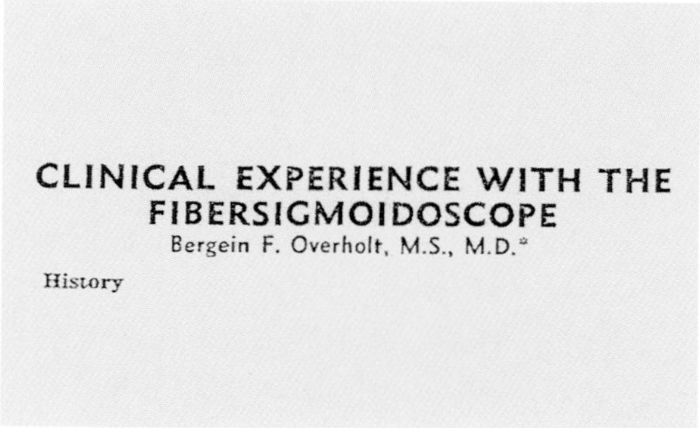

CLINICAL EXPERIENCE WITH THE FIBERSIGMOIDOSCOPE
Bergein F. Overholt, M.S., M.D.[a]

History

Fig. 17. Heading of the first paper by Overholt on flexible sigmoidoscopy (1968).

TOTAL COLONOSCOPY BY TRANSINTESTINAL INTUBATION

The anatomical structure of the colon with its plicae and flexures together with the similar flexibility of the fibrescopes meant progression of the instrument beyond the reach of a rigid sigmoidoscope was difficult. Flexible instruments bent, twisted and made loops causing problems that even today are not completely solved. Several clinicians attempted to use some kind of a guide to facilitate the progression of the colonoscope and the inspection of as great a length of the colon as possible.

Two Italian teams, working independently, came up with the same idea: the possibility of using a thin plastic tube or a strong thread as a guide for the progression of the endoscope. This would be attached distally to a weight which would be previously swallowed and which could be attached to the endoscope once it began to be expelled by the rectum. Torsoli and his associates[37] in Rome used the Blankenhorn tube[1] used to retrieve samples of intestinal contents. In 1964, they used this tube to obtain biopsies of the right colon by means of a Crosby-Kugler capsule[4]. Their technique consisted of having the patient swallow a thin

1.5 mm polyvinyl tube attached to a mercury bag. Once the bag appeared in the anus, traction was performed on the polyvinyl tube attached to the colonoscope so that the different colonic segments could be straightened in some way. The Roman clinicians controlled the progression of the colonoscope by fluoroscopy, employing an average of 5 very short exposures (about 20 seconds in all, 0.15 mA/per second). Their technique was reminiscent of that used by Eduard Rehn in 1920 to introduce his semiflexible metal rectoscope guided by a previously swallowed thread (see Chapter 10).

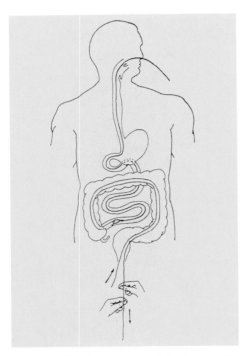

Fig. 18. The Provenzale and Revignas pulley traction and double intubation system to achieve total colonoscopy (ref. 32).

At around the same time, Provenzale and Revignas, working at Catania University[32], employed an original but more complex technique which apparently allowed them to perform the first total colonoscopy. They used the same type of soft polyvinyl tubes employed by Torsoli's team. They were rendered radiopaque by filling them with a liquid contrast medium. The tubing had two parts. The proximal segment was 4.5 m long and ended in a loop a few centimetres in diameter. The distal part was about 3 m. long and was threaded through the loop of the first tube and folded on itself so that it could be run through the loop in both directions like a pulley *(Fig. 18, 19).*

Transintestinal intubation was done by either the oral or the nasal route. When the first tubing had appeared through the anus, usually 24 to 48 hours later, the second tube was attached to its oral end. Intermittent traction on the tube emerging from the anus pulled the double tube downwards in an isoperistaltic direction. When both extremities of distal tube had appeared outside the body, one of them was pulled so that the colonoscope could be attached to the other end. Further pulling resulted in the antiperistaltic progress of the endoscope guided by the second extremity of the tube working like an intraluminal pulley. The loop through which the tubes were manipulated usually rested 30-40 cm above the ileocaecal junction.

AN ORIGINAL METHOD FOR GUIDED INTUBATION OF THE COLON

(Technique and Applications for Different Types of Transanal Examination of the Large Bowel)*

Luciano Provenzale, M.D., Antonio Revignas, M.D.

Fig. 19. Heading of the paper in English by Provenzale and Revignas on total colonoscopy (1969).

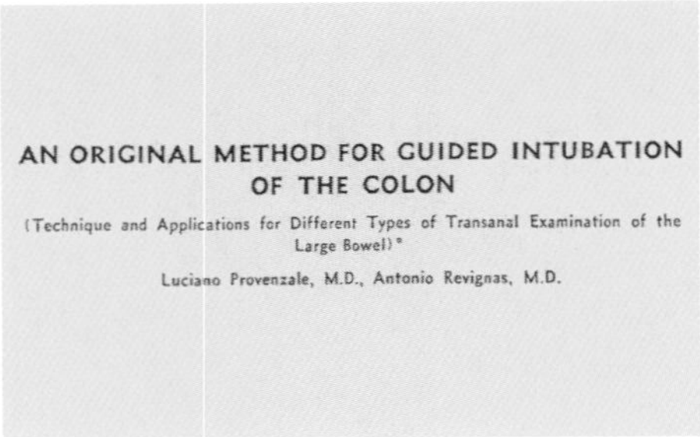

In 1969, Provenzale and Revignas published their experience based on 167 colonoscopies[33]. In 10 per cent of patients they could not penetrate through the rectosigmoid flexure and there were no accidents.

Other endoscopists, such as Deyhle, Ottenjann and other members of Demling's department in Erlangen[7, 8], as well as Fox in the United Kingdom, also employed transintestinal intubation. Fox[12] managed to perform colonoscopies up to part of the transverse colon by previously introducing a relatively large polyvinyl tube in the rectum under fluoroscopic control and then sliding a 7.5 mm A.C.M.I. colonoscope through its lumen.

RETROGRADE COLONOSCOPY WITHOUT GUIDING DEVICES

Little by little, improvements in the proximal control knobs of the colonoscope as well the increasing experience of the operators, who showed a considerable amount of patience, decreased the need for auxiliary devices and complicated techniques such as the ones that we have described. Colonoscopists, especially in Japan and Germany, succeeded in performing total colonoscopies, introducing the endoscope in the left lateral position with the help of only a guide wire to straighten the instrument and progress through the descending colon. Starting in 1969, other flexible sigmoidoscopes, manufactured by the firm Richard Wolf could easily reach a distance of 44 cm. One of the pioneers of this technique was Ewe[11] at Mainz University. He used a tube similar to the one employed by Fox[12] in 1969 *(Fig. 20)*.

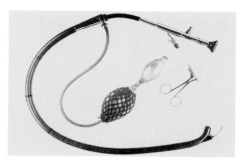

Fig. 20. Guiding tube for the introduction of the colonoscope according to Ewe's technique. Presented at the 2nd World Congress of Digestive Endoscopy in Rome-Copenhagen (ref. 20).

In 1970, this technique was employed by Demling's group. They used a long colonoscope[8] which enabled them to reach the middle section of the transverse colon in 93 percent of cases and the caecum in 80 percent of 59 patients. In 17 percent of cases they were able to penetrate through the ileocaecal valve. In 1970, Matsunaga and Tajima[20] had done colonoscopies in 188 patients; they succeeded in inspecting the transverse colon in 86 percent of instances, the ascending colon in 42 percent of cases and the ileocaecal region in 16 percent of patients. However, learning the technique was still difficult and the majority of endoscopists utilised fluoroscopy to push the endoscope through the colonic flexures and to avoid loop formation in the sigmoid. In 1970, Nagasako and his associates[22, 23] were able to visualise the ileo-caecal valve and for the first time, aided by deep abdominal palpation, they pushed a colonoscope into the terminal ileum in three patients. They employed a 2.13 metre long FCS colonoscope made by the Machida company, featuring prograde vision and a distal tip which could be bent in four directions. In 1971, the same authors described three types of ileo-caecal valve configuration: labial, papillary and intermediate[24] *(Fig. 21)*.

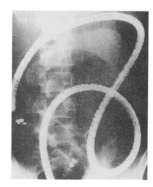

Fig. 21. Radiographic demonstration of the first total colonoscopy performed by Nagasako and associates in 1970. (courtesy of Prof. M. Classen, Editor of Endoscopy).

In 1970, the Olympus company presented its new colonoscope CM-FB with a movable four-directional tip. In 1971, Wolff and Shinya[44] examined 241 patients, without complications, using the colonoscope CF-SB and later the CF-LB from Olympus, and by 1972 they had performed more than 1,600 diagnostic colonoscopies. In 1972, at Saint Mark's Hospital in London, Christopher

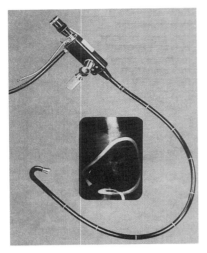

Fig. 22. Prototype of the A.C.M.I. F91S colonoscope (courtesy of A.C.M.I.-Zircon).

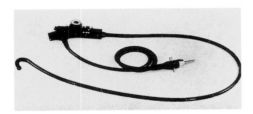

Fig. 23. Control knobs of the Machida FCS colonoscope (courtesy of Machida Inc.).

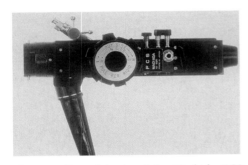

Fig. 24. Machida's FSW colonoscope of variable stiffness (courtesy of Machida Inc.).

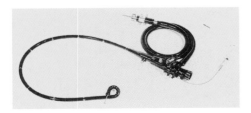

Fig. 25. Olympus CMFB-3 colonoscope featuring a very flexible tip (courtesy of Olympus Inc.).

Williams began to practice total colonoscopy routinely[40] and Jerry Waye did the same in New York[39]. The firm A.C.M.I., led at that time by Reinhold Wappler Jr., introduced the colonoscopes F9 and F1S with movable tips *(Fig. 22)*.

However, Japanese instruments slowly displaced other makers. Handling of their colonoscopes was easier because the disposition of the control knobs left the right hand free. According to Elewaut[10], this was necessary if manoeuvres such as biopsies were to be performed. On the other hand, image definition was better with the Japanese instruments because of the superior quality of the fibres employed.

The Machida colonoscopes FCS and FCS-W, of variable stiffness, were used extensively in Japan, while the Olympus colonoscope CMFB –3, which was even easier to handle, later became the most popular[2] *(Figs 23, 24, 25)*.

In 1977, image amplification provided by some Japanese prototypes allowed a 10-fold magnification of the colonic mucosa with a standard colonoscope and in 1979 it was possible to increase magnification 30-fold[36]. Colonoscopy became a widespread examination and today total colonoscopy is a standard examination that must be performed in all gastroenterology centres. The new endoscopes, such as the VS Olympus model of variable stiffness, will help in achieving total colonoscopy in all cases. However, some 25 percent of patients who undergo colonoscopy still find the examination unpleasant even after adequate deep sedation[21].

POLYPECTOMY WITH THE FIBRESCOPE

As already discussed in chapter 10, polypectomy was performed at the end of the 19th century with the appearance of rigid metal rectoscopes. Clamps and pincers of different types were introduced into the rectum to take biopsies and to excise small polyps. Gottstein, Kelly, Bouie and Schreiber employed diathermic loops and electrocoagulation for the removal of polyps.

Until the advent of flexible colonoscopy, the usual therapeutic rule consisted of endoscopically excising polyps below the rectosigmoid junction and to proceed with open surgery in polyps implanted above the junction unless a long sigmoidoscope could reach them and remove the growth if the polyps had a long thin stalk[3]. The emergence of colonoscopy has been hailed as extraordinary progress in the management of colonic polyps; the new instruments and the perfected techniques allow the treatment of the great majority of polyps by the endoscopic route without having to resort to surgical excision *(Figs. 26, 27)*.

The first colonoscopic polypectomies were performed in the United States and in Germany. In 1971, in their first paper on sigmoidoscopy, Wolff and Shinya[45] mention the successful removal of pedunculated polyps. Since then, Shinya's experience has possibly become the largest in the world. However, the first group to perform polypectomy in the right colon was that of Demling in Erlangen. In their first communication, also dated 1971, Deyhle[9], an associate of Demling', described how he introduced a 2.5 m. long flexible steel probe bearing a diathermic snare at the tip of the diathermic loop through the biopsy channel of either Machida or Olympus 2 m. colonoscopes. The snare was connected to an insulated handle of the colonoscope by means of a flexible wire. Wire and diathermic loop were incorporated in an insulated Bowden cable. By pushing forward a handle, the polypectomy snare protruded from the Bowden cable and opened to a diameter of some 3 cm. Polypectomy was performed after CO_2 insufflation to prevent methane-oxygen explosions in the colon due to the heat generated by the diathermy loop. In their first communication, they showed the results of 6 polypectomies, three of which were done on lesions of less than 1.5 cm of diameter in the proximal colon. In spite of the technological advances and the increasing experience of endoscopists, in 1983 it was thought that 2 - 5 per cent of polyps escaped endoscopic detection[25, 35]. Christopher Williams at London's Saint Mark's Hospital devised the so-called "hot biopsy"[41] for the elimination of small polyps which could be destroyed by electrocoagulation, while a portion of the tumour remained in the biopsy clamp, usually a sufficient amount for the pathologist.

By 1973, Wolff and Shinya[44] had carried out 1,500 colonoscopies and had endoscopically excised 303 polyps, varying from 0.5 to 5.0 cm in diameter, without mishaps (20 polyps were greater than 3 cm in diameter). By 1979, Shinya and Wolff[45] had performed more than 7,000 polypectomies, an awe-inspiring figure, and had established the efficacy and the risk of endoscopic polypectomy on solid grounds[42] *(Figs. 28, 29, 30)*.

In 1980, Gilbertsen suggested the prevention of colon cancer through polypectomy[14]. More recent data from 1993 confirm the value of colonic endoscopy and polypectomy for the protection of patients as in the National Polyps Study chaired by Sidney Winawer[43]. However, systematic colonoscopic examination of individuals without associated risk factors is still under discussion.

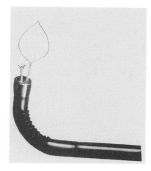

Fig. 26. Polypectomy snare of the A.C.M.I. F9A colonoscope (courtesy of A.C.M.I.-Zircon).

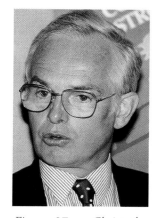

Fig. 27. Christopher Williams, gastroenterologist and endoscopist at Saint-Marks' hospital in London. He devised the "hot biopsy" technique to excise polyps, providing biopsy material at the same time (World Gastroenterology News).

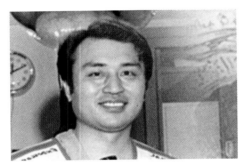

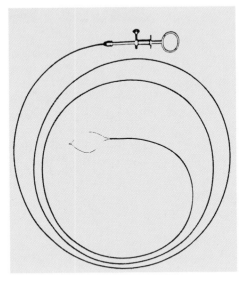

Fig. 28. *Hirumi Shinya, who together with William Wolff made the first fibrescopic polypectomies in the United States (courtesy of Prof. H. Niwa).*

Fig. 29. *Title page of the first paper by Wolff and Shinya on colonoscopy and polypectomy (1971).*

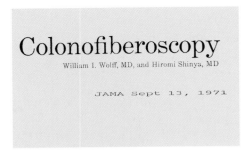

Fig. 30. *The first polypectomies of the right colon were performed by Peter Deyhle and Lydwig Demling in Demling's Department at the University of Erlangen (1971). Picture of the long polypectomy snare employed by the authors (courtesy of the late Prof. L. Demling).*

ACCIDENTS AND COMPLICATIONS OF THE FIRST COLONOSCOPIES

In possibly the most comprehensive review of the subject, Frühmorgen and Demling[13] made a survey in Germany in 1979 that comprised 27 hospitals with a total of 35,892 colonoscopies and 7,365 polypectomies. They reported 0.008 percent of haemorrhages and 0.13 percent of perforations for colonoscopy, while among patients who underwent polypectomy, haemorrhage occurred in 2.24 percent of cases and perforation in 0.34 percent, with a mortality of 0.1 percent. There was a direct relationship between the number of complications and the expertise of the endoscopists. Thus there were 18.7 percent of accidents among operators who had only performed 200 colonoscopies, while the figure was only 0.4 percent for those who had done more than 1,000 examinations. A large series from the United States gave comparable results[34].

REFERENCES

1 Blankenhorn D.H., Hirsch J, Ahrens E.H. Transintestinal intubation: technique for measuring the gut length and physiologic sampling at known loci. Proc Soc Exp Biol Med 1955; 88: 356-362.

2 Brooker JC., Saunders B.P., Shah S.G., Williams C.B. A more variable stiffness colonoscope makes colonoscopy easier; a randomized controlled study. Gut 2000; 48: 801-805.

3 Clain J.E. Endoscopy of the colon. in The Large Intestine: Physiology, Pathophysiology and Diseases. S.F.Phillips, J.H. Pemberton, R.G. Shorter (eds) New York, Raven Press, 1991

4 Colagrande C., Arullani P. La biopsia del colon. Arch Ital Mal Appar Dig 1964; 31: 369-374.

5 Cook GB., Margulis AR. Silicone foam diagnostic enema. I. Assessment with surgical specimens of human sigmoid colon. Surgery 1961; 50: 513-518.

6 Dean A.C.B., Shearman D.J.C. Clinical evaluation of a new fiberoptic colonoscope. Lancet 1970;1: 550-551.

7 Deyhle P., Ottenjann R. Zur transintestinale Intubation. Fortschritte der Endoskopie Band 2, Stuttgart, Schattauer Verlag, 1969: 205-212

8 Deyhle P., Demling L. Coloscopy. Technique, results, indication. Endoscopy 1971; 3: 143-151.

9 Deyhle P., Seuberth K., Jenny S., Demling L. Endoscopic polypectomy in the proximal colon. Endoscopy 1971; 3: 103-105.

10 Elewaut A., Cremer M. The history of gastrointestinal endoscopy. The European perspective. in Gastroenterological Endoscopy. M.Classen, G.N.J. Tytgat, C.J. Lightdale (eds.) Stuttgart, Thieme, 2002.

11 Ewe K., Wanitschke R. Coloscopy as a routine procedure. Advances in Gastrointestinal Endoscopy. Proceedings 2nd World Congress of Gastrointestinal Endoscopy. G.Marcozzi, M.Crespi (eds) 1970: 849-850.

[12] Fox J.A. A fibreoptic colonoscope. Brit med J 1969; 2: 50-51.

[13] Frühmorgen F., Demling L. Complications of diagnostic amd therapeutic colonoscopy in the Federal Republic of Germany. Result of an enquiry. Endoscopy 1979; 11: 146-150.

[14] Gilbertsen V.A., Nelms J.M. The prevention of invasive cancer of the rectum. Cancer 1978; 41: 1137-1139.

[15] Hirschowitz B.J., Modlin I.M. The history of endoscopy. the American perspective. in Gastroenteroloigcal Endoscopy, M.Classen, G.N.J. Tytgat, C.J. Lightdale (eds.) Stuttgart, Thieme, 2002.

[16] Kanazawa T., Tanaka M. Endoscopy of colon. Gastroenterol Endosc (Tokyo) 1965; 7: 398-400.

[17] Kawai K., Niwa H., Fujita R., Shimizu S. The history of endoscopy: the Japanese perspective. In Gastroenterological Endoscopy, M.Classen, G.N.J. Tytgat, C.J.Lightdale (eds). Stuttgart, Thieme, 2002.

[18] Lemire S., Cocco A.E. Visualization of the left colon with the fiberoptic gastroduodenoscope. Gastrointest Endosc 1966;13: 29-30.

[19] Matsunaga F. Clinical studies in ulcerative colitis and its related diseases in Japan. Proceedings First World Congress of Gastroenterol, Washington 1958. Williams & Wilkins. Vol II. Baltimore 1959: 955-963.

[20] Matsunaga F. Colonofiberscopy. Advances in Gastrointestinal Endoscopy. Proceedings 2nd World Congress of Gastrointestinal Endoscopy. G.Marcozzi, M.Crespi (eds) 1970:161-16 and 833-839.

[21] Morfoisse JJ., Grasset D., Seineuric C. Opinion des malades après coloscopie. Gastroenterol Clin Biol 2000; 24: 279-283.

[22] Nagasako K. Endo M., Takemoto T. The insertion of fibercolonoscope into the cecum and the direct observation of the ileo-cecal valve. Endoscopy 1970; 2: 123-126.

[23] Nagasako K. Fibercolonoscopy of the terminal ileum. Advances in Gastrointestinal Endoscopy. Proceedings 2nd World Congress of Gastrointestinal Endoscopy. G.Marcozzi, M.Crespi (eds), 1970: 861-864.

[24] Nagasako K., Yazawa C., Takemoto T. Observation of the terminal ileum. Endoscopy 1971;3: 45-51.

[25] Neugut A.L., Forde KA Screening colonoscopy: has the time come? Am J Gastroenterol 1983; 78: 295-297.

[26] Niwa H. Endoscopy of colon. Gastroenterol Endosc (Tokyo) 1965: 7: 402-408.

[27] Niwa H., Utsumi Y., Nakamura T., Yoshitoshi Y. Endoscopy of the colon. Proc. 1st World Congress Int Soc Endoscopy, Tokyo 1966: 425-430.

[28] Niwa H., Utisumi T., Kaneko E. Clinical experiences of colonic fiberscope. Jpn J Gastroenterol 1969; 66: 907-911.

[29] Oshiba S., Watanabe A. Endoscopy of colon. Gastroenterol Endosc (Tokyo) 1965; 7:400-402.

[30] Overholt B.F. Clinical experience with the fibersigmoidoscope. Gastrointest Endosc 1968;15, 27.

[31] Overholt B.F. The history of colonoscopy. In Colonoscopic Techniques, Clinical Practice and Colour Atlas. Junt R.H, Waye J.D. (eds) London, Chapman Hall, 1981.

[32] Provenzale I., Camerada P., Revignas A. la coloscopia totale transanale. Una metodica originale. Rassegna Medica Sarda 1966; 69: 149-156.

[33] Provenzale I., Revignas A. An original method for guided intubation of the colon. Gastrointest Endosc 1969; 16: 11-17.

[34] Rogers BH., Silvis SE., Nebel OT., Sugawa Ch., Mandelstam I, Complications of flexible colonoscopy and polypectomy 1975; 22: 73-76.

[35] Shinya H., Wolff W.I. Anatomic distribution and cancer potential of colonic polyps. Ann Surg 1979; 190: 679-683.

[36] Tada M., Suyama Y., Shimizu T., Inatomi I., Fujii H., Mioshi M. Magnifying observation of the colonic mucosa by means of a newly developed colonoscope. type CF-HM. Gastroenterol Endosc 1979; 21: 527-537.

[37] Torsoli A., Arullani P., Casale C. An application of transintestinal intubation in the study of the colon. Gut 1967; 8: 192-194.

[38] Turell R. Fiber optic colonoscope and sigmoidoscope Am J Surg. 1963; 105: 133-136.

[39] Waye J. Colonoscopy. Surg Clin North Am 1972; 52:1013-1024.

[40] Williams C.B., Muto T. Examination of the whole colon with fiberoptic colonoscope. Br Med J 1972; 3: 278-281.

[41] Williams C.B. Diathermy-biopsy —a technique for the endoscopic management of small polyps. Endoscopy 1973; 5: 215-218.

[42] Williams C.B. The logic and logistics of colon polyps follow-up. in Progress in Gastroenterology (GBJ Jerzy Glass, P Sherlock (eds) vol. IV New York, Grune & Stratton, 1983: 513-525.

[43] Winawer S.J., Zauber A.G., Nah Ho M: O'Brien M.J., Gottlieb L.S, Sternberg S.S. Prevention of colorectal cancer by colonoscopic polypectomy. New Engl J Med 1993; 329: 1977-1995.

[44] Wolff W.I., Shinya H. Colonofiberoscopy. J.A.M.A. 1971; 217: 1509-1512.

[45] Wolff W.I., Shinya H. Polypectomy via fiberoptic colonoscope: removal of neoplasms beyond the reach of the sigmoidoscope. N Engl J Med 1973; 288: 329-332.

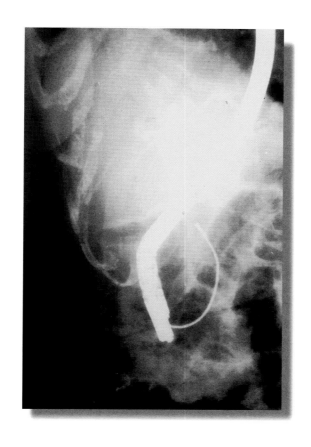

CHAPTER 12

The evolution of bilio-pancreatic endoscopy

GALLSTONE VISUALISATION AND CHOLECYSTOGRAPHY

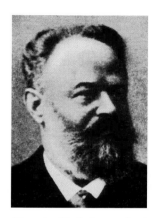

THE MODERN HISTORY OF BILIARY DIAGNOSIS BEGINS WITH CARL Johann Langenbuch (1810-1901), a German surgeon[21], who in 1882 performed the first successful cholecystectomy at the long since disappeared Sankt Lazarus hospital in Berlin[41]. A few years later, in 1888, a Swiss, Louis Bard (1857-1930), professor of medicine in Geneva and later in Lyon where he directed the medical service at the Hôtel-Dieu hospital together with his intern Adrien Pic,[4] described in detail the clinical features of malignant obstructive jaundice and noted how often in these patients the gallbladder became palpable *(Figs. 1, 2, 3)*. A Frenchman, Jean Martin Charcot, better known for his studies on neurological disease and the first to identify intermittent claudication, described the clinical symptoms of choledocal lithiasis, emphasising the diagnostic triad of fever, chills and jaundice[12] *(Fig. 4)*.

In 1890, Ludwig Courvoisier, a surgeon from Basel (Switzerland),[14] published a treatise on biliary surgery which achieved widespread diffusion. In it he described

Fig. 1. Karl Langenbuch (1810-1901), a German surgeon who, in 1882, performed the first cholecystectomy in Berlin (collection Dr. Jacinto Vilardell).

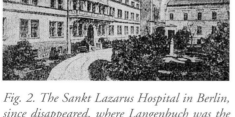

Fig. 2. The Sankt Lazarus Hospital in Berlin, since disappeared, where Langenbuch was the head of the surgical service (unknown copyright).

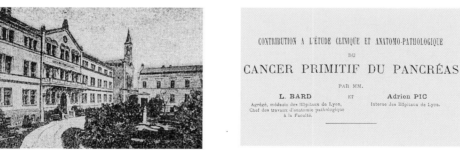

Fig. 3. Title page of the paper (1888) by Louis Bard (1857-1930) and his intern Adrien Pic, on cancer of the pancreas. They described in detail the features of obstructive jaundice and the dilatation of the gallbladder the so-called "Bard and Pic sign", misnamed as "Courvoisier's sign" by some authors.

239

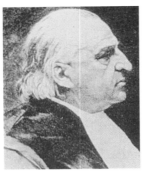

Fig. 4. Jean Martin Charcot (1825-1893), famous clinician at La Salpetrière Hospital in Paris, known for his studies on neurological disease, hysteria and for the first description of intermittent claudication. He described the clinical features of common duct biliary stones: pain, fever with chills and dark urine in his "Leçons sur les Maladies du Foie des Voies Biliaires et des Reins" (Paris 1880) (collection Dr. Jacinto Vilardell).

the famous "Courvoisier sign", often erroneously interpreted in the medical literature: what Courvoisier really said is that in cases of obstructive jaundice, whether malignant or not, the gallbladder could not be palpated if it had undergone scleroatrophy from previous chronic calculous cholecystitis *(Figs. 5, 6).*

The first paper dealing with the x-ray visualisation of radiopaque gallbladder calculi is usually attributed to Carl Beck from New York[5] who, in January 1901 at a session of the New York Academy of Medicine, presented radiographs showing gallstones. However, as we have repeatedly noticed, priorities are always difficult to establish and in 1899, A. Buxbaum from Karlsbad (today Karlovy Vary in the Czech Republic, then part of the Austrian Empire) presented several plain radiographs of gallstones at the Wiener Medizinischen Club[9] in Vienna. Unfortunately, the journals and the illustrations of these publications did not stand the test of time and are today practically uninterpretable *(Fig. 7).*

Clinicians then took advantage of the development of biliary duodenal drainage by Max Einhorn in New York (see Chapter 1) and by his disciple Henry Bockus and his associates in Philadelphia. Anatole Chauffard (1855-1932), an eminent clinician at the Hospital Saint-Antoine in Paris, and the head of his laboratories Adrien Grigaut, had shown that biliary calculi were mostly made of cholesterol and calcium bilirubinate[12] *(Figs. 8, 9, 10).*

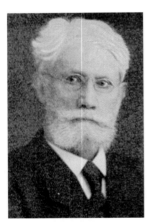

Fig. 5. Ludwig Georg Courvoisier (1843-1918), professor of surgery at Basel University, author of an important treatise on biliary surgery He described the "Courvoisier sign" (see text) He was also a great collector of butterflies (kindness of Dr. Heinz Affolter, Basel).

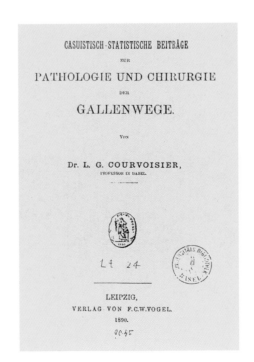

Fig. 6. Frontispiece of Courvoisier's treatise on Pathology and Surgery of the Biliary Tract (1890).

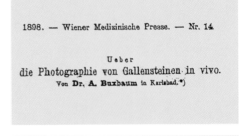

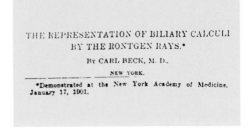

Fig. 7. a and b. Title pages of the papers published a: in 1889 by A. Buxbaum (above) and b: in 1901 by Carl Beck (below) in which they independently presented radiographs of biliary stones.

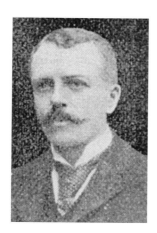

Fig. 8. Anatole Chauffard (1855-1932), professor of clinical medicine at the Saint-Antoine hospital in Paris. He became famous for his studies on gallstones and the correlation between hypercholesterolaemia and cholelithiasis (collection of Dr. Jacinto Vilardell).

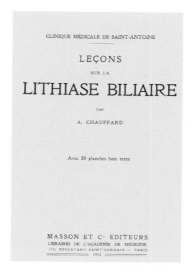

Fig. 9. Frontispiece of Chauffard's book "Leçons sur la Lithiase Biliaire" of 1914 which became a classic. For the first time he studied the composition of gallstones in detail.

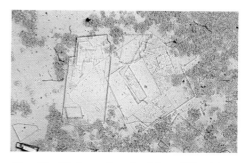

Fig. 10. Cholesterol and calcium bilirubinate crystals obtained by biliary drainage which according to Chauffard, Einhorn and Bockus were diagnostic of gallstones (archives of the Gastroenterology Postgraduate School, Hospital de Sant Pau, Barcelona.)

The simultaneous finding of both cholesterol and bilirubinate crystals in the bile sediment after gallbladder stimulation with magnesium sulphate was considered pathognomonic of cholelithiasis and even today this finding is valued positively to affirm the biliary etiology of some cases of pancreatitis in which imaging techniques are inconclusive.

However, in 1924 the major breakthrough in biliary diagnosis was the work of two surgeons from Saint Louis, Evarts Graham and Warren Cole[28] (Figs. 11, 12, 13), who demonstrated that a radiopaque substance (tetrabromephtalein) given intravenously was excreted in the bile and stored in the gallbladder which then became opacified. In this way, they introduced the first contrast medium which would show and delineate the gallbladder and part of the bile ducts and could reproduce their image radiographically. Soon the brome of the molecule which was shown to be very toxic was replaced by iodine (tetraiodophtalein). Being less dangerous, it was soon commercialised, although sometimes accidents still occurred. Years later, other contrast media, which could be absorbed orally and excreted by the bile, were synthetised. For nearly the next fifty years, oral cholecystography has been the preferred technique for the visualisation of the gallbladder and, in lucky instances, of the cystic duct and the proximal hepatic duct. An American physiologist and radiologist, Edward Boyden from Minneapolis[7], who published several papers on the physiology of biliary excretion, perfected the technique of oral cholecystography using a fatty meal to stimulate gallbladder contraction and facilitate its emptying, thus allowing better visualisation of

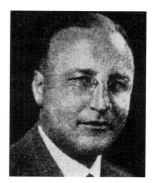

Fig. 11. Evarts Graham, the American surgeon from Saint Louis who in 1924 with his associate Warren Cole, performed intravenous cholangiography for the first time, first in dogs and then in humans. (courtesy of the late Dr. J. Puig LaCalle).

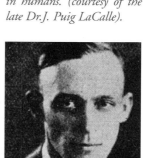

Fig. 12. Warren Cole, who later became a distinguished professor of surgery (courtesy of the late Dr. J. Puig LaCalle).

ROENTGENOLOGIC EXAMINATION OF THE GALLBLADDER

PRELIMINARY REPORT OF A NEW METHOD UTILIZING THE INTRAVENOUS INJECTION OF TETRABROMPHENOLPHTHALEIN *

EVARTS A. GRAHAM, M.D.

AND

WARREN H. COLE, M.D.

ST. LOUIS

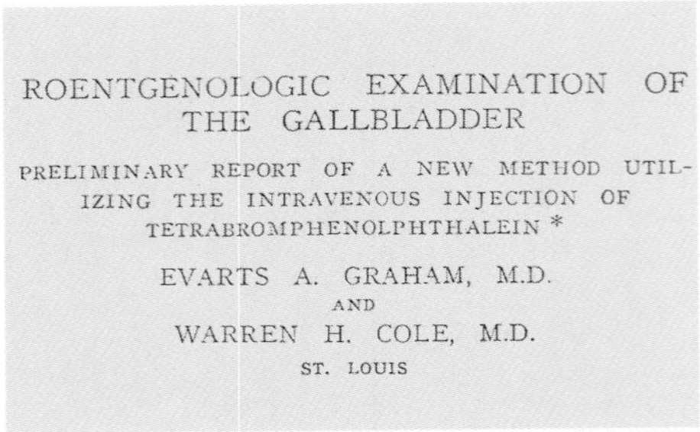

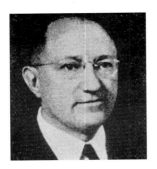

Fig. 13. Title of the paper by Graham and Cole on intravenous cholecystography (1924).

gallstones as well as the detection of abnormalities of the infundibulum and the cystic duct *(Fig. 14).*

Around 1950, a new contrast medium which could be injected intravenously was developed to replace oral products that were sometimes poorly absorbed and excreted. This new product (Cholegraphin, Biligrafin) had been researched in Germany and became relatively popular for the imaging of the common bile duct, for measuring its size and for detecting the presence of stones in its lumen. In spite of the advantages of this procedure, which included the possibility of tomography, accidents due to the large intravenous concentration of iodine were reported in the literature. As of 1960, oral as well as intravenous cholecystography practically disappeared with the emergence of harmless imaging techniques.

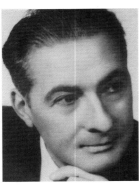

Fig. 14. Edward Boyden, American physiologist and radiologist who studied gallbladder emptying after different stimuli. The Boyden test was used extensively in clinical radiology (courtesy Dr.A.Sierra, Ed. Científico-Médica).

However, the main contribution of cholecystography with contrast media was the principle that the bile ducts could be visualised with radiopaque substances able to be excreted in the bile and attempts were therefore made to inject the contrast media directly into the biliary tree.

THE FIRST SURGICAL CHOLANGIOGRAPHIES

The first peroperative cholangiography was performed by Pablo Mirizzi[45, 46], a surgeon from Córdoba (Argentina) *(Fig. 15).* Mirizzi used lipiodol as a radiological contrast and injected it through the cystic duct during cholecystectomy. The technique rapidly became popular in Latin America and in Europe where it has been performed for many years using water soluble contrast media instead of lipiodol which was dense and viscous and could produce artifacts. Its use in the Anglo-Saxon world took time and never reached the popularity that it had in other countries, perhaps because most European and Latin American publications on the subject were written either in French or Spanish rather than in English.

Fig. 15. The Argentinian surgeon Pablo Mirizzi (1893-1969), professor of surgery of Cordoba University, who performed peroperative cholangiography around 1930 for the first time (courtesy of the late Dr. A. Llauradó).

The main indication of operative cholangiography was the detection of stones in the main duct and their extraction by cholechotomy or later through a Kehr T tube (Kehr, 1862-1916) placed for the drainage of the bile ducts. Many surgeons performed control postoperative cholangiographies through the T tube and used various manoeuvres to retrieve residual gallstones. In France, Jacques Caroli[10], a clinician from Paris, and Pierre Mallet-Guy[42], a surgeon from Lyon, completed the cholangiographic examination by measuring pressures in the biliary tree by means of intraductal manometers *(Figs. 16, 17).* They measured the pressure necessary to pass through the sphincter of Oddi in order to detect possible anomalies, either organic (Odditis) or functional (hypertonic sphincter).

However, peroperative biliary manometry was seldom used outside France. A revival in the technique has taken place in recent times since intraductal pressures can be taken directly during endoscopic cholangiography.

PEROPERATIVE CHOLEDOCHOSCOPY

While clinicians perfected radiographic techniques, surgeons began to explore the common duct during operation in search of stones and other lesions. The first attempts to visualise the choledochal lumen were made by the Czech surgeon Jaroslav Bakes (1871-1930)[3] who was well known for the design of several instruments used to dilate the ampulla of Vater and the main bile duct during surgical interventions (Bakes serial dilators). Bakes *(Fig. 18)* was born in a small village near Brünn (today Brno in the Czech republic). He was appointed chief of surgery at the Brno hospital and he was soon interested in biliary surgery and the possibility of inspecting the main duct by means of an endoscope. He asked Joseph Leiter, the well-known instrument maker from Vienna, to manufacture a "choledochoscope" which consisted of a hollow tube provided with a lighting system and a distal mirror in which the lumen of the main biliary duct was indirectly reflected. With his "choledochoscope", Bakes succeeded in detecting the presence of stones and in dilating stenosed papillae of Vater using his own dilators.

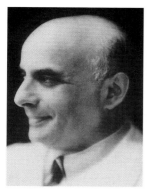

Fig. 16. Jacques Caroli (1903-1979), a successor of Chauffard at the Saint-Antoine hospital in Paris. For more than twenty years, he was the leader of a renowned hepatology group. He devised biliary peroperative and postoperative radiomanometry and described the clinical features of "Odditis" (author's colecction).

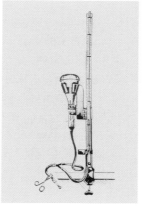

Fig. 17. Caroli's water manometer used during operation or through a postoperative T tube (Kehr tube) to perform cholangiography and biliary radiomanometry (ref. 9).

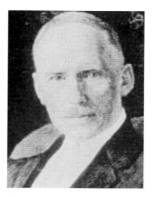

Fig. 18. Jaroslav Bakes (1871-1930), a Czech surgeon from Brno who used a modified cystoscope to explore the lumen of the biliary ducts for the first time. He also designed several kinds of probes to dilate the sphincter of Oddi, frequently used in open biliary surgery (Bakes dilators) (from ref. 17).

AN INSTRUMENT FOR VISUALIZING THE INTERIOR OF THE COMMON DUCT AT OPERATION

Preliminary Note

Monroe A. McIver, M.D., Cooperstown, N. Y.

(From the Surgical Service of the Mary Imogene Bassett Hospital)

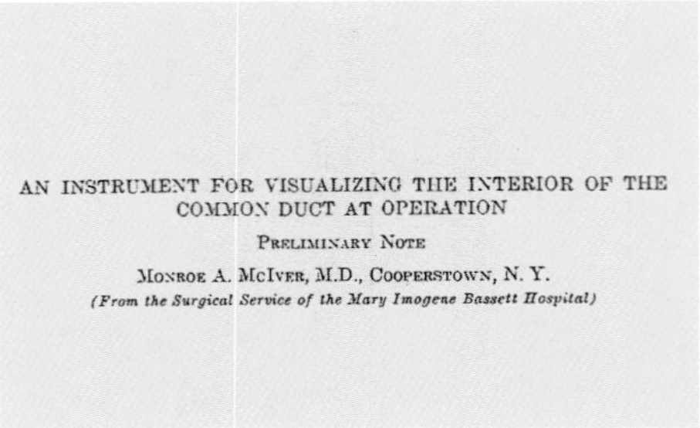

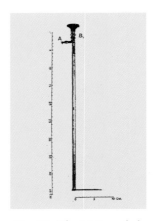

Fig. 19. Title of a paper by the American surgeon Monroe McIver on choledochoscopy, using an instrument which he had designed in 1941. The optical system was manufactured by Frederick Wappler from the Reinhold Wappler firm (A.C.M.I.)

The American surgeon Monroe Mac Iver[44], working at the Mary Imogene Bassett Hospital, perfected Bakes' choledochoscope and in 1941 he designed a telescopic endoscope ending in a right angle to inspect the main duct through an incision in its wall. The horizontal portion of the instrument, which was introduced into the duct, was 5 cm in diameter and 7 cm long. The optical system of the endoscope was designed by Frederick Wappler, a relative of Reinhold Wappler, the founder of American Cystoscope Makers (A.C.M.I.) *(Figs. 19, 20).*

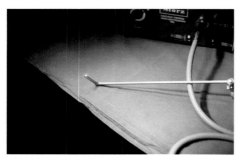

Fig. 20. The McIver choledochoscope: A) connection for lavage. B) connection to electrical source. Diameter of the main tube 10 mm. Diameter of the choledochoscope: 5 mm. (redrawn from ref. 43).

Other more perfected instruments were later made in the United States and in Germany. Perhaps the best known was Wildegans choledochoscope[70], designed in 1953. Essentially, it consisted of a rigid angular probe including an optical system and an irrigation device. A set of lenses allowed magnification of the image 2-4 times the real size at a distance 2.5 cm from the object. Wildegans and his associates made 54 choledochoscopies, mostly associated with an operative cholangiography *(Fig. 21).* Their main achievement was the identification of pathologic findings which would otherwise have gone unnoticed. Nevertheless, rigid choledochoscopy was not devoid of risk as can be inferred from the discussion which took place after the presentation that McCune later made on fibrescopic cholangiography in which an instance of biliary perforation with the choledochoscope was presented.

As in other fields of endoscopy, rigid instruments were gradually replaced by fibreoptics. In the mid-1960s, the American surgeon Clarence Schein[61, 62] suggested the possibility of using fibrescopes to explore the bile ducts and several surgeons started to do so in 1970. Manny and Ernest Shore[63] in Los Angeles performed 100 fibrescopic examinations of the common duct in one-hundred consecutive patients. Their fibrescope was 50 cm long and 6 mm in diameter; it was inserted through a choledochotomy and in the majority of cases a cholangiography was also done. The Shores judged that the examination had given important information in 13 patients in whom main duct stones had not been previously detected.

Fig. 21. The Wildegans choledochoscope frequently used for exploring the common duct during open surgery (courtesy of the late Dr. J. Puig LaCalle).

THE FIRST OPERATIVE PANCREATOGRAPHIES

Starting in the 1950s, a few surgeons, among then Henry Doubilet (1955), described operative pancreatography in detail, directly injecting liquid contrast through the papilla of Vater or by puncturing a dilated pancreatic duct[20]. However, the technique was complex and required considerable technical skill. It did not become popular and complications (acute pancreatitis) occasionally occurred. It is performed today in selected cases only.

PERCUTANEOUS TRANSHEPATIC CHOLANGIOGRAPHY (P.T.C.)

Eighty years have elapsed since clinicians first tried to inject a liquid contrast medium directly into the gallbladder or a liver biliary duct. In 1921, Hans Burckhardt and Walter Müller[8], respectively chief resident (oberartz) and assistant at the Surgical Clinic of Marburg University in Germany, performed punctures of the gallbladder in cadavers under fluoroscopic guidance and obtained radiographic images of the gallbladder and the bile ducts, using a 0.7 mm in diameter cannula guided by a 0.4 mm wire. Once bile had been aspirated, they injected a radiopaque silver nitrate solution (Kollargol). After a number of tests in rabbits and in cadavers, they performed their technique in a patient (using local anaesthesia) and punctured the gallbladder. They went on to examine other patients, under general anaesthesia, just prior to cholecystectomy, apparently without mishaps. Although they published their findings in a German surgical journal their paper received little attention and is barely mentioned in the literature *(Figs 22, 23)*.

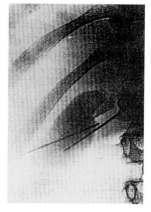

Fig. 22. First cholecystographies obtained by blind transhepatic puncture by Hans Burckhardt and Walter Müller in 1921, first in cadavers and later in patients before surgery. A needle inside the gallbladder and another near the gallbladder bed are clearly seen. They were used to check the technique during the surgical intervention (see fig. 23).

In 1937, Pierre Huard, a Parisian surgeon working at the Lanessan Hospital in Hanoi (Indochina, today Vietnam), together with a local colleague, Do-Xuan-Hop, succeeded in delineating the biliary tree by blindly injecting lipiodol in a biliary duct after aspirating bile through a percutaneous transhepatic route[32]. They reported instances of biliary obstruction due to Clonorchis Sinensis and also a case of cancer of the pancreas. Their paper was published in French in the Bulletin of the Medico-Surgical Society of Indochina and although it is sometimes quoted, the original Bulletin can be found only with great difficulty *(Fig. 24)*.

In 1952, R. Franklin Carter and George M. Saypol[11] of New York performed preoperative transhepatic cholangiographies in several patients with a trocar and a needle of the type used for lumbar puncture. At a later date, under general anaesthesia, they blindly punctured the liver, greatly enlarged, of a patient with obstructive jaundice, demonstrating a complete biliary obstruction. The patient died a few days later from massive haemorrhage and at autopsy, cirrhosis of the liver and an apparently primary liver cancer with metastatic lymph nodes that were compressing the main bile duct was found *(Fig. 25)*.

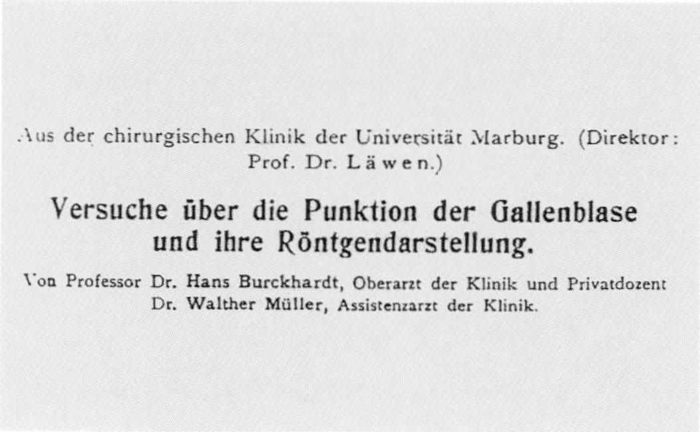

Aus der chirurgischen Klinik der Universität Marburg. (Direktor: Prof. Dr. Läwen.)

Versuche über die Punktion der Gallenblase und ihre Röntgendarstellung.

Von Professor Dr. Hans Burckhardt, Oberarzt der Klinik und Privatdozent Dr. Walther Müller, Assistenzarzt der Klinik.

Fig. 23. Title of the article by Burckhardt and Müller (1921).

The case was published in a well known journal which helped in disseminating their technique internationally. However, accidents were reported and only the advent of Kunio Okuda's[54] thin caliber Chiba needle, which allowed punctures with little risk of haemorrhage or bile leaks, provided a safe way to visualise the biliary tree. It was used in many centres until it was displaced by the new imaging techniques and the E.R.C.P. *(Figs. 26, 27).*

One procedure derived from percutaneous cholangiography is the percutaneous direct cholangioscopy.

PERCUTANEOUS TRANSHEPATIC CHOLANGIOSCOPY

In the 1970s, the manufacturing of 7 mm in diameter choledocoscopes, which were easy to insert into the main duct through a choledochotomy or through a T tube, encouraged Japanese clinicians to attempt visualisation of the bile ducts by the percutaneous route, prompted by the frequency of obstructive jaundice due to intrahepatic stones and parasitic infestations in the liver in the Far East. The method consisted of previously performing a percutaneous cholangiography through an intrahepatic duct leaving an external drain in place. The drain orifice was dilated with a probe and a flexible tube 6-7 mm in diameter

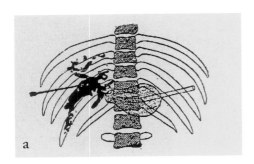

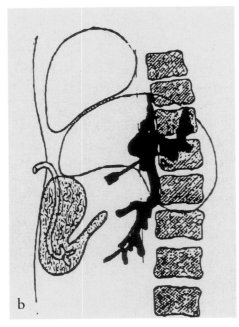

Fig. 24. Drawings made from x-rays of the dilated bile-ducts injected with lipiodol by the transhepatic route in 1937 by Huard and Do-Huan-Xop in Hanoi. (A) above: a reproduction of a frontal radiograph. (B) below: a profile view showing a cholecystostomy tube for drainage of the obstructed bile ducts.

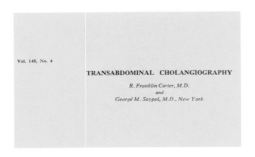

Vol. 148, No. 4

TRANSABDOMINAL CHOLANGIOGRAPHY

R. Franklin Carter, M.D.
and
George M. Saypol, M.D., New York

Fig. 25. In 1952 Franklin Carter and George Saypol, unaware of Huard's work, published their experience on "Transabdominal cholangiography".

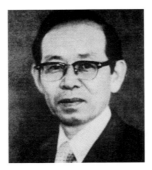

Fig. 26. Kunio Okuda (1921-2003), professor of Medicine at Chiba University, haematologist and hepatologist of international reputation, who designed the thin "Chiba needle" for percutaneous cholangiography (courtesy of the late Prof.K.Okuda).

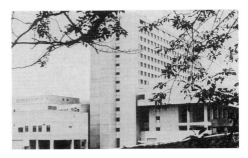

Fig. 27. The Chiba University Hospital where Okuda designed his well-known needle (courtesy of the late Prof.K.Okuda).

was then inserted into the duct and kept inside the channel opened by the dilating probe for a minimum of three weeks. Thereafter, a sort of a solid intrahepatic fibrous tract had formed through which a fibrecholedocoscope could be introduced *(Fig. 28)*.

The main indication of this rather complex technique was the identification of intrahepatic stones and parasites which could sometimes be removed by this route[25, 26, 28, 50].

MARCELO ROYER AND LAPAROSCOPIC CHOLANGIOGRAPHY

The development of laparoscopy in Germany (see Chapter 13) and later in the rest of the European Continent and in South America and the ease with which the gallbladder could be inspected, prompted several endoscopists to attempt its puncture and to obtain cholangiographies under direct vision. In 1935, according to Harald Henning[30], Heinz Kalk tried to puncture the gallbladder, withdraw bile and inject air so that radiographs could be taken to demonstrate gallstones by some kind of double contrast technique. Around 1940, Marcelo Royer, a distinguished gastroenterologist from Buenos Aires[58], was the first to perform cholangiographies by injecting a soluble contrast medium into the gallbladder under laparoscopic guidance *(Fig. 29)*.

Royer standardised the technique which was not without risk especially because of the danger of leaks of infected bile into the peritoneum and the occurrence of bile peritonitis, an extremely serious complication. In 1942, Royer began to report his results in various publications[59, 60].

Around 1950, Kalk[33] and Norbert Henning[31] attempted laparoscopic cholangiography either by direct gallbladder puncture or through the adjacent liver parenchyma, a less risky undertaking. Laparoscopic cholangiography was also performed in Japan. In 1966, at the First World Congress of Digestive Endoscopy in Tokyo, Yamagata and his associates[72] presented a new instrument for laparoscopic cholangiography. They had employed their device in 20 patients by punctioning the gallbladder with a thin 1 mm needle and placing a small clip to seal the orifice of the puncture *(Figs. 30, 31)*.

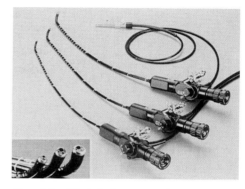

Fig. 28. Choledochoscopes of various sizes employed by Koji Gocho of Santa Marianna University in Kawasaki (Japan) for percutaneous transhepatic choledochoscopy (courtesy of Machida Inc).

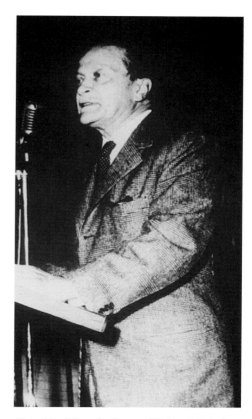

Fig. 29. Marcelo Royer (1899-1980) from Buenos Aires, probably the most respected Latin-American gastroenterologist. Of French origin, he worked in Paris where he published a book, "La Urobiline", which gave him an international reputation. He was the first to perform laparoscopic cholangiography (author's collection).

In 1970, at the Second World Congress of Digestive Endoscopy (Rome-Copenhagen), a team of endoscopists led by Kiyonaga from Osaka[38] reported the astonishing figure of 1,100 laparoscopic cholangiographies but gave no details of the technique or any accidents that may have occurred.

A safer procedure was employed by some laparoscopists by puncturing the gall-bladder or a visibly dilated bile duct through the adjacent liver tissue using a technique similar to that of Yamagata. Laparoscopic cholangiography was performed in some centres outside Japan and Germany but was soon replaced by simpler techniques which employed ultrasonographic guidance.

NON-SURGICAL CHOLANGIO-PANCREATOGRAPHY

The first direct radiological attempts

In 1965, Keith Rabinov and Morris Simon[56] of the Radiology Department of Harvard University, succeeded in introducing a double lumen tube by via oral through the ampulla of Vater, using fluoroscopy for orientation *(Fig. 32)*.

The external hollow tube was made of flexible coils like those used in intestinal biopsy instruments and a thinner tube was inserted inside its lumen which could be orientated independently from the outer cylinder. Very patiently, they tried to introduce the inner tube in the papilla and then slowly injected small amounts of a soluble contrast medium ("renografin") until the biliary duct became opacified. Apparently they succeeded in completing the injection on two different occasions in a single patient but failed in another seven patients. However, their paper includes radiographs in which a dilated main duct with stones in its lumen is clearly seen.

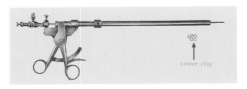

Fig. 30. Instrument for laparo-cholangiography designed by Yamagata and presented at the first World Congress of Digestive Endoscopy (Tokyo 1966) (ref. 71).

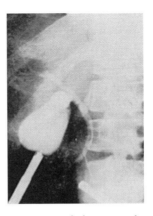

Fig. 31. Cholangiography performed by Yamagata with his method (ref. 71).

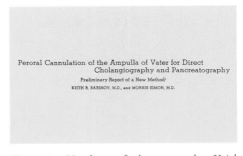

Peroral Cannulation of the Ampulla of Vater for Direct
Cholangiography and Pancreatography
Preliminary Report of a New Method[1]
KEITH R. RABINOV, M.D., and MORRIS SIMON, M.D.

Fig. 32. Heading of the paper by Keith Rabinov in which he described a blind radiological method for catheterisation of the ampulla of Vater by manipulation of a flexible tube, an outstanding technical "tour de force!".

DUODENOSCOPIC CHOLANGIOPANCREATOGRAPHY (ERCP)

The papilla of Vater was easily identified thanks to the progress in instrumentation and particularly in the ease of new duodenoscope manoeuvres in the duodenal lumen. In 1968, William S. McCune (1909-1998)[43], a respected surgeon at George Washington University (Washington DC), was apparently able to insert a probe in the ampulla of Vater with the aim of obtaining pancreatograms. He employed an experimental Eder fibrescope fitted with forward and side view lenses and the cannula was strapped to its side. In a preliminary communication *(Fig. 33)*, McCune reported that he had visualised the ampulla of Vater in "approximately 50 patients" and that in 50 percent of these he had been able to cannulate the ampulla, injecting a contrast medium ("Hypaque"). He reported that he had been able to obtain a successful pancreatography in half of them, that is in about 25 percent of the cases in which it was attempted (some 12 patients). Rather surprisingly, his paper does not mention whether or not he also obtained cholangiograms during his procedure. The illustrations of his paper are unsatisfactory and difficult to interpret. McCune attributed this to the excessive dilution of the contrast medium. He obtained better documents using a 40 percent concentration of Hypaque. The paper does not include a detailed account of his results. Years later, he acknowledged that in his presentation he was able to show "only one very good radiograph"[64].

The Eder fibrescope was not ideal for this endeavour as it was necessary to attach a balloon at the tip of the instrument. This had to be inflated to keep a distance from the duodenal mucosa which had a tendency to stick to the instrument. The distended balloon helped in inserting the catheter which was strapped outside the duodenoscope and could be directed under vision provided by the lateral lens.

The McCune procedure did not seem to have many adepts in the United States and apparently he did not pursue this project, perhaps because simpler procedures had been developed, largely in Japan. Several teams of endoscopists in Japanese centres used the Machida duodenoscope, which provided limited vision but could be bent in two directions, or the JF Olympus duodenoscope which could be deflected in four directions. The technique was not exempt of difficulties, such as crossing the pylorus, keeping the endoscope oriented into the duodenum, and managing to identify the papilla of Vater, which varied greatly in morphology from one individual to another.

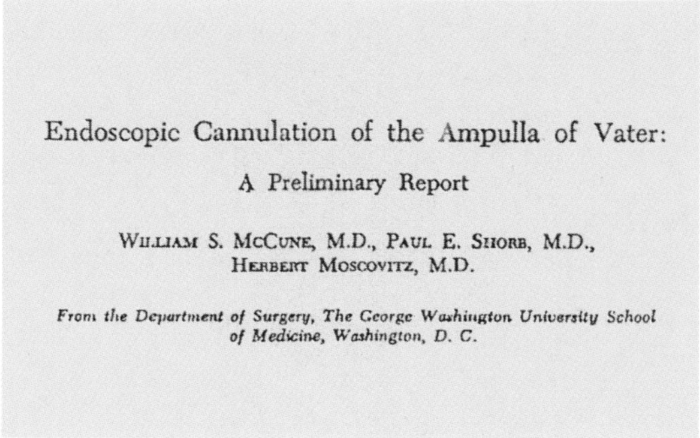

Endoscopic Cannulation of the Ampulla of Vater:

A Preliminary Report

WILLIAM S. McCUNE, M.D., PAUL E. SHORB, M.D.,
HERBERT MOSCOVITZ, M.D.

From the Department of Surgery, The George Washington University School of Medicine, Washington, D. C.

Fig. 33. Title of the preliminary communication by W. McCune on endoscopic pancreatography (see text).

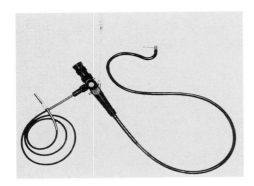

Fig. 34. Machida FDS1 duodenoscope which allowed visualisation of the ampulla of Vater (1970).

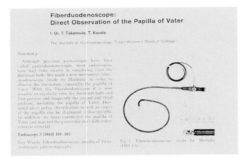

Fig. 35. Title page of Oi, Takemoto and Kondo's paper on visualisation of the papilla of Vater (1970).

Japanese endoscopists were the first to publish their findings in detail. In 1969, using a Machida duodenoscope, Itaru Oi, Takayoshi Takemoto and Taigoro Kondo[51] at the Tokyo Women's Medical College, documented their first endoscopic observations of the ampulla of Vater *(Fig. 34)*. With the FDS-1b Machida duodenoscope they were able to carefully examine the duodenal bulb and the second and third portions of the duodenum, including the papilla.

In 1970, Oi and associates published the first cholangiograms obtained by means of the Machida duodenoscope[52, 53] while Kunio Takagi and his team[67] did similar work with the JFB Olympus instrument. Many of us still remember with awe the presentation by Oi, Kobayashi and Kondo on endoscopic cholangio-pancreatography at the World Congress of Digestive Endoscopy in 1970 (Rome-Copenhagen) *(Figs. 35, 36)*. Oi employed the Machida instrument which we have already referred to. In April 1969 in Japan, the same team had demonstrated their first duodenoscopic pancreatograms. With the patient lying in the left lateral position and using only pharyngeal anaesthesia, they identified the papilla which they catheterised with a cannula especially designed for that purpose. The contrast medium ("Urografin 60 %) was injected under fluoroscopic control in the pancreatic duct, radiographs were taken and the biliary duct was then cannulated *(Figs. 37, 38, 39)*.

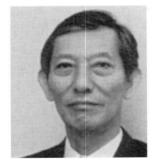

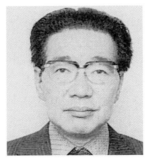

Fig. 36. Itaru Oi, pioneer of E.R.C.P. (courtesy of Prof. R.Fujita)

Fig. 37. Takayoshi Takemoto, of Tokyo University and The Women's Medical College, another founding father of E.R.C.P. (courtesy of Prof. R.Fujita).

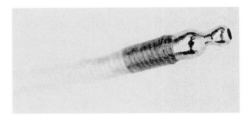

Fig. 38. Tip of the probe employed by Oi and Takemoto for cholangio-pancreatography (courtesy of Machida Inc.).

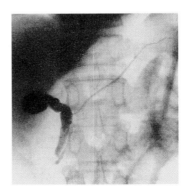

Fig. 39. Cholangio-pancreatography of the original paper by Oi, Takemoto and Kondo (1970) (courtesy of Prof. M.Classen, editor of Endoscopy).

Using a similar technique but under general anaesthesia, Kunio Takagi and his associates[67] at the Tokyo Cancer Center Hospital *(Fig. 40, 41),* identified the papilla of Vater in 13 patients and were able to catheterise it in nine of them. In every case they found gall-stones in the common duct. They had no accidents but they noticed an increase in serum amylase after the examination. They also presented their results at the Second World Congress of Endoscopy in 1970. Starting from 1970, the JFB Olympus duo-denoscpe became the instrument of choice in the majority of endoscopic centres and in 1971 Tatsuzo Kasugai[34] *(Fig. 42)* and his team at the Aichi Cancer Center in Nagoya also published their findings, while in 1972, Takuo Fujita[22] presented his own results at the A.S.N.E.M.G.E. Congress in Paris (see Chapter 14).

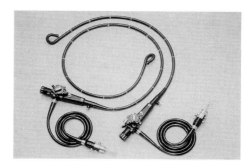

Fig. 40. The Olympus duodenoscope JF-B which replaced the Machida endoscope and was employed by K. Takagi and R.Fujita (courtesy of Olympus Inc.)

At the World Congress of Gastroenterology and Endoscopy in Mexico City in 1974, endoscopic cholangiography was unanimously termed E.R.C.P. (endo-scopic retrograde choledoco-pancreatography).

ENDOSCOPIC MANOMETRY OF THE SPHINCTER OF ODDI

Since Ruggero Oddi (1884-1913) described in detail the anatomic structure of the sphincter that bears his name *(Fig. 43),* many anatomic and functional studies have been performed to evaluate its role in biliary physiology and in biliary disease. The first investigations were done by measuring biliary flow stimulated during duode-nal drainage. Intravenous cholecystography demonstrating the absence of bile in the duodenum and operative cholangiography and radiomanometry which were practiced in France, as well as biliary radiocinematography, all contributed to con-firm that the Oddi sphincter was a real entity. The term "Odditis", indicating inflam-mation of the sphincteric area, was employed mostly in countries where operative cholangiography began, that is, in South American and Mediterranean countries. However, correlation between surgical anatomical findings and the results of the first biliary manometries done by Caroli and Mallet-

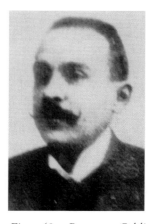

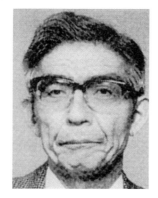

Fig. 41. Kunio Takagi, one of the first to perform endos-copic cholangiographies at the Tokyo Cancer Institute.

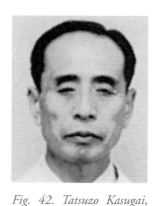

Fig. 42. Tatsuzo Kasugai, from Nagoya, a well-known endoscopist for his studies on gastric carcinoma (see Chapter 8). He was also a developer of duodenoscopic ERCP (courtesy of Dr. Gabriel Nagy)

Fig. 43. Ruggero Oddi (1884-1913), Italian phy-siologist and clinician who described the functional anatomy of the sphincter at the terminal bile duct in the ampulla of Vater (courtesy of the Italian Society of Gastroenterology).

Guy was not always good. In the course of time it was shown that many semiological findings such as "hypertony of the Oddi sphincter" were often artefacts caused by unreliability of the manometric techniques or other variables such as the effects of general anesthesia and the use of muscle relaxants.

The emergence of fibreduodenoscopy, the easy identification of the papilla and its catheterisation soon induced many endoscopists to take pressures of the sphincter in a retrograde fashion during duodenoscopy. In 1974, the first measurements of intraductal pressure were apparently made by P. Vondrasek and G. Eberhardt[68, 69] in Bad Driburg (Westfalia, Germany) using a catheter 1.67 mm in diameter provided with a semiconductor element used in haemodynamic laboratories (microtip sensor PC-350 Millar). It was inserted in the papilla under direct duodenoscopic control *(Fig. 44)*. They obtained graphic pressure data in the basal state as well as after injecting glucagon and pancreozymin.

In 1977, using a much more sophisticated and precise perfusion system consisting of open catheters of minimal compliance, Joseph Geenen, Walter Hogan and associates[23, 24] succeeded in clearly demonstrating contractile waves originated in the Oddi sphincter. The system that they kept improving, consisted of a triple catheter, 1.6 mm in external diameter that included three tubes, each 0.5 mm in diameter, manufactured by the firm Medi-Tech. These were introduced through the accessory channel of the duodenoscope. With their method they were able to measure pressures in the Oddi sphincter, the bile ducts and the main pancreatic duct. Other authors have employed pressure transducers for the same purpose. As Geenen himself acknowledges, time will tell regarding the practical relevance of biliary manometric studies in clinical practice *(Fig. 45)*.

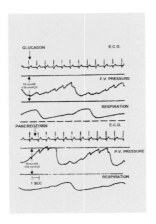

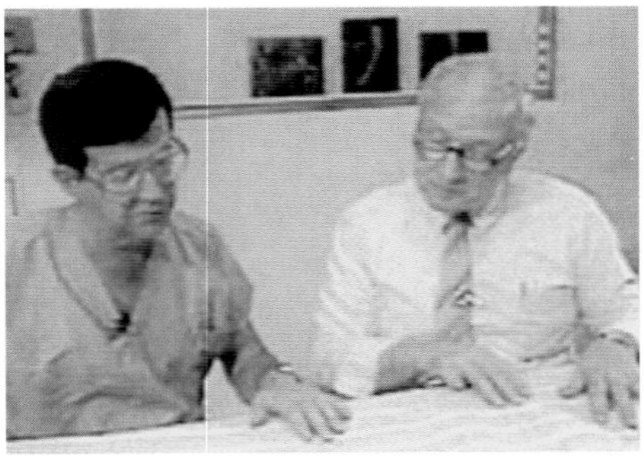

Fig. 44. Endoscopic manometries of the sphincter of Oddi performed in Germany by Vondrasek, Eberhardt and Classen showing the effects of glucagon amd pancreozymine on sphincteric pressures (modified from references 67,68).

Fig. 45. Joseph Geenen (left) and Walter Hogan (right), professors at Wisconsin University, the first to perform standardised endoscopic biliary manometry. (courtesy of Dr. J.Geenen).

CHOLANGIO-PANCREATOSCOPY WITH THE CHOLANGIOSCOPE ("BABYSCOPE")

This already "modern" technique probably represents the uttermost refinement in biliary diagnosis. The standard tubing used for contrast injection is replaced by a minimum calibre fibrescope which can be introduced through the papilla. According to Nakajima from Kyoto, in 1975[48], Takekoshi and Takashi published their first experiences with retrograde endoscopic pancreato-cholangioscopy in a Japanese journal (Gastroenterol Endosc Jpn). This was followed by those of Nakamura and associates as well as by Nakajima and Kawai in the same journal in 1976[47]. The first choledochoscopes were very fragile; visibility was poor and they were soon replaced by an instrument designed by Kawai and Nakajima in collaboration with Olympus engineers[35]. They employed JF-B or JF B2 Olympus duodenoscopes.

Yamakawa[73] with Nakajima and Kawai designed another duodeno-scope provided with a 2.8 mm wider channel, through which they could insert an endoscope 1.7 to 2.3 mm in diameter. This "baby scope" could be introduced under direct vision in the main bile duct as well as in the pancreatic duct *(Fig. 46)*.

Nakajima managed to examine thirteen patients with only one failure. He was able to inspect the bile and pancreatic ducts in seven instances, the bile duct only in three and the main pancre-atic duct in two.

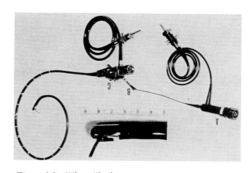

Fig. 46. The "babyscope", a minifibrescope which can be inserted in the channel of the duodenoscope and which allows visualisation of the lumen of the biliary ducts (courtesy of Olympus Inc.).

The instrument had some drawbacks: the thin calibre allowed the introduction of a bundle of only 3000 fibres resulting in reduced visibility and poor illumination. The fibres were very brittle as the length of the babyscope was 1.85 m. and on the other hand, the lumen of the ducts often contained bile or pancreatic secretion. The result was often a blurred view[18]. The technique has been used successfully in many centres, and in Spain particularly by J.R. Armengol-Miró[2], but it is usually only employed as a complement of ERCP. Peroral endoscopic cholangiogra-phy is slowly being replaced by imaging tecniques, in particular by nuclear magnetic resonance which often delineates the biliary and pancreatic ducts with great accuracy and detail as well as being devoid of any significant risk *(Figs. 47, 48, 49)*.

RISK OF ENDOSCOPIC CHOLANGIOPAN-CREATOGRAPHY

In 1976, an important survey col-lected data on 10,000 examinations performed in American centres[6]. The authors of the survey separately analysed examinations done by endo-scopists with different degrees of expe-rience. Among experts, the percentage of complications was 3 per cent, while among trainees it was 7 percent when they were unable to catheterise the ampulla, rising to 15 percent if they had completed the examination. In another survey in which 400 members of the American Society of Gastrointestinal Endoscopy (ASGE)

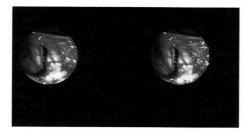

Fig. 47. Introduction of the choledochoscope in the papilla of Vater (courtesy of Dr. J.R. Armengol-Miro).

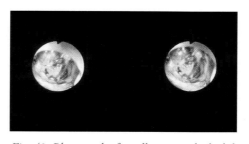

Fig. 48. Photograph of a gallstone inside the bile duct (courtesy of Dr. J.R. Armengol-Miro).

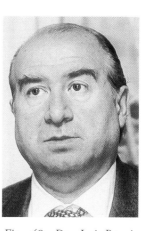

Fig. 49. Dr. José Ramón Armengol-Miró, who gave great impulse to digestive fibrescopy in Spain, in par-ticular for the treatment of acute bleeding and for biliary sphincterotomy and choledochoscopy (authors'-personal collection).

had been questioned, the percentage of complications among experts was 2.16 per cent[49].

In the entire series, the complication that caused the greatest morbidity and mortality was secondary infection and sepsis, which occurred in some 1 per cent of cases. Other reported accidents were isolated instances of instrumental perforation and acute pancreatitis after pancreatography (near one per cent risk) although raised levels of serum amylase were observed in as many as 50 per cent of cases in some series, albeit without any clinical consequences. The prophylaxis and the treatment of this complication are still not entirely solved.

THERAPEUTIC BILIARY ENDOSCOPY

Endoscopic sphincterotomy.

The possibility of endoscopically identifying the ampulla of vater and inserting a probe in its orifice to obtain cholangiographies, prompted gastroenterologists to attempt the extraction of biliary calculi which were obstructing the biliary tree and had been previously identified radiologically. Once again, urologists led the field as they had done in the early days of endoscopy, and provided invaluable indirect help (see Chapter 3). The first attempts to extract renal calculi from a ureter date back to 1896 when the Viennese urologist Gustav Kolischer (1863-1942), who later emigrated to the United States, was able to retrieve a stone from the ureter of a lady patient by inserting a catheter followed by the injection of sterilised oil[39]. Using various instrumental techniques urologists had succeeded in extracting small ureteral calculi and fragments of larger ones by catheterising the ureters during cystoscopy. They performed ureteral dilations with great caution as the dangers of cysto-ureteral reflux were already recognised and occasionally they succeeded in retrieving stones by means of clamps and various types of baskets.

The basket designed by Enrico Dormia from Milan has been very popular but several methods for lithotripsy had to be employed for the complete extraction of fragmented stones. A complete description of these instruments can be found in the splendid history of endoscopy by Hans and Matthias Reuter[57].

Gastrointestinal endoscopists tried to do the same through the papilla of Vater during duodenoscopy. The problems, however, were quite different: urologists had little chance of performing ureteral dilations or meatotomies because of the already men-

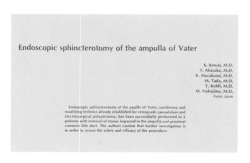

a

b

Fig. 50. Publication in 1974 of the first endoscopic sphincterotomies A) above: by Meinhard Classen in Erlangen and B) below: by Keiichi Kawai in Kyoto.

tioned danger of cystopyelic reflux. The situation was different in biliary disease as surgeons already had plentiful experience in the practice of sphincterotomy and sphincteroplasty of Oddi's sphincter, interventions often needed to extract gallstones lodged in the terminal main biliary duct. As we have seen repeatedly in the history of endoscopy, two teams of endoscopists working in distant countries, one in Erlangen[13] (Germany) and the other in Kyoto[36] (Japan), very amicably contended for the priority of endoscopic sphincterotomy. Both began their experiments using diathermic loops fitted to a probe of a calibre that allowed passage into the papillary orifice, taking as a model the instrumentation used for endoscopic polypectomy *(Fig. 50 a and b)*. Keiichi Kawai in Kyoto experimented first in animals and as of 1973 published his first results in Japanese journals. In October 1973, however, Kawai also read a paper at the Honolulu convention of the American College of Gastroenterology and in 1974 he published a detailed account of his technique in the journal "Gastrointestinal Endoscopy"[36]. His group had performed endoscopic sphincterotomies in 3 patients with calculi obstructing the area of the papilla of Vater. The patients were given an antispasmodic drug parenterally (40 mg. Buscopan) as well as local pharyngeal anaesthesia. The electrode employed by Kawai featured two small 2.0 mm in length diathermic loops shaped like a triangular surgical knife. The device was made by the Olympus company and introduced through an independent channel of a specially insulated Olympus duodenoscope. The other end of the electrode was connected to a diathermic device (ACOMA type E2).

Two kinds of electrical current were used intermittently, one for cutting and the other one for electrocoagulation. In October 1973, they were able to retrieve stones in two of the three patients without any untoward effects *(Figs. 51, 52)*.

Around the same dates, in Erlangen, Meinhard Classen also accomplished his first endoscopic sphincterotomies using a high frequency diathermic device. The Erlangen papillotome, designed by Demling and Classen, consisted of an outer Teflon catheter containing a thin flexible steel wire which exits the catheter about 3 mm from its distal end and reenters it about 3mm from its tip. Tension applied to the wire produces a bow string which once placed in the papilla, functions as a knife when high frequency current is applied[16]. The teflon tube enables injection of a radiopaque contrast medium and correct positioning of the papillotome. Like his Japanese colleagues, Classen began by experimenting in dogs without encountering bleeding or perforations. In 1974, they published the case of a seventy-year-old patient in whom they performed a papillotomy by first introducing the closed loop, opening it inside the bile duct and slowly withdrawing it. The cut was 10 mm in length and allowed the introduction of a Dormia basket and the extraction of a single stone.

The Erlangen and the Kyoto techniques were thus dissimilar. Kawai pushed the papillotome inwards, while Classen and his mentor Demling, proceeded to make the cutting while withdrawing the snare. Neither technique, whether

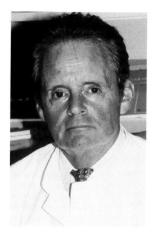

Fig. 51. Meinhard Classen, disciple of L. Demling in Erlangen and later director of the leading endoscopy centre in Germany at the Technische Universität in Munich (courtesy of Prof. M.Classen).

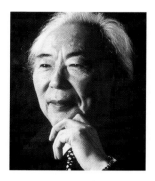

Fig. 52. Keiichi Kawai, professor of preventive medicine at Kyoto University, who performed the first endoscopic sphincterotomies in Japan, simultaneously with Meinhard Classen in Germany (courtesy of Prof. K.Kawai).

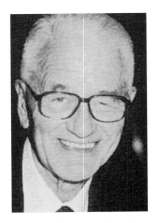

pushing or pulling, was devoid of risk and sphincterotomy took longer to be accepted than standard cholangiography. However, many endoscopists tried one of the techniques and a variety of clamps, baskets, small balloons and other tools were devised to retrieve biliary stones, most being miniature versions of the instruments used by surgeons in urological and biliary operations[19]. The Erlangen papillotome and lithotryptor became very popular in Europe while the Kyoto version did the same in Japan and Asiatic countries *(Figs. 53, 54, 55)*. A modification of the instrument designed by Fujita and Sohma[22] became the technique of choice in Japan. Ten years later, about 2,000 endoscopic sphincterotomies had been performed in 10 countries. In Spain, one of the largest sphincteromy series was published by Armengol-Miró[1]. Professor Michel Cremer from Brussels succeeded in performing a biliary sphincterotomy in a nine-month-old baby *(Fig. 56, 57)*.

In large series, the risk of pancreatitis post-sphincterotomy may be estimated between 1.2 and 2.1 per cent, that of secondary cholangitis at 0.9 to 2.7 per cent, and that of haemorrhage between 1.2 and 2.6 per cent.

INNOVATIONS AFTER 1980

Still later, stone fragmentation using mechanical lithotryptors such as those designed by Demling in 1982[15], or hydraulic instruments[40], were also in use.

The insertion of protheses in the biliary tract and the pancreas[29, 65] pertain to the present day activity of the endoscopist and are not within the scope of a historical review. Another useful innovation has been the palliative treatment of malignant stenoses and postoperative lesions by means of naso-biliary drainage procedures which were started in 1975 in Germany[55, 71]. The first protheses were placed by Soehendra and Reynders-Frederix[65] and by Hagenmüller and

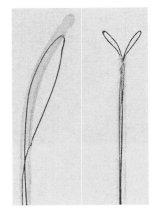

Fig. 54. Papillotome designed by Ludwig Demling for biliary sphincterotomy (courtesy of the late Prof. L. Demling).

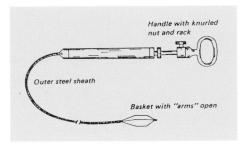

Fig. 55. Lithotriptor devised by Demling to be employed by the duodenoscopic route (courtesy of the late Prof. L. Demling).

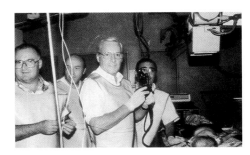

Fig. 56. Prof. Michel Cremer of Brussels, performing a sphincterotomy in a nine month old infant (courtesy of Prof. Michel Cremer).

Classen[29]. Since then, many new prototypes of protheses and drainage tubes have been manufactured including devices for the endoscopic drainage of pancreatic pseudocysts. Ultrasound endoscopy[17, 66] is discussed in Chapter 6.

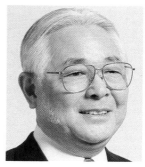

Fig. 57. Rikya Fujita of Showa University, Director of the International Learning Center of Digestive Endoscopy. Together with S. Sohma, he modified Kawai's papillotome which has been frequently employed in Japan. (from a book in honour of Prof. R. Fujita, Showa University, September 2001).

REFERENCES

1 Armengol-Miró J.R. Endoscopic sphincterotomy. Hepatogastroenterology 1992; 39 (suppl 1): 56-61.

2 Armengol-Miró J.R. Terapéutica endoscópica bilio-pancreática. in F.Vilardell, J.Rodés, J.Malagelada, J.M.Pajares, A.Perez-Mota, E.Moreno Gonzalez y J.Puig-Lacalle (eds). Enfermedades Digestivas. vol.III, 2 edition, Madrid, Aula Médica, 1998.

3 Bakes J.- Die Choledocopapilloskopie nebst Bemerkungen über Hepaticusdrainage und dilatation der Papilla Arch Klin Chir 1923; 126: 473-483.

4 Bard L., Pic A.- Contribution à l'etude clinique et anatomopathologique du cancer primitif du pancreas Rev Med (Paris) 1888; 8: 257-282.

5 Beck C.- The representation of biliary calculi by the roentgen rays. N.Y. Med J. (mar 16) 1901; 446-448.

6 Bilbao M.K., Dotter C.T., Lee T.G. y cols. Complications of endoscopic retrograde cholangiopancreatography (E.R.C.P.). A study of 10,000 cases. Gastroenterology 1976; 70: 314-320.

7 Boyden E.A. Behavior of human gallbladder during fasting and in response to food. Proc. Soc Exper Biol & Med 1926; 24: 157-162.

8 Burckhardt H., Müller W.- Versuche über die Punktion der Gallenblase und ihre Röntgendarstellung. Deutsch Zeitschr f. Chir 1921;162: 168-197.

9 Buxbaum A.- Über die Photographie von Gallensteinen in vivo. Wiener med Presse 1898; 14: 534-538.

9 Caroli J.- les ictères par rétention. Diagnostic medico-chirurgical, Paris, Masson, 1956.

10 Carter R.F., Saypol G.M.- Transabdominal cholangiography. J.A.M.A. 1952; 148: 253-255.

11 Chauffard A. Leçons sur la Lithiase Biliaire. Paris, Masson, 1914.

12 Classen M., Demling L.- Endoskopische Sphinkterotomie der Papilla Vateri und Steinextraction aus dem Ductus Choledocus. Deutsch Med Wschr 1974; 99: 496-497.

13 Courvoisier L.J.- Kasuistische Beiträge zur Pathogenese und Chirurgie der Gallenwege. Leipzig, Vogel, 1890.

14 Demling L., Seuberth K., Riemann J.F.- A mechanical litotriptor. Endoscopy 1982; 14: 100-101.

15 Demling L.- Operative endoskopie. Die Medizinische Welt 1973; 24: 1253-1255.

16 DiMagno E.P., Buxton J.L., Regan P.T. y cols. Ultrasonic endoscope. Lancet 1980; 1: 629-631.

17 Dittrich H.- Zur Geschichte der Cholangioskopie. in Meilensteine der Endoskopie. 2. Symposium der Internationalen Nitze-Leiter Forschungsgesellschaft für Endoskopie. Wien, Literas Universitätsverlag, 2000: 339-344.

18 Dormia E.- Due nuovi apparecchi per la rimozione dei calcoli dall'uretere. Urologia 1958; 25: 225-233.

19 Doubilet H., Poppel M.H.,Mulholland J.H.- Pancreatography: technics, principles and observations. Radiology 1955; 64: 325-339.

20 Editorial: Langenbuch, master surgeon of the biliary system. Arch Surg (Chicago) 1932;178: 25-26.

21 Fujita R., Sohma S.- Endoscopic sphincterotomy Gastroenterol Endosc 1974; 16: 446-453.

22 Geenen J.E., Hogan W.J., Schaffer R.D. y cols. Endoscopic electrosurgical papillotomy and manometry in biliary tract disease. J.A.M.A. 1977; 237: 2075-2078.

23 Geenen J.E., Hogan W.J., Dodds W.J. Sphincter of Oddi. In M.V.Sivak (ed.) Gastroenterologic Endoscopy. Philadelphia, W.B. Saunders, 1987: 735-751.

24 Gocho K., Hiratsjuka H, Hasegawa M. et al.- Percutaneous intrahepatic fistula dilation for nonoperative cholechoscopy in intrahepatic stones. Jpn J Gastroenterol 1974; 71: 526-527.

25 Gocho K., Hiratsuka., Yamakawa T.- Endoscopic management of intrahepatic calculi using the choledochofiberscope. Proceedings of the Second Asian-Pacific Congress of Endoscopy. Singapore 1976: 214-218.

26 Gocho K., Kameya S., Iljima N. Choledochofiberscopy. en M.V. Sivak (ed) Gastroenterologic Endoscopy, Philadelphia, W.B. Saunders, 1987: 732-769.

27 Graham E.A., Cole W.H.- Roentgenological examination of the gallbladder. Preliminary report of a new metod utilizing the intravenous injection if tetrabromophenolphtalein J.A.M.A. 1924; 82: 613-614.

28 Hagenmüller F.,Dammermann R, Wurbs M, Classen M. Directe Cholangiographie und biliäre Drainage beim Ikterus. en H.Henning (ed.) Fortschritte der gastroenterologischen Endoskopie Band 10. Baden-Baden, Witzstock, 1979: 65-70.

29 Henning H., Look D.- Laparoskopie. Atlas und Lehrbuch, Stuttgart, Georg Thieme, 1985.

30 Henning N., Demling L., Gigglberger H.- Über die laparoskopische Cholezysto-cholangiographie. Münch med Wschr 1952; 94: 830-834.

31 Huard P, Do-Xuan-Hop.- La ponction transhépatique des canaux biliaires. Bulletin de la Société de Médecine et Chirurgie d'Indochine. 1937; 28: 1090-1100.

32 Kalk H.- Laparoskopische Colezysto und Colangiographie. Dsch med Wschr 1952; 77: 590-591.

33 Kasugai T., Kuno N., Kobayashi S. et al.- Endoscopic pancreatocholangiography I.the normal endoscopic pancreatocholangiogram. Gastroenterology 1972; 63: 217-226.

34 Kawai K., Niwa H., Fujita R., Shimizu S.- The history of endoscopy: the Japanese perspective in Gastroenterological Endoscopy M.Classen, G.N.J.Tytgat, CJ Lightdale (eds) Stuttgart, Georg Thieme 2002: 32-45.

35 Kawai K., Akasaka Y., Murakami M., Tada M., Kohli Y., Nakajima M.- Endoscopic sphincterotomy of the ampulla of Vater. Gastrointest Endosc 1974; 20: 148-151.

36 Kawai K., Akasaka Y., Nakajima M.- Preliminary report on endoscopic papillotomy. J Kyoto Pref Univ Med 1973; 82: 53-55.

37 Kiyonaga G., Shinji Y., Kakiuchi Y., Nakajima K., y cols. Experience of 1100 cases examined by direct cholecystography with special apparatus under laparoscopic control. Advances in Gastrointestinal Endoscopy, Proceedings 2nd World Congress of Gastrointestinal Endoscopy 1970. G.Marcozzi, M.Crespi (eds) Padua, Piccin Medical Books 1972: 925-926.

38 Kolischer G. Der Katheterismus der Ureteren beim Weibe. Wien Klin Wschr 1896; 9: 1155-1156.

39 Koch H., Rösch W., Valz V.- Endoscopic lithotripsy in the common bile duct. Gastrointest Endosc 1980; 26: 16-18.

40 Langenbuch C.J.A. Ein Fall con Extirpation der Gallenblase wegen chronische Cholelithiasis Berlin Klin Wschr 1882; 725-728.

41 Mallet-Guy P.Jean-Jean R, Marion P. La chirurgie biliaire sous contrôle manométrique et radiologique per-opératoire. Paris, Masson, 1947.

42 McCune W.S., Shorb P.E., Moscovitz H.- Endoscopic cannulation of the Ampulla of Vater. A preliminary report. Ann Surg 1968; 167: 752-756.

43 McIver M.A.- An instrument for visualizing the interior of the common duct at operation. Surgery 1941; 9: 112-114.

44 Mirizzi P.L. La colangiografía durante las operaciones de las vias biliares. Boletines y Trabajos Soc Cir Buenos Aires 1932; 16: 1133-1141.

45 Mirizzi P.L. Operative cholangiography Surg Gynecol Obstet 1937; 65: 702-705.

46 Nakajima M, Akasaka Y, FukumotoK, Mitsuyoshi Y, Kawai K. Peroral cholangiopancreatoscopy (PCPS) under duodenoscopic guidance. Am J Gastroenterol 1976; 66: 241-247.

47 Nakajima M., Mukai H, Kawai K. Peroral cholangioscopy and pancreatoscopy. en Gasrtroenterologic Endoscopy. M.Sivak (ed), 2nd edition, Philadelphia, WB Saunders, 2000.

48 Nebel O.T., Silvis S.E., Rogers B.H-G. y cols. Complications associated with retrograde cho-

langiopancreatography. Results of the 1974 A.S.G.E. survey. Gastrointest Endosc 1975; 22: 34-36.

49 Nimura Y., Hayakawa M., Toyoda S.et al. Percutaneous transhepatic cholangioscopy (PTCS) Stomach and Intestine 1981; 16: 681-689.

50 Oi I., Takemoto T., Kondo T.- Fiberduodenoscopoe: direct observation of the papilla of Vater. Endoscopy 1969; 3: 101-103.

51 Oi I., Kobayashi S., Kondo T.- Endoscopic pancreatocholangiography Endoscopy 1970; 2: 103-106.

52 Oi I.- Fiberduodenoscopy and endoscopic pancreaticocholangiography Gastrointest Endosc 1970;17: 59-62.

53 Okuda K., Tanikawa K, Emura S. y cols. Nonsurgical, percutaneous transhepatic cholangiography —diagnostic significance in medical problems of the liver. Dig. Dis 1974; 19: 21-27.

54 Ottenjann R.- Choledochusverweilsonde nach endoskopischer Papillotomie. Münch med Wschr 1976; 118: 114-118.

55 Rabinov K., Simon M.- Peroral cannulation of Ampulla of Vater for Direct Cholangiography and pancreatography. Radiology 1965; 85: 693-697.

56 Reuter M.A.- Geschichte der Endoskopie. Handbuch und Atlas Band 1-4. Stuttgart-Zürich, Karl Krämer Verlag, 1998.

57 Royer M., Solari A.V., Cottero-Canari R.- La colangiografía no quirúrgica: nuevo método de exploración de las vías biliares. Arch Argent Enferm Apar Dig 1942: 17: 368-382.

58 Royer M., Solari A.V.- Cholangiography performed with the help of peritoneoscopy. Gastroenterology 1947; 8: 586-591.

59 Royer M. La colangiografía laparoscópica. Buenos Aires, El Ateneo, 1952.

60 Schein C.J., Stern W.Z., Hurwitt E.S., Jacobson H.G.- Cholangiography and biliary endoscopy as complementary methods of evaluating bile ducts Am J Roentgenol 1963; 89: 864-875.

61 Schein C.J.- Biliary endoscopy: an appraisal of its value in biliary lithiasis. Surgery 1969; 65: 1004-1007.

62 Shore J.M., Shore E.- Operative biliary endoscopy: experience with flexible choledocoscope in 100 consecutive cholecocholithotomires Ann Surg 1970; 171: 269-276.

63 Sivak M. ERCP at thirty years an interview with Dr. William S. McCune (1909-1998) Gastrointest Endosc 1998; 48: 643-644.

64 Soehendra N., Reynders-Frederix V.- Palliative Gallengangsdrainage. Eine neue Methode zur endoskopischen Einführung eines inneren Drains. Dtsch Med Wschr 1979; 104: 206-207.

65 Strohm W.D., Phillip J., Hagenmüller F., Classen M.- Ultrasound tomography by means of an ultrasound fiberendoscope. Endoscopy. 1980; 12: 241-244.

66 Takagi K., Ikeda S., Nakagawa Y., Kumakura K., Maruyama M., Someya N., Takada T., Takekoshi T., Kin T.- Endoscopic cannulation of the Ampulla of Vater Endoscopy 1970; 2: 107-115.

67 Vondrasek P., Eberhardt G., Classen M. Endoscopic semiconductor manometry. Int J. Med. 1974; 3: 188-192.

68 Vondrasek P., Eberhardt G. Endoskopische Druckmessungen mittels Halbleitertechnik. Z. Gastroenterologie 1974; 12: 453-458.

69 Wildegans H. Die operative Gallengangenendoskopie. München, Urban & Schwarzenberg, 1960.

70 Wurbs D., Classen M.- Transpapillary longstanding tube for hepatobiliary drainage. Endoscopy 1977; 9: 192-194.

71 Yamagata S., Miura K., Tadaki H., Kohyama K., Komatsu K. A new instrument for peritoneoscopic cholangiography. Proceedings First World Congress of Endoscopy, Tokyo 1966: 516-519.

72 Yamakawa T., Komako F., Shikata J.- Biliary tract endoscopy with an improved choledochoscope. Gastrointest Endosc 1978; 24: 110-113.

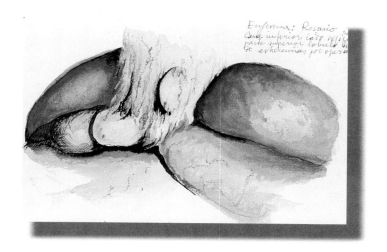

CHAPTER 13

History of diagnostic and therapeutic laparoscopy

INTRODUCTION

THE EMERGENCE OF LAPAROSCOPY OWES MUCH TO THE TALENTED urologist Max Nitze from Berlin (1848-1906) and the instrument maker Joseph Leiter from Vienna (1839-1892) who together designed the first optical cystoscope (see Chapter 3). A few years later, some daring surgeons attempted to introduce cystoscopes, somewhat modified, inside the abdominal cavity. The procedure developed slowly as it was more complex and dangerous than endoscopy of the digestive tract, the indications were not so clear-cut and patients with acute conditions were often included.

Laparoscopy developed above all in Germany and neighbouring countries, thanks to internists and surgeons interested in abdominal disease. The first examinations were mostly done in patients with ascites; the abdominal fluid helped the introduction of the instrument and air insufflation. Pneumoperitoneum slowly gained adepts. It was often done in patients with "dry" abdomens and laparoscopy became a greatly valued examination for the diagnosis of liver disease, especially once biopsy needles were invented as these samples could then be taken under visual control.

Through the years, imaging techniques such as ultrasonography, nuclear magnetic resonance and the CAT scan have replaced many of the classical indications for laparoscopy[11]. However, starting from the late 1970s, the apparent loss of popularity of diagnostic laparoscopy was amply compensated for by the increasing usage of the method by gynaecologists who employed it extensively for diagnosis and surgical interventions which usually required laparotomies, such as tubal ligations.

As we will discuss later, it was a gynaecologist, Kurt Semm[97] who first performed a surgical laparoscopic intervention on the digestive tract, an appendectomy (1983). Since then, the interest of surgeons for laparoscopy has turned it into the elective method for a great variety of abdominal operations and at the same time it has allowed a resurgence of laparoscopy as a diagnostic tool.

PARACENTESIS AND PNEUMOPERITONEUM AS DIAGNOSTIC PROCEDURES.

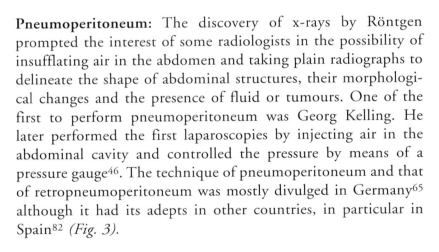

Paracentesis: Paracentesis was the first diagnostic and therapeutic procedure employed for the examination of the abdominal cavity. The use of a trocar (derived from the old French expression "trois-quarts") for punction and drainage seems to be rather an old procedure[98]. The first "modern" instrument for abdominal punction was devised by Pierre Charles Edouard Potain (1825-1901), a famous French cardiologist[3]. Potain was born in Paris into a family of physicians. He studied at the Sorbonne, graduated in 1853 and invented the first device to measure arterial pressure (the sphingomanometer). He was also one of the first to graphically document cardiac murmurs. Potain designed his trocar to perform pleural and abdominal punctures in patients with serous effusions at the Necker Hospital in Paris where in 1875 he was chief of the medical service and professor of Clinical Medicine. His instrument, not very different from those used today, consisted of a metal sheath in which a sharp probe was introduced and then withdrawn after puncture, allowing the drainage of fluid through the outer sheath. The tube was connected to a vacuum-aspirating device of his invention, particularly useful in the case of pleural punctures *(Fig.1, 2).*

Fig. 1. Pierre Charles Potain (1825-1901). Cardiologist, inventor of the sphyngomanometer, physician to the Hospital Necker in Paris (courtesy of Dr. F.J.Cortada, Buenos Aires).

Fig. 2. Trocar used by Potain for abdominal paracentesis (ref. 84).

Pneumoperitoneum: The discovery of x-rays by Röntgen prompted the interest of some radiologists in the possibility of insufflating air in the abdomen and taking plain radiographs to delineate the shape of abdominal structures, their morphological changes and the presence of fluid or tumours. One of the first to perform pneumoperitoneum was Georg Kelling. He later performed the first laparoscopies by injecting air in the abdominal cavity and controlled the pressure by means of a pressure gauge[46]. The technique of pneumoperitoneum and that of retropneumoperitoneum was mostly divulged in Germany[65] although it had its adepts in other countries, in particular in Spain[82] *(Fig. 3).*

VON OTT'S "VENTROSCOPY"

Most authors attribute the first attempts at laparoscopy, or peritoneoscopy as it was called for many years in the Anglo-Saxon world, to Dimitri Oskarovich Ott, a well-known gynaecologist from Saint Petersburg. The author is mentioned as simply "Ott" in the Soviet Encyclopaedia but as Demetrius von Ott or Edler von Ott in articles which he published in German medical journals. Ott was born

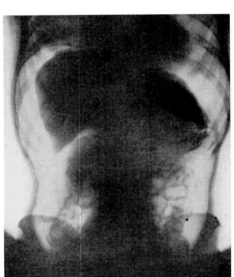

Fig. 3. Diagnostic Pneumoperitoneum (Lorey, 1914) (ref. 65).

in 1855 in Ulianovo and was director of the department of obstetrics and gynae-cology at the Saint Petersburg University Hospital *(Fig. 4)*.

Ott examined the abdominal cavity in several female patients by means of a speculum introduced into the abdomen by the transvaginal route. He named his method "ventroscopy" and also, according to the Soviet Encyclopaedia, "vaginal laparotomy", but unfortunately all his early papers were published in Russian and therefore were little read in other countries. In 1902, he published a paper with several illustrations –in a German journal which had a wide diffusion– on the direct inspection of the abdominal cavity, the bladder and the colon[76]. Ott made a section in the posterior vaginal fornix, introduced a speculum and a lighting system. This could be either external by means of a frontal lamp or internal, using a lamp attached to his speculum. He then insufflated air filtered through sterile cotton pads, to separate the bowel. Ott claimed that by properly positioning the patient, in the majority of cases he was able to visualise not only the pelvis but also the navel, the gallbladder, a portion of the liver, the caecum and the appendix *(Figs. 5, 6, 7, 8)*.

In 1929, Ott died in Leningrad (then the new name for Saint Petersburg), apparently unmolested by the Soviet Government in spite of his German name (von Ott) and his probably noble origin. He did not seem to have any followers in spite of his assertion that thanks to "ventroscopy" the number of laparotomies in his service had decreased by half[77].

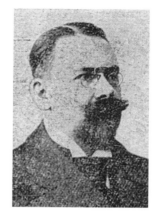

Fig. 4. Dimitri Oskarovich Ott or von Ott, (1855-1929) professor of gynaeco-logy in Saint Petersburg. (redrawn from Bubibchenko, Akud Ginek 1958;34:120).

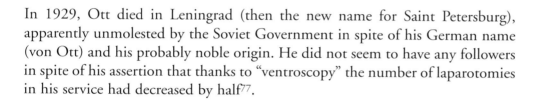

Fig. 5. Title page of the most extensive article on "ventroscopy" published in German by von Ott one hundred years ago (1902) (ref. 76).

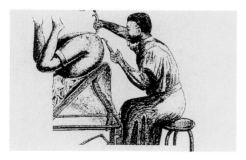

Fig. 6. Position of the patient for the perfor-mance of ventroscopy. (ref. 76).

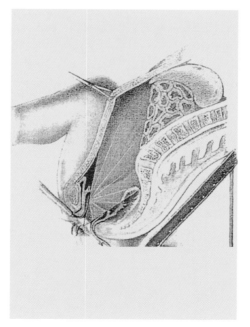

Fig. 7. Visual field of von Ott's speculum after pneumoperitoneum. (ref. 76).

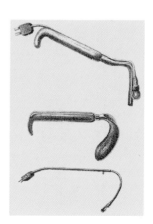

Fig. 8. Set of instruments employed by von Ott for "ventroscopy" (ref. 76).

GEORG KELLING'S "COELIOSCOPY"

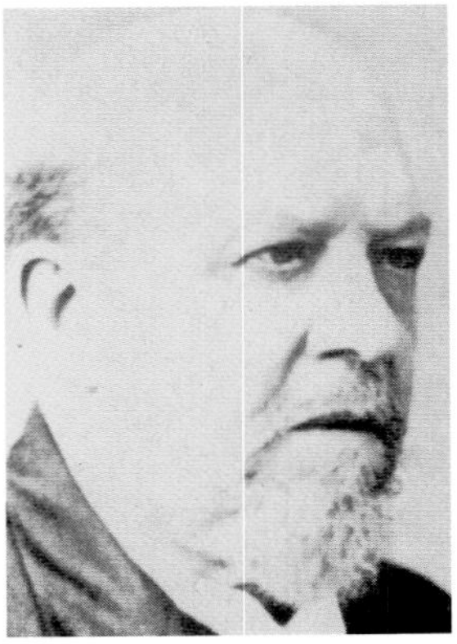

The first to examine the peritoneal cavity through an external abdominal incision was Georg Kelling (1866-1945). Kelling was born in Dresden and died there —one of the thousands of victims of the aerial bombings that destroyed the city at the end of World War Two (1945). After studying medicine in Leipzig and later in Berlin he then returned to Leipzig where he passed his medical licensure examinations. His doctoral thesis on "the measurement of the capacity of the stomach" was probably written in Ewald's laboratory in Berlin. He was later appointed professor of surgery in Dresden *(Fig. 9)*.

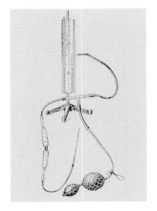

Fig. 9. Georg Kelling (1866-1845), surgeon, disciple of von Mikulicz, inventor of a gastrocamera, and a gastroscope and pioneer of laparoscopy. He died during the Dresden bombings in 1945. (courtesy of Dr. Harald Henning).

Kelling was a pioneer in many endoscopic examinations, as we have seen in other chapters of this book, and he created original instruments for oesophagoscopy, gastroscopy and intragastric photography (chapters 4 and 7). After starting his career as a clinician, he changed to surgery after an internship in Mikulicz's service in Breslau. Another subject which Kelling studied in depth was the technique of pneumoperitoneum. As of 1901, after experiments in dogs, he employed this technique to control intraabdominal haemorrhage by means of a tamponade, injecting air into the abdomen under pressure and controlling the operation by means of a mercury manometer ("Lufttamponade") *(Fig. 10)*.

To observe the effects of introducing air under pressure into the peritoneum, Kelling decided to use a cystoscope. In experiments in dogs he introduced a small Nitze cystoscope (6 mm in diameter) after previous insufflation with a Fiedler trocar. In 1901 in Hamburg he presented his observations at the 73rd Congress of the German Society for Biology and Medicine. He even gave a demonstration of "coelioscopy" on a living dog and suggested the possible use of the technique in humans. His Hamburg presentation in which he also reported his observations on oesophagoscopy and gastroscopy, was published in 1902 with the title: "Uber Oesophagoskopie, Gastroscopie und Kölioskopie"[46]. Although he announced his intention to publish his results of coelioscopy in humans, a review of later literature does not include any further mention of this method by Kelling. Neither did he insist, it seems, in his attempts to stop intraperitoneal bleeding by means of air tamponade, a technique apparently poorly tolerated by the patients.

Fig. 10. Manometer employed by Kelling for pneumoperitoneum, also utilized for abdominal "tamponade" in intraperitoneal haemorrhage (in Gumprecht F. Die Technik der speziellen Therapie, Jena, Fischer, 1906).

HANS CHRISTIAN JACOBAEUS AND "LAPARO-THORACOSCOPY"

Ten years later, the famous Swedish clinician Hans Christian Jacobaeus (1879-1937), unaware of Kelling's work, also used a cystoscope to examine the pleural, abdominal and even the pericardial cavities in patients with serous effusions. As an aid he injected air through a trocar which he used to insert the cystoscope. In 1910, he published his first experiences in the "Münchener Medizinische Wochenschrift", a weekly medical journal from Munich, perhaps the most prestigious in Germany at the time[31, 32] *(Figs. 11, 12)*.

Jacobaeus was mainly interested in the treatment of tuberculosis and the dissemination of the infection through the serosal cavities. He had performed thoracocentesis and then insufflated air, creating an artificial pneumothorax, following the method of the Italian pneumologist, Forlanini, of whom he considered himself an intellectual disciple. Jacobaeus noticed that one could inject air into the pleural cavity without danger and that the space created was sufficient for the insertion of a cystoscope. He then thought that it would be even easier to insufflate the peritoneum (a technique which had been employed therapeutically in cases of tuberculous peritonitis) and thus easily explore the abdominal cavity with an endoscope.

For the abdominal puncture, Jacobaeus employed a trocar size 17 and a cystoscope diameter nº 15 of the same Charrière gauge. Later on he used a nº 13[33].

In his first paper, Jacobaeus reported cases of pleuroscopy after thoracocentesis and of abdominal endoscopy after withdrawal of ascites and inducing a pneumoperitoneum. He published a study comprising seventeen patients with ascites and two more patients without peritoneal effusion in whom he performed pneumoperitoneum and laparoscopy. It is interesting to remark that already at that time Jacobaeus predicted that "laparoscopy will be useful for the examination of the upper abdominal cavity, particularly of the liver". The Swedish clinician gave wide publicity to his method and published papers in several languages; he gave a lecture in London and he made laparoscopic demonstrations in Germany, in particular at the Hamburg-Eppendorf Hospital where diagnostic pneumoperitoneum had been used extensively by radiologists[33, 65]. In 1912, Jacobaeus published a monograph *(Fig. 13)* which made him famous and in which he described in great detail 97 laparoscopies performed over two years. Among the diagnoses reported in his book were cases of cirrhosis, hepatic syphilis and tuberculous peritonitis. The beneficial effect of air insufflation in the clinical course of tuberculous peritonitis was also confirmed[34].

Jacobaeus did very few examinations in patients without ascites, probably for fear of perforating an intestinal loop during the examination, and he suggested that in the future laparoscopy would possibly compete with diagnostic laparotomy in the

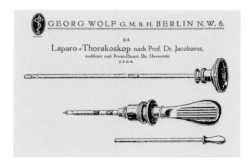

Fig. 11. Jacobaeus performing thoracoscopy (courtesy of the late Dr. Laurits Lauridsen).

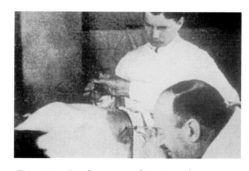

Fig. 12. Trocar and laparoscope manufactured by the firm Georg Wolf employed by Jacobaeus (from a press advertisement by the firm G. Wolf).

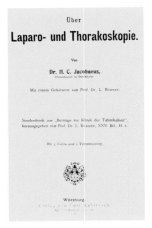

Fig. 13. Front page of the book "Laparo-und Thorakoskopie" by Jacobaeus which gave him great prestige (1913).

investigation of abdominal disease. His monograph was the first of its kind and apparently until 1927 there was no other book published on the subject[49].

After reading Jacobaeus paper, Kelling reacted violently and published a note, also in Münchener Medizinische Wochenschrift, claiming the paternity of laparoscopy based on his communication of 1901 and on two other laparoscopies which he had performed in patients during the following years. He wrote " I am happy to know that Mr. Jacobaeus has reintroduced the question of the visualisation of serosal cavities which he has done with such success. However, you will easily understand that I cannot accept his priority claim on a method which I performed first"[47]. There followed an acerbic discussion between the two authors, and Kelling continued to insist on the matter of his paternity of laparoscopy. Years later, he was still complaining because neither Korbsch nor Kalk quoted his work in their monographs on laparoscopy[48]. Kalk, who was not an accommodating man either, sent a harsh rebuttal to the journal: "if over nine years Kelling has only performed two laparoscopies in human beings it follows that he did not value the method very much, as he would not have limited himself only to two examinations.... laparoscopy would exist today even without Kelling's coelioscopy"[39].

An impartial observer, Litynski[60] summarised the controversy as follows: "Kelling was no doubt the first to conceive the idea of examining the peritoneum with a cystoscope, but there is no doubt either that Jacobaeus was the first to employ laparoscopy for the diagnosis of abdominal disease, that he published the results of 19 observations and that he was the first to use the term "laparoscopy". Curiously enough, in the following years, Jacobaeus apparently lost interest in laparoscopy and his name became mostly associated with an intervention which he preconised for endoscopically resecting pleural adhesions in patients with tuberculosis, the so-called "Jacobaeus operation".

BERNHEIM, RENON, MEIRELLES, ROCCAVILLA, STOLKIND, TEDESCO

Other physicians became interested in Jacobaeus' publications[89, 94]. Bertram Bernheim (1911)[8] from the Johns Hopkins Hospital in Baltimore was the first in the United States to employ a cystoscope to examine the abdominal cavity. He called his method "organoscopy". Somewhat later, in 1913, Louis Renon[84] from France published two papers on the technique and the value of laparoscopy, while in 1913 in Brazil, E.A. Meirelles[67] also employed Jacobaeus instruments. In 1914, a paper on laparoscopy appeared in Italy. It was signed by Andrea Roccavilla from Modena[86] and described an instrument for the direct vision of the abdomen through a tube without any optical system, using a trocar that he had devised. This was made by the firm Fischer from Freiburg in Brisgau and was fitted to the Brünings electroscope employed by oesophagoscopists *(Figs. 14, 15)*.

The trocar was provided with a fawcet for the withdrawal of ascites and a valve to avoid fluid leaks during the examination. However, when judged necessary, a cystoscope could also be inserted through the trocar[87]. The instrument did not represent a step forward and was little used because of the difficulty in observation through a hollow instrument and the poor illumination. In an English journal in 1919, the Russian E.J. Stolkind[102] published his own laparoscopic technique which he had apparently been using since 1912 according to the references (in Russian) which were included in his paper. He employed Nitze's cystoscope and before the examination performed a pneumoperitoneum in patients without ascites using a blunt needle with distal and lateral holes and insufflating air very slowly *(Fig. 16)*.

Another follower of Jacobaeus was F. Tedesco, who in 1912 published an article on laparoscopy based on a communication which he presented at the Viennese Society for Internal Medicine and Paediatrics[103].

THE FIRST GERMAN LAPAROSCOPIST: ROGER KORBSCH

As of 1921, Korbsch promoted the Jacobaeus techniques more than any other physician in Germany. He was already known as an expert in oesophago-gastroscopy and designer of a rigid gastroscope which was very easy to insert because of its thin calibre (see Chapter 3). In 1927, he published an important textbook and atlas on laparoscopy in which he reported 300 observations of laparoscopy as well as 200 thoracoscopies done in 6 years[49]. Korbsch was chief of medicine at the St Elizabeth Hospital in Oberhausen (Westphalia). After local anaesthesia of the skin, he performed a pneumoperitoneum with a Götze or a Schmidt needle and then introduced a trocar provided with a small valve to control the injection of air. The trocar was marked with signs at 3 and 5 cm. to control the depth of penetration. He used a straight cystoscope fitted with Ringleb's optical system (made by the firm Georg Wolf in Berlin) and a calibre n. 13 of Charrière which pro-

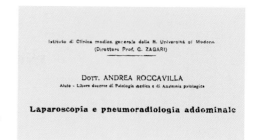

Fig. 14. Title page of the article by Andrea Roccavilla from Modena on Laparoscopy and diagnostic pneumoperitoneum (1914).

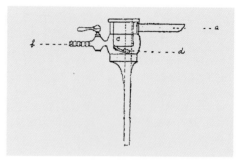

Fig. 15. Roccavilla's trocar provided with a lateral arm (a) for fitting the electroscope. A fawcet on the opposite side which is conected to the endoscopic tube and allows air insufflation or withdraw ascitic fluid. A valve (c) closes the instrument hermetically. A Nitze's cystoscope can be introduced through it when necessary (ref. 86).

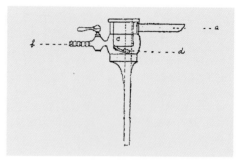

Fig. 16. Title page of the paper by the Russian E. Stolkind on laparoscopy (1919).

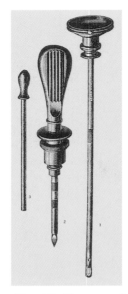

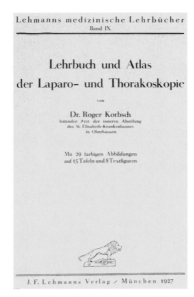

Fig. 17. Trocar and laparoscope designed by R. Korbsch and made by the firm Georg Wolf from Berlin (ref. 49).

Fig. 18. Front page of Roger Korbsch's book on laparoscopy, published in 1927 (courtesy of Dr. Tomas Pinós Desplat).

vided an angle of vision greater than the 90º given by Jacobaeus' instruments *(Figs.17, 18, 19)*.

His laparoscope was 22 cm long. The atlas included a series of watercolours of the abdominal cavity (the work of the artist Elfriede Hähndels) and may be considered a classical work on diagnostic laparoscopy. In 1923, another distinguished laparoscopist was Unverricht[105]. He too performed thoracoscopy.

Although Jacobaeus had established the general indications of the laparoscopic examination, Korbsch wrote that " laparoscopy should be used when the diagnosis cannot be established by any other means and there are good possibilities to visualise the lesion", a statement which seems perfectly valid today. Korbsch also mentioned the possibility of performing laparoscopy at the bedside, a prediction which has not been fulfilled.

HEINRICH-OTTO KALK (1895-1973)

Possibly Heinz Kalk (as he is usually named) was the greatest clinical laparoscopist of all times. His detailed biography is the work of his old disciple and close associate, Egmont Wildhirt[108]. Kalk was born in Frankfurt, the son of a school master. He studied medicine in Freiburg, Marburg and Frankfurt.

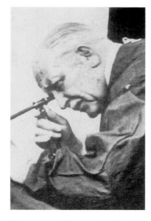

Fig. 20. Heinz Kalk, the most famous laparoscopist of his era, performing laparoscopy (courtesy of the Falk Foundation).

Upon graduation, he began to practice surgery as an assistant of von Schmieden. He then worked in internal medicine for 4 years with von Bergmann whom he followed to Berlin, first as an assistant and then as an Oberartz (chief resident) of his chair at the renowned La Charité Hospital *(Fig. 20)*.

Von Bergmann's clinic was not short of attending physicians who acquired great reputations: Hans Heinrich Berg later went on to Hamburg and became world known for his work on the early diagnosis of gastric cancer, and

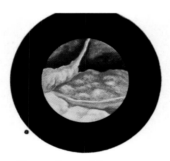

Fig. 19. Watercolour of liver metastases (author: Elfriede Hähndels) (ref.49).

Gerhard Katsch became chief of medicine in Greifswald where he studied gastric and pancreatic secretion. There Kalk initiated his endoscopic experience, mainly in rectoscopy and gastroscopy and in 1934 he was appointed chief of medicine at the Hospital Friederichshain in Berlin, where he established a great reputation. One of his patients was Cardinal Pacelli, the Vatican Nunzio, who became Pope under the name of Pius XII and with whom he developed a lasting friendship[108]. His success in Berlin led him to turn down a chair in Erlangen (later taken up by Norbert Henning). After World War Two, in 1949, Kalk was able to move to Kassel where he was appointed chief of medicine at the City Hospital (Stadtkrankenhaus). He remained there until his official retirement in 1963, ending his days in Bad Kissingen where he had first started his private practice.

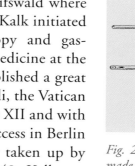

Fig. 21. First laparoscope employed by Kalk, made by the firm Heynemann (ref. 38).

KALK AND THE BOOM OF LAPAROSCOPY

Kalk's interest in laparoscopy was prompted by Georg Katsch, von Bergmann's associate. He had invented a method for the internal examination of the abdomen of animals "in vivo" by means of a celluloid window through which the peristaltic movements of the bowel could be observed[108]. Kalk did laparoscopies using an instrument of his own design made by the firm Heynemann (also known also for its rectoscopes). The endoscope had an oblique 135 º lens system and was introduced through a trocar 6 mm in diameter. By 1929 he had examined 100 patients[38] *(Figs. 21, 22)*.

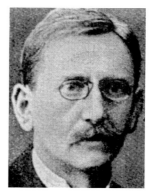

Fig. 22. C.J. Heynemann, optical instruments maker. Among them N. Henning's gastroscope and the first Kalk laparoscope (courtesy of Prof. H.J. Reuter).

A few years earlier, in 1924, the Swiss physician Zollikofer started using CO_2 instead of air for pneumoperitoneum insufflation[109]. Later, in 1940, Kalk started taking liver biopsies with needles made by Georg Wolf, under direct vision, introducing the needle through a second abdominal puncture *(Figs. 23, 24, 25)*.

In 1942 Kalk made the first colour photographs with a photo-laparoscope[42]. His influence in Europe was immense[54, 69]. Between 1950 and 1963 Kalk welcomed more than 357 visitors

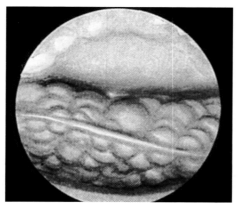

Fig. 23. Liver cirrhosis according to Kalk (courtesy of Editorial Alhambra).

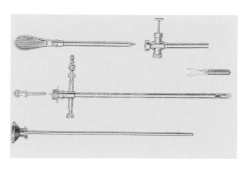

Fig. 24. The improved Kalk laparoscope manufactured by the firm Sass-Wolf (ref. 41).

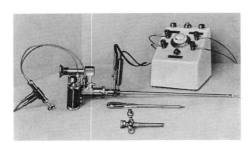

Fig. 25. Kalk's photolaparoscope made by the firm Sass-Wolf (leaflet by Sass Wolf, archives Hospital de Sant Pau).

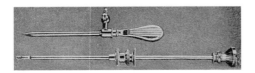

Fig. 26. Laparoscope designed by Norbert Henning and made by Richard Wolf (ref. 27).

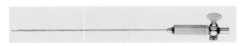

Fig. 27. Veres needle for pneumoperitoneum which was an improvement over other instruments (Hospital de Sant Pau).

to his service[108], these including H. Popper, G.Martini, H. Thaler, F. Hofstetter, J.Findor, L. de Laserna, and T.A.Pinós[83]- who would organise laparoscopy in Spain – and especially Giorgio Menghini who later invented a practical needle biopsy which was universally used.

Thanks to his enormous experience Kalk established the laparoscopic semiology of liver disease on solid grounds and was able to make long term follow-ups of many conditions, confirming his visual impressions by means of targeted biopsies[44, 45]. In his time, laparoscopy was probably the most important test to differentiate jaundice from various causes (red liver in hepatitis, green liver in obstructive jaundice). In 1952, as we have already described in chapter 9, Kalk attempted cholangiographies by directly puncturing the gallbladder under laparoscopic guidance[43].

THE DEVELOPMENT OF LAPAROSCOPIC INSTRUMENTATION

The first laparoscopists, such as Jacobaeus and others, used endoscopes derived from the original Nitze's cystoscope. All these instruments had an optical angle of 90º. The diagnostic laparoscope has not changed much through the years. It essentially consists of:

1) a needle provided with a guide for pneumoperitoneum, such as the one designed by Veres (this is the correct name of the author who is named Verres or Veress in some publications; even in the paper in which he introduced his needle, the name is mispelled!)[26, 73].
2) a trocar with a handle and a distal conical sharp end for the puncture of the abdomen, which may vary somewhat in design according to the instrument maker. The puncture is usually done through a small cutaneous incision.
3) an external sheath provided with a pressure valve to avoid loss of the insufflated air and at the same time to allow injection of either air or gas.
4) a rigid straight tube which is introduced into the hollow sheath once the trocar is withdrawn and which contains the optical system –not unlike that of a rigid cystoscope.

The development of the optical system owes a great deal to Kalk. In earlier times he used an instrument which was designed for him by the firm Heinemann from Berlin. It had an oblique (130º) optical lens which eliminated most blind areas[41]. Norbert Henning also designed a foroblique optical system manufactured by Georg Wolf *(Figs. 25, 26, 27)*.

After World War Two, Kalk designed a more perfected instrument for the Sass-Wolf company, one of the successors of the old Georg Wolf firm, known for its cystoscopes and for the semi-flexible Schindler gastroscope. In spite of the fact that Kalk had performed more than 3,000 laparoscopies with the first Heynemann laparoscope[42], his new instrument was longer (25 cm) to allow visualisation of the lower aspect of the diaphragm and the pelvic area. The diameter was somewhat greater and the trocar thinner (9 mm) with an optical rod 6.6 mm in diameter. The objective had a 135° angle, somewhat greater than that of the first model, giving a greater magnification of the image[45].

In 1952, Norbert Henning ordered a new laparoscope from the firm Richard Wolf, in Knittlingen, another successor of the original Georg Wolf firm. The trocar of this instrument was very sharp and smooth. The optical rod was inserted through a sheath 7.5 mm in caliber. The optical system, like Kalk's, was designed by the firm Zeiss-Kollmorgen with an angle deviation of 135° from the axis of the instrument, comparable to the Kalk version, and a somewhat smaller visual angle - 60°. The instrument's major drawback was the very short life of the distal lamps which had to be removed and changed quite frequently[27]. Henning, like Kalk, also tried to perform laparoscopic cholangiography, aided by Ludwig Demling who was his assistant at that time[28].

FIRST ATTEMPTS AT THERAPEUTIC LAPAROSCOPY: CARL FERVERS

Another innovator in laparoscopy was the German Carl Fervers (1898-1972) who was medical associate (Secundärarzt) at the City Hospital in Solingen. Fervers performed more than fifty laparoscopies with a cystoscope and he possibly did the first endoscopic liver biopsy in 1933, although he did not show much enthusiasm for the procedure. Apparently he was also the first to try therapeutic measures with the laparoscope. By means of a cautery, he sectioned suture threads which apparently caused abdominal pain in some operated patients. For this purpose, he employed light inhalation anaesthesia followed by local injections of novocaine and he described his technique in detail[15].

LAPAROSCOPY IN THE UNITED STATES. JOHN RUDDOCK (1891-1964)

We have already mentioned[8] the contributions of Bertram Bernheim (1911) who coined the term "organoscopy", those of B.H. Orndorff[75] in 1920, and those of Steiner in 1924, who used an angular cystoscope with a movable tip which was introduced after pneumoperitoneum. He first used oxygen and then air for insufflation. O.P. Steiner named his method "abdominoscopy" and he

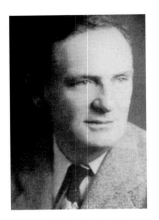

Fig. 28. John Ruddock (courtesy of Dr.G.S.Lytinski)

apparently believed that he had been the first to employ a cystoscope to visualise the inside of the abdomen. As one can readily guess by reading his paper, he was completely unaware of any previous work on the subject[101].

However, the greatest advocate of laparoscopy in the United States was John Ruddock. According to Litynski[59], Ruddocks' career after his military service in the Navy developed in the field of internal medicine which he practiced privately in California. His major interest was cardiology and he was successful to the point of being elected president of the California Heart Association. During the 1930s, he became interested in laparoscopy which he performed with a McCarthy cystoscope, made by the firm Wappler (later A.C.M.I.) in patients with ascites, selected as others had done before him, because of the ease with which pneumoperitoneum could be carried out *(Figs. 28, 29, 30)*.

In 1934, he introduced his own peritoneoscope with which he had performed 200 examinations[90]. In 1937, with a better instrument, he published a series of 500 cases[91]. His laparoscope was employed by American laparoscopists for several decades. It consisted of a trocar ending in a knife, a metal sheath, an optical system 35 cm long and a biopsy clamp that could be fitted to the optical tube and could be used for electrocoagulation without having first to withdraw the tissue obtained by biopsy. Ruddock used air for insufflation. His was the only instrument that allowed biopsies to be taken under direct visual control until Jacobs and Palmer designed their own operative laparoscope.

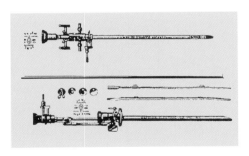

Fig. 29. McCarthy's cystoscope employed by Ruddock in his first examinations (1923). (ref. 90).

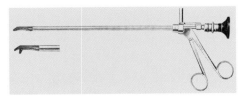

Fig. 30. Ruddock's clamp for laparoscopic biopsy made by the firm A.C.M.I. (courtesy of A.C.M.I.).

Ruddock used the laparoscope mostly for the differential diagnosis between cirrhotic ascites and neoplastic effusions, and performed peritoneal as well as liver biopsies. He considered that one of the main indications of laparoscopy was the investigation of liver metastases in patients suspected to be harbouring gastric carcinoma. He also described the endoscopic diagnosis of gynaecological tumours and ectopic pregnancies. In 1944, during World War Two, Ruddock was appointed chief of medical services at the San Diego Naval Hospital. After the war, he returned to his clinical practice. His last paper dates from 1957 and in it he reported on 5,000 laparoscopic examinations[92]. He analysed the accuracy of the procedure in detail and stated that in his hands the percentage of errors was around 6 per cent, while the clinical diagnosis could be wrong in as many as 48 per cent of instances. However, Ruddock always insisted that laparoscopy was not a substitute for laparotomy.

Ruddock demonstrated the relatively harmlessness of laparoscopy. He described eight accidents during his first 900 examinations, including three deaths, two from haemorrhage and the third because of a perforated viscus. In contrast with Kalk who used general anaesthesia, Ruddock used only local anaesthesia and recommended a brief hospitalization of 24 hours for his patients. However, laparoscopy was never much in demand among his American colleagues.

By 1941, more than 3,500 laparoscopies had been done in the entire United States. However, in 1966, two years after Ruddock's demise, a survey[79] carried out among 600 internists and 600 surgeons revealed that fewer than 10 per cent had done a single laparoscopy and fewer than one per cent had performed more than fifty examinations. The great majority of those who did were surgeons who did not find much practical application for the technique. However, there were exceptions, such as Edward Benedict from Boston –author of a popular book on endoscopy[5]– who had designed an operative gastroscope for taking biopsies based on Schindler's instrument, Steigmann and Villa in Chicago[100] and also William Lee in Philadelphia who even did a laparoscopic cholecystography[52]. On the other hand, laparoscopy established itself on much more solid grounds in continental Europe. Laparoscopy became quite popular in Spain thanks to Laserna[51], Gironés[24] and Pinós with his collaborators, Serés and Martí Vicente[66, 82].

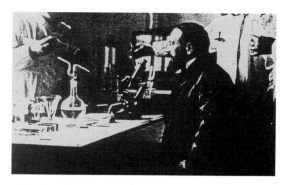

Fig. 31. Luigi Lucatello (1863-1926), professor of medicine and Rector of the University of Padova, who first sampled liver tissue with an aspiration needle for cytologic studies (courtesy of Ms. Maria Crapulli, Universitá Campus Bio-Medico, Rome).

LAPAROSCOPIC LIVER BIOPSY

According to Giorgio Menghini[68], the first to suggest the use of a needle for puncturing the liver tissue was Paul Ehrlich around 1885. However, in 1895, the versatile Italian pathologist Luigi Lucatello, professor of medicine at Padova University, was the first to recognise the potential diagnostic possibilities of the method. He employed a needle for the aspiration of liver tissue and obtained samples of cells in cases of cirrhosis. He described fatty degeneration and anysocytosis in these cells and also reported the resistance of the fibrotic liver tisssue to the puncture[83]. However, aspiration liver biopsy as such was probably first carried out in Denmark in 1939 by P. Iversen and K. Roholm[38] who led the way for other more practical and less dangerous devices. Laparoscopists usually employed longer needles which allowed sampling in spite of the greater distance between the abdominal wall and the liver surface caused by the presence of pneumoperitoneum (Figs. 31, 32, 33).

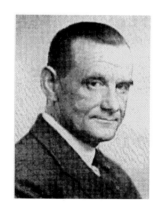

Fig. 32. Poul Iversen (Copenhagen) a pioneer with K.Roholm of aspiration biopsy of the liver and later, with C.Brun, of kidney biopsy (courtesy of the National Library of Medicine, copyright unknown).

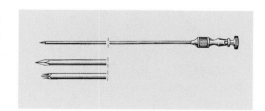

Fig. 33. The Iversen-Roholm aspiration needle, showing its jagged distal end and the pointed trocar. The needle was rotated after aspiration (courtesy of Dr. Harald Henning).

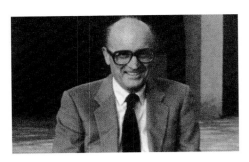

Fig. 34. Giorgio Menghini (1916-1984), a distinguished Italian clinician, designer of the so-called "Menghini needle" and of the Storz photolaparoscope (courtesy of Mr. M.G. Lorenzatto).

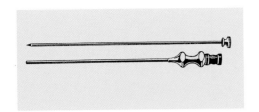

Fig. 35. Menghini's needle (courtesy of Dr. Harald Henning).

In general, liver biopsy was done through a separate incision by an assistant and visually guided by the laparoscopist[56]. Aspiration biopsy was first performed with Iversen and Roholm needles about 18 cm. long and 2 mm. in diameter[30, 88], while longer Vim-Silverman needles were used by French laparoscopists in Caroli's service in Paris. Iversen's and Vim-Silverman's needles were gradually replaced by Menghini's needle which was later used in most centres[74] (Figs. 34, 35).

The Pinós needle was also widely used in Spain[107] (Figs. 36, 37, 38). The Richard Wolf laparoscopes and those manufactured by the firm Karl Storz became universally employed for laparoscopy and biopsy. Nowadays, it is the "Tru-cut" type needle which is most employed for liver biopsy.

RISKS AND COMPLICATIONS IN THE EARLY DAYS

In 1966, Brühl[9] thoroughly reviewed the data on accidents of diagnostic laparoscopy in 63,845 examinations. The frequency of complications was 2.5 per cent and mortality was 0.03 per cent. Later series collected by Harald Henning[26] include 94,382 laparoscopies with a frequency of complications of 0.87 per cent and a mortality of 0.064 per cent. The most dangerous complications reported were, and still are, intestinal perforations and haemorrhage, the latter usually related to the performance of biopsy[40]. The frequency of complications, as expected, was lower in statistics featuring large

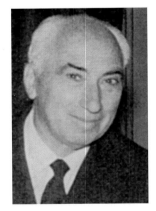

Fig. 36. Professor Tomás A. Pinós (1892-1974), Director of the postgraduate School of Gastroenterology, Hospital de Sant Pau, Barcelona. He designed a useful liver biopsy needle and he established laparoscopy as a routine procedure in Spain.

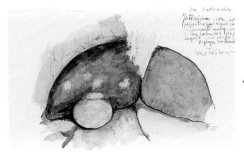

Fig. 37. Original drawing by T.A. Pinós of a laparoscopic examination in malignant obstructive jaundice (circa 1945) (courtesy Dr. Tomás Pinós Desplat).

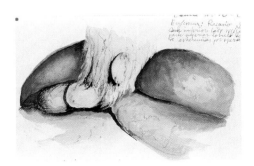

Fig. 38. Original drawing by T.A. Pinós: laparoscopy in hydatid disease of the liver (circa 1945) (courtesy of Dr. Tomás Pinós Desplat).

numbers of examinations, indicating a close relationship with the expertise of the endoscopist.

As of 1970, laparoscopy was employed most frequently in the diagnosis of acute abdominal conditions and a special mention should be made of the great experience gathered in Havanna by the Cuban clinician Raimundo Llanio and his co-workers who did thousands of examinations in patients of this kind[63, 64]. The great boom in laparoscopic surgery has turned emergency laparoscopy into a routine technique in many centres, mainly practiced by surgeons.

LAPAROSCOPIC DOCUMENTATION: THE FOURÈS LAPAROSCOPE.

Although Kalk in Germany[41] and Horan and Eddy[29] as well as Hancock[25] in the United States had begun to take colour laparoscopic photographs in the 1940s, the contributions of André Fourès deserve a special mention as he was one of the main contributors to the progress of photography using an electronic flash[17]. Fourès, who had been trained as a pneumologist, was interested in bronchoscopy, and he also owned a small factory of medical instruments. He became acquainted with Jacques Caroli, a chief of service at the Saint-Antoine Hospital in Paris and a prestigious hepatologist. Caroli had a good knowledge of liver pathology and he was one of the few French hepatologists who knew German well. He once told me himself that while in hiding during World War Two because of his Jewish origin, he spent several years in seclusion translating the volume on liver pathology of the famous treatise edited by Hencke-Lubarsch into French. He was aware of the German contributions to laparoscopy and in 1950 he convinced Fourès to design an instrument with which he could photograph his observations. The Fourès laparoscope, virtually hand-made, consisted of a trocar with three lateral orifices. With this design, the bowel could be separated with ease to gain access to the liver, which was Caroli's interest *(Figs. 39, 40)*.

The technique for pneumoperitoneum was similar to that of pneumothorax with which Fourès had gained experience in his own practice as a pneumologist[18].

The Fourès laparoscope (made by his own firm S.F.C.A.M. of Paris) was of a very small calibre. Of only 5 mm in diameter it was less dangerous than other instruments. The optical system

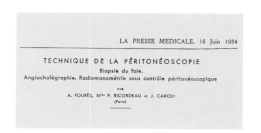

Fig. 39. Title page of the paper by André Fourès, Jacques Caroli and Paulette Ricordeau on laparoscopy technique used extensively in Caroli's service at Hospital Saint Antoine around 1950.

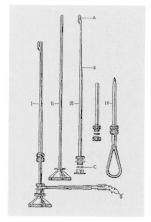

Fig. 40. The Fourès laparoscope manufactured by his own firm S.F.C.A.M. in Paris (1954) (ref. 16).

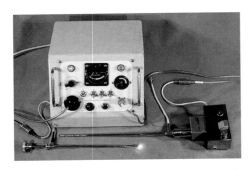

Fig. 41. The Fourès laparoscope showing the light source for the electronic flash and the lamp for the conventional examination (courtesy of Dr. A.Marti Vicente, Hospital de Sant Pau).

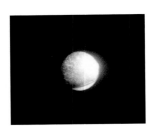

Fig. 42. One of the first pictures obtained with the intraabdominal flash of the Fourès laparoscope. The image (biliary cirrhosis) was of such small diameter that it had to be projected on a screen for evaluation (courtesy of Dr. A.Marti Vicente).

was prograde and also allowed oblique vision. The angle of vision was 120º. The optical system was independent from the lighting system which was fitted to a rod attached to the sheath of the instrument. The rod could be pushed 2-3 cm. beyond the optical lens so that it could separate intestinal loops and the epiplon. It was sturdy enough for the liver edge to be lifted and its inferior aspect examined. The lamp was protected to avoid burning the adjacent abdominal tissues. Fourès always stressed the simplicity of his instrument and its low cost in comparison with those of his competitors.

As of 1955, Fourès was able to introduce a carefully isolated electronic flash at the distal tip of the laparoscope. For a few tenths of a second this provided a brilliant light (160 volts) and pictures of excellent quality and detail –although very small– could be taken. Some of these pictures made with a reflex camera were presented at the First World Congress of Endoscopy (Tokyo 1966). I am not aware of any accidents occurring with the Fourès intra-abdominal flash which was used extensively in our Hospital de Sant Pau in Barcelona. The instrument was not authorised in Germany for fear of the excessive voltage of the flash light[18, 85] (Figs. 41, 42). André Calame, a distinguished surgeon from Geneva, also employed a laparoscope similar to that of Fourès. It too included an intraabdominal flash independent from the laparoscope which had to be introduced into the abdomen by a separate puncture[10].

The Italian Giorgio Menghini, already known for his liver biopsy needle, designed, with contributions by Egmont Wildhirt, an excellent photolaparoscope for the Storz company[69]. The trocar was wider, 12 mm in diameter. At the distal end of the instrument, a lamp was screwed on for abdominal inspection. For photography, an external electronic flash transmitted its light by means of a quartz rod which was inserted inside the sheath of the laparoscope. Pictures were taken with a robot camera attached to the proximal end of the laparoscope. This system without an internal flash, was devoid of danger and became extremely popular. The quality of the pictures with Fourès instrument required magnification but gave even more faithful details.

"Cold light" illumination began to be employed in laparoscopy at about the same time as in urology. In its initial phase, proximal light was transmitted to the tip of the laparoscope by means of a quartz rod as with Fourestier instruments dating from 1952[19] and in that of Menghini which we have already described. Quartz rods transmitted a much more potent light than any light bulb and pictures could be taken without any kind of flash light. Quartz rods eliminated distal illumination and replaced it by proximal light systems. However, optical fibres further improved the quality of the lighting systems (Figs. 43, 44).

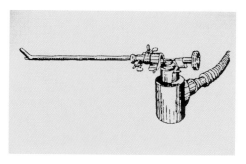

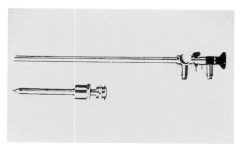

Fig. 43. The Fourestier endoscope provided with a quartz rod which allowed transmission of external "cold light". Manufactured by the firm Gentile, successor of Charrière-Collin in 1951) (Catalogue Maison Gentile, 1951).

Fig. 44. Photolaparoscope designed by Giorgio Menghini in collaboration with Edmund Wildhirt, manufactured by Karl Storz in Tuttlingen (Germany) (Hospital de Sant Pau).

Possibly the most widely employed instrument at that time was Kalk's photolaparoscope provided with a double lighting system: one standard lamp for simple inspection and another featuring a much thicker filament used for photography. Transformers provided the electrical source (one for each lamp). Increasing the voltage to 24 v. one could obtain enough intermittent light for photography. The last Kalk prototypes were 19.2 cm long with a diameter of 6.8 mm. The best photographic camera was the "Endovisoflex" from the Leica company[4, 45].

OPERATIVE LAPAROSCOPES

As we have already mentioned, the first laparoscopic liver biopsy was probably done by Carl Fervers. Following Jacobaeus, who often resected pleural adhesions, Kalk had asked Heynemann to manufacture a laparoscope provided with a channel coupled to the sheath of the instrument which would allow the introduction of pincers, clamps, knives and small scissors in a similar way as was done in cystoscopy. An Albarrán lever (Joaquin Albarrán, a famous urologist from Paris) placed at the tip of the endoscope allowed the accessory tool to be directed to the chosen spot. The instrument was later improved by the firm Sass-Wolf. However, to perform biopsies or cholangiographies, Kalk employed a second puncture.

A practical laparoscope which we frequently used in our own hospital was the laparoscope by Jacobs-Palmer (1966). This instrument bears the name of the Belgian gastroenterologist, Edouard Jacobs, and that of the French gynaecologist, Raoul Palmer[35, 36]. The instrument, in the shape of a bayonet, was (Fig. 45, 46) con-

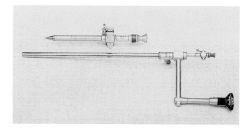

Fig. 45. The Jacobs-Palmer operative laparoscope (1966) often used at Hospital de Sant Pau.

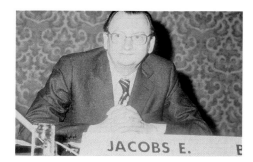

Fig. 46. Edouard Jacobs, chief of the gastroenterology service, Université Libre de Bruxelles who designed the operative laparoscope with Raoul Palmer (courtesy of Dr. E. Jacobs).

structed including a channel along its principal axis. Probes, biopsy needles and electrodes for electro-coagulation could be introduced under guidance of the objective placed at the distal end of the bayonet. The instrument was most useful as it enabled all kinds of instrumentation without the need for an additional puncture.

HAROLD HOPKINS, COLD LIGHT AND LAPAROSCOPY

Laparoscopes, which in reality were modified cystoscopes, were provided with a distal light through a more or less potent lamp. As early as 1908, the German urologist Ringleb together with technicians of the Zeiss company, improved the illumination of the Nitze-Leiter cystoscope which had been designed by the optician Louis Benèche from Berlin at the end of the 19th century. Images were of better quality, were not deformed and were not inverted as with the first instruments. With his own designs, Ringleb was able to produce excellent black and white photographs of the urinary bladder[23] (see Chapter 7).

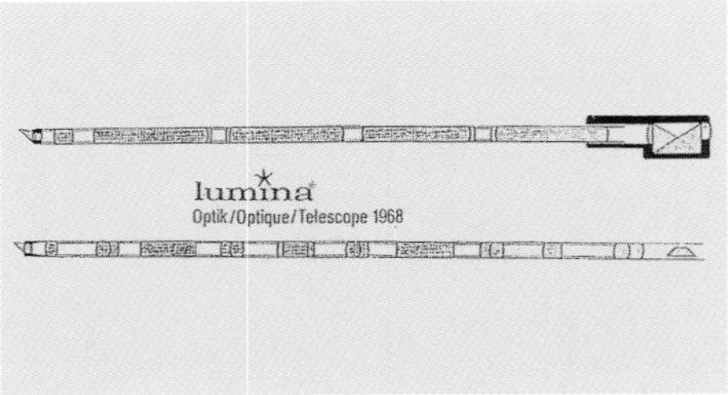

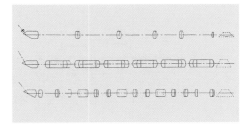

Fig. 47. Above: drawing made by H. Hopkins for a "cold light" system patent (1968). Below: "lumina" optics devised by Lent (1969).

Fig. 48. Schematic drawings of different lighting systems for laparoscopy: Above: the standard optical system derived from the cystoscope. Centre: the Hopkins optical system used in the Storz laparoscopes (Stablinsen). Below: optical system according to Lent, employed in the Richard Wolf laparoscopes. The lenses are much more spaced ("Lumina" optics) (courtesy of the late Prof. L.Demling).

Besides being one of the most innovative researchers in the field of fibre optics, Harold Hopkins invented –and perhaps this was his greatest achievement– an original optical system. Using cold light", it greatly improved the quality of images. In 1959, Hopkins applied for a patent for his invention but this was not awarded until 1964. The principle of his design is quite different from the previous models: the large empty spaces between the inner lenses were substituted by cylindrical glass rods placed in succession and separated by short annular air spaces: the so-called "Stablinsensystem" in German (from the German "Stab": rod). The inside of the instrument was coated with an anti-refringent substance[26] *(Figs. 47, 48)*.

Hopkins, who did not find economic support for his projects in Great Britain, gave a lecture in Germany where he met Karl Storz, the instrument maker, who was in the audience. As a result of this event, the optical system which we have described became a reality and Karl Storz manufactured it for his endoscopy instruments. The Storz laparoscope, with the Hopkins lens system consisted of a 7.0mm trocar while the diameter of the laparoscope itself was only 5.8 mm. The instrument, lit by means of optical fibres, could be attached to a reflex camera with a "zoom" lens for close-ups. Storz also manufactured a paediatric laparoscope with a trocar 4 mm in diameter and an optical system of only 2.7 mm wide[55] *(Fig. 49)*.

Some time later a team of physicists and opticians who worked for the firm Richard Wolf of Knittlingen, designed, together with an endoscopist, H. Lent[53] another optical system, called "Lumina". It was less compact than the Hopkins prototype, and was based on shorter rods and larger air spaces. This alternative optical system has also been used in many centres. From 1977 onwards, it was possible to add a magnification lens to both the Storz and the Wolf instruments, allowing photography at 2-3 cm of distance and providing images of astonishing detail but, in our opinion, of little practical value *(Fig. 50)*.

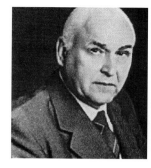

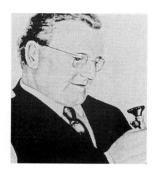

Fig. 49. Karl Storz (1910-1996), founder in Tuttlingen (Germany) of the medical instrument firm that bears his name. He was the first to correctly assess the importance of Hopkins' research on the transmission of "cold light" (courtesy of Karl Storz GmbH.)

Fig. 50. Richard Wolf ((1906-1958), successor of Georg Wolf from Berlin, manufacturer among other instruments of the photolaparoscope with the "Lumina" optical system (courtesy of the Richard and Annemarie Wolf Foundation).

ATTEMPTS AT LAPAROSCOPIC FIBRESCOPY

In the 1970s, several attempts were made to employ a paediatric laparoscope through the trocar of a standard instrument or the Jacobs-Palmer endoscope so as to visualise abdominal lesions when adhesions made the examination difficult *(Figs. 51, 52, 53)*. The firms Machida and also Olympus made prototypes of flexible instru-

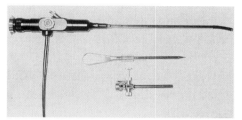

Fig. 51. Prototype of laparo-fibrescope of the firm Machida featuring a flexible tip (courtesy of Machida Inc.).

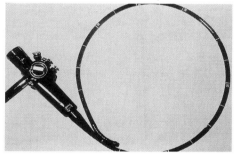

Fig. 52. Prototype of flexible laparo-fibrescope (courtesy of Olympus Inc.).

ments or rigid endoscopes with flexible tips. The Olympus prototype (A3635) was 22 cm long with a flexible distal portion of 11.5 cm in length which could be tilted to an angle of 100º. A biopsy instrument could be introduced through an additional channel. As far as we know, none of these instruments have been introduced commercially[93, 107]. However, it should be mentioned that in 1972, showing unusual skills, Meyer-Burg was able to visualise and biopsy areas of the pancreas with a standard laparoscope[70].

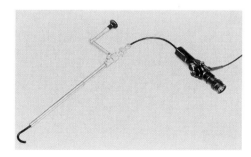

Fig. 53. Introduction of a mini-fibrescope (5 mm.) through the Jacobs-Palmer operative laparoscope (courtesy of Dr.Harald Henning).

CINELAPAROSCOPY AND TELEVISION *(Fig. 54, 55)*

The beginnings of cinelaparoscopy were technically difficult because of the great differences in the absorption and reflection of light by solid structures such as

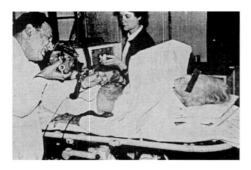

Fig. 54. Sacha Segal from Reims (France), a pioneer of televised endoscopy and laparoscopic cinematography (courtesy of Dr. Sacha Segal).

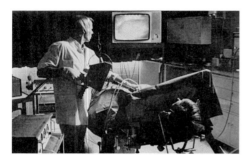

Fig. 55. Televised laparoscopy (courtesy of Dr.Harald Henning).

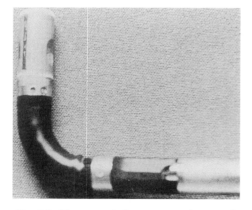

Fig. 56. Olympus echolaparoscope, showing the flexible distal tip (courtesy of Dr. Giorgio Dagnini).

the liver or the spleen or the brilliant serosal and peritoneal reflections. One of the pioneers of cinelaparoscopy in the United States was George Berci. He used a 16 mm Beaulieu camera and other prototypes that he himself developed[6, 7]. In France, Debray's associates, and in particular Sacha Segal from Reims who had great experience in cinegastroscopy, also used Beaulieu or Bolex cameras for cinelaparoscopy[12].

Endoscopic television had been experimentally tried in 1957 by French bronchoscopists, such as Soulas[99], using an Orthicon camera and closed circuit television. However, the instrument was very bulky and of little practical interest. Later on Dubois de Montreynaud[14] employed a Vidicon camera. Miniature cameras such as the Mark II were designed by Berci[6]. As always, the main problem with laparoscopic cinematography was the need to obtain enough light. That had to wait until the advent of the various optical systems provided with cold light.

Attempts at televised laparoscopy were initiated by Harald Lindner from Hamburg in 1968, using magnetic videotapes in colour with a Phillips TV LDK 13 instrument[57].

As expected, the universal diffusion of videoendoscopy has completely transformed communications in the visual field as it has done with the daily activities of the endoscopists. Current indications of diagnostic laparoscopy were recently reviewed by the American Society for Gastrointestinal Endoscopy[1].

ECHOLAPAROSCOPY

Starting in the mid-1960s, the idea of introducing a minute ultrasound sensor under laparoscopic control in the abdomen soon attracted the interest of Japanese laparoscopists and surgeons[37], although the method has not been widely employed. During the 1990s, it was still considered experimental and echolaparoscopy should not be considered as a purely "historical" procedure. According to Dagnini[11], echolaparoscopy has decreased the number of accidents caused by the introduction of needles and trocars, as any vascular abnormality of the abdominal wall can be readily detected *(Fig. 56)*.

In spite of these improvements in laparoscopic techniques, it has become obvious that imaging methods have replaced diagnostic laparoscopy in the majority of its indications. This has occurred in our own hospital, as well as in many other centres *(Fig. 57)*.

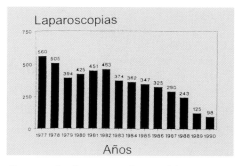

Fig. 57. Declining incidence of laparoscopies done at the Gastroenterology Service, Hospital de Sant Pau, Barcelona from 1977 to 1990 (courtesy of Dr. A.Martí-Vicente).

GYNAECOLOGISTS: THE PIONEERS OF SURGICAL LAPAROSCOPY

Before attempting to describe this last section on the history of laparoscopy, I would like to render a public tribute to Dr.Grzegorz S. Lityinski, author of an outstanding investigation on the beginnings of laparoscopy and its evolution towards the most modern surgical techniques. This part of the chapter owes much to his tremendous work and to his unfailing courtesy in providing me with many documents of great interest[59].

More than fifty years ago, several French and American gynaecologists gave a great boost to the gynaecologic laparoscopic diagnosis which had been started by von Ott in Saint Petersburg. Gynaecologists were the first to realise the great therapeutic possibilities which some clinicians such as Jacobaeus, Fervers or Kalk had already grasped. These clinicians had sectioned adhesions to improve visibility but also in some instances, to alleviate pain which they attributed to strictures caused by adhesions or badly placed suture threads. Among these originators the names of Raoul Palmer in France, Hans Frangenheim in Germany and Patrick Steptoe in the United Kingdom, deserve special praise[59].

RAOUL PALMER *(Fig. 58)*

Raoul Palmer began his medical studies in Paris in 1929. He was an intern of Noël Fiessinger's a reputed internist specialised in liver disease. Palmer wrote a doctoral thesis on the physiopathology of liver surgery and the liver blood supply. Later on, he was an assistant at the service of a gynaecologist, Dr. R. Proust, brother of the famous novelist Marcel Proust, and in 1938 he worked at the Hospital Broca in Paris where gynaecology and obstetrics were prominent specialities. In 1943, during World War Two, Palmer started his first laparoscopies using a cystoscope, as others had already done. He employed a rheostat to obtain a light intensity of 4.5 V for his lamps, which unfortunately blew out easily. For peritoneal insufflation, Palmer recommended CO_2 which was easily absorbed[78].

HANS FRANGENHEIM *(Fig. 59)*

Frangenheim, the son of a professor of surgery in Cologne, studied medicine in Münster and began to specialise in gynaecology in Wuppertal. He slowly began to practice gynaecologic endoscopy through the Douglas pouch under

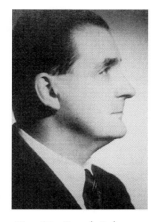

Fig. 58. Raoul Palmer, a distinguished French gynaecologist one of the introducers of laparoscopic gynaecology, he designed with E.Jacobs the operative laparoscope (courtesy of Dr. G.S.Lytinski).

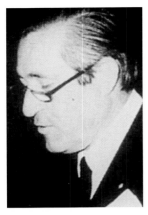

Fig. 59. Hans Frangenheim, pioneer of diagnostic and surgical laparoscopy in gynaecology in Germany (courtesy of Dr. G.S.Litynski).

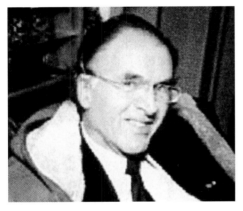

Fig. 60. Kurt Semm, German gynaecologist, he designed instruments for electrocoagulation and laparoscopic suture. This paved the way for his first laparoscopic appendectomy in 1980 (courtesy of Dr. G.S.Litynski).

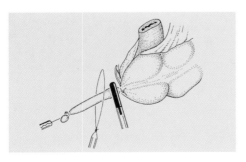

Fig. 61. Drawing of the first laparoscopic appendectomy done by K.Semm (courtesy of the editor of Endoscopy, Prof. M.Classen).

the name "douglascopy" or "culdoscopy". In 1952, Frangenheim began to perform laparoscopy using Kalk's technique with instruments modified for gynaecological work. In 1955 he visited Raoul Palmer who had been performing laparoscopies in Paris for some years. This was the beginning of a lasting friendship and mutual collaboration between the two gynaecologists. By 1958, Frangenheim had done more than 350 laparoscopies and had published his findings[20].

From the diagnostic point of view, laparoscopy represented enormous progress in gynaecologic diagnosis especially because of the frequent use of magnification lenses. These allowed a detailed analysis of ovarian and tubal pathology and provided excellent photographic documentation. Some years later, Frangenheim, who had acquired a great reputation, listed the indications for laparoscopy in gynaecology. In many aspects, they are of interest to the gastroenterologist[22].

In 1959, he published a book[21] on gynaecological laparoscopy, the first of its kind, in which he stressed the advantages of abdominal endoscopy over culdoscopy.

The laparoscopic operations proposed by Frangenheim led the way to modern laparoscopic digestive surgery. From the first operations such as tubal ligation, an easy and simple technique which required relatively little technical skill, surgical laparoscopy progressed rapidly with video-endoscopy, which freed the eyes and the hands. Nowadays, at least 40 to 50 percent of gynaecological operations are performed by laparoscopy[7].

KURT SEMM AND THE FIRST APPENDECTOMY

In 1983, the journal "Endoscopy" published an article by Kurt Semm,[96] a German gynaecologist, in which he gave details –including drawings– of a laparoscopic technique he had employed to perform appendectomy. This was the beginning of abdominal surgery through the laparoscope. The early pioneers would not have dreamt of the popularity it has since acquired. The article was not entirely devoid of surprise as Semm had already performed gynaecological surgery, especially tubal ligation, an operation widely done for sterilisation[95] *(Figs. 60, 61).*

Semm had studied medicine in Munich, where he was awarded a Summa Cum Laude for his doctoral thesis[61]. Starting from 1951 he began his training as a gynaecologist at Munich University. His attention was attracted by a film by Raoul Palmer that he saw at a congress and instigated him to start laparoscopy. He began by designing a special automatic insufflator for pneumoperitoneum but not until 1967 did he begin his first laparoscopies. He named these "pelviscopies" to distinguish his procedures from those of the internists. Semm became a distinguished innovator in his gynaecology service at Kiel University where he created a series of new instruments for gynaecological operations with the help of his father and a brother who was the owner of a firm specialised in manufacturing surgical instruments[62]. Among these instruments, an "endocoagulator" and other devices to perform ligations deserve special mention. He used a magnifying lens of the Hopkins type and a pneumoperitoneum insufflator controlled electronically. In 1977, Semm performed sutures through the laparoscope and on 13th September 1980, the first appendectomy. Once again, the history of endoscopy repeats itself: Semm's report was presented at several meetings where it was received with great hostility by clinicians and by surgeons, so much so that his article was not published until 1983! Laparoscopic appendectomies were judged dangerous by the majority of surgeons and also by gynaecologists, including Frangenheim, who sharply critisised Semms' temerity. Semm retorted in strong terms (both oral interventions were later published)[2]. Semm's possible lack of "diplomacy" does not obviate the fact that he should be considered father of digestive laparoscopic surgery.

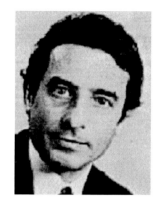

Fig. 62. Eric Mühe, a German surgeon who performed the first laparoscopic cholecystectomy using an instrument of his invention, the "galloscope" (courtesy of Dr. G.S.Litynski).

ERIC MÜHE AND THE FIRST LAPAROSCOPIC CHOLECYSTECTOMY

Semm's achievements led the way to other surgical endoscopic interventions that could rule out the need for laparotomy. In some papers, the paternity of the first laparoscopic cholecystectomy has been attributed to Philippe Mouret from Lyon, but other publications have revealed that the priority of laparoscopic cholecystectomy should be awarded to the young German surgeon, Eric Mühe[58]. Mühe received his surgical training at Erlangen University where he worked closely with the members of the famous gastroenterological endoscopy centre created by Norbert Henning and greatly expanded by his successor Ludwig Demling, where laparoscopy had been done years before World War Two (Figs. 62, 63).

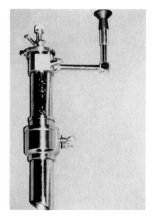

Fig. 63. Eric Mühe's "galloscope", later replaced by a more conventional instrument (courtesy of Dr. G.S.Litynski).

Mühe acquired experience in diagnostic laparoscopy in Erlangen in spite of some opposition on the part of anaesthetists who thought the procedure too long for a simple diagnostic test. Mühe then went to Konstanz where he designed an instrument which he named "galloscope" (from Galle: gallbladder in German), in order to perform pneumoperitoneum and surgical procedures. The instrument resembled a short rectoscope with proximal illumination, a lateral vision optical system, a channel for instrumentation and another for

insufflation. On September 1st 1985, using Semm's technique for appendectomy as a guide, Mühe performed a pneumoperitoneum with a Veres needle,
inserted a trocar and introduced his "galloscope" through the umbilical region.
Two hours later, he had resected a gallbladder by the laparoscopic route[72] for
the first time.

Mühe presented his operation at the Congress of the German Society of Surgery
where he fared no better than Semm did years beforehand. He was received by
the audience, which included many prestigious professors, with perhaps even
more opposition than Semm. Once more, this confirms the long repetitive history of enmity and malevolence which illustrates the appearance of new endoscopic techniques and instruments and which started with the rejection of
Bozzini's Lichleiter by the illustrious professors of Vienna University (see
Chapter 2). As a consequence, Mühe's written paper was not published in the
proceedings of the congress, and only an abstract was printed. However, Mühe
persisted in performing laparoscopic cholecystectomies. Between September
1985 and March 1987 he had done 97 operations, although after an accident
ending in death, he had to stop surgical practice for some time[58].

PIONEERS IN FRANCE: MOURET, DUBOIS AND PERISSAT *(Figs 64, 65, 66)*

In 1972, in France, Philippe Mouret[71], a gynaecologist and general surgeon,
who trained from 1968 to 1987 in Clermont-Ferrand with former associates of
Raoul Palmer, began to do laparoscopic surgery in cases of intestinal occlusion

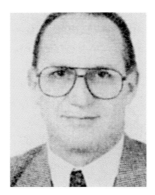

Fig. 64. Philippe Mouret from Lyon, general surgeon and gynaecologist who, unaware of Mühe's contri-butions, did the first lapa-roscopic cholecystectomy in France (courtesy of Dr. E.Laporte).

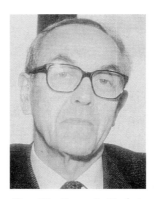

Fig. 65. François Dubois, a Parisian surgeon who after doing cholecystectomy through minilaparotomy, was one of the first to start laparoscopic cholecystec-tomy (courtesy of Dr. G.S.Litynski).

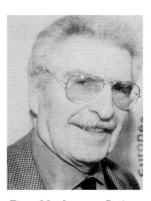

Fig. 66. Jacques Perissat, Professor of Surgery in Bordeaux. He performed laparoscopic intraabdomi-nal lithotripsy followed by cholecystectomy by the same route (courtesy of Dr. G.S.Litynski).

sectioning post-operative adhesions. In 1983 he did his first laparoscopic appendectomy. In March 1987, unaware of Mühe's work, Mouret, who at that time had his practice in Lyon, performed his first cholecystectomy. In 1988, François Dubois[13], a well-known Paris surgeon who employed a technique of open cholecystectomy using a very small cutaneous incision and who had seen a video made by Mouret, did his first cholecystectomy by laparoscopy. Together with Mouret they presented their combined experience at the European Congress of Surgery the same year.

Laparoscopic cholecystectomy took time to be accepted by internists and many surgeons, among other reasons, because of the discovery of biological methods for the dissolution of bile stones, either with biliary acids or by direct puncture of the gallbladder. Biliary extracorporeal lithotripsy had also appeared on the market and even endoscopic lithotripsy had been attempted by directly cannulating the biliary tract. Cholecystectomy also took some time to be accepted in the Anglo-Saxon world as most early publications were either in German or French.

The third pioneer of surgical laparoscopy in France was Jacques Perissat[80], a surgeon from Bordeaux who had been one of the first to perform extracorporeal biliary lithotripsy and was dissatisfied with its results. He then invented a technique of intraabdominal lithotripsy, introducing an ultrasonic lithotriptor in the gallbladder, irrigating its lumen, aspirating its contents and leaving a cholecystostomy drain. After seeing a demonstration by Dubois, Perissat decided to complete his own intervention by performing a cholecystectomy combined with the lithotripsy. His operation was technically complex and I remember very well a video that Perissat showed at a Congress of the French Society of Gastroenterology which was received by the majority of the audience with clear demonstrations of disapproval. However, the evident advantages of the operation, such as the avoidance of laparotomy and the shortened hospital stay, made laparoscopic cholecystectomy the method of choice for removing the gallbladder. It was rapidly divulged in the European Continent[50, 81, 104] and soon among young surgeons everywhere. It must be stressed that French surgeons and particularly Mouret[71] always recommended great caution in the indications and the practice of laparoscopic cholecystectomy. Laparoscopy is now being employed for all kinds of abdominal surgery well beyond the scope of a history book.

REFERENCES

[1] American Society for Gastrointestinal Endoscopy.- Diagnostic laparoscopy guidelines for clinical application. Gastrointest Endosc 2001; 54: 818-820.
[2] Bach H.G.- Bemerkungen zur Frangenheim-Semm Kontroverse. Geburst Frauenheilk 1980; 40: 429-433.

[3] Bailey H., Bishop, W.J.- Pierre C.E. Potain. in Notable Names in Medicine and Surgery, 2nd edition, London, H.K.Lewis, 1946.

[4] Beck K.- Farbatlas der Laparoskopie. Stuttgart, Schattauer, 1968.

[5] Benedict E.B.- Endoscopy as related to Diseases of the Bronchus, Esophagus, Stomach and Peritoneal Cavity. Baltimore, Wiliams & Wilkins, 1951.

[6] Berci G.- Television and Endoscopy. en Endoscopy, G.Berci (ed) New York, Appleton, Century-Crofts, 1976:271-279.

[7] Berci G., Forde K.A.- History of endoscopy. What lessons have we learned from the past? Surg Endosc 2000;14: 5-15.

[8] Bernheim B.- Organoscopy: cystoscopy of abdominal cavity. Ann Surg 1911; 53: 764-767.

[9] Brühl W.- Zwischenfalle und Komplicationen bei der Laparoskopie und gezielten Leberpunktion. Dtsch Med Wschr 1966; 91: 2297-2299.

[10] Calame A.- La photographie laparoscopique. Presse Med 1955; 63: 1848-1850.

[11] Dagnini G.- Laparoscopy and Imaging Techniques. Berlin, Springer Verlag, 1990.

[12] Debray Ch., Housset P., Segal S., Paolaggi A., Pette F.- la photographie et la cinématographie endoscopiques digestives. État actuel en France. Sem Hôp Paris 1961; 37: 963-969.

[13] Dubois F., Berthelot G., Levard H.- Cholécystectomie par coelioscopie. Presse Med 1989;18: 980-982.

[14] Dubois de Montreynaud J.M., Bruneau Y., Jomain J.- Traité Pratique de Photographie et de Cinématographie Médicales. Paris, Paul Montel, 1960.

[15] Fervers C.- Die Laparoskopie mit dem Cystoskop. Ein Beitrag zur Vereinfachung der Technik und zur endoskopischen Strangdurchtrennung in der Bauchhöhle. Med Klin 1933; 29: 1042-1045.

[16] Fourès A., Ricordeau P., Caroli J.- Technique de la péritoneoscopie, biopsie du foie, angiocholegraphie et radiomanométrie sous contrôle péritoneoscopique Presse Med 1954; 62: 929-933.

[17] Fourès A., Ricordeau P., Caroli J.- La laparophotographie. Sem Med. (Paris) Suppl. Sem Hôp. 1956; 46: 37-38.

[18] Fourès A., Ricordeau P.- Possibilités actuelles de la photographie endopéritoneale. Proc. 1st World Congress of Endoscopy. Tokyo, 1966: 439-441.

[19] Fourestier M., Gladu A., Vulmière J.- Perfectionnements à l'endoscopie médicale. Presse Med 1952; 60: 1292-1293.

[20] Frangenheim H.- Die Bedeutung der Laparoskopie fur die gynäkologische Diagnostik. Fortschr Med 1958; 76: 451-452.

[21] Frangenheim H.- Die Laparoskopie und die Kuldoskopie in der Gynäkologie. Stuttgart, G.Thieme, 1959.

[22] Frangenheim H.- Welche Möglichkeiten gibt es für die endoskopischen Untersuchungen in der Gynäkologie? Endoscopy 1969: 1: 9-14.

[23] Fromme F., Ringleb O. Lehrbuch der Kystophotographie. Wiesbaden, I.F.Bergmann, 1913.

[24] Gironés Navarro L., Sánchez-Lucas J.- Sobre Laparoscopia. Rev Esp Enf Apar Dig 1945; 11:165-181.

[25] Hancock A.F.- Peritoneoscopic photography. J Bio Photogr Ass 1946; 14: 163-165.

[26] Henning H.,Look D.- Laparoskopie. Atlas und Lehrbuch. Suttgart, Georg Thieme, 1985.

[27] Henning N.- Ein neues Laparoskop. Dtsch Zeitschrft Verdauu- Stoffwechselkr 1950; 10: 49-52.

[28] Henning N., Demling L., Gigglberger H.- Über die laparoskopische Cholezysto-cholangiographie. Münch med Wschr 1952; 94: 830-834.

[29] Horan T.N., Eddy C.G.- Intra-abdominal photography in color. Surg Gynec Obstet 1941; 73: 273-276.

[30] Iversen P., Roholm K.- On aspiration biopsy of the liver with remarks on its diagnostic significance. Acta Med Scand 1939; 102:1-16.

[31] Jacobaeus H.C.- Über die Möglichkeit, die Zystoskopie bei Untersuchung seröser Höhlungen anzuwenden. Münch med Wschr 1910; 57: 2090-2092.

[32] Jacobaeus H.C.- Kurze Übersicht über meine Erfahrungen mit der Laparothorakoskopie. Münch med Wschr 1911; 58: 2017-2019.

[33] Jacobaeus H.C.- Über Laparo- und Thorakoskopie. Beitr Klin Tuberk 1912; 25: 183-254.

34 Jacobaeus H.C.- Laparo- und Thorakoskopie. Würzburg, Curt Kabitsch, 1913.

35 Jacobs E.- Principes d'un nouveau laparoscope-opérateur. Rev Internat Hepatol 1966;16: 1345-1346.

36 Jacobs E., Morobe J.- Apports et limites de la laparoscopie. Expérience basée sur 3000 laparoscopies. Acta Gastroenterol Belgica 1969; 32: 279-286.

37 Japan Society of Ultrasonics in Medicine. Ultrasonics in Medicine, principle, research and practice. Tokyo, Igaku-Shoin, 1966.

38 Kalk H.- Erfahrungen mit der Laparoskopie (zugleich mit Beschreibung eines neuen Instrumentes). Zeitschrft Klin Med 1929;111: 303-348.

39 Kalk H.- Schlusswort zu der Stellungnahme von Prof. G.Kelling zu dem Artikel von Kalk über Laparoskopie. Med Klinik 1932; 28: 1747.

40 Kalk H.- Indikationsstellung und Gefahrenmoment bei der Laparoskopie. Dtsch Med Wschr 1935; 61: 1831-1832.

41 Kalk H.- Fortschritte der Laparoskopie. Dtsch Med Wschr 1942; 68: 677-681.

42 Kalk H., Brühl W.- Leitfaden der Laparoskopie und Gastroskopie, Stuttgart, G.Thieme, 1951.

43 Kalk H.- Laparoskopische Cholezysto- und Cholangiographie Dtsch med Wschr 1952; 77: 590-592.

44 Kalk H.- Cirrhose und Narbenleber, Stuttgart, Enke, 1954.

45 Kalk H., Wildhirt E.- Lehrbuch und Atlas der Laparoskopie und Leberpunktion, Stuttgart, Thieme, 1962.

46 Kelling G.- Über Oesophagoskopie, Gastroskopie und Kölioskopie. Münch med Wschr 1902; 49: 21-24.

47 Kelling G.- Über die Möglichkeit, die Zystoskopie bei Untersuchung seröser Höhlungen anzuwenden. Bemerkungen zu dem Artikel von Jacobäus. Münch med Wschr 1910; 57: 2358.

48 Kelling G.- Zu dem Artikel von Kalk über Laparoskopie. Med Klinik 1932; 28: 1747.

49 Korbsch R.- Lehrbuch und Atlas der Laparo- und Thorakoskopie, Munich, J.F.Lehmann Verlag, 1927.

50 Laporte Roselló E.- Cirugía Laparoscópica. Barcelona, Pulso Ediciones S.A., 1993.

51 Laserna y Espina L. de -. Laparoscopia. Un método para la visión directa de los órganos del abdomen en el vivo. Rev Esp Enf Apar Dig. 1936;11:11-21.

52 Lee W.Y.- Evaluation of peritoneoscopy in intraabdominal diagnosis. Rev Gastroenterol 1942; 9:133-141.

53 Lent H.- Diagnostische Möglichkeiten mit modernen Laparoskop-optiken. in Fortschritte der Endoskopie, R.Ottenjann (ed.) Bd. II, Stuttgart, Schattauer, 1969.

54 Lenzi G., Cavassini G.B., Lenzi E.- La laparoscopie, Paris, Masson, 1960.

55 Lindner H.- Grundlagen und Fortschritte der Laparoskopie. Verhandlungsband n.2; Z.Gastroenterol. München, Karl Demeter, 1969.

56 Lindner H. Die Perkutane Leberbiopsie. Verhandlungdband n.3; Z.Gastroenterol. München, Karl Demeter, 1970.

57 Lindner H., Fintelmann V.- Peritoneoscopic photographic documentation in the present and the future. Advances in Gastrointestinal Endoscopy. Proceedings, 2nd World Congress of Gastrointestinal Endoscopy. G.Marcozzi, M.Crespi (eds), Padova, Piccin Medical Books, 1971: 895-897.

58 Litynski G.S.- Eric Mühe and the rejection of the laparoscopic cholecystectomy. A surgeon ahead of his time. J Soc Laparoendosc Surg 1988; 2: 341-346.

59 Litynski G.S.- Highlights in the History of Laparoscopy. Frankfurt, Barbara Berners Verlag, 1996.

60 Litynski G.S.- Georg Kelling –die Anfänge der Laparoskopie. en Meilensteine der Endoskopie. Wien, Literas, Universitätsverlag, 2000: 324-333.

61 Litynski G.S.- Endoscopic surgery –The History, the Pioneers. World J Surg 1999; 23: 745-753.

62 Litynski G.S.- Kurt Semm and the fight against skepticism. Endoscopic hemostasis, laparoscopic appendectomy snd Semm's impact on the laparoscopic revolution. J Soc Laparoendosc Surg 1998; 2: 309-313.

63 Llanio R., Sotto A., Jimenez C., y cols.- La laparoscopie d'urgence (étude portant sur 1265 cas) Sem Hôp Paris 1973; 49: 873-875.

64 Llanio R.- Laparoscopia en Urgencias. La Habana, Editorial Científico-Técnica, 1977.

65 Lorey W.- Über das Einblasen von Luft in die Bauchhöhle als diagnostisches Hilfsmittel bei der röntgenologischen Untersuchung der Bauchorgane nebst Bemerkungen über die zur Darstellung des Magendarmkanals verwandten Kontrastmittel. en Festschrift dem Eppendorfer Krankenhause zur Feier seines 25 jährigen Bestehens Gewidmet. L.Brauer (ed) Leipzig, Verlag Leopold Voss, 1914: 84-93.

66 Martí-Vicente A.- Laparoscopy in Spain (data pending publication), 2003.

67 Meirelles E.A.- Laparoscopia. Tribuna Medica (Rio de Janeiro) 1913; 19: 199-205.

68 Menghini G., Ghergo G.F.- Needle biopsy of the liver. in Gastroenterology (H.L.Bockus ed.) Third edition, vol. III Philadelphia, W.B. Saunders 1976: 88-112.

69 Menghini G., Benda N.- Un nuovo complesso per laparofotografia a colori. In Studi e Ricerche in Epatologia. Roma, ed.Pensiero Scientifico, 1958.

70 Meyer-Burg J., Ziegler U., Palme G.- Zur supragastralen Pankreaskopie. Ergebnisse aus 125 Laparoskopien. Dtsch med Wschr 1972; 97: 1969-1971.

71 Mouret P.- La cholecystectomie laparoscopique a 4 ans. La coeliochirurgie tient une solide tête de pont. Lyon Chir 1991; 87/2 bis: 179-182.

72 Mühe E.- Die erste Cholecystectomie durch das Laparoskop. Langenbecks Arch Chir 1986; 369: 804.

73 Nord H.J. Technique of laparoscopy. in Gastroenterologic Endoscopy. M.Sivak (ed) 2ª edición. Philadelphia, W.B. Saunders, 2000:1476-1503.

74 Orlandi F. Just a needle. Ital J Gastroenterol 1986; 18: 174-175.

75 Orndorff B.H.- The peritoneoscope in the diagnosis of diseases of the abdomen. J Radiol (Iowa City) 1920; 1: 307-325.

76 Ott v. D.O. - Die Beleuchtung der Bacuhhöhle (Ventroskopie) als Methode bei Vaginales Köliotomie. Centralblatt Gynäkologie 1902; 26: 817-820.

77 Ott v. D.O. - Die Resultate der Anwendung der direkten Beleuchtung der Bauchhöhle des Dickdarms und der Harnblase bei der Operationen und zu diagnostische Zwecken. Centralblatt Gynäk1 1909; 33: 131-135.

78 Palmer R.- Instrumentation et technique de la coelioscopie gynecologique. Gynécol Obstet 1947; 46: 420-431.

79 Parker G., Hitzelberger A.L.- The status of peritoneoscopy in the United States. A query to 1020 American Physicians. Gastrointest Endosc 1966; 13: 11-14.

80 Perissat J., Collet D., Belliard R.- Gallstones:laparoscopic treatment –cholecystectomy, cholecystostomy and lithotripsy. Our own technique. Surg Endosc 1990; 4: 1-5.

81 Perissat J.- Laparoscopic cholecystectomy. The European experience. Am.J.Surg 1993; 165: 444-449.

82 Pinós Marsell T.A.- Neumoperitoneo y Laparoscopia in "Patología Abdominal Clínica, F.Gallart-Monés (ed.), Barcelona, Editorial Salvat, 1943: 580-620.

83 Premuda L. Luigi Lucatello a cinquant'anni della morte. Padova, "La Garangola", 1976.

84 Renon L.- Technique et indications de la laparoscopie (présentation d'instruments) Bull Mem Soc Hôp Paris 1913; 3s. 35: 510-513.

85 Ricordeau P.- La laparoscopie dans les maladies de l'appareil digestif. A propos de 6.000 cas. Proc. 1st World Congress of Endoscopy. Tokyo, 1966: 466-472.

86 Roccavilla A.- L'endoscopia delle grandi cavitá sierose mediante un nuovo apparecchio ad illuminazione diretta. Riforma Medica 1914; 30: 991-996.

87 Roccavilla A.- Laparoscopia e pneumoradiologia addominale. La Radiologia Medica 1920; 7: 411-419.

88 Roholm K., Iversen P.- Changes in liver in acute epidemic hepatitis (catarrhal jaundice) based on 38 aspiration biopsies. Acta Path Microbiol Scandinav 1939; 16: 427-442.

89 Rosenthal G.- Le laparothoracoscope de Jacobaeus. Bull Gen de Thérapie 1913; 165: 804.

90 Ruddock J.C.- Peritoneoscopy. Western J Surg 1934; 42: 392-405.

91 Ruddock J.C.- Peritoneoscopy Surg Gynec Obstet 1937; 65: 623-639.

92 Ruddock J.C.- Peritoneoscopy: a critical review. Surg Clin N Am 1957; 37: 1249-1260.

93 Sanowski R.A., Kozarek R.A., Prtyka E.K.- Evaluation of a flexible endoscope for laparoscopy. Am J Gastroenterol 1981; 76: 416-419.

94 Schmidt A.- Laparoskopie und Thorakoskopie nach Jacobaeus. Münch med Wschr 1914; 61:1882-1884.

95 Semm K.- Pelviskopische Chirurgie in der Gynäkologie. Geburst u. Frauenheilk. 1977; 37: 909-920.

96 Semm K.- Endoscopic appendectomy. Endoscopy 1983; 15: 59-64.

97 Semm K.- Operationslehre für endoskopische Abdominal-Chirurgie., Stuttgart, Schattauer, 1984.

98 Seydl G.- The history of trocars in De Historia Urologiae Europaeae. Mattelaer J.J., Schultheiss D. (eds) Historical Committee, European Association of Urology. 1999.

99 Soulas A.- Bronchoscopie televisée. Presse Med 1956; 64: 97-98.

100 Steigmann F., Villa F.- Peritoneoscopy. in Gastroenterologic Medicine, M.Paulson (ed.) Philadelphia, Lea & Febiger, 1969.

101 Steiner O.P.- Abdominoscopy. Surg Gynec Obstet 1924; 38: 266-269.

102 Stolkind E.- The value of pleuroscopy (thoracoscopy) in the diagnosis of pulmonary disease and laparoscopy in the diagnosis of abdominal diseases. Med Press (London) 1919; 107: 46-48.

103 Tedesco F.R.- Über Endoskopie des Abdomens und des Thorax. Mitt Gesell Inn Med Kinderh (Wien) 1912; 13: 323-327.

104 Troidl H.- First step: the idea. World J Surg 1999; 23: 754-767.

105 Unverricht W.- Die Thorakoskopie und Laparoskopie. Klin Wschr 1923; 2: 502-504.

106 Veres J.- Ein neues Instrument zur Aufführung von Brust-oder Bauchpunktionen und Pneumothoraxbehandlung. Dtsche Med Wschr 1938; 64: 1480-1481.

107 Vilardell F., Marti-Vicente A.- Peritoneoscopy (laparoscopy) in Gastroenterology, HL Bockus (ed) 3rd edition, Philadelphia, W.B. Saunders, 1976.

108 Wildhirt E.- Heinrich-Otto Kalk (1895-1973). Lebensbild eines Gastroenterologen und Hepatologen. Freiburg, Falk Foundation, 1996.

109 Zollikofer R.- Zur Laparoskopie. Schweiz med Wschr 1924;104: 264-267.

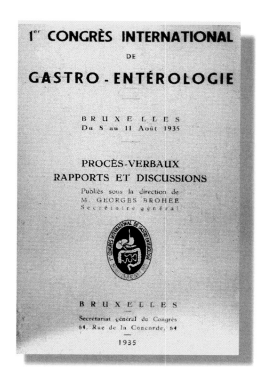

Ier CONGRÈS INTERNATIONAL

DE

GASTRO - ENTÉROLOGIE

BRUXELLES
Du 8 au 11 Août 1935

PROCÈS-VERBAUX
RAPPORTS ET DISCUSSIONS
Publiés sous la direction de
M. GEORGES BROHÉE
Secrétaire général

BRUXELLES
Secrétariat général du Congrès
64, Rue de la Concorde, 64
1935

CHAPTER 14

The emergence of digestive endoscopy organisations

THE DEVELOPMENT OF MEDICAL SPECIALITIES

DURING THE 19TH CENTURY, MEDICAL SPECIALITIES DEVELOPED IN A rather haphazard way, perhaps as an answer to the needs of medical care, but mostly because of the personality and the creativity of professional groups. Nosologic systems and diagnostic techniques were identified and differentiated, and certain types of patients were set apart. New specialities were created and needs that did not seem to exist previously were established. Today, such developments seem to be in operation in a similar fashion, although clearly in a much more sophisticated manner.

The mechanisms that guided the development of medical specialities varied a great deal: some were centred on organs, such as cardiology or ophthalmology while others depended on technical skills, such as surgery or on the invention of more or less complex instruments such as imaging. The creative stimulus for any speciality was often prompted by a respected scientific personality who was interested in some particular aspect of medicine; through his own initiative, he became the leader of a group of interested colleagues, organised working teams, seminars and meetings to discuss clinical cases, published their reports in medical journals and finally decided to create an organisation which would be responsible for the supervision of these activities, a society assembling those interested in this "new" speciality.

From a functional point of view, specialities may be divided into "traditional" areas, such as internal medicine, general surgery, paediatrics or obstetrics, and "relative" ones such as all sub-specialities of internal medicine (cardiology, gastroenterology, neurology, etc.) or surgery (orthopaedics, vascular and digestive surgery and so on). But there may also be "absolute" specialities in which the tasks of specialised personnel cannot be done by other physicians with a more general education unless they undergo a long, specialised training, as these unique specialities are the consequence of the emergence of new technologies: endoscopy, NMR, ultrasound, microsurgery and so forth.

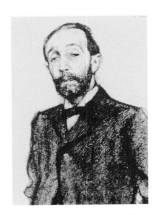

Fig. 1. Bartolomé Robert, Professor of Medicine at Barcelona University, author of the first Spanish treatise on "Diseases of the Digestive System" (1889).

Gastroenterology and hepatology grew around the study of digestive organs while digestive endoscopy developed through the invention of instruments able to explore these organs. These circumstances may have created competition among several specialists: surgeons, clinicians or radiologists may claim the exclusivity of the use of a given technique or a field of action: Thus, oesophagoscopy was performed by otolaryngologists until the invention of fibre-optics which allowed the examination of the entire upper gastrointestinal tract; gastroscopy has been done by internists and surgeons; proctosigmoidoscopy has also been a medical or a surgical technique, and laparoscopy in recent years has mostly become a procedure practiced by surgeons.

THE BIRTH OF GASTROENTEROLOGY

The first books describing digestive diseases, in particular those of the stomach, and the appearance of treatises on the "Diseases of Digestion" were first published around the second half of the 19th century, mostly in Germany and Great Britain. The first Spanish book on Digestive Diseases was written by Bartolomé Robert in 1889[25]. Clinicians were stimulated by the work of physiologists such as Claude Bernard in France, Ivan Pavlov in Russia or William Bayliss and Ernest Starling in the United Kingdom. The names of many great clinicians of that time have already appeared in this book (see Chapters 1 and 2). After Kussmaul's observations, many of them became interested in endoscopy. A new path in the field of surgery also began thanks to great surgeons and scholars such as Billroth, Péan, Hartmann, Mikulicz and others. The discovery of x-rays by W. Röntgen (1845-1923) represented an extraordinary step forward and enabled precise diagnosis of many gastrointestinal conditions. Endoscopy, as an accepted diagnostic method, is barely mentioned in books until the last decade of the 19th century *(Fig. 1)*.

THE FIRST JOURNALS AND THE FIRST SOCIETIES

Little by little clinicians specialising in gastroenterology started organising official meetings where digestive diseases were discussed. The earliest society on record was the American Gastroenterological Association (A.G.A.) which is still the most prestigious and dates back to 1897. The first society to appear in Europe was the Polish Society in 1907 when Poland was still part of the Empire of the Czars. The German Society had its origins in 1911 with the publication of the "Archiv für Verdauungskrankheiten". For a long time this was the most famous journal and it is still of great historical interest. The Netherlands Society was founded in 1913 and the French Society began its activities in 1922 under the name "Societé de Gastroenterologie de Paris", although a journal "Archives Français des Maladies de l'Appareil Digestif" had already appeared many years earlier. The Belgian Society dates from 1928, the Spanish Society from 1933[11, 17] (although a Journal entitled "Archivos Españoles de Enfermedades del Aparato Digestivo" had been created in 1918)[4], the Italian Society from 1934, the Swiss Society from 1935 and the British Society was founded in 1937. In South America the first association, the Argentinian Society of Gastroenterology, was created in 1927 in Buenos Aires.

THE FIRST GENUINELY SPECIALISED GASTROENTEROLOGY SERVICES

In the early years of the 20th century (1910-1930), there were very few specialised gastroenterology centres. In most cases there were internal medicine units in which a head of a service who was interested in digestive diseases orientated the work of his associates towards the speciality and admitted to his wards a majority of gastroenterology patients. I still remember how in a single hospital in Paris around 1950 (Saint-Antoine) there were at least four medical services doing mostly gastroenterology work.

In other hospitals, gastroenterologists acted as consultants to surgical services and there were also clinicians who would practice medical as well as surgical gastroenterology. Many of them did their own radiological examinations. Examples of this double activity were relatively frequent: Georges Brohée, founder of the First International Society of Gastroenterology, was a surgeon and a clinical radiologist. Medico-surgical gastroenterologists usually thrived in small cities in many countries, such as Spain. Current opinion favours the creation of multidisciplinary gastroenterological units in which internists, surgeons, endoscopists and radiologists work together dealing with complex patients such as those admitted with acute haemorrhage, with pancreatitis or for transplantation.

Many clinicians and surgeons were well known thanks to their publications and both radiology and endoscopy favoured the diffusion of the speciality. There were internists doing nothing but gastroenterology in Germany, Austria, France but also in Scandinavia, Italy, Belgium and Spain. The most prestigious German and Austrian centres were visited by American and British physicians while Latin-American and southern Europeans mainly visited Paris, probably because their education included French as a second language.

There were many contacts among specialists from both continents as can be readily verified by the similarities found in bibliographical references in books published on both sides of the Atlantic. American gastroenterology received a great boost after 1930 with the arrival of many prominent German specialists of Jewish origin who had to leave their country because of the Nazi persecutions.

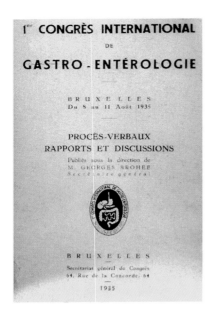

Fig. 2. Proceedings of the First International Congress of Gastro-enterology, Brussels 1935.

THE FIRST INTERNATIONAL CONGRESS OF GASTROENTEROLOGY *(Figs 2, 3, 4)*

All these scientific exchanges hastened the development of international meetings for exchanging technical information and for discussing the progress of the speciality. The international origins of gastroenterology are strongly linked to the personality of Georges Brohée (1887-1957), a Belgian surgeon and radiologist who, according to his excellent biographer Ludovic Standaert[26] who has dealt repeatedly with the origins of European gastroenterology, was an untiring individual, with tremendous enthusiasm and an authoritarian manner which allowed him to preside over a divided Europe. He started by founding the Belgian Society of Gastroenterology and the journal "Acta Gastroenterologica Belgica" which he believed were necessary tools for his aim to internationalise gastroenterology. His name is remembered thanks to the Brohée Medal which is awarded at each World Congress to an invited Brohée Lecturer.

In 1935, Brohée and a group of enterprising friends organised the First International Congress of Gastroenterology (Brussels 8-11 August 1935) under the presidency of the famous Dutch surgeon Ian Schoemaker from the Hague. Among other operative procedures, he was the author of a brilliant modification of the Billroth II gastrectomy. The congress was attended by the presidents of the ten already active national societies of gastroenterology as well as by 600 delegates from 35 countries. Official languages were French, English and German[6] *(Fig. 5, 6, 7)*.

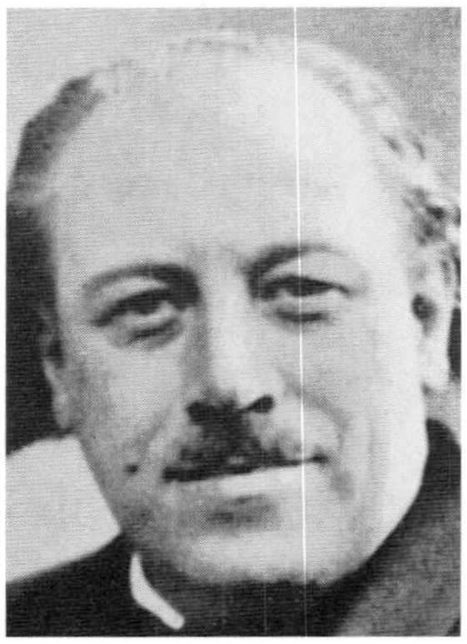

The two main subjects at the congress were gastritis and non-amoebic colitis, conditions which 70 years later continue to puzzle many investigators. The contributions of endoscopy to both reports are noteworthy, in particular one by François Moutier from Paris on gastroscopy of gastritis (see Chapter 4). The proceedings of the congress were later published in Brussels and include all the invited reports, among them one by Drs F. Gallart-Monés and P. Domingo (Spain) on the etiology of ulcerative colitis, and others from Sir Arthur Hurst (U.K.) on achlorydria (see Chapter 9) and from Georg Konjetzny from Hamburg on the pathology of gastritis. These reports include concepts which remain valid even today. In the proceedings, Brohée also published the provisional statutes of the International Society of

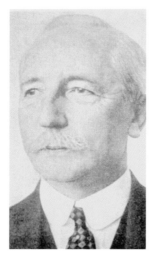

Fig. 3. Georges Brohée, a surgeon from Brussels, who created the first international society of gastroenterology (SIGE). Secretary of the First International Congress held in 1935 in Brussels (author's collection).

Fig. 4. Ian Schoemaker, Professor of Surgery at the Hague, President of the First International Congress of Gastroenterology (Brussels, 1935). (from ref. 6).

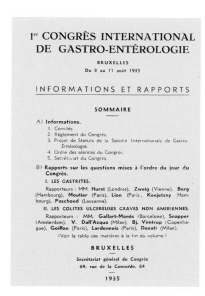

1ᵉʳ CONGRÈS INTERNATIONAL
DE GASTRO-ENTÉROLOGIE

BRUXELLES
Du 8 au 11 août 1935

INFORMATIONS ET RAPPORTS

SOMMAIRE

A) **Informations.**
   1. Comités.
   2. Règlement du Congrès.
   3. Projet de Statuts de la Société Internationale de Gastro-
      Entérologie.
   4. Ordre des séances du Congrès.
   5. Secrétariat du Congrès.

B) **Rapports sur les questions mises à l'ordre du jour du Congrès.**
   I. LES GASTRITES.
   Rapporteurs : MM. **Hurst** (Londres), **Zweig** (Vienne), **Berg** (Hambourg), **Moutier** (Paris), **Lion** (Paris), **Konjetzny** (Hambourg), **Paschoud** (Lausanne).
   II. LES COLITES ULCEREUSES GRAVES NON AMIBIENNES.
   Rapporteurs : MM. **Gallart-Monès** (Barcelone), **Snapper** (Amsterdam), **V. Dall'Acqua** (Milan), **Bj. Vimtrup** (Copenhague), **Goiffon** (Paris), **Lardennois** (Paris), **Donati** (Milan).
   (Voir la table des matières à la fin du volume.)

BRUXELLES

Secrétariat général du Congrès
64, rue de la Concorde, 64
—
1935

Fig. 5. *Index of the programme of the First International Congress, with reports by François Moutier on Gastritis and by Francisco Gallart on ulcerative colitis in which there are numerous endoscopic observations.*

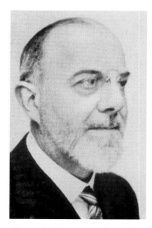

Fig. 6. *François Moutier, eminent gastroscopist from Paris. His name is honoured by a Moutier Lecture at the Congresses of O.M.E.D. (collection Dr. Jacinto Vilardell).*

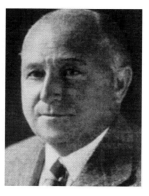

Fig. 7. *Francisco Gallart-Monès (1880-1960), founder of the Postgraduate School of Gastroenterology at the Hospital de Sant Pau in Barcelona where in 1913 he organised the first postgraduate course in gastroenterology which has been held annually from that date. He was the last president of S.I.G.E. (author's collection).*

Gastroenterology. The volume may be consulted at the Library of the Wellcome Institute of the History of Medicine in London.

THE SECOND INTERNATIONAL CONGRESS OF GASTROENTEROLOGY

The Second International Congress of Gastroenterology took place in Paris on 13-15 September 1937 under the presidency of the surgeon Pierre Duval. In attendance were delegates of 35 countries in numbers comparable to those of Brussels two years earlier in spite of the absence of Spanish delegates because of the Spanish Civil War. The main themes of the Congress were "Early diagnosis of gastric cancer" to which the most outstanding contributions were made by René A. Gutmann (Paris) and by Hans Heinrich Berg (Hamburg) who described signs and presented radiographic documents of early cancers of the stomach which went unsurpassed until the advent of fibrescopy thirty or more years later *(Fig. 8)*.

Other participants were Norbert Henning (Germany) and François Moutier (France) on gastroscopic aspects of early cancer, as well as Dr. C. Garin (France) on intragastric photography with a gastrocamera (see Chapter 7). The second topic of the congress was a surgical theme, on acute and chronic obstruction of the small bowel[26].

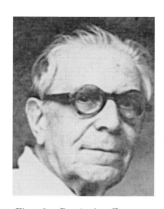

Fig. 8. *René A. Gutmann (1885-1982) (Paris). Lecturer on early gastric cancer at the Second International Congress of Gastroenterology (Paris 1937). President of S.I.G.E. and one of the founders of O.M.G.E. (author's collection).*

The Third Congress had been planned for London in 1940 under the presidency of Sir Arthur Hurst, the founder of the British Society of Gastroenterology, but World War Two prevented its venue. The congress took place eight years later in 1948 in Lausanne.

SOCIETÉ INTERNATIONALE DE GASTROENTÉROLOGIE (S.I.G.E.)

On the 10th of August 1935 before the closing ceremony of the First Congress, it was decided to create an international society of gastroenterology based on individual membership. Members would have to pay a small fee to run a permanent secretarial office in Brussels. According to the provisional statutes, each country had to establish a national committee including an internist, a surgeon, a radiologist and a biochemist (endoscopists were not yet considered!). In the proceedings of the foundation of the Society there is a list of national committees from sixteen different nations.

It was agreed to organise a congress every two years and that the main themes of the meeting would be selected by the general assembly of delegates. Reports would be presented by members of the local organising national society as well as by other gastroenterologists elected by the general assembly.

The Organising Committee of the "Societé Internationale de Gastroentérologie" (S.I.G.E.) was presided by Professor Leopold Mayer from Brussels and the Secretary-General was Georges Brohée who in 1936 founded a journal "Archives de la Societé Internationale de Gastroentérologie". According to L. Standaert, copies of this very short-lived journal are extremely difficult to come across in medical libraries. The first issue was published in 1936 and four more followed in 1937 when the journal ceased to exist due to the impossibility to find financial backing. However, Georges Brohée's interest in achieving an adequate international status for gastroenterology in spite of the tremendous political and material difficulties caused by a divided Europe did not lose impetus[26].

THE FOUNDATION OF A.S.N.E.M.G.E.

After a series of meetings of European delegates convened by Brohée after the war, it was resolved to organise the Third International Congress in 1948 in Lausanne and to create a new association with the exclusive aim of organising congresses independently from the S.I.G.E. It was named A.S.N.E.M.G.E. ("Association des Societé Nationales Européennes et Mediterranénnes de Gastroentérologie") and continues to exist today as part of the general organisation of the "United European Digestive Disease Week". A.S.N.E.M.G.E. differed from S.I.G.E., a society made up of individual members, in that it was a federation of gastroenterology societies, without individual members, practically without statutes and functioning on the basis of a few rules orientated toward the organisation of biennial congresses. The administrative structure was very simple: the president and the secretary of the Association were the president and secretary of the past congress, although a permanent secretariat was operating in Dr Brohée's office in Brussels.

A.S.N.E.M.G.E. was officially founded on 11 October 1947. Starting in 1949, congresses were organised in Madrid (1950), Bologna-Montecatini (1952)and Paris (1954) with scientific programmes very similar to that of the first congress: one or two main topics presented by designated speakers (rapporteurs) and free papers on the subject of the main reports.

CREATION OF THE INTERAMERICAN ASSOCIATION OF GASTROENTEROLOGY

The first Panamerican Congress of Gastroenterology took place in Buenos Aires in 1948, under the presidency of the distinguished Argentinian gastroenterologist Carlos Bonorino Udaondo (1884-1951). The Interamerican Association of Gastroenterology (AIGE) was created with the same administrative and scientific features as those of A.S.N.E.M.G.E, probably following the advice of Dr. Georges Brohée. A.I.G.E. was established as a federation of national societies; the Argentinian Society –founded back in 1927– played a leading role. A.I.G.E. today continues its periodical meetings and the "Instituto Carlos Bonorino Udaondo" is still a leading institution in gastroenterology in Latin America[3].

A NEW CONTINENTAL ASSOCIATION OF GASTROENTEROLOGY: A.P.A.G.E.

The Asian-Pacific Association of Gastroenterology A.P.A.G.E. was founded in Tokyo in 1961, following the lines of A.S.N.E.M.G.E. It is also based on a Federation of National Societies established in Asia and the Pacific Area. The organisation includes a president, a vice-president, a secretary and a treasurer (all officers of the previous congress) as well as a general assembly constituted by the presidents or delegates of each of the member societies. In 1986, "The Journal of Gastroenterology and Hepatology", official journal of A.P.A.G.E. and of the Asian-Pacific Association for the Study of the Liver was published. Since the first congress in 1961 in Tokyo, other meetings have taken place in 1964 in

Chandigarh (India), in 1968 in Melbourne (Australia), in 1972 in Manila (Philippines), in 1976 in Singapore. In all, 11 APAGE congresses have been organised[5].

O.M.G.E. REPLACES S.I.G.E.

According to Ludovic Standaert who described the history of A.S.N.M.G.E. in detail, for many years there was an uncertain relationship between S.I.G.E., the international society of gastroenterology and A.S.N.E.M.G.E., a federation of societies created with the exclusive aim of organising European congresses. Dr. Brohée was responsible for the secretariat of both organisations and this added to the confusion. The fact that S.I.G.E. was composed of individual members did not help its development. The Fourth European Congress (Paris 1954) which was presided by René A. Gutmann, of world fame because of his radiological investigations on early gastric cancer, helped to clarify matters *(Fig. 8)*. At a business session during the congress which was attended also by representatives from American countries, it was decided to transform the S.I.G.E. into a World federation, based on the existing European (A.S.N.E.M.G.E.) and the American (A.I.G.E.) associations, constituting an organisation at world scale of existing national societies of gastroenterology. The decision was made by a committee whose members were, among others: Dr. R.A. Gutmann, president of A.S.N.E.M.G.E., Dr. Francisco Gallart Monés (President of S.I.G.E.) and Georges Brohée. The Fifth A.S.N.E.M.G.E. Congress took place in London in 1956 under the presidency of Dr. Thomas Hunt, and was attended by large numbers of participants from both sides of the Atlantic. There the decision was finally made to hold a world congress of Gastroenterology in Washington in 1958[26] *(Fig. 9)*.

THE FIRST WORLD CONGRESS OF GASTROENTEROLOGY

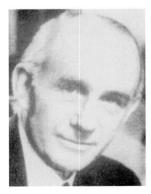

Fig. 9. Thomas Hunt, (1901-1980). London gastroenterologist, President of the International Congress (London 1956), during which the programme of the First World Congress and the preliminary statutes for a World Society were established. He was the second president of O.M.G.E. (courtesy of the British Society of Gastroenterology).

The congress was presided by Dr. Henry L. Bockus of Philadelphia, well-known author of an outstanding treatise of gastroenterology. It was attended by more than 1,500 specialists from 51 countries and caused admiration for its excellent organisation as well as for the high scientific quality of the selected papers that were presented. There were panel discussions, symposia, poster sessions, audiovisual demonstrations and distribution of abstracts before the sessions. Visits to leading American gastroenterology centres were also organised[29]. *(Figs. 10, 11, 12)*.

The congress was very successful and became a model in which new ways of presenting scientific material were tried and perfected later at the following congresses. The main symposia and lectures were recorded by the firm RCA and published on several L.P. records. They are available for study at the Wellcome Institute for the History of Medicine in London.

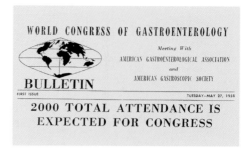

Fig. 10. First News Bulletin published during the First World Congress of Gastroenterology (Washington 1958).

ENDOSCOPY IN THE FIRST WORLD CONGRESS OF GASTROENTEROLOGY

A perusal of the index of the two volumes of Proceedings of the Congress which were published in 1959 by Williams & Wilkins shows that there were no specific papers on endoscopy presented at the meeting[22]. However, there was a presentation on gastric photography and the gastrocamera by Dr. Tazaki from Japan, another on the sigmoidocamera by Prof. Matsunaga and two British studies on ulcerative colitis and another on polyposis in which endoscopic findings were extensively described. There were no papers on either oesophagoscopy or on laparoscopy. Eight years later, in 1966, in Tokyo where the third World Congress took place, the situation had changed considerably.

THE DEVELOPMENT OF O.M.G.E.

During the 2nd World Congress of Gastroenterology (Munich 1962) presided by Norbert Henning, a clinician often referred to in this book, the first O.M.G.E. President, Henry L. Bockus succeeded in convincing the General Assembly to approve preliminary Statutes of the World Organisation in spite of vigorous opposition from some member societies. After several amendments[28] the essential points of the OMGE statutes were and still are, the following *(Figs. 13, 14)*:

1. O.M.G.E. at a difference with S.I.G.E. is a federation of societies based on the three existing continental associations, A.S.N.E.M.G.E., A.I.G.E., A.P.A.G.E.
2. O.M.G.E. not only would organise congresses every four years, but it would also foster research, organise multicentric stud-

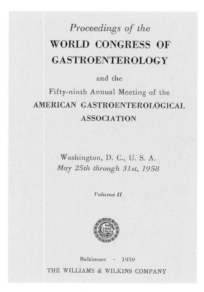

Proceedings of the
WORLD CONGRESS OF GASTROENTEROLOGY
and the
Fifty-ninth Annual Meeting of the
AMERICAN GASTROENTEROLOGICAL ASSOCIATION

Washington, D. C., U. S. A.
May 25th through 31st, 1958

Volume II

Baltimore · 1959
THE WILLIAMS & WILKINS COMPANY

Fig. 11. Front page of the Proceedings of the First World Congress of Gastroenterology (Washington 1958). The two volumes were published in 1959.

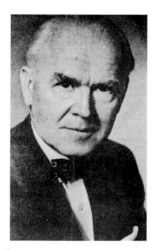

Fig. 12. Henry Leroy Bockus (1894-1982), professor of gastroenterology at the University of Pennsylvania in Philadelphia, President of the Organising Committee of the First World Congress of Gastroenterology and first president of O.M.G.E. A Bockus Medal and a Lecture commemorate his name at each World Congress. (author's collection).

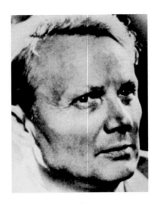

Fig. 13. Norbert Henning, one of first pioneers of digestive endoscopy. His name is associated to originally designed oesophagoscopes, gastroscopes and laparoscopes. His service at Erlangen University became a reference point for gastroenterological endoscopy. He presided over the Second World Congress of Gastroenterology (author's collection).

ies and establish the basis for the education of the gastroenterologist through committees created for that purpose. Another important aim was to solicit funds to achieve the necessary economic stability of the organisation.

TABLE I. O.M.G.E. PRESIDENTS

1958 - 1962	Henry L. Bockus	United States
1962 - 1966	Thomas Hunt	United Kingdom
1966 - 1970	Heliodoro G. Mogena	Spain
1970 - 1974	Marvin H. Pollard	United States
1974 - 1978	Geoffrey Watkinson	United Kingdom
1978 - 1982	Joel Valencia P	Venezuela
1982 - 1990 *	Francisco Vilardell	Spain
1990 - 1998 *	Ian A.D. Bouchier	United Kingdom
1998 - 2002	Meinhard Classen	Germany
2002 - 2005	Guido Tytgat	The Netherlands

(*) reelected for four years.

THE FIRST DIGESTIVE ENDOSCOPY ASSOCIATION: THE "AMERICAN GASTROSCOPIC CLUB"

In the same way that the American Gastroenterological Association (A.G.A.) was the first official gastroenterology society, the "American Gastroscopic Club" became the first endoscopic national association. Rudolf Schindler, who had left Germany and was working at the University of Chicago, took a leading role[9, 13]. (Fig. 15, 16, 17).

In the April 1942 issue of the "American Journal of Digestive Diseases", the first official meeting of the club, which took place at the Claridge Hotel in Atlantic City where the A.G.A. met very often, was announced[12]. The meeting took place on Sunday 7th of June 1942, and was convened by Dr. Joseph Kirsner from Chicago, secretary-treasurer of the Club. The programme included a symposium on chronic gastritis, its clinical and endoscopic aspects and perhaps more importantly, its repercussions on the health of Army and Navy personnel. Among others there were presentations by Schindler (who probably suggested the subject), Edward Benedict from Boston, George Eusterman from the Mayo Clinic and the Boston physiologist Seymour Gray.

According to Irvin Modlin[19], a group of interested gastroenterologists had met a few months earlier at the home of Dr.Schindler to discuss the founding of an endoscopy organisation. They finally agreed on naming it "American Gastroscopic Club", with Rudolf Schindler as the first president. In 1946, the name was changed to "American Gastroscopic Society" and in

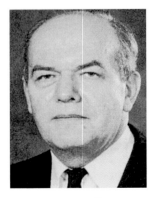

Fig. 14. Geoffrey Watkinson, British gastroenterologist, secretary-general of O.M.G.E. during 12 fruitful years and then president (OMGE Newsletter).

1962 the current name "American Society for Gastrontestinal Endoscopy" appeared for the first time.

The Club published a "Bulletin of the American Gastroscopic Club", which later became the "Bulletin of the American Gastroscopic Society". The name was changed again to "Bulletin of Gastroscopy and Oesophagoscopy" and in 1961 it appeared as the "Bulletin of Gastrointestinal Endoscopy". In 1964, due to the outstanding development of fibrescopy, the name was changed yet again to "Journal of Gastrointestinal Endoscopy", shortened later to "Gastrointestinal Endoscopy". Although the great majority of society members were gastroenterologists, there was a general feeling that the society should be kept independent from the American Gastroenterological Association, which was more inclined to clinical research and to basic science although many endoscopists were also often prominent clinicians who were doing research[16].

The progressive expansion of endoscopy not only in diagnosis but also in therapy, as well as the necessity to include endoscopic training in all gastroenterology residency programmes, has resulted in the very close participation of clinicians in both societies. The meetings of both groups thus take place simultaneously or in succession, as we have also witnessed in international gastroenterology congresses.

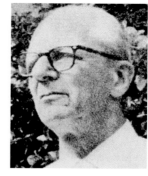

Fig. 15. Rudolf Schindler, possibly the best known digestive endoscopist (see Chapter 4), one of the founders of the American Gastroscopic Club. At each O.M.E.D. Congress his name is honoured by a "Schindler lecture". (author's collection).

BIRTH OF THE "EUROPEAN ENDOSCOPIC CLUB"

In the early 1960s, gastrointestinal endoscopy was growing fast although fibrescopy was not yet on the market; however, gastroscopists and laparoscopists were playing a bigger and bigger role in meetings. During the 6th A.S.N.E.M.G.E. Congress (Leiden 1960), there was a symposium on several endoscopy subjects in which many already reputed endoscopists took part: Adolf Wiebenga (Amsterdam), Edouard Jacobs (Brussels) Zdenek Maratka (Prague), Sacha Segal (Reims, Sandu Stoichita (Bucarest). They decided to create a "European Gastroscopic Club" along the lines of the American counterpart. The name "European Endoscopic Club" was finally agreed upon, as several participants such as E. Jacobs and S. Segal were outstanding laparoscopists. At the next European congress which took place in Brussels in 1964 the "European Society of Gastrointestinal Endoscopy" was officially created (E.S.G.E.)[14] *(Fig. 18).*

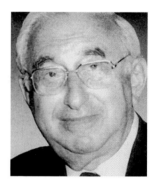

Fig. 17. Joseph B Kirsner, Emeritus Professor of Gastroenterology at the University of Chicago, who welcomed R. Schindler to his service when he had to leave Germany. He was one of the founders of the American Gatroscopic Club and of the American Society for Gastrointestinal Endoscopy (courtesy of Dr. J.B.Kirsner).

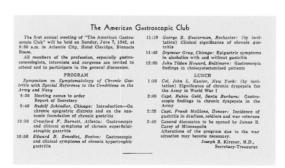

Fig. 16. Announcement of the first meeting of the American Gastroscopic Club (Atlantic City 1942). The meeting was convened by Dr. Joseph Kirsner.

ENDOSCOPY EARNS AN INDEPENDENT VOICE AT CONGRESSES

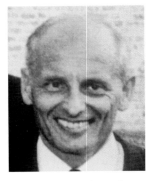

At the 1962 World Congress in Munich, Klaus Heinkel, an associate of the president Norbert Henning, was asked to organise a session on endoscopy which, as in Leiden, consisted mostly of papers on gastroscopy.

At the A.S.N.E.M.G.E. Congress in 1964 in Brussels, Digestive Endoscopy reached maturity. The Congress was presided by the surgeon Prof. L. Deloyers and the Secretary General was Dr. P. Massion. A full day session on endoscopy was programmed on the 2nd of June 1964. The moderators of the session were Drs R.Le Cluyse, E. Jacobs and F.Vilardell[7]. There was no simultaneous translation and papers were given in English, French, German and in Italian. Twenty-three papers were read from France, Germany, Spain, Italy, Hungary, Rumania, Australia, the United States, Japan, the Netherlands and Argentina. There were discussions after each presentation and films were also shown. Seven papers dealt with endoscopic documentation (photography, cinematography, television), one on laser experimentation, four on gastrocamera and fibrescopy, a paper on suction gastric biopsy, five on laparoscopy and two on rectosigmoidoscopy, which completed the session.

These were the beginnings of fibrescopy and the ingenuity and the creativity of endoscopists in order to provide objective documentation were clearly apparent at the meeting (Fig. 19, 20).

Fig. 18. Adolf Wiebenga (1920-1977). Professor of gastroenterology at Amsterdam University and later of Hospital Organisation. Founder of the "European Gastroscopic Club" which then became the E.S.G.E. of which he was president (1968-1970) (author's collection).

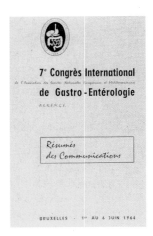

Fig. 19. Title page of the proceedings of the International Congress of Gastroenterology (Brussels 1964) during which an entire day session was devoted to digestive endoscopy.

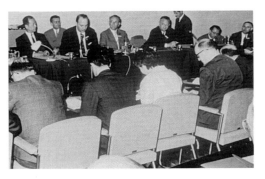

Fig. 20. View of the hall where the endoscopy session took place during the Brussels Congress (see text). The moderators were Raymond le Cluyse (Belgium) and Francisco Vilardell (Spain) accompanied by Drs. Yamagata (Japan) and Wittman (Hungary) (author's collection).

THE BIRTH OF E.S.G.E.

During the 1964 Brussels Congress a meeting was convened by A. Wiebenga, in which the original members of the European Endoscopic Club met with other invited endoscopists. As a result of diplomatic efforts by Adolf Wiebenga —who had been the promoter of the Club— by Sandu Stoichita and Edouard Jacobs, the attending endoscopists unanimously agreed upon the creation of a European society which received the name which still prevails: the European Society of Gastrointestinal Endoscopy (E.S.G.E.). The provisional governing board of the society included a President: Charles Debray (France), three Vice-Presidents: E.Jacobs (Belgium). S.Segal (France). A. Wiebenga (The Netherlands), a Secretary: Sandu Stoichita (Rumania), Treasurer: Klaus Heinkel (Germany) and an Editor, Raymond Le Cluyse (Belgium). Prof. Norbert Henning (Germany) was elected Honorary President. The minutes of this meeting are not available, but the data have kindly been given to me by Edouard Jacobs.

The first official appearance of the new society, E.S.G.E. took place in 1968 in Prague during the A.S.N.E.M.G.E. Congress presided by Prof. Kojecki. Dr. Zdenek Maratka took the presidency of this First Congress of Digestive Endoscopy and Dr. J.Setka acted as secretary.

TABLE 2. E.S.G.E. PRESIDENTS

1964-1968	Ch. Debray	Paris
1968-1970	A.Wiebenga	Amsterdam
1970-1974	F.Vilardell	Barcelona
1974-1976	K.Heinkel	Stuttgart
1976-1980	Z.Maratka	Prague
1980-1984	R.Cheli	Genova
1984-1988	L.Demling	Erlangen
1988-1992	M.Crespi	Rome
1992-1994	M.Cremer	Brussels
1994-1996	J.R.Armengol	Barcelona
1996-1998	F.Hagenmüller	Hamburg
1998-2000	A.Montori	Rome
2000-2002	A.Axon	Leeds
2002-2004	A.Nowak	Katowice
2004-2006	J.F.Rey	St. Laurent du Var

FIRST CONGRESS OF THE INTERNATIONAL SOCIETY OF ENDOSCOPY (1966)

During the Second World Congress of Gastroenterology (Munich 1962), Japanese gastroenterologists proposed the creation of an international society of endoscopy and the organisation of a congress which would take place jointly with the Third World Congress of Gastroenterology to be held in Tokyo in 1966. The Congress, which was very successful, was organised by Sadataka Tasaka (President), Takeo Hayashida (Vicepresident), Tadeo Takahashi and Shoichi Yamagata (Secretaries), Yawara Yoshitoshi (Secretary-treasurer) and Masasuke Masuda (Secretary for International Relations). In 1966, the Proceedings were edited by Prof. Yoshitoshi in a beautifully printed volume[23] (Fig. 21, 22, 23).

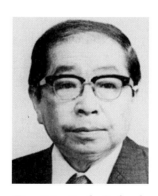

Fig. 21. Prof. Sadataka Tasaka, President of the First World Congress of Endoscopy and first President of O.M.E.D. (courtesy of Olympus Inc.).

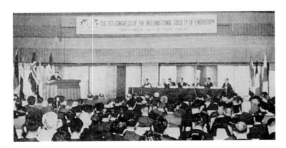

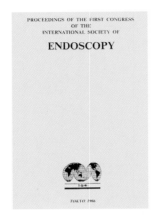

Fig. 22. Plenary session at the First World Endoscopy Congress (Tokyo 1966) (courtesy of Prof. H. Niwa).

The 629 pages of the Proceedings confirm the importance of the contributions made by endoscopists to this First World Congress. The book is headed by messages from the Honorary President of the Congress, Norbert Henning, and by Rudolf Schindler, considered by many as the father of digestive endoscopy. The working sessions were divided into the following themes (with the number of papers in each session in brackets): 1) oesophagoscopy (13) 2) gastrointestinal endoscopy (70), 3) rectosigmoidoscopy and coloscopy (8), 4) laparoscopy (20), 5) technical advances (16) 6) cine-endoscopy (8). The total number of papers and films presented was 135.

Fig. 23. Proceedings of the First World Congress of Digestive Endoscopy (Tokyo, 1966).

The new fibrescopes were of course the exciting novelties along with the massive use of the gastrocamera in Japan, the developments and refinements of photography, television and cinematography as well as the importance of diagnostic laparoscopy.

At the end of the congress on September 15, 1966, an assembly of delegates was chaired by Professors Y. Yoshitoshi and M. Masuda. Among those in attendance were many European and American delegates. It was resolved to establish a World Organisation of Digestive Endoscopy with a structure similar to that of O.M.G.E., based on a federation of societies from the three continental areas, European, Asian-Pacific and American. According to the provisional statutes, the future O.M.E.D. (Organisation Mondiale d'Endoscopie Digestive) in each continental association would include in its membership the societies of its own geographic area, each one co-ordinated by a secretary. It was also decided that congresses would be organised jointly with those of O.M.G.E. and that the second congress would take place in the "European Zone". As we will explain later, the organisation of this second congress suffered many setbacks. In the meantime, most European countries were busy setting up their own endoscopic societies so that they could actively participate in future congresses as well as in their organisational structures. The Spanish Association of Digestive Endoscopy was founded in 1969[2].

ROME AND COPENHAGEN: 2ND WORLD CONGRESS OF DIGESTIVE ENDOSCOPY.

During the E.S.G.E. Congress in Prague (1968) which we have already reported, Adolf Wiebenga from Amsterdam was elected the second president of ESGE and was given the task to organise the Second World Congress. The few endoscopic societies active in Europe at that time and the lack of effective organisations in other countries created serious difficulties for the organisation of the congress. There were two options: either to make the endoscopy congress independent from the O.M.G.E. meeting, or to include endoscopy in the larger clinical congress. In the end, both options had to be carried out and between 1-3 July 1970 a first independent part of the congress took place in Rome under Prof. G.Marcozzi (president) and M.Crespi (Secretary). On 9-10 July a second part was held in Copenhagen in connection with the World Congress of Gastroenterology, presided by A.Wiebenga and with Drs Birsgard-Pedersen and J.Mosbech as local secretaries.

Both congresses were attended by large audiences and the Proceedings were published by Drs M.Crespi and G.Marcozzi in a large volume of 929 pages! No further proof was needed of the interest of gastroenterologists for endoscopy which had developed immensely since the previous congress four years earlier in Tokyo[1] *(Fig. 24).*

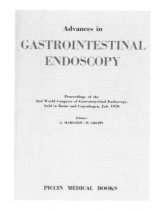

Fig. 24. Proceedings of the Second World Congress of Digestive Endoscopy (Rome-Copenhagen 1970).

The papers presented in Rome were organised according to the following headings (number of papers in brackets):

1) Papers comparing endoscopy with other diagnostic procedures (12).
2) Limits between normal and pathologic findings in endoscopic biopsy (9).
3) New instruments (8).
4) New research procedures with the aid of endoscopy (10).
5) Digestive cytology (5).
6) Endoscopy in acute gastrointestinal bleeding (9).
7) New indications for endoscopic procedures (10).
8) Endoscopy in digestive cancer and precancerous lesions (11).
9) Laparoscopy (10).
10) Recent advances in gastrointestinal electronic microscopy (5).
11) Endoscopy of the duodenum and the colon (12).

In all, 101 presentations.

The congress programme for Copenhagen was simply distributed into areas as follows:

1) Oesophagoscopy: 8 papers.
2) Gastrocamera: 9 papers.
3) Gastroscopy: 14 papers.
4) Gastrobiopsy and cytology: 10 papers.
5) Duodenoscopy: 6 papers.
6) Colonoscopy: 7 papers.
7) Laparoscopy: 16 papers.

In all, 70 communications. The total number of papers presented between Rome and Copenhagen was 171.

For the first time, invited lectures were given at a World Congress, honouring two outstanding personalities of digestive endoscopy: 1) The "Schindler Lecture" given by Dr. S.Tasaka from Japan on "The future of the technical development of the endoscope"; 2) The "Moutier lecture" given by Charles Debray from France, in collaboration with J.A.Paolaggi and P. Housset on "The future of gastrointestinal endoscopy from the point of view of the clinician". Both lectures are given regularly in all World Congresses of Digestive Endoscopy today.

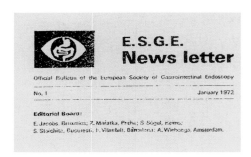

Fig. 25. Title page of the first Newsletter of the E.S.G.E. (European Society for Gastrointestinal Endoscopy). (January 1972).

STRENGTHENING THE E.S.G.E.

At the closure of the 2nd World Congress of Digestive Endoscopy in Copenhagen, after protracted discussions, a general assembly elected a new E.S.G.E. governing board with the following composition:

— President: F.Vilardell (Spain)
— Vicepresident: K.Heinkel (Germany)
— Administrative Secretary: G.Miller (Switzerland)
— Scientific Secretary: R.Cheli (Italy)
— Editorial Secretary: M.Crespi (Italy)

A committee was appointed to revise the statutes of the society and a bulletin (ESGE Newsletter) was edited by Gaudenz Miller. The first issue appeared in January 1972, the official editors were G.Miller, K.Heinkel, R.Cheli and M.Crespi and the Newsletter was distributed to all European societies[10] *(Fig. 25)*.

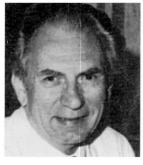

Fig. 26. Klaus Heinkel (1921-1982), a leading endoscopist in Germany, a close associate of Norbert Henning especially interested in teaching endoscopy, author of several endoscopy teaching devices. President of E.S.G.E. and of O.M.E.D. (author's collection).

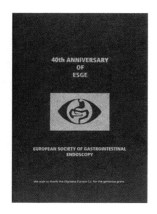

Fig. 27. Title page of the book commemorating forty years of E.S.G.E., edited by Dr. J. Kotrik. November, 2000.

The ESGE Statutes were again amended and definitely approved at the assembly that took place in 1972 in Paris during the A.S.N.E.M.G.E. Congress. A new Governing Board was elected as follows:

— President: F.Vilardell (Spain)
— President Elect: K.Heinkel (Germany)
— Vicepresidents: A.Cornet (France), Z.Maratka (Czechoslovakia), S.Stoichita (Rumania)
— Scientific secretary: R.Cheli (Italy)
— Administrative Secretary: G.Miller (Switzerland). *(Figs. 26, 27).*

FOUNDATION OF S.I.E.D. IN 1973

The foundation of the Interamerican Society of Digestive Endoscopy (SIED) took place during the

Panamerican Gastroenterology Congress which was held in Buenos Aires in September 1973, and ratified during the Third World Congress of Digestive Endoscopy in 1974 in Mexico City[3] *(Fig. 28).*

Dr. Horacio Rubio from Argentina was elected as the first president and the First Interamerican Congress took place in Caracas in November 1975. At this meeting, three vice-presidents were elected: Raimundo Llanio (Cuba), Marcos Matos Villalobos (Venezuela), and Joseph Sidorov (Canada). At the following congress, Dr.Henry Colcher (U.S.A.) replaced Dr. Horacio Rubio as president *(Fig. 29, 30).*

AIGE
ASOCIACION INTERAMERICANA DE GASTROENTEROLOGIA
BOLETIN INFORMATIVO
AÑO 1974
XIV Congreso Panamericano y
II Congreso Venezolano de Gastroenterologia
Y
I Congreso Interamericano de Endoscopia Digestiva
Caracas - Venezuela
23-28 de Noviembre de 1975

Fig. 28. Front page of the A.I.G.E. Bulletin in which an announcement is made of the First Interamerican Congress of Digestive Endoscopy (Caracas 1973).

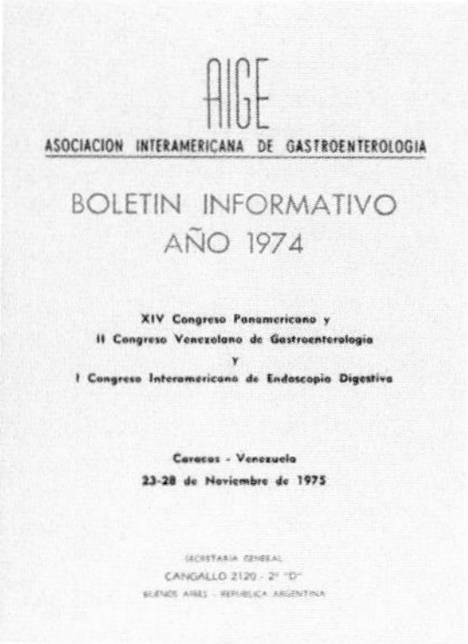

THE ASIAN-PACIFIC SOCIETY OF DIGESTIVE ENDOSCOPY (APSDE)

This society was founded in Tokyo during the Third World Congress of Gastroenterology[5]. An ad-hoc committee was appointed which consisted of S.Tasaka as President, T.Hayashioda as Vice-President and Dr. Y.Yoshitoshi as Secretary-General. Seventeen other members of this interim committee included delegates from the Philippines, Korea, Australia, Turkey, Hong Kong, Thailand, India, Taiwan, Sri-Lanka and New Zealand. At the APAGE Congress that took place in 1972 in Manila, the composition of this committee was ratified. Dr. Tasaka continued as President until 1976, followed by Prof. M.Masuda (1976-1982). Other presidents have been Drs Yoshitoshi, Kidokoro, Takemoto and Niwa all from Japan. Successive meetings took place in Kyoto (1973), Singapore (1976), Taipei (1980), Jakarta (1984), Seoul (1988), Bangkok (1992).

O.M.E.D. REPLACES THE INTERNATIONAL SOCIETY OF ENDOSCOPY

During the World Congress in Copenhagen (1970) a meeting was arranged including participants of the three continental associations of Digestive Endoscopy. Among those attending were Drs Tasaka, Yamagata, Masuda and Sakita for the Asian-Pacific Zone, Drs. Rumball, Wolff, Valencia-Parparcén and Berk for the American zone and Drs Wiebenga, Heinkel, Stochita, Miller, Maratka, Cheli and Vilardell for the E.S.G.E. A draft of provisional statutes was presented by Dr. J.E.Berk and ratified in Paris in 1972 at a second meeting by the same group *(Figs. 31, 32, 33).*

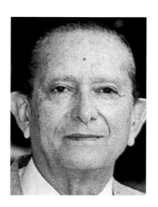

Fig. 29. Dr. Horacio Rubio, a distinguished gastroenterologist from Buenos Aires (Argentina), first president of the Interamerican Society for Digestive Endoscopy (S.I.E.D.) (courtesy of Dr. Horacio Rubio Jr.)

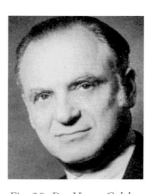

Fig. 30. Dr. Henry Colcher, American gastroenterologist of Belgian origin, pioneer of endoscopic cinematography (see chapter 7). The second president of S.I.E.D. succeeding Dr. Horacio Rubio (author's collection).

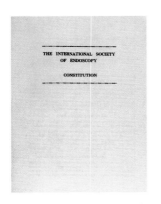

The definitive statutes of O.M.E.D. were approved during the 1974 World Congress in Mexico City. A Governing Body was elected including the following delegates:

TABLE 3. FIRST O.M.E.D. GOVERNING COUNCIL
(Elected on 19th October 1974)

Honorary Members
Charles Debray (France), Norbert Henning (Germany), Joseph B.Kirsner (USA), Marcelo Royer (Argentina) Hermon Taylor (United Kigdom)

President
Sadataka Tasaka (Japan)

Vicepresidents
Henry Colcher (USA), Klaus Heinkel (Germany), Yawara Yoshitoshi (Japan)

Councillors
Asian-Pacific
Masasuke Masuda (Japan), Gabriel S.Nagy (Australia)

America
José Ramirez-Degollado (Mexico), Horacio H.Rubio (Argentina)

Europe
Francisco Vilardell (Spain), Adolph Wiebenga (Netherlands)

Secretaries
José M.Job (Brazil), Hirohumi Niwa (Japan), Gaudenz Miller (Switzerland)

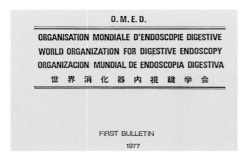

Fig. 32. Front page of the first O.M.E.D. Bulletin, edited in Japan (1977).

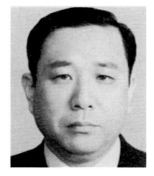

Fig. 33. Prof. Hirohumi Niwa, a distinguished Japanese endoscopist, pioneer of the gastrocamera and of the colonoscope, author of a book on the History of Digestive Endoscopy. Current president of O.M.E.D. (2002). (courtesy of Prof. H.Niwa).

Since then, the OMED has followed a progressive and fruitful course including the quatriennal congresses in close association with OMGE[20, 21] *(Fig. 34).*

THE DEVELOPMENT OF ENDOSCOPIC TERMINOLOGY

Since the first international meetings dealing with endoscopy it was soon felt that there was a need to unify the terminology employed by endoscopists in their reports. A pioneer in this field has been Professor Zdenek Maratka from Prague who presided the 1968 International Congress of Digestive Endoscopy in the same city. In the following year, he also organised in Prague the first congress on "Urgent

TABLE 4. WORLD CONGRESSES OF DIGESTIVE ENDOSCOPY

Year	City	President
1966	Tokyo	S. Tasaka
1970	Rome	G. Marcozzi
	Copenhagen	A. Wiebenga
1974	Mexico City	J. Ramirez-Degollado
		R. Tinajero Ayala
1978	Madrid	L. Gándara
1982	Stockholm	H. Reichard
1986	Sao Paulo	J.S. Meirelles Filho
1990	Sydney	J. St John
1994	Los Angeles	H. Worth Boyce
1998	Vienna	A. Gangl
2002	Bangkok	P. Luengrojanakul
2005	Montreal	R. Bailey

TABLE 5. O.M.E.D. PRESIDENTS

1974 - 1978	Sadataka Tasaka	Japan
1978 - 1982	Henry Colcher	U.S.A.
1982 - 1982	Klaus Heinkel	Germany
1982 - 1982	Masasuke Masuda	Japan
1983 - 1986	Wilfred Sircus	U.K.
1986 - 1990	Horacio Rubio	Argentina
1990 - 1994	Takao Sakita	Japan
1994 - 1998	Rodolfo Cheli	Italy
1998 - 2002	Glaciomar Machado	Brazil
2002 - 2006	Hirohumi Niwa	Japan

Drs Heinkel and Masuda both died in 1982. After a mail-vote, Dr. Wilfred Sircus (Edinburgh) was elected President.

Endoscopy". During the 1980s, with the help of a large number of contributors, Maratka edited successive editions of "Endoscopic Terminology" in several languages[27], based on strictly objective descriptions. It was recently complemented by a CD-Rom version edited by Prof. Maratka and Dr. J.R. Armengol-Miró which provides useful material for teaching purposes. O.M.E.D. has organised a committee for the evaluation of minimal standards of endoscopic nomenclature which are revised periodically (Figs. 35, 36).

DIGESTIVE ENDOSCOPY IN THE MUSEUMS

For those interested in the history of digestive endoscopy, it might be useful to briefly review some of the opportunities

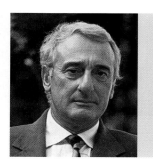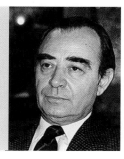

Fig. 34. Two distinguished Italian endoscopists: Left: Massimo Crespi, Secretary-General and editor of the Proceedings of the 2nd World Congress of Digestive Endoscopy, President of E.S.G.E. (1988-1992). Right: Alberto Montori, Senior editor of O.M.E.D. and "World Gastroenterology News", President of E.S.G.E. (1998-2000) (courtesy of World Gastroenterology News).

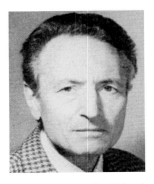

Fig. 35. Prof. Zdenek Maratka, Czech gastroenterologist, he presided the first International Congress on Emergency Endoscopy in Prague (1969). Editor of the Endoscopic Terminology in which many well-known endoscopists have collaborated. (courtesy of Z.Maratka).

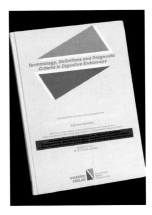

Fig. 36. Front page of the Terminology which lists definitions and objective diagnostic criteria in digestive endoscopy. Editions in several languages have appeared, including a CD-Rom.

that are offered to inspect the early first instruments employed in endoscopy. Besides the well-known collections at the Wellcome Institute for the History of Medicine in London and those assembled at the Smithsonian Institution in Washington, there is an excellent museum for the History of Medicine in Paris in the building of the old Faculté de Medecine in which one can admire the Désormeaux endoscope as well as a collection of rigid and semi-flexible instruments for gastroscopy which were the property of Dr. François Moutier[15]. The Steno Museum in Ahrus (Denmark), the Heilkunde Museum/Johann Winter in Andernach (Germany), the William O. Didusch in Baltimore and the Ditrick Medical History Center in Cleveland also include early endoscopes among their collections (Figs. 37, 38, 39, 40).

However, the most complete and unique collection of endoscopy instruments is unquestionably that of the Institute for the History of Medicine in Vienna, which is lodged at the old Josephinum, the famous Military Medical School (see Chapter 2). A few years ago I had the chance to admire there the earliest rigid and semiflexible endoscopes, among them the Nitze-Leiter oesophago-gastroscope provided with a "lobster-tail" end. But the main contribution to the Endoscopy museum, which is part of the Institute, is the large collection of instruments donated by Professor Hans Joachim Reuter from Stuttgart. For years he had collected all kinds of urologic endoscopes as well as instruments used in gastroenterol-

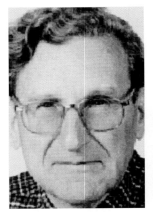

Fig. 37. Hans Joachim Reuter, famous German urologist, author with his son Matthias A. Reuter of a monumental history of endoscopy, and creator of the Max Nitze Endoscopy Museum, currently lodged at the Institute for the History of Medicine in Vienna (courtesy of Prof. H.J.Reuter).

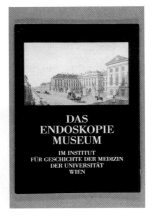

Fig. 38. Illustrated publication of the Museum for the History of Medicine of Vienna University at the Josephinum, the old Military Medical School. (see Chapter 2) (courtesy of the Institute for the History of Medicine).

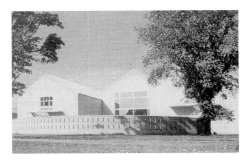

Fig. 39. View of the Steno Museum for the History of Medicine in Aarhus (Denmark). (courtesy of the Institute for the History of Medicine in Vienna).

ogy, starting with the first instruments designed by Max Nitze and produced by Joseph Leiter (see Chapter 3). He created the Max Nitze Museum honouring the famous urologist, which now constitutes the main part of the Endoscopy Museum in Vienna. The Museum contains more than 3,000 instruments and is an essential visit for anyone interested in endoscopic history. Together with the Institute for the History of Medicine of Vienna University, Professor Reuter has organized symposia on the history of endoscopy, and he and his son Matthias have edited a huge volume in four parts on the history of endoscopy, a true historical milestone which includes a very large and admirable iconography as well an exhaustive bibliography[24].

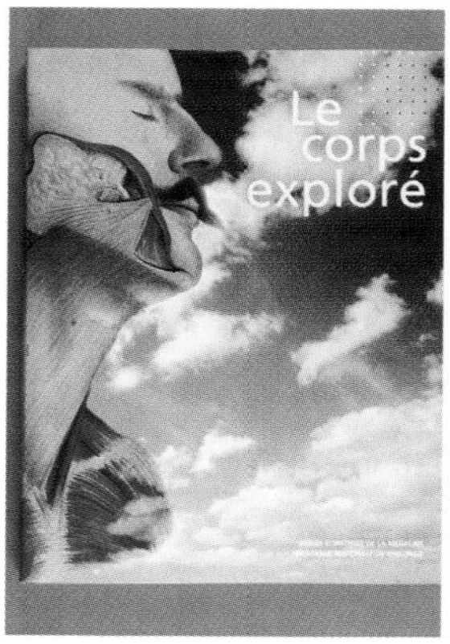

Fig. 40. Front page of "Le Corps Exploré", an outstanding publication illustrated with many examples of old endoscopic instruments which are exhibited at the Medical Museum of the Faculté de Médecine de Paris.

REFERENCES

1 "Advances in Gastrointestinal Endoscopy" Proceedings of the Second World Congress of Gastrointestinal Endoscopy. Editor M.Crespi, Padova, Piccin 1971.

2 Asociación Española de Endoscopia Digestiva. Website: www.aeed.org

3 Asociación Interamericana de Gastroenterología, Boletín Informativo, Buenos Aires, 1974.

4 Archivos Españoles de Enfermedades del Aparato Digestivo y de la Nutrición. R.Luis y Yagüe, Fidel F.Martinez, Luis Urrutia editores, Tomo 1, Madrid, 1918.

5 Asian-Pacific Society for Digestive Endoscopy, third Bulletin, 1996.

6 1er Congrès International de Gastroenterologie. Rapports. G.Brohée editeur, Bruxelles, 1935.

7 7ème Congrès International de Gastroentérologie. Resumés des Communications. Bruxelles, 1-4 Juin 1964.

8 Das Wiener Endoskopie Museum. Eröffnungssymposium 1966. Wien. Literas Universitätsverlag, 1997.

9 Edmonson J.M., McCray R.S. Past tense: history of ASGE. Gastrointest Endosc 1998; 47: 91-93.

10 ESGE NewsLetter, Gaudenz Miller Executive Editor, (Jan) n° 1, 1972.

11 Gallart-Esquerdo A. Historia de la Gastroenterología Española. Discurso de Ingreso en la Real Academia de Medicina de Barcelona 1955.

12 Kirsner J.B. The American Gastroscopic Club. Am J Dig Dis. 1942; 9: 146.

13 Kirsner J.B. The Development of American Gastroenterology, Nwe York, Raven Press, 1990: 283-285.

14 Kotrik J. History of E.S.G.E. 40th Anniversary of ESGE. European Society of Gastrointestinal Endoscopy, November 2000.

15 Le Corps Exploré. Avec la collaboration de Georges-Alfred Cremer, M.V. Clin, M.Bonduelle, A.Cornet, P.Lefebvre, D.Pellerin, A.Ségal. Musée d´Histoire de la Médecine, Académie Nationale de Chirurgie. Paris, La Compagnie d'Hauteville, 1997.

16 Lightdale C.J. Notes on the development of the American Society for Gastrointestinal Endoscopy. Gastrointest Endosc 1983; 29: 51-53.

17 Martinez Pérez F., Neira-Reina F., Ortega-García J.L. Historia de la Sociedad Española de Patología Digestiva y de la Nutrición, Madrid, Editores Médicos S.A., 1997.

18 Meilensteine der Endoskopie. 2. Symposium der Internationalen Nitze-Leiter Forschunggesellschaft für Endoskopie, Wien, Literas Universitätsverlag, 2000.

19 Modlin I.M. A Brief History of Endoscopy. Milano. Multi-Med, 2000:117-122.

20 O.M.E.D. Organisation Mondiale d'Endoscopie Digestive, World Organization of Digestive Endoscopy, Organización Mundial de Endoscopia Digestiva. First Bulletin, 1977.

21 O.M.E.D. Organisation Mondiale d'Endoscopie Digestive. Website:

22 Proceedings First World Congress of Gastroenterology, Vols I and II, Washington 1958. Baltimore, Williams & Wilkins, 1959.

23 Proceedings of the First Congress of the International Society of Endoscopy, Y.Yoshitoshi (editor), Tokyo, Hitachi Printing Co, 1966.

24 Reuter M., Reuter H.J. Geschichte der Endoskopie Band 1-4. Stuttgart-Zürich, Karl Kramer, 1998.

25 Robert B., Roig i Bofill E. Enfermedades del Aparato Digestivo, Madrid, Administración de la Revista de Medicina y Cirugía Prácticas, 1889.

26 Standaert L. History of ASNEMGE. Gastroenterology International. 1993; 6: 180-186.

27 Terminology, Definitions and Diagnostic Criteria in Digestive Endoscopy, Z.Maratka (ed.) Normed Verlag, (several editions in various languages).

28 Vilardell F. Origins of the OMGE. World Gastroenterology News 1993; 1: 1-7.

29 World Congress of Gastroenterology Bulletin, First Issue, Tuesday May 27, Washington, 1958.

Index of names

Index of Subjects

Index of hospitals, medical instruments and instrument makers

Medical Instruments

Instrument makers

James A. DiSario, M.D.

SYMBIOSIS the benjamin cummings custom laboratory program for the biological sciences

Principles of Ecology Laboratory
ENV 1020
Department of Natural Science
Baruch College
City University of New York

Pearson Custom Publishing

New York   Boston   San Francisco
London   Toronto   Sydney   Tokyo   Singapore   Madrid
Mexico City   Munich   Paris   Cape Town   Hong Kong   Montreal

Senior Vice President, Editorial and Marketing: Patrick F. Boles
Senior Sponsoring Editor: Natalie Danner
Executive Marketing Manager: Nathan L. Wilbur
Operations Manager: Eric M. Kenney
Development Editor: Kelly Harris
Editorial Assistant: Jill Johnson
Database Product Manager: Jennifer Berry
Art Director: Renée Sartell
Cover Designer: Kristen Kiley

Cover Art: Courtesy of Michael R. Martin, Darryl Johnson, and Photodisc.

Pyrex, pHydrion, Chem3D Plus, Apple, Macintosh, Chemdraw, Hypercard, graphTool, Corning, Teflon, Mel-Temp, Rotaflow, Tygon, Spec20, and LambdaII UV/Vis are registered trademarks.

Chem3D Plus is a registered trademark of the Cambridge Soft Corp.

The information, illustration, and/or software contained in this book, and regarding the above mentioned programs, are provided "as is," without warranty of any kind, express or implied, including without limitation any warranty concerning the accuracy, adequacy, or completeness of such information. Neither the publisher, the authors, nor the copyright holders shall be responsible for any claims attributable to errors, omissions, or other inaccuracies contained in this book. Nor shall they be liable for direct, indirect, special, incidental, or consequential damages arising out of the use of such information or material.

The authors and publisher believe that the lab experiments described in this publication, when conducted in conformity with the safety precautions described herein and according to the school's laboratory safety procedures, are reasonably safe for the students for whom this manual is directed. Nonetheless, many of the described experiments are accompanied by some degree of risk, including human error, the failure or misuse of laboratory or electrical equipment, mismeasurement, spills of chemicals, and exposure to sharp objects, heat, body fluids, blood or other biologics. The authors and publisher disclaim any liability arising from such risks in connections with any of the experiments contained in this manual. If students have questions or problems with materials, procedures, or instructions on any experiment, they should always ask their instructor for help before proceeding.

This special edition published in cooperation with Pearson Custom Publishing.

Printed in the United States of America.

Please visit our web site at *www.pearsoncustom.com/symbiosis*.

Attention bookstores: For permission to return unused stock, contact us at *pe-uscustomreturns@pearson.com*.

**Pearson
Custom Publishing**
is a division of

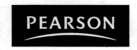

www.pearsonhighered.com

ISBN 10: 0-558-28056-0
ISBN 13: 978-0-558-28056-7

Laboratory Safety: General Guidelines

1. Notify your instructor immediately if you are pregnant, color blind, allergic to any insects or chemicals, taking immunosuppressive drugs, or have any other medical condition (such as diabetes, immunologic defect) that may require special precautionary measures in the laboratory.

2. Upon entering the laboratory, place all books, coats, purses, backpacks, etc. in designated areas, not on the bench tops.

3. Locate and, when appropriate, learn to use exits, fire extinguisher, fire blanket, chemical shower, eyewash, first aid kit, broken glass container, and cleanup materials for spills.

4. In case of fire, evacuate the room and assemble outside the building.

5. Do not eat, drink, smoke, or apply cosmetics in the laboratory.

6. Confine long hair, loose clothing, and dangling jewelry.

7. Wear shoes at all times in the laboratory.

8. Cover any cuts or scrapes with a sterile, waterproof bandage before attending lab.

9. Wear eye protection when working with chemicals.

10. Never pipet by mouth. Use mechanical pipeting devices.

11. Wash skin immediately and thoroughly if contaminated by chemicals or microorganisms.

12. Do not perform unauthorized experiments.

13. Do not use equipment without instruction.

14. Report *all* spills and accidents to your instructor immediately.

15. Never leave heat sources unattended.

16. When using hot plates, note that there is no visible sign that they are hot (such as a red glow). Always assume that hot plates are hot.

17. Use an appropriate apparatus when handling hot glassware.

18. Keep chemicals away from direct heat or sunlight.

19. Keep containers of alcohol, acetone, and other flammable liquids away from flames.

20. Do not allow any liquid to come into contact with electrical cords. Handle electrical connectors with dry hands. Do not attempt to disconnect electrical equipment that crackles, snaps, or smokes.

21. Upon completion of laboratory exercises, place all materials in the disposal areas designated by your instructor.

22. Do not pick up broken glassware with your hands. Use a broom and dustpan and discard the glass in designated glass waste containers; never discard with paper waste.

23. Wear disposable gloves when working with blood, other body fluids, or mucous membranes. Change gloves after possible contamination and wash hands immediately after gloves are removed.

24. The disposal symbol indicates that items that may have come in contact with body fluids should be placed in your lab's designated container. It also refers to liquid wastes that should not be poured down the drain into the sewage system.

25. Leave the laboratory clean and organized for the next student.

26. Wash your hands with liquid or powdered soap prior to leaving the laboratory.

27. The biohazard symbol indicates procedures that may pose health concerns.

The caution symbol points out instruments, substances, and procedures that require special attention to safety. These symbols appear throughout this manual.

Measurement Conversions

Metric to American Standard

Length

1 mm = 0.039 inches

1 cm = 0.394 inches

1 m = 3.28 feet

1 m = 1.09 yards

Volume

1 mL = 0.0338 fluid ounces

1 L = 4.23 cups

1 L = 2.11 pints

1 L = 1.06 quarts

1 L = 0.264 gallons

Mass

1 mg = 0.0000353 ounces

1 g = 0.0353 ounces

1 kg = 2.21 pounds

Temperature

To convert temperature:

$$°C = \frac{5}{9}(F - 32)$$

American Standard to Metric

Length

1 inch = 2.54 cm

1 foot = 0.305 m

1 yard = 0.914 m

1 mile = 1.61 km

Volume

1 fluid ounce = 29.6 mL

1 cup = 237 mL

1 pint = 0.474 L

1 quart = 0.947 L

1 gallon = 3.79 L

Mass

1 ounce = 28.3 g

1 pound = 0.454 kg

Temperature

$$°F = \frac{9}{5}C + 32$$

°F | °C

230 — 110
220
210 — 100 ← Water boils
200
190 — 90
180
— 80
170
160
— 70
150
140 — 60
130
120 — 50
110
— 40
98.6°F — 100
Normal human body temperature — 90 ← 37.0°C Normal human body temperature
80 — 30
70
— 20
60
50 — 10
40
30 — 0 ← Water freezes
20
10 — −10
0
— −20
−10
−20 — −30
−30
−40 — −40

Centimeters | Inches

20 — 8
19
18 — 7
17
16 — 6
15
14
13 — 5
12
11
10 — 4
9
8 — 3
7
6
5 — 2
4
3 — 1
2
1
0 — 0

Contents

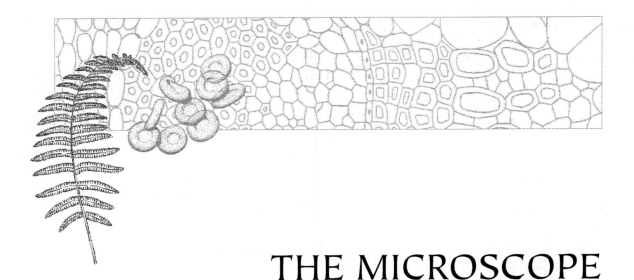

THE MICROSCOPE

PURPOSE

- Introduce the microscope, microscope protocol, and microscope skills.
- Learn the terms associated with the use of the microscope.

MATERIALS

Microscope
Lens tissue
Lens cleaner
Permanent slide with letter "e"
Permanent slide with colored fibers
Clean microscope slides
Cover slips
Eyedroppers
Clear plastic millimeter ruler

PART A — LEARNING TO USE THE MICROSCOPE

1. MAKE A PRELIMINARY STUDY OF FIGURE 1. Be able to identify the **arm, stage**, and **base**.

2. OBTAIN A MICROSCOPE. Carry it to your worktable with two hands. One hand should be on the arm, the other under the base. Always carry it upright, with stage level.

Written by the editors with Ed Perry, James H. Faulkner State Community College, Bay Minette, AL.

3. WITH MICROSCOPE IN FRONT OF YOU, RETURN TO FIGURE 1.

Find all of the parts labeled in the drawing on your instrument.

4. READ ALL OF THE EXPLANATIONS FOR THE LABELS FOLLOWING FIGURE 1.

What you fail to absorb will return to haunt you.

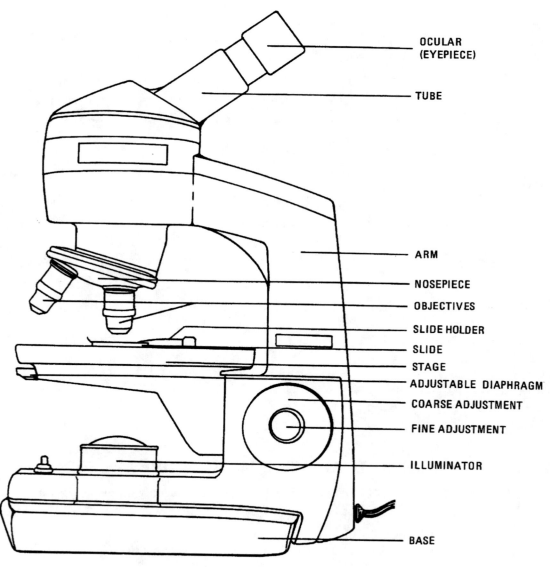

Figure 1. Typical student microscope.

Functions of Parts on the Microscope Drawing

OCULAR or EYEPIECE. The lens into which you look. It magnifies the image received from the objective lens below. Some oculars have an internal pointer that you can use when asking questions.

TUBE. Part of microscope body that holds ocular at the proper distance from other lenses.

HEAD. Not labeled on the diagram, it is the movable section that holds the tube. It can be rotated in its housing 180 degrees when needed.

SET SCREW. Not labeled on the diagram, it locks the head in place. It should always be snug when microscope is in use or stored.

ARM. Support for the head and ocular and also convenient handle for carrying. In some microscopes the arm contains cams and levers for moving the nosepiece.

NOSEPIECE. Rotating mounting for the objective lenses. It has detents so that you feel a click when lens is in place.

OBJECTIVES. These lenses are named for being next to the objects being viewed. Increase the length of lens to increase the magnification. They need to be cleaned frequently with lens tissue and lens cleaner, especially when used by students.

SLIDE HOLDER. These fixed and movable parts secure the slide on stage.

MECHANICAL STAGE. Includes slide holder. It has graduated markings to help relocate slide.

MECHANICAL STAGE CONTROLS. Not shown in Figure 1. Knob for moving slide around on stage. Knobs may be on the stage or beneath the stage on side at diaphragm level.

SLIDE. 1" x 3" piece of glass that supports specimen. Only transparent objects can be viewed.

STAGE. Flat surface on which slide is placed. Center hole allows light transmission through slide.

ADJUSTABLE DIAPHRAGM. A device for controlling light to slide. Some have a series of different sized holes; others have an iris.

COARSE ADJUSTMENT. The fast focusing knob. Used only with 4x and 10x objective

FINE ADJUSTMENT. The fine focusing control. Allows delicate adjustment. On some microscopes these controls raise or lower the stage. On others they move the barrel and nosepiece.

ILLUMINATOR. Sends light through the diaphragm. Switch may be on microscope itself or on the cord.

BASE. Supports the instrument. Usually weighted to add stability. Always use a two-handed carry.

5. DETERMINE THE MAGNIFICATION CAPABILITIES of your instrument.

    The total magnification is determined by multiplying the magnifying power of the eyepiece by the magnifying power of the objective in use.

    You will find the power, such as 4x or 10x, on the side of each lens. Your eyepiece is 10x.

Calculate the total magnification for the following objectives. You may not have four objective lenses on your microscope.

Objective	Power	Eyepiece	Total Magnification
Shortest (red)	_____	x 10 =	_____
(yellow)	_____	x 10 =	_____
(blue)	_____	x 10 =	_____
Longest (white)	_____	x 10 =	_____

PART B — USE THE MICROSCOPE WITH A SLIDE

Always make sure your microscope is clean. Clean the ocular, objectives, illuminator, diaphragm, and stage before you begin. Use only lens paper for this purpose.

1. OBTAIN A PREPARED SLIDE CONTAINING A LETTER "e". Make sure the slide is clean. Wipe carefully with tissue.

    Turn the nosepiece so that the lens marked 4x clicks in place over hole. ALWAYS START WITH THE SHORTEST OBJECTIVE.

    Place the slide on stage in holder. Adjust mechanical stage knobs to place the letter "e" over the center of hole.

    Adjust the diaphragm so that you see light on the letter "e".

    Adjust the focus while watching lens and slide from the side. If you have focusing stage, raise to highest point with coarse knob. If you have a focusing nosepiece, use the coarse knob to lower to the lowest point.

    Look through the eyepiece. You should see a uniform, circular field of light. This is called the field of view.

    If the light is dim or you just see a partial circle:

    > Check your illuminator. You may need a new bulb.

    > Check the alignment of the objective; make it click.

    > Practice aligning the pupil of your eye with the eyepiece.

    While looking through the eyepiece, turn the coarse knob to focus. A movable stage should move slowly down, away from the objective. A movable nosepiece should move slowly up, away from the stage. If you don't see anything, try centering the "e" better.

    Make the image appear more crisp with the fine focus.

2. PRACTICE MOVING THE SLIDE ON THE STAGE. Look through ocular at focused image and move the slide to the right.

What do you learn about direction of movement of the image?

Use several minutes to move the slide in all directions, enough so that your movements are smooth, controlled, and always in the direction you want.

3. COMPARE WORKING DISTANCES AND SIZES OF FIELDS OF VIEW. **Working distance** is the space between the objective and the slide. **Field of view** is the amount of the slide visible at one time.

Before you start examining slides with more powerful objectives, please study Figure 2 and answer the questions.

Why can you use coarse focus with the 4x and 10x objectives but not with the 40x or the oil immersion lens?

OBJECTIVE LENS MAGNIFICATION

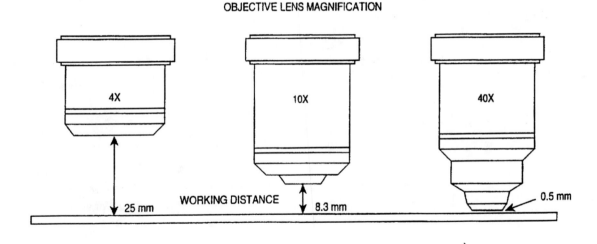

**RELATIVE DIAMETER OF FIELD
(ENLARGED)**

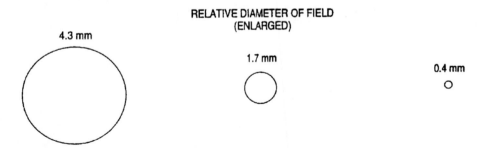

Figure 2. Working distances and fields of view.

All of the dry lenses on your nosepiece should be parfocal. That means that if one of them is in sharp focus, the others will be within one turn of the fine focus adjustment, when brought into place.

Why is it easier to find an object on the slide with the 4x objective than with the 10x, and easier with the 10x than the 40x?

Give two reasons why we insist that you always start with 4x.

4. EXPERIMENT WITH THE HIGHER POWERED OBJECTIVES. Exactly center the letter "e" in the field of view. If you do this poorly, you may not find the "e" in the next field of view.

Without changing the focus, turn nosepiece to bring 10x lens in place. Don't touch the slide either, or you will have to start again with 4x. Adjust the fine focus. If your microscope is not parfocal, tell your instructor.

What happened to your field of view?

Look at lens from the side. What happened to your working distance?

Center your letter "e" again. Make sure the center includes both light and dark areas. Edges and lines are easier to find and focus on than open space. Make sure it is precisely focused.

Again without changing focus, turn the nosepiece to bring 40x lens in place. Do not touch the slide. You will find it a very close fit. Adjust the focus. What happened to your field of view?

Move the slide so as to find the edge of printed image. Does the image move faster than with 10x?

What has happened to your working distance?

REMEMBER: Cover slips are fragile.

The mounting medium under the cover slip is permanently sticky.

The medium is difficult to remove from objective lenses.

Some of the permanent slides you will study cost many dollars each.

What is an economic reason for always starting with 4x?

RETURN THE LETTER "E" SLIDE TO ITS SOURCE.

PART C — MEASURING WITH A MICROSCOPE

1. FIND THE DIAMETER OF THE FIELD OF VIEW. Obtain a millimeter ruler. One made of thin flexible transparent plastic is ideal.

Make sure 4x objective is in place for viewing.

Place the edge of the rule across the center of the hole in stage.

Look through the eyepiece, adjust the focus and ruler placement. Estimate the diameter of the field of view on low power. Express answer in millimeters, to one decimal point.

Follow same procedure with the 10x objective. Express diameter of field in millimeters, to one decimal.

Compare your answers with the numbers given in Figure 2. Microscopes vary, but the proportions should be the same.

This procedure will not work with the 40x objective.

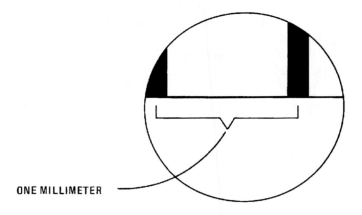

ONE MILLIMETER

Figure 3. Size of microscope field.

Calculate the field of view diameter of the 40x objective. You will need to make a few other calculations first.

The diameter of the field is inversely proportional to the magnification. That means, if the magnification goes up, the diameter goes down.

For example, the magnification of the 4x lens is .4 of that of the 10x lens. But the field of view of the 10x lens is .4 of that of the 4x lens. Check that statement by dividing your measurements into each other as appropriate. (Remember a little sixth grade arithmetic.)

If we use the numbers from Figure 2 we can divide 1.7 mm by 4.3 mm. The answer is .395. Considering that our measurements are not precise our answer is very close to .400.

The magnification of the 10x lens is 1/4 that of the 40x lens and the field of view of the 40x lens is 1/4 that of the 10x lens.

If the diameter of the field of view of the 10x lens is about 1.7 mm, what is the approximate diameter of the field of view of the 40x lens?

Express in millimeters.

Compare to the number given in Figure 2. Remember, we are not measuring precisely.

2. INTRODUCE YOURSELF TO A MICROMETER. Cytologists, people who study cells, and Histologists, people who study tissues, express measurements in terms of the micrometer. A micrometer is 1/1000 of a millimeter, or 1/1,000,000 of a meter.

    Express the field of view diameter of your lenses in micrometers.

    4x _____   10x _____   40x _____

    Try making estimates of sizes of things. Assume you were looking at an *Amoeba* with your 40x objective. By moving your slide around and using your imagination, you estimate that you could fit about eight of them into your field of view. Express the estimated length of one *Amoeba* in micrometers.

    Assume that your are looking at the alga *Spirogyra* with your 40x objective. This alga is colonial and forms long chains of cells. You count two and about a third of another cell in your field.

    Express the estimated length of one cell in micrometers.

PART D — DEPTH OF FIELD

Depth of field is the amount of vertical space on slide actually in focus at any given moment.
With microscope lenses, this vertical space is very small. It gets progressively smaller with increased magnification.

OBTAIN A PERMANENT SLIDE WITH CROSSED COLORED FIBERS. These slides may be coded so your instructor can tell the order in which the fibers are stacked.

Examine the slide. Begin with the 4x objective.

Move the slide so the crossing of the fibers is centered in your view.

Work the fine focus. Can you determine which fiber is on top?

Rotate nosepiece to bring 10x objective in place. Work the fine focus. Can you be more precise about the top fiber?

Rotate nosepiece to bring 40x objective in place. Be very careful. Colored fiber slides are often quite thick. Work the fine focus.

Which fiber is on top?

Which fiber is in the middle?

Which fiber is on the bottom?

Compare the depth of field of the three objectives.

RETURN THE CROSSED FIBER SLIDE TO ITS SOURCE.

PART E — ANOTHER LOOK AT MAGNIFICATION

You are now familiar with the figures for total magnification of your microscope.
You should know that these figures apply to a virtual image; that is, to an image in your mind.

When you look into your microscope, you see a nice round lighted field of view. Where is that field?

The eyepiece projects an image that is focused on your retina. Your brain interprets that image.

Keep both eyes open when looking into the microscope. After a while you will be able to superimpose both images in your head. The white field is at about the same level as the table top, or somewhere between it and the level of the stage.

Assume the field of view with the 10x objective is 1.7 mm. The total magnification, including the eyepiece, is 100x.

Draw a circle on white paper. Make the diameter 170 mm or 17 cm. Keep both eyes open, look into microscope again. Hold the paper along side the stage on the side of your free eye. How does the size of the circle compare with the size of the view in your head?

This may suggest other ways for you to measure objects under the microscope.

PART F — LOOK AT SOME OTHER OBJECTS

1. OBTAIN A BLANK MICROSCOPE SLIDE AND A COVER SLIP. Tear off a very small piece of notepaper from a piece of newspaper or notebook. You want at least one edge ragged, one edge smooth.

   Place the scrap of paper on the slide. Add a drop of water. The water will improve the image. Add the cover slip. Remove the excess water with paper towel. The cover slip will keep the paper flat so you can focus on the specimen (the scrap of paper).

   Examine with the 4x objective in place. The paper will be almost opaque. Only the edges will show detail.

   Examine with 10x objective. Again only the edges will hold interest.

   DO NOT TRY THE 40X. The slide is too thick, and has no biological information anyway. Clean and dry the slide. Deal with the cover slip as directed by your instructor.

   If you have time, make another slide with another type of paper, such as facial tissue.

2. PLACE A FEW SALT CRYSTALS IN THE CENTER OF A DRY SLIDE. Do not get the crystals wet. Try to keep them one layer thick.

   Hold slide level and place on stage in proper location.

   Crystals should show that they are illuminated.

   Examine with 4x and then with 10x. You may scratch the objective lenses if you try 40x. If you find them interesting, draw some pictures of what you see.

   Are the crystals uniform in size and shape? Describe their size and shape.

Exercise — The Microscope

NAME _____ DATE _____

1. _____ Another name for eyepiece is __.

2. _____ The movable part of the microscope on which objectives are mounted is the __.

3. _____ The total magnification of your microscope when the low power objective is locked in place is __.

4. _____ If you moved the slide with the letter "e" to the right and away from you, the image moved __.

5. _____ Whenever you examine a slide you always begin with the __ power lens.

6. _____ At what magnification do you see the largest area from your slide?

7. _____ Assume that your instructor gave you a 15x ocular that fit your microscope. What would be the total magnification if it were used with the third longest objective?

8. _____ The diameter of the field of view of your slide is approximately __ when the 40x objective is in use.

9. _____ If after a 10x lens is carefully focused, the 40x lens is swung into place and it is also in focus with only minor adjustments, the two lenses are considered __.

10. _____ Which objective should be in place when the microscope is put away for the day?

EXERCISE: The Metric System

OBJECTIVES

1. ... Students will be able to correctly convert from one unit to another within each of the three main measurements: length, volume, and mass.

2. ... Students will be able to accurately use a balance.

3. ... Students will be able to accurately measure liquids in the laboratory setting.

4. ... Students will be able to convert from Fahrenheit to Centigrade and vice versa.

5. ... Students will be able to change very large or very small numbers into scientific notation.

INTRODUCTION

The metric system is used as the standard form of measurement around the world. The reason it has gained such widespread popularity is that it is easy to use. The metric system is based on the number 10, and as you move between one metric unit to the next, all one has to do is move the decimals. For example, if you have 3.45 meters, that is equal to 345 centimeters or 3450 millimeters. On the other hand, if you have 3.45 yards, that is equal to 10.35 feet or 124.2 inches. In the case of the metric example, only the decimal was moved, while the original number stayed the same. While using American units one has to know and then convert the number of yards into the appropriate units.

Below are listed the basic metric units for length, volume, and mass. Notice that as you change units it is usually by an order of magnitude of 1000; the only exception below is the centimeter. Also, notice that the prefix of the units does not change from length to volume or mass. This is another way the metric system prevents confusion.

Length

1 Kilometer (km) = 1000 Meters (m)
1 m = 100 Centimeters (cm)
1 m = 1000 Millimeters (mm)
1 mm = 1000 Micrometers (μm)
1 μm = 1000 Nanometers (nm)

Volume

1 Liter (L) = 1000 Milliliters (ml)
1 ml = 1000 Microliter (μl)
1 μl = 1000 Nanoliters (nl)

Mass

1 Kilogram (kg) = 1000 Grams (g)
1 g = 1000 Milligrams (mg)
1 mg = 1000 Micrograms (μg)
1 μg = 1000 Nanograms (ng)

From *Reflections in Biology: A Laboratory Manual,* Third Edition, Volume 1, Greg Phillips and Eric Winkler. Copyright © 2006 by Pearson Education. Published by Pearson Custom Publishing. All rights reserved.

Conversion

When converting between American units and metric units one needs a conversion factor to efficiently make the shift between the two forms of measuring. Listed below are several conversion factors that will help you during the exercise.

2.54 cm = 1 inch	1 lb = 16 oz
29.57 mL = 1 Oz	3 ft = 1 yd
1 gram = .035 oz	8 oz = 1 cup
2 cups = 1 pint	2 pints = 1 quart

Below are a few problems to give you practice at converting from one unit to the next.

1. How many μl are in 2.45 liters? _____

2. How tall are you in cm? Measure to the nearest .1cm_____

    Convert the answer to meters. _____

    Convert the answer to inches. _____

3. Which is larger, 10 meters or 1,000,000 micrometers?

    _____

4. What is the width of the room in centimeters? _____

    Convert it to millimeters. _____

Doing a Balancing Act

Using a balance is another key skill in a science laboratory. Everything is weighed in metric units of mass, the basic unit being the gram. Weighing accurately is an acquired skill and takes a bit of practice. You will be taking measurements from a quadruple beam balance. It is called a quadruple beam balance because of the three main weighing crossbars. One weighs in 100 gram increments, the second in 10 gram increments, and the third in 1 gram increments. Sometimes there is a fourth bar which measures in 1/10 of gram increments. Observe the diagram on the following page. Can you determine the weight shown on the balance?

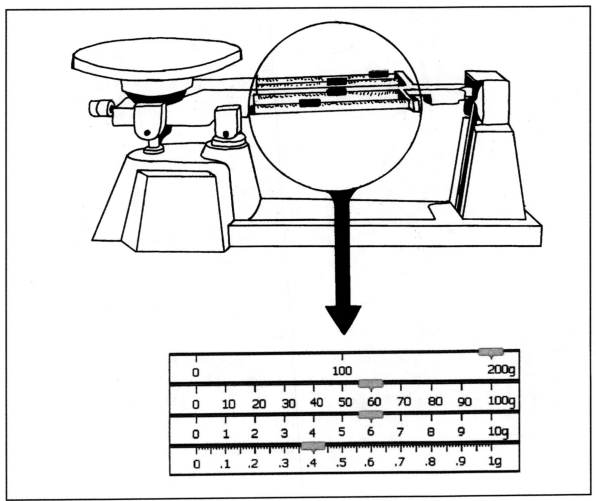

FIGURE 1: Diagram of Quadruple Beam Balance.
(Copyright © drawing of scale by Keith Neumann, drawing of metric measure by Shawn Albright)

Weight displayed on balance is _____.

The large weight is on 200 grams, the medium weight is on 60 grams, the small weight rests on 6 grams, and there is an additional .4 grams shown on the 4th beam. That means the substance weighs 266.4 grams.

Another important thing to remember about weighing items in the laboratory is to never place your substance directly onto the pan. Always place it in a weighing dish. This keeps your substance from contaminating the balance or becoming contaminated from other substances previously weighed. However, since you are using a weighing dish, you must **tare** the balance. Taring a scale means to rezero or account for the weight of your weighing dish. For example, if you want exactly 135.5 grams of a substance and you weigh it out precisely in a weighing dish but forgot to account for the weight of the dish you will be short some material.

To check your accuracy on the balance, do the following problems.

1. Get a candy bar and read the weight of the contents from the package. _____ Have one lab partner cut the bar in half, the other gets to choose which half is whose. *Caution* Do not place unwrapped food on weighing dish or balance pan. Weigh the candy while it is still in the wrapper. Weigh out the two sides of the candy bar _____ and _____. Who came out ahead? Combine the two weights _____. Did you get your money's worth? _____

2. Dr. Pepper gives you your cold medicine and warns you not to take too much, as the side effects could be hazardous. He reminds you to take only half a gram, no less and no more. However, when you get home and read the directions it says:

   Mr. D. Rink Pibb   Cold medication
                        Use caution when taking and follow
                        doctor's advice
                        Each spoonful contains 50 mg

   How many spoonfuls are you to take? _____

3. Read the nutritional facts table on the side of a can of soda. How many grams of sugar are in the can? _____

   Weigh out the amount of sugar found in that can:

   a. weight of weighing dish _____

   b. weight of dish + sugar _____

   c. Instructors initials _____

VOLUME

In a laboratory one also needs to know how to accurately measure volume. The basic metric unit of measurement is a liter. However, in a science laboratory one measures most often in milliliters. When measuring liquids, remember to read from the bottom of the **meniscus**.

You should be able to identify the basic pieces of glassware used to take these measurements. Identify in your laboratory the following pieces of glassware:

- Beaker
- Erlenmeyer Flask
- Graduated Cylinder
- Pipette

Neither the beaker nor the Erlenmeyer are extremely accurate. They are used when one doesn't have to be precise. Whereas the graduated cylinder and pipettes are used when it is necessary to be accurate.

Measure 100 ml's of H_2O in a beaker.

A. Pour it into an Erlenmeyer flask. Is it still accurate? _____

B. Pour it into a graduated cylinder. How many ml's were you off? _____

C. Why? _____

_____

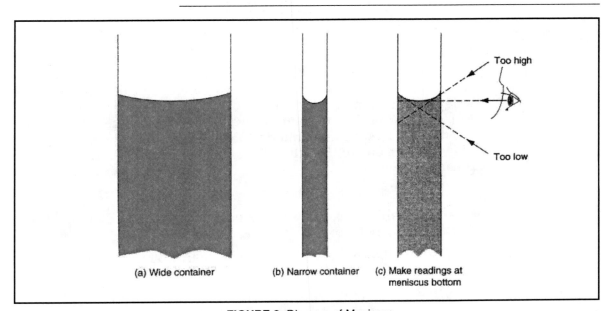

FIGURE 2: Diagram of Meniscus.
(From *Safety-scale Laboratory Experiments for General Organic and Biochemistry,* 3rd Edition,
by Spencer L. Seager and Michael R. Slabaugh, 1997, Brooks/Cole Publishing Company.)

PIPETS

There are many kinds and sizes of pipets. We will be using graduated pipets in this exercise. There are two kinds of graduated pipets: deliver by blow and deliver /by drain. ***Caution*** *Never use your mouth to draw liquids into or to blow out of a pipet. Always use a pipet pump.*

Procedure:

1. Obtain a small bottle of red food coloring, a 1.0 mL graduated pipet, a pipet pump, and a 10 mL graduated cylinder.

2. Following the technique described by your instructor use the pipet pump to obtain 0.8 mL of the red liquid and transfer it to the graduated cylinder.

3. Leave the liquid in the graduated cylinder and repeat Step 2, **four** more times.

4. What is the total volume of liquid in the graduated cylinder now?_____

5. Calculate how much liquid should be in the graduated cylinder if you moved 0.8 ml five times. _____

6. Are the calculated and actual amount volumes the same? _____

   If they are not, give an explanation as to why not. _____

   _____

TEMPERATURE

Another important measurement that is taken in a science laboratory is temperature. There are two different scales for taking temperature. Centigrade/Celsius which is based on the freezing (0°) and boiling (100°) points of water, and Fahrenheit which is most often used in the United States. Occasionally one needs to convert from one to the other. Below you will find the formulas to do so.

$$°C = (°F - 32) \times 5/9 \qquad °F = (°C) \times 9/5 + 32$$

It is important to take care of the parenthesis first, otherwise the formulas will not work.

Do the following exercise to check your ability to use a thermometer and the formulas.

What is the temperature of the following in degrees Celsius, then convert it to Fahrenheit:

	°C	°F
a. ice water	_____	_____
b. tap water	_____	_____
c. salted ice water	_____	_____
d. room temperature	_____	_____
e. body temperature	_____	_____

(hold the thermometer under your arm for two minutes)

SCIENTIFIC NOTATION

Scientific notation is a way of expressing extremely large or small numbers in a simplified manner so they can be more easily managed. As you convert these large or small numbers into scientific notation you must move the decimal to the right or left. When completed there should be only one number to the left of the decimal, and two numbers to the right of the decimal, drop all of the others. Multiply the number by 10^N where N = the number of places you moved the decimal. For example, if you have the number 9,765,432,810.64 which is difficult to repeat and use, it can be converted into scientific notation by moving the decimal place over 9 places to the left. The number then becomes 9.77×10^9. On the other hand, if you have an extremely small number like .000000721 scientific notation converts it into 7.21×10^{-7} by moving the decimal 7 places to the right. Notice the negative sign; the negative sign must be used if the number is small, and the decimal is moved to the right.

Practice on the following several problems by converting them into scientific notation or turning the numbers from scientific notation back into real numbers.

1. 822,375,163,987.63 _____

2. .0000000000787643 _____

3. 3.92×10^{-5} _____

4. 2.83×10^8 _____

REVIEW QUESTIONS

1. What is the temperature in °C if it is 54°F? _____

2. How many ounces are there in 12 liters? _____

3. Which is more accurate, a graduated or a volumetric pipette?

_____

4. How many cm are there in 15 feet? _____

5. You have just opened your new European cookbook and are ready to create an Epicurean delight, but the recipe says to set the oven at 192° centigrade. At what temperature should you set your oven (which reads in °F)? _____

6. How many micrograms are found in a half pound? _____

Population Genetics

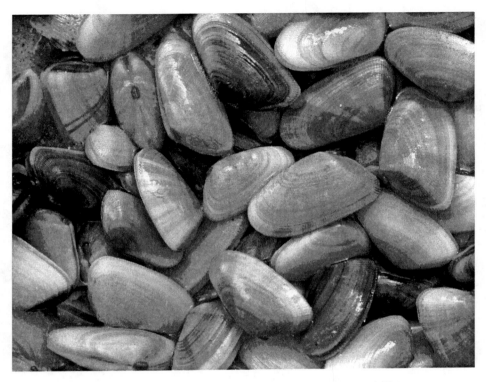

Figure 1 Genetic variation in the coquina clams, *Donax variabilis*.

INTRODUCTION

Coquina clams (Figure 1) live in dense populations on sandy beaches of the Atlantic and Gulf coasts of the United States. They occupy the active surf zone, constantly digging in against the action of the waves, filter feeding on **plankton**, and providing food for a variety of shore birds. As their scientific name *Donax variabilis* implies, these little bivalves exhibit noticeable variations in color and pattern among members of the same species found on the same beach. Ecologists call this a **polymorphic** population, because genetic differences among individuals create more than one common local phenotype. Although polymorphism often involves biochemical traits less easily observed than the colors of coquina shells, genetic variation among individuals is a widespread and ecologically relevant feature of natural populations of plants and animals.

Population genetics pioneer Ernst Mayr pointed to polymorphism as an essential, but frequently unappreciated source of difference between the life sciences and physical sciences (Lewin, 1982). The study of life, Mayr said, requires "**population** thinking," because life scientists always have to consider genetic variations among subjects of their research. While the chemist may assume one oxygen atom reacts in pretty much the same way as any other, biologists cannot assume all black bears exhibit similar feeding behavior, or that all Douglas fir trees respond identically to climate change. Genetic diversity is a driving force in populations, affecting all sorts of ecological processes from competition for resources to the formation of new species. Emerging theory in conservation ecology relies heavily on population genetics to develop effective strategies for protecting vanishing organisms (e.g., Loew, 2002). Ecologists are therefore wise to investigate how much genetic variation exists in the species they study, and how this variation is distributed within and among populations.

Genetics: A Brief Review

We will begin with a brief review of the basic principles of genetics. If you are confident that you understand and remember the concepts covered in the next two "Check your Progress" boxes, you may wish to skip to the next section on genetics and probability.

Every organism in every population carries a set of genetic instructions called its **genome**. In multicellular species, the genome is replicated in every cell, encoded by the DNA in each cell's nucleus. **Diploid** organisms have two sets of chromosomes, one set inherited from each parent. As a result, each gene is represented twice in the genome. We call the two chromosomes carrying copies of the same genes a **homologous pair**. Prior to reproduction, a specialized kind of cell division called meiosis divides the homologous chromosomes, sending them into separate **haploid** cells called **gametes** (Figure 2). Gametes are the sex cells, either sperm or eggs. Any given chromosome carries a predictable sequence of genetic instructions from one end of its DNA code to the other. For example, a particular gene for flower color would be found in a predictable place on a particular chromosome of a given plant species. That place is called the gene's **locus**. If you examined the corresponding locus on the other homologous chromosome, you would find the other copy of the flower color gene.

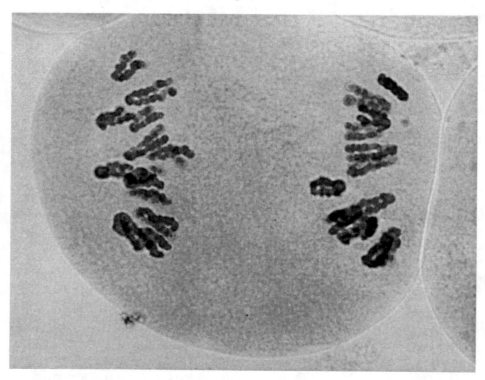

Figure 2   Homologous chromosomes separating during gamete formation in lily cells.

If a gene comes in more than one form, we say there are two **alleles** at this locus. For example, a gene for flower color in snapdragons can carry instructions to make a red pigment or a white pigment (Figure 3). Let's use the symbol C^R to represent the red allele and the symbol C^W to represent the white allele. The genes a plant carries for this trait are called its **genotype**; the actual flower color we see when we look at the plant is its **phenotype**. Snapdragon plants with two copies of the same allele for red pigment, designated as genotype $C^R C^R$, have red flowers as their phenotype. Snapdragon plants with two copies of the allele for white pigment, designated as genotype $C^W C^W$, have white flowers as their phenotype. Whether red or white, any snapdragon having two copies of the same allele is said to be **homozygous**. If the snapdragon inherits one allele from its male parent and a different allele from its female parent, the plant is said to be **heterozygous**. These plants have the genotype $C^R C^W$ and their phenotype is pink—intermediate between red and white.

The phenotype of a heterozygote is not always intermediate between the homozygous types. For many genetic traits, the instructions on a **dominant allele** override the instructions on a **recessive allele** so that the heterozygous phenotype looks just like the homozygous dominant. The recessive allele is still present in the genome, and is inherited by half the offspring, but its presence is "masked" or hidden in heterozygous individuals. Note that dominant genes are *not* necessarily better or more prevalent than recessive genes. Dominance refers *only* to the way one allele overrides the other in determining the phenotype in the heterozygous condition.

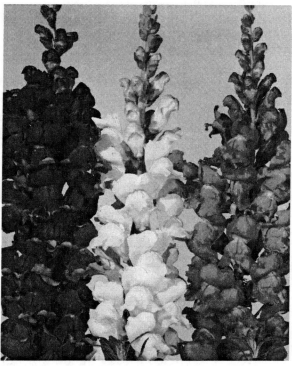

Figure 3   Snapdragons.

Within a population, there can be more than two alleles for the same gene. For example, for the **ABO blood groups** in the human genome, there are three alleles: I^A, I^B, and i. All three of these alleles can be found in a typical human population, but any individual in the population can have a maximum of two—one on each homologous chromosome. Individuals having the homozygous $I^A I^A$ genotype produce a molecule on the surface of the red blood cells called the A **antigen**. Their phenotype is "type A blood." (See Table 1.) Individuals with the $I^B I^B$ genotype produce a type B antigen on their blood cells, so their phenotype is "type B blood." Homozygous i i individuals have neither type A antigens nor type B antigens, so their phenotype is called "type O blood." The i allele is recessive to both of the others, so the I^A i genotype produces type A antigens, resulting in type A blood. The recessive i allele is still present on the chromosome, and can be inherited by offspring, but is masked by its dominant counterpart. Similarly, the I^B i genotype results in type B blood. The I^A and I^B alleles express no dominance over one another, so persons with the genotype $I^A I^B$ produce both kinds of antigens, and their phenotype is "type AB."

Table 1

GENOTYPES	PHENOTYPES
$I^A I^A$ or I^A i	Type A blood
$I^B I^B$ or I^B i	Type B blood
$I^A I^B$	Type AB blood
i i	Type O blood

Check your progress:

Make sure you can explain the difference between the following pairs of terms:

1. Genome and chromosome
2. Haploid and diploid
3. Locus and allele
4. Genotype and phenotype
5. Homozygous and heterozygous
6. Dominant and recessive
7. ABO blood groups and Rh factor

Hint: Consult the glossary if terms are not clear.

You may have heard the words "positive" and "negative" along with A, B, and O in reference to blood types. These descriptors refer to a totally different trait that was first found in rhesus monkeys, appropriately named "**Rh factor.**" Since the human genome and the genomes of other primates contain many DNA sequences in common, it is not surprising that the Rh gene was later discovered in humans as well. The Rh locus has two alleles, (+) and (−). This is where the "positive" and "negative" terms come from. Rh factor is important for matching blood types, but its inheritance is independent of the ABO system.

The preceding generalizations about chromosomal pairs are true of 22 of the 23 pairs of human chromosomes, but there is one exception. Human **sex chromosomes** come in two types: X and Y. Females have two X chromosomes, while males have an X and a Y. The **X chromosome** is quite large, and contains lots of information, some of which is essential for normal growth and development. The **Y chromosome** is much smaller, and carries few genetic instructions. Even though it is small, the Y chromosome is important for male development, because one of its genes triggers hormonal changes resulting in a male child. Thus, XY babies develop as males; XX babies develop as females.

Because the X chromosome contains many genes, we need a system for tracking the inheritance of these characters, which are called **sex-linked traits**. We can indicate a gene on the X chromosome with a superscript. The most common form of **color blindness**, for example, is caused by a recessive gene that resides on the X chromosome. X^B symbolizes an X chromosome carrying the dominant allele for normal color vision, and X^b represents an X chromosome carrying the recessive allele for color blindness. Since females have two X chromosomes, a woman can be homozygous for either trait, or heterozygous (having genotype $X^B X^b$). Since the allele for color blindness is recessive, heterozygous females have full color vision. Males, however, have only one X chromosome, so they are either color-blind (genotype $X^b Y$), or not color-blind (genotype $X^B Y$). Note that no superscript is attached to the Y chromosome, since it carries no genetic information about color vision.

Check your progress:

If a man is color-blind, which of his parents passed the allele for color blindness to him?

Hint: Men inherit their Y chromosome from their fathers.

The familiar fruit fly, **Drosophila melanogaster,** is a useful model for the study of sex-linked traits, because it also has the XX chromosomal arrangement in females and an XY arrangement in males. Although the developmental mechanism for sex determination in fruit flies is not the same as for humans, inheritance of sex chromosomes and sex-linked traits works in a similar fashion. In fruit flies, a gene for eye color resides on the X chromosome. Most fruit flies have the dominant allele for red eyes, but the recessive allele at this locus produces white eyes. The following table shows all possible genotypes and phenotypes with regard to the white or red eye color gene.

Table 2

DROSOPHILA GENOTYPES	*DROSOPHILA* PHENOTYPES
$X^B X^B$ or $X^B X^b$	Red-eyed Female
$X^b X^b$	White-eyed Female
$X^B Y$	Red-eyed Male
$X^b Y$	White-eyed Male

Genetics and Probability

Genetic inheritance is a **stochastic** process. This means that some of the mechanisms controlling the inheritance of genes follow predictable laws, but others operate in a random fashion. **Random events** cannot be predicted in individual cases, but if we look at a large group of random events, we can make reliable observations about outcomes for the group as a whole. For example, the gender of a baby is unpredictable before conception. If a family has one baby girl, and the mother becomes pregnant with a second child, no one can say in advance whether to expect a baby sister or a baby brother. Determination of sex in each child is an independent random event with the probability of having a girl roughly equal to $\frac{1}{2}$, and the probability of a boy $\frac{1}{2}$. (The ratio is actually more like 1.06 boys for every girl at birth, but we will adopt $\frac{1}{2}$ as a reasonable approximation for this example.)

Even though gender outcome is unpredictable for individual pregnancies, the process becomes predictable at the population level. If you checked records for the past 1000 births at your local hospital, you could predict with some confidence 50% girls and 50% boys, or 500 of each sex in the sample of 1000. An outcome of 495 to 505 would not be surprising, but the prediction holds true within limits determined by sample size. If you expanded your study to include the past 100,000 babies born in your state or province, the predicted 50:50 ratio would be even more accurate. This is an important scientific principle misunderstood by most people: *random events are subject to natural laws, and can be predicted in the aggregate.* To the scientist, the word "random" does *not* mean "without cause." It refers instead to events that are more easily predicted at the level of the population than at the level of the individual.

Check your progress:

When 1 kg of 50° water is mixed with 1 kg of 40° water, we can accurately predict the resulting mixture will have a temperature of 45°. Water temperature is defined as the average kinetic energy of the H_2O molecules. Since individual water molecules move at random, we cannot say what the kinetic energy of any individual molecule will be at a given time. How can we know the outcome of a series of random events with such certainty?

Hint: Consider the sample size.

Population ecologists have found a few simple probability laws quite powerful in explaining inheritance at the population level. To introduce these useful principles, let's begin with some symbols and terms.

Let (A) represent an event that may or may not happen. The symbol f(A) stands for the frequency of A's occurrence from past experience. We can also use f(A) to represent the probability that A will occur under the same set of conditions in the future. We can use a number between 0 and 1 to represent the range of all possible frequencies of occurrence, from f(A) = 0 if the event is impossible, to f(A) = 1 if the event is absolutely certain. Between these end points, we can designate probabilities much more accurately with fractions between 0 and 1 than we could using English phrases such as "possibly," "maybe," or "in most cases."

Check your progress:

Match each numerical probability with a verbal description by writing in a phrase from the following list: "Always," "Half the time," "Never," "Rarely," "Pretty often," "Usually."

f(A) = 0 _____*never*_____   f(A) = 0.5 _____*pretty often*_____

f(A) = 0.01 _____*rarely*_____   f(A) = 0.9 _____*usually*_____

f(A) = 0.3 _____*half*_____   f(A) = 1.0 _____*always*_____

Hint: A higher number means greater likelihood.

In our example of the sex of a baby, two outcomes are possible. To examine this in probability terms, f(female) = frequency of female births, and f(male) = frequency of male births. Since we define no third outcome, the frequencies must sum to one. Assuming equal likelihoods for girls and boys,

$$f(male) = 0.5, \qquad f(female) = 0.5, \text{ and} \qquad f(male) + f(female) = 1.0$$

What if we wanted to describe more than one characteristic of these children? Handedness, here defined as the hand we choose to write with, is influenced by culture and training, but has innate biological causes as well. Right-handedness occurs in about 90% of the North American population. We may therefore designate f(right-handed) = 0.9 and f(left-handed) = 0.1, assuming for the purpose of this exercise that ambidextrous people will favor one hand or the other for writing. To calculate the likelihood that a randomly selected child will be female *and* left-handed, we can simply multiply the probability fractions together:

$$f(female) = 0.5$$

$$f(left\text{-}handed) = 0.1$$

Thus, $\quad f(female \textit{ and } left\text{-}handed) = (0.5)(0.1) = 0.05$

This means that we could expect 5% of the population to be made up of left-handed females. It is important to note that this demonstration assumes left-handedness is equally common among females and males. If this is true, we could say determination of gender and of handedness are **independent events**. If this were not the case, we would have to change the handedness probability to the frequency of left-handedness *given that the child is female.*

The product rule makes intuitive sense if you remember that frequencies (or probabilities) are expressed as fractions. The probability of two uncertain events happening at the same time has to be smaller than the probability of either event by itself. Since the product of fractions is always a smaller fraction, multiplying probabilities gives us the smaller probability of a joint occurrence.

PRODUCT RULE: (Calculating joint occurrence of two independent events)

$$f(A \text{ } and \text{ } B) = f(A) * f(B)$$

f(A and B) = frequency of both events happening together
f(A) = frequency of event A
f(B) = frequency of event B

Check your progress:

Apply the product rule to predict the frequency of right-handed male babies.

Answer: f(male and right-handed) = 0.45

Often in biology, outcomes are grouped so that we need to know how often either of two events occurs. For our example, we could ask how often would a randomly selected child be *either* female *or* right-handed? Since this pooled frequency will be larger than the frequency of either females or right-handed children considered separately, it makes sense to add the frequencies together. However, simple addition would overestimate the frequency of children either female or right-handed. Adding f(female) + f(right-handed) would yield a frequency of 0.5 + 0.9 = 1.4, which would amount to 140% of the entire population!

Figure 4 shows how we obtained a fraction over 100%. The rectangle shaded with vertical stripes represents the frequency of right-handed children in the population, and the rectangle shaded with horizontal stripes represents the frequency of girls. By adding the frequency of all girls to the frequency of all right-handed children, we counted right-handed girls twice. (The overcounted individuals are represented by the cross-hatched area in the figure.) To calculate the area covered by the two rectangles without double-counting right-handed girls, we could add the areas of the two rectangles, and then subtract the area of overlap. By analogy, the frequency of children either female or right-handed would be calculated as follows:

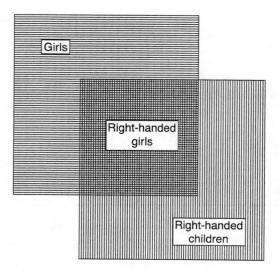

Figure 4   Adding frequencies of all right-handed children and of all girls in a population results in double-counting all the right-handed girls, who fit into both groups.

f(female *or* right-handed) = f(female) + f(right-handed) – f(female *and* right-handed)

Since we have already calculated f(female and right-handed) to be (0.5 * 0.9), the equation can be solved as follows:

f(female *or* right-handed) = 0.5 + 0.9 – (0.5 * 0.9) = 0.95 of all children.

This method for finding either/or probabilities is called the sum rule. Stated generally:

SUM RULE: (Calculating the frequency of either event A or event B)

f(A *or* B) = f(A) + f(B) – f(A *and* B)

      f(A *or* B) = frequency of either one event or the other
      f(A) = frequency of event A
      f(B) = frequency of event B
      f(A *and* B) = frequency of both events happening together
         This last term can be dropped if the two events never occur together.

Check your progress:

Apply the sum rule to find the expected frequency of children who are either male or left-handed.

Answer: f(male *or* left-handed) = 0.55

It is worth noting that if the two events never occur at the same time, the third term in the sum rule equation is equal to zero and can be dropped. For example, f(male *or* female) = f(male) + f(female) = 0.5 + 0.5 = 1. Since children are not both male and female, there is no "overlap" to subtract in this case. In this situation, we say the two events are **mutually exclusive**, because the occurrence of one excludes the possibility of the other.

Always remember to use the product rule to find f(A and B), and use the sum rule to find f(A or B).

Population Genetics

Predicting distributions of genes in populations can be accomplished with a straightforward application of the two probability rules. You have already done this kind of calculation in introductory biology if you have used a Punnett square to generate frequencies in a genetics cross. For a cross of two pea plants heterozygous for plant height, where T is the dominant allele for tall plant size, and t the recessive allele for dwarf size:

	T f(T eggs) = 0.5	**t** f(t eggs) = 0.5
T f(T pollen) = 0.5	**TT** f(TT offspring) = (0.5)(0.5) = 0.25	**Tt** f(Tt offspring) = (0.5)(0.5) = 0.25
t f(t pollen) = 0.5	**Tt** f(Tt offspring) = (0.5)(0.5) = 0.25	**tt** f(tt offspring) = (0.5)(0.5) = 0.25

Because a heterozygous plant produces dominant (T) and recessive (t) pollen in equal proportions in its stamens, f(T pollen) = 0.5 and f(t pollen) = 0.5, as seen on the left side of the Punnett square. Similarly, since the other parent produces eggs in equal proportions in its ovaries, f(T eggs) = 0.5 and f(t eggs) = 0.5, as seen across the top of the square. Inside the Punnett square are expected offspring frequencies. To calculate the probability of a dwarf plant, for example, we first acknowledge that an offspring must inherit the t allele from both its male parent and its female parent. Since two events must co-occur to make a dwarf offspring, we apply the product rule as follows:

Check your progress:

Consider a genetic cross between a man with type B blood (genotype I^B i) and a woman with type A blood (genotype I^A i). Use the probability rules to calculate the expected frequency of female offspring with type O blood from this type of cross.

Answer: f(female *and* ii) = 1/8

$$f(tt \text{ offspring}) = f(t \text{ pollen}) * f(t \text{ egg}) = (0.5)(0.5) = 0.25$$

The equation predicts that 1/4 of the offspring are expected to exhibit the recessive phenotype in a cross between two heterozygous parents. The frequency of **TT** homozygous tall offspring can be calculated in the same way:

$$f(TT \text{ offspring}) = f(T \text{ pollen}) * f(T \text{ egg}) = (0.5)(0.5) = 0.25$$

To calculate the frequency of heterozygotes, we can use the sum rule:

$$f(Tt \text{ offspring}) = f(T \text{ pollen meets } t \text{ egg}) + f(t \text{ pollen meets } T \text{ egg}) = (0.25) + (0.25) = 0.5$$

Note that the two ways to make a heterozygous offspring are mutually exclusive, so we do not have to worry about subtracting a third term in this case.

In summary, we use the probability rules every time we calculate frequencies for a genetic cross. Think of a Punnett square as a graphic representation of the probability rules, applied to inheritance in one "nuclear family" of two parents and their immediate offspring. Having mastered that analysis, you are ready to calculate expected genotypic frequencies for the whole population.

The Hardy-Weinberg Rule

To illustrate the Hardy-Weinberg calculation in a natural population, let's return to our polymorphic population of coquina clams (Figure 1). Coquinas reproduce by releasing eggs and sperm into the sea. Fertilization occurs when sperm meet eggs, and the resulting larvae drift with the currents before settling down on a beach to lead their adult lives. Because mating in coquinas is a random event, probability rules can be realistically applied to predict the genetic structure of its populations.

Assume for the sake of illustration that a dominant allele R produces purple rays (radiating stripes) on the coquina's shell. We will assume that rr genotypes are solid white clams with no purple rays. If the **gene pool**, defined as all the genes in all the members of a population, contains 70% R alleles and 30% r alleles, we would say that the **gene frequencies** are f(R) = 0.7 and f(r) = 0.3 in this population. Given this information, we could use the probability laws to predict the proportions of RR, Rr, and rr genotypes. These proportions, called **genotypic frequencies**, determine the ratio of shell phenotypes we could actually observe if we dug up a bucket of coquinas from the sand.

Imagine our population of coquinas releasing their eggs and sperm into the ocean, where they combine at random to produce the next generation. Frequencies of offspring genotypes can be predicted using the product rule. The following table illustrates frequencies of eggs and sperm cells as column and row headings, and probabilities for offspring genotypes in the cells. The resulting diagram resembles a Punnett square, but notice that the frequencies of R and r gametes are unequal in this case. To generalize this model, let p = f(R) and q = f(r). As long as there are only two alleles, p + q = 1.0 because the gene frequencies must add up to 100%.

	f(R eggs) p = 0.7	f(r eggs) q = 0.3
f(R sperm) p = 0.7	f(RR offspring) $p^2 = (0.7)(0.7) = 0.49$	f(Rr offspring) $pq = (0.7)(0.3)$ $= 0.21$
f(r sperm) q = 0.3	f(Rr offspring) $pq = (0.7)(0.3) = 0.21$	f(rr offspring) $q^2 = (0.3)(0.3)$ $= 0.09$

Following the rules of probability,

$$f(\text{RR offspring}) = f(\text{R sperm meets R egg}) = p^2 = (0.7)(0.7) = 0.49$$
$$f(\text{Rr offspring}) = f(\text{R sperm meets r egg}) + f(\text{r sperm meets R egg}) = 2pq = 2(0.7)(0.3) = 0.42$$
$$f(\text{rr offspring}) = f(\text{r sperm meets R egg}) = q^2 = (0.3)(0.3) = \underline{0.09}$$
$$\text{Total} = p^2 + 2pq + q^2 = 1.00$$

THE HARDY-WEINBERG CALCULATION

To determine genotypic frequencies from frequencies of alleles R and r:

$$f(RR) = p^2 \qquad f(Rr) = 2pq \qquad f(rr) = q^2$$

To sum genotypic frequencies in the population:

$$p^2 + 2pq + q^2 = 1.0 \qquad \text{where: } p = f(\text{R allele})$$
$$q = f(\text{r allele})$$

This set of equations is known as the Hardy-Weinberg law, named after a mathematician and a biologist who both came up with the same idea in 1908. Apparently, great minds do sometimes think alike!

Check your progress:

If p = f(R) = 0.6, and q = f(r) = 0.4, what proportion of the population would you expect to be heterozygous under Hardy-Weinberg rules?

Answer: 2 pq = 0.48

Genetic Equilibrium

For our coquina clam population having 70% R alleles and 30% r alleles, the Hardy-Weinberg equations predict that a collection of 1000 coquinas from the surf will be made up of 490 coquinas homozygous for purple rays, 420 heterozygous coquinas, and 90 plain white coquinas with the rr genotype.

Since we have generated these genotypic frequencies from the gene pool of gametes in the ocean, have the gene frequencies changed as a result of reproduction? No, they have not. When coquinas reproduce again, for every 1000 individuals, all of the gametes coming from the 490 RR clams and half of the gametes coming from the 420 heterozygous Rr clams will carry the R allele. Similarly, all of the gametes from the 90 rr clams and half of the gametes from 420 Rr clams will carry the r allele. If we divide observed numbers of clams by 1000 to convert these expected numbers of clams to genotypic frequencies f(RR) = 0.49, f(Rr) = 0.42, and f(rr) = 0.09, we can generate the next gamete pool as follows.

To calculate genotypic frequencies from gene frequencies

$$p = f(RR) + 1/2\ f(Rr) = 0.49 + 0.5\ (0.42) = 0.7$$

Similarly,

$$q = f(rr) + 1/2\ f(Rr) = 0.09 + 0.5(0.42) = 0.3$$

Note that the gene frequencies remain *exactly where they were at the beginning of our calculation*: at 70% R and 30% r allelic frequencies. This is why we say the genes are in equilibrium. In each generation, the two alleles are separated by meiosis, and recombine according to the rules of probability, but neither (R) nor (r) changes its proportional representation in the gene pool.

Check your progress:

In a population of 1000 coquinas, if 360 are RR, 480 are Rr, and 160 are rr, what are the gene frequencies of R and r?

Answer: f(R) = 0.6 and f(r) = 0.4

Violating Hardy-Weinberg Equilibrium

The Hardy-Weinberg formula is what ecologists call a **neutral model**. It shows what to expect if no biological forces are changing gene frequencies in the population. In nature, gene frequencies are not always held in equilibrium. **Evolution**, defined as changes in a population's genetic makeup over time, happens constantly and has been demonstrated across a full range of biological species from bacteria to humans. To understand the origins of evolutionary change, we need to consider the following biological factors that can push gene frequencies out of Hardy-Weinberg equilibrium.

1. **Small population size:** Just as the sex ratio of newborn babies can depart from an expected 50:50 ratio in a small group of children, genotypic frequencies can depart from the expected proportions of p^2, $2pq$, and q^2 in a small population. Remember that genetic inheritance is a random process that becomes less predictable as the number of events decreases. A population reduced to a "bottleneck" of a few survivors can experience significant genetic change due to the small sample size represented in its gamete pool. The longer the population stays very small, the more significant are potential shifts in gene frequencies. Change of this type is called **genetic drift** because frequencies go up or down at random. If one allele or the other ever drifts to a frequency of 100%, we say the allele is **fixed** in the population. The other allele cannot drift back up from a frequency of 0, after it has been pushed to extinction. This is why very small populations tend to lose genetic variation over time.

2. **Non-random mating:** Coquina gametes combine at random in the sea, but many organisms are more selective in their choice of mates. For example, chemical reactions in the female tissues of many flowers block the passage of pollen too similar in genetic composition to the female parent. This promotes outcrossing to unrelated pollen donors, and also results in more heterozygosity than would be expected under the Hardy-Weinberg rule. On the other hand, some bird species tend to select mates that look like themselves. This kind of **"assortative mating"** reduces heterozygosity below Hardy-Weinberg expectations, because (AA) and (aa) genotypes do not mate with one another to produce (Aa) offspring as often as predicted.

3. **Immigration or emigration:** Imagine a coquina population that is primarily of the (rr) genotype. If (RR) larvae are brought in by ocean currents from another population down the coast, then the frequency of the R allele will increase, and more purple-rayed shells will appear than we would have predicted based on the genotypes of adult clams on the beach. Emigration (or outward migration) can also affect some animal species if one genotype tends to migrate out of the population with greater frequency than another. Movement of genes via gametes, juveniles, or breeding adults is called **gene flow**, and these movements have a large potential influence on genotypic frequencies.

4. **Mutation:** Although mutation is a rare and usually deleterious event, it is important to realize that all new alleles arise by mutation from a pre-existing gene. Mutation makes a small initial impact on gene frequencies, but in conjunction with other factors, mutation can be the beginning of significant genetic changes in the population.

5. **Natural Selection:** Many shore birds feed on coquinas. What would happen if the purple-rayed coquina shells were a little harder for predatory birds to see in the surf than the pure white shells? In this case, we would say the **fitness** of the white coquinas is smaller than the fitness of the purple-rayed shells. If white shells are taken by birds at a disproportionately high rate, then we would expect a shift in gene frequencies away from Hardy-Weinberg equilibrium as clams producing (r) gametes declined, and the proportional representation of (R) gametes increased. Depending on the environment and the adaptive advantage of one genotype over another, natural selection can exert measurable effects on the gene pool. Whether selection occurs among sperm competing to reach the eggs, among juveniles competing to survive, or among adults competing to produce more offspring, any advantage of one allelic type over another will alter the genetic balance that Hardy and Weinberg described.

In summary, a population is expected to remain in Hardy-Weinberg equilibrium only if there is no natural selection, no mutation, no immigration or emigration, and only as long as mating is random and population size is very large.

Check your progress:

If RR and rr genotypes are more common in a large coquina population, and Rr genotypes are less common than we would expect under Hardy-Weinberg equilibrium, what biological causes could explain this observation?

Hint: You can rule out mutation, non-random mating, and selection.

METHOD A: POPULATION GENETICS SIMULATION
[Laboratory activity]

Research Question
How do population size and natural selection influence gene frequencies?

Preparation
In a craft store, find beads of two colors having holes large enough to slip over a toothpick. For convenience, styrofoam blocks can serve as toothpick holders.

Materials (per laboratory team)
Calculator

1500-ml beaker

100 light-colored beads

100 dark-colored beads

10 toothpicks

Procedure 1: Modeling Genetic Drift
1. Select 10 toothpicks to represent a population of 10 animals.
2. Place 50 dark-colored beads and 50 light-colored beads into a beaker. These represent genes in a gamete pool with allelic frequencies 0.5 A and 0.5 a. Stir up the beads to ensure random genetic recombination.
3. Calculate expected frequencies of AA, Aa, and aa individuals, based on Hardy-Weinberg expectations. Multiply these expected frequencies by 10 and round off to the nearest whole numbers to calculate how many AA, Aa, and aa individuals to expect in your population.
4. Without looking at the beaker, draw out two beads and slip them onto a toothpick. If you draw two dark beads, this animal has genotype AA. Two light beads means aa. One of each means Aa. Repeat this process, placing two beads on each of the 10 toothpicks. How do your actual genotypic frequencies compare to the expected frequencies calculated in step 3? Can you explain the reason for any discrepancies?

5. Calculate gene frequencies in your population by counting "genes" in your population of 10 animals: p = f(A) = (# dark beads)/20, and q = f(a) = (# light beads)/20. Record your result for p and q on the calculation page.
6. Take all of the beads off your 10 toothpicks, and generate a new gamete pool by changing the ratio of light and dark beads in the beaker to match the p and q values you calculated in step 5. Keep the size of the gamete pool constant at 100 beads, but take out or put in beads to create the correct proportions. For example, if your population has values p = 0.55 and q = 0.45, you would fill the beaker with 55 dark-colored beads and 45 light-colored beads. Since you started with 50 of each, return all beads to the beaker, then take out five light-colored beads and replace them with 10 dark-colored ones to make a new p = 55/100 and q = 45/100.
7. Repeat steps 4 through 6 a total of 10 times to simulate 10 generations of genetic drift. Record p and q values on the calculation page each time you recalculate them. Since departures from original gene frequencies are random, you cannot predict which way genetic drift will take your small population. If p becomes 1.00, we say that the A gene has gone to fixation and the a gene to extinction. Fixation of the a gene could also happen.
8. Plot changes in p on the graph at the end of this section. The first point, showing p = 0.5, is already entered on the graph. Draw similar points for p in each generation, and connect the points with a line to show how p changes over time due to genetic drift. Then compare your results with those of other lab groups. Do you find different results in different groups?

Table of Genetic Drift Results (Method A, Procedure 1)

Generation number	Observed f(RR)	Observed f(Rr)	Observed f(rr)	p value = (# dark beads) (total # beads)	q value = 1 – p
				0.50	0.50
1	4	3	3	.55	.45
2	3	6	1	.60	.40
3					
4					
5					
6					
7					
8					
9		3			
10					

(handwritten margin notes)
12/20
4/20
Wild – dominant
silver – recessive
14/20 = .7
12/20
18 silver
22 gold

Graph of Genetic Drift Results

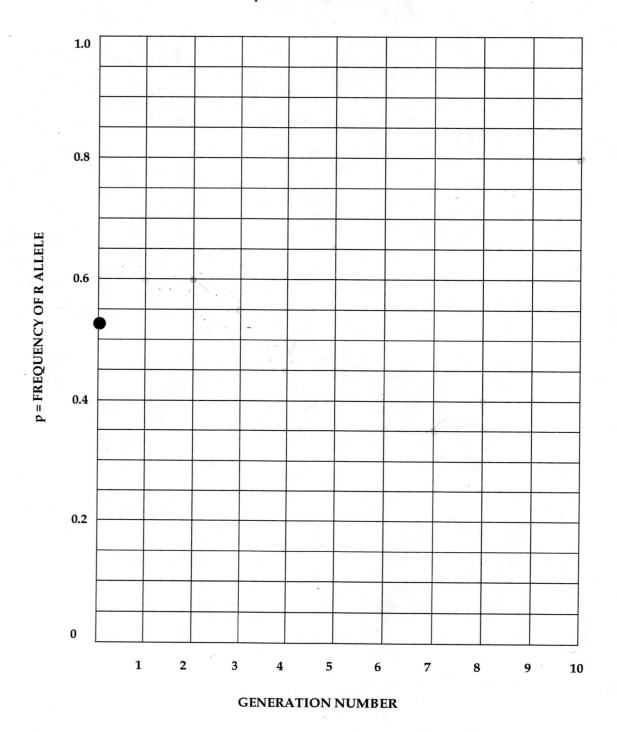

GENERATION NUMBER

Questions (Method A, Procedure 1)

on exam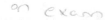

1. In horses, the genes for white coat color and red coat color are codominant. Heterozygotes have a light red coloration, called roan. If you located a population of wild mustangs in a valley that had 476 red horses, 323 roan horses, and 51 white horses, could you say the population is in Hardy-Weinberg equilibrium? First calculate p and q, then use the Hardy-Weinberg formula to calculate expected genotypic frequencies.

$$R \rightarrow \frac{952 + 323}{1700} = .75 \qquad p = .75$$

RR   476 red
Rr   323 roan $850 \times 2 = 1700$ compare
rr   51 white   alleles

$\frac{102 + 323}{1700} = .25$

$p^2 = .5625 \times 850 = .478 \mid 476$
$2pq = .37.5 \times 850 = 318 \mid 323$
$q^2 = 6.25 \times 850 = 53 \mid 51$

2. If we look at Rh factor genes in the United States, the dominant Rh⁺ allele makes up about 60% of the gene pool and the recessive Rh⁻ allele makes up 40%. If the U.S. population were in Hardy-Weinberg equilibrium, what portion of people in the country would you expect to have Rh positive blood? What factors might result in departures from expected frequencies in this example?

$p = .6$ $p^2 = .36$ domin
$q = .4$ $2pq = .48$ domin
                      $q^2 = .16$ recessive

$\begin{array}{r} .36 \\ + .48 \\ \hline .84 \end{array} = 84\%$

3. Based on this exercise, can you explain why zoos go to so much trouble to exchange rare animals such as tigers or gorillas rather than maintaining small separate breeding populations?

They went to expand the gene pool.
Small populations can lose an allele
Avoid genetic drift

4. In a classic study of blood types in Italy, Dr. Luigi Cavalli-Sforza (1969) found that small, isolated towns in mountain regions had reduced genetic diversity within populations, but showed significant genetic differences from one town to the next. In valley regions with more movement of people from place to place, he found more diversity within the population of any given town, and fewer differences between towns. If you consider your genetic simulation to represent one mountain town, and other lab groups to represent different mountain towns, can you explain Cavalli-Sforza's results? How could you alter this lab procedure to simulate what happens in the valley towns?

In a isolated town, you lose alleles. In between the towns there is alot more gene poll population for new genetic mederrals.

5. Gene frequencies for the ABO alleles vary geographically. For example the I^A allele makes up nearly 50% of the genes for blood type among Australian Aborigines, about 25% in Central Asian populations, and 0% in peoples native to South America. No blood type has sufficient selective advantage over another to explain these regional differences. From these facts, what can you infer about the history of our species? Did humanity develop as a large and continuous population spreading out across the planet, or did we disperse while still living in small scattered groups?

Small scattered groups are different. If humanity developed as large & continuous population we would expect the same genes.

Procedure 2: Modeling Selection

In this simulation, we will assume that a is a recessive lethal gene. It causes no harm in heterozygotes, but is fatal to aa individuals. Rather than a random change in gene frequency, here we will see how natural selection against one allele can make a directional change in gene frequencies.

1. Select 10 toothpicks to represent a population of 10 animals as you did in the first simulation.
2. Begin the simulation, as you did in Procedure 1, with 50 dark-colored beads and 50 light-colored beads in the beaker. These represent genes in a gamete pool with allelic frequencies 0.5 A and 0.5 a. Stir up the beads to ensure random genetic recombination.
3. Draw two beads to place on each toothpick as you did before. Look at the resulting genotypes. In this simulation, assume that aa genotypes produce a fatal genetic illness. Since A is dominant, Aa individuals do not have this disease. Record frequencies for all three genotypes in the table, then remove the aa toothpicks to represent selection against the aa genotype.
4. Calculate p and q for the surviving population. This time,
   p = f(A) = (# dark beads)/(all beads in surviving animals), and
   q = f(a) = (# light beads)/(all beads in surviving animals).
   Check your accuracy by confirming that p + q = 1. Record your values of p and q in the data table for natural selection results.
5. Remove beads from toothpicks and refill the beaker with dark and light beads to generate a gamete pool of 100 total beads, in the proportion of p and q that you just calculated. Mix the beads thoroughly.
6. Repeat steps 3 through 5 for 10 generations, recording the p and q values each time.
7. Complete graph 2 for the results of selection against a recessive lethal gene. The first point, showing p = 0.5, is already entered on the graph. Draw similar points for p in each generation, and draw a line connecting the dots to show the changes in p over time.

Table of Natural Selection Results (Method A, Procedure 2)

Generation number	Observed f(RR)	Observed f(Rr)	Observed f(rr)	p value $= \dfrac{(\text{# dark beads})}{(\text{total # beads})}$	q value $= 1 - p$
				0.50	0.50
1					
2					
3					
4					
5					
6					
7					
8					
9					
10					

Graph of Natural Selection Results

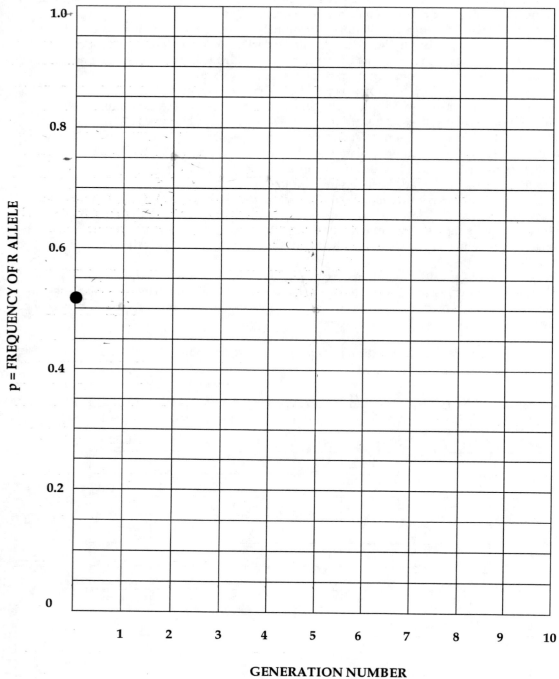

Questions (Method A, Procedure 2)

1. Most serious genetic diseases are caused by recessive alleles rather than dominant alleles. Based on this exercise, can you explain why a recessive lethal gene could persist in a population, while a dominant lethal gene could not?

_____

_____

_____

_____

_____

_____

2. Suppose your model of selection represents the change in frequency of plain white coquina clams because predatory birds see and remove them more quickly from a beach with dark-colored sand. If larval offspring from this population drift to a different beach made of light-colored sand, could selection go the other way? What does this say about fitness of a particular gene?

_____

_____

_____

_____

_____

_____

_____

3. In this simulation, you established the fitness of the aa allele as 0, removing all aa individuals from the breeding population. This may be realistic in the case of a serious genetic disease, but selection is not always so drastic. In the case of coquinas on the beach, white shells may suffer a measurable disadvantage due to higher bird predation, but their fitness is obviously not zero. Some white clams do survive to reproductive age. Suppose predation rates on white clams were not total, but did occur at twice the rate of predation on purple-rayed clams. How would you alter this procedure to simulate a 50% survival rate of the aa genotype? How would you expect this change in the simulation rules to affect the outcome?

_____

_____

_____

_____

_____

_____

_____

4. Many people incorrectly think of evolution as a completely random process. Based on the changes you observed in frequencies of alleles in this simulation, would you say natural selection is totally predictable, totally unpredictable, or something in between? Explain.

_____

_____

_____

_____

_____

_____

5. In this simulation, you sampled the gene pool without replacing beads in the beaker after you drew each one. Thus, f(A) and f(a) in the gene pool changed slightly after each bead was drawn. For example, if you begin with 50 light and 50 dark beads, the probability of drawing a dark bead the first time is $50/100 = 0.500$. The beaker would then contain 49 dark beads and 50 light beads, so the probability of drawing a second dark bead becomes $49/99 = 0.495$. Does this make your simulation slightly less realistic? In small natural populations, does one mating change the gene pool available for the next mating, or not? What biological factors must be considered in answering this question?

_____

_____

_____

_____

_____

_____

METHOD B: POPULATION GENETICS IN A FRUIT FLY CULTURE

[Laboratory activity]

Research Question

Do white and red eye color alleles exhibit Hardy-Weinberg equilibrium in a fruit fly population?

Preparation

Obtain a culture of wild-type (red-eyed) *Drosophila melanogaster* and a culture of the sex-linked white-eyed genotype. At least a month before this laboratory exercise, fill a large culture bottle to a depth of 4–5 cm with *Drosophila* medium. Add a few grains of dried baker's yeast if your growth medium does not already include it. You will need one culture bottle for each laboratory group. To each culture, introduce the same number of white-eyed and wild-type flies, making sure both males and females of both genotypes are included. You now have a polymorphic population with equal representation of the wild type and white alleles. Keep the cultures at room temperature (about 21° C) through two generations (about four weeks). If necessary, replace the culture medium by making up new bottles and moving all the adult flies from the old culture to the new.

Materials (per laboratory team)

A large fruit fly culture of mixed white-eyed and red-eyed genotypes

Dissecting microscope, preferably with 15 × magnification

Small paintbrush for manipulating flies

5 × 7 index card for holding flies

Anesthetic for flies

Small fly vial for anesthesia

Calculator

Background

In this exercise, we will investigate frequencies of a sex-linked gene for eye color called white. The dominant allele, X^+, codes for a tomato-red pigmentation in the prominent compound eyes of the fruit fly. The recessive allele, X^w, produces a white eye. Since males have only one X chromosome, males are either X^+Y with red eyes or X^wY with white eyes. Assuming that males inherit X chromosomes in proportion to their frequency in the gene pool, the fraction of male flies exhibiting the white-eyed phenotype should indicate $f(X^w)$ in the population as a whole. Similarly, the proportion of males exhibiting the red-eyed phenotype should be a good indicator of $f(X^+)$.

Females, on the other hand, have two X chromosomes so they have three possible genotypes. Females with the X^+X^+ genotype are homozygous red-eyed flies. Females with the X^+X^w genotype are carriers of the white allele, but have red eyes, and X^wX^w females have white eyes. If you use the frequencies of X^+Y males vs. X^wY males to determine $p = f(X^+)$ and $q = f(X^w)$, you should be able to use the Hardy-Weinberg equations to calculate the frequencies of homozygous red, heterozygous, and homozygous white genotypes among the females.

Procedure

1. Get as many flies as you can out of the large culture and into an empty *Drosophila* vial. This is a critical step, because you do not want to introduce bias in your sample. You can place the vial over the mouth of the larger culture, tip both containers, and tap flies into the vial. Be careful, however, not to dislodge the *Drosophila* medium from the bottom of the culture. Alternatively, you can take advantage of fruit flies' tendency to walk upward and toward a light source. Cover the large container with paper or foil, place an empty vial over its mouth, and place the combined vessels, empty vial on top, under a laboratory lamp. With patience, you should be able to collect a large number of flies from the culture.

2. Use commercial fly anesthesia to put the flies to sleep. Although timing is critical for anesthesia if you want to revive the flies later for genetics crosses, it is not necessary for the purpose of this experiment to keep the flies alive. Make sure they are sufficiently anesthetized so that they do not awaken and fly away before you have time to count them.

3. When all the flies are well anesthetized, tap them out onto the 5×7 index card and place the card on the stage of the dissecting scope. Using your paintbrush, separate the flies by sex. Refer to Figure 5 to see differences between male and female *Drosophila*. The dark patches of bristles, called sex combs, on the front feet of males provide a good way to separate younger adult flies. Older males have sex combs too, but they also have a darker tip of the abdomen which makes them easier to distinguish from females.

4. When you have separated flies by sex, count the numbers of white-eyed vs. red-eyed males. Enter those numbers in the data table. Then count the numbers of white-eyed vs. red-eyed females. Enter those numbers as well.

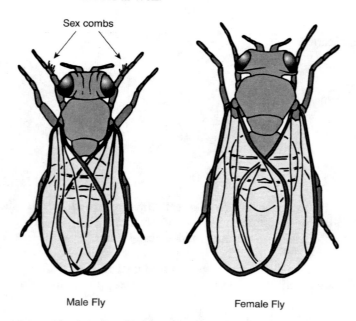

Male Fly   Female Fly

Figure 5   Fruit fly male (left) and female (right). Note differences in overall body size, banding pattern on the abdomen, and bundles of black bristles, called sex combs, on the front legs of the male.

5. Complete the data table for Method B, using frequencies of males to generate p and q. Then use the Hardy-Weinberg formula to calculate expected frequencies of red-eyed and white-eyed females.
6. Compare your observed frequencies of red-eyed and white-eyed females to the expected frequencies, based on values of p and q you calculated from the male data.

Table of Fruit Fly Population Genetics Results (Method B)

MALES	FEMALES
Number of red-eyed males collected from the population:	**Number of red-eyed females collected from the population:**
Number of white-eyed males collected from the population:	**Number of white-eyed females collected from the population:**
$p = f(X^+) =$ **red-eyed males/total males**	**Observed frequency of red eyes in females = (red-eyed females/total females)**
$q = f(X^w) =$ **white-eyed males/total males**	**Observed frequency of white eyes in females = (white-eyed females/total females)**
Use p and q from male data to calculate expected frequency of red-eyed females. ⇒	**Expected frequency of red eyes in females = $f(X^+X^+) + f(X^+X^w) = p^2 + 2pq$**
Use q from male data to calculate expected frequency of white-eyed females. ⇒	**Expected frequency of white eyes in females = $f(X^wX^w) = q^2$**

Questions (Method B)

1. How did your expected frequencies of red-eyed vs. white-eyed females compare with observed frequencies? Do your observations support the assumption that the female flies exhibit Hardy-Weinberg equilibrium? Explain.

_____

_____

_____

_____

2. Of the female red-eyed flies, how many would you expect to be homozygous X^+X^+ genotypes, and how many heterozygous X^+X^w, based on Hardy-Weinberg expectations? Show your calculations.

3. Consider each of the biological factors that can force a departure from Hardy-Weinberg equilibrium. Based on what you know about the fly culture, the behavior of fruit flies, and your observed phenotypic frequencies, which factors could have major effects on population genetics in this system? Which factors are less likely to exert a significant influence?

_____

_____

_____

_____

4. The Hardy-Weinberg model assumes no selection for or against the X^w allele. This may or may not be the case. Did you observe a 50:50 sex ratio in all flies? Was the number of white-eyed males equal to the number of red-eyed males? Based on initial frequencies of p and q = 0.5, these statements would be true in the absence of selection or drift. If these statements are not consistent with your observations, develop a hypothesis to explain what you see.

_____

_____

_____

_____

5. Based on the frequencies you calculated for heterozygous and homozygous females, what is the probability that a red-eyed female randomly chosen from this population and bred to a white-eyed male will produce a white-eyed offspring from the very first egg she lays? (Hint: list all statements that must be true for this to happen, along with the separate probability of each. Then using the sum rule, multiply the probabilities together to calculate the joint probability.)

FOR FURTHER INVESTIGATION

1. Repeat the genetic drift simulation in Method A with a population of 20 animals, represented by 20 toothpicks. Bear in mind that you will now need to divide the number of dark beads by 40 when calculating p. What difference do you see in the rate of genetic drift when the population size is doubled?

2. Sickle cell anemia, represented by the symbol (s), is a genetically determined change in the hemoglobin molecule, which carries oxygen in the blood. The sickle-cell trait is a good example of an allele whose selective value depends on the environment. Before modern medical therapies, the gene was often fatal in the homozygous ss condition, but Ss heterozygotes were protected from malaria. In many tropical regions, malaria is historically so serious that most SS genotypes would be too sick to survive and reproduce. In extreme cases, heterozygous Ss people would be the only survivors. Heterozygote advantage, also called **heterosis**, results in stable **polymorphism**. You can model this kind of natural selection using your toothpick animal system. Run the selection model as you did in Method A, Procedure 2, but remove both the homozygous recessive and the homozygous dominant individuals. You will need only a couple of generations to see what happens to gene frequencies. Do you think this kind of selection for heterozygotes could explain why so much polymorphism exists in natural populations?

3. As an independent study project, anesthetize flies carefully, and perform the above analysis as described. After sexing and counting your flies, select a random sample of 20 of the red-eyed female flies for further testing. You will need 20 culture vials, each with *Drosophila* medium prepared according to supplier's directions. Place each red-eyed female in a separate fly vial along with a white-eyed male. Allow several days for the flies to mate and for the females to lay eggs. As soon as you see larvae in the vials, remove the adults. The offspring will indicate the genotype of the female parents: X^+X^+ females will produce all red-eyed offspring, while X^+X^w females will produce half red-eyed and half white-eyed offspring. Draw out Punnett squares to demonstrate the two outcomes. After you have progeny in all 20 vials, use the data to calculate the proportion of X^+X^+ to X^+X^w females in the original population. Do these proportions conform to Hardy-Weinberg expectations?

4. For a long-term experiment, keep the polymorphic fly culture alive for several more weeks. Collect samples of flies periodically to see whether p and q shift due to drift or selection over time. Consider maintaining more than one culture for comparison so that you can determine whether genetic change is due to selection (where all bottles would be expected to change in the same direction) or drift (where the direction of change should vary at random).

FOR FURTHER READING

Cavalli-Sforza, L. L. 1969. Genetic drift in an Italian population. *Scientific American* 221(2):30–38.

Edgren, Richard A. 1959. Coquinas (*Donax variabilis*) on a Florida beach. *Ecology* 40(3): 498–502.

Lewin, Roger. 1982. Biology is not postage stamp collecting. *Science* 216:718–720.

Loew, S. 2002. Role of genetics in conservation biology. *Quantitative Methods for Conservation Biology* (Ferson, S. and M. A. Burgman eds.) Pp. 226–258. Springer-Verlag, N. Y.

EXERCISE 4
ENVIRONMENTAL CHEMISTRY

Chemistry is the scientific discipline concerned with the structure, composition, and properties of substances and of their transformations. Chemists have discovered that all living things are constructed of some combinations of chemical elements. Nutrients, air, water, the sun and other factors required by living things are all composed of such chemicals. Thus a fundamental knowledge of chemistry is vital to understanding ecology.

The science of chemistry organizes matter at the simplest non-living and living levels into three classes of materials--mixtures, compounds, and elements. The basis for this classification system is our ability to identify a homogeneous material and to distinguish between physical and chemical changes. The identity of a homogeneous or uniform material is specified by a set of properties or characteristics that are independent of the quantity of material. Color, physical state, density, boiling point, and freezing point are examples of such identifying properties. Materials also undergo changes and from our ability to identify materials, a change may be defined as a chemical or physical change. In a physical change, the identity of the starting material(s) does not change while in a chemical change or chemical reaction, the identity of the starting material(s) changes and new materials are produced. For example, if the starting material is a colorless liquid and heating changes the liquid to a colorless gas, the evidence indicates no change in identity of the starting material and a physical change. However, if the starting material is a colorless liquid and heating produces a colored gas, then the evidence indicates a chemical change has occurred. (Note for this example we must use identifying properties which do not depend on temperature.) Studies of the changes that a homogeneous material can undergo have found that, depending on the material, the material may or may not be separated into two or more simpler substances. Now, by definition, a mixture is a material that can be separated into two or more simpler materials by physical changes, a compound can be separated into two or more simpler materials by chemical change, and an element cannot be separated into simpler materials by either a chemical or physical change.

As defined in the previous paragraph, elements are the simplest materials and all matter on earth is either an element or combination of elements. Today, 105 elements have been identified and 92 of these elements occur naturally in our environment. Some familiar examples of elements from our environment are oxygen, nitrogen, aluminum, and iron. Approximately 96.3% of the matter on earth is composed of the

- 21 -

six elements--iron, oxygen, silicon, magnesium, nickel, and sulfur. Atoms are the smallest submicroscopic division of an element and to speak about an atom of a specific element, chemists will use an atomic symbol. Atomic symbols for the naturally occurring elements consist of a single capital letter or a capital letter and a lower case letter. For example, O is the atomic symbol for oxygen while Fe is the atomic symbol for iron. These quantities are more clearly defined in Figure 4-1 which gives the structure of an atom. It should be noted that the mass of the atom is contained almost entirely in the nucleus of the atom (protons and neutrons) and that the volume of the atom is principally filled by the electrons. An interesting consequence of atomic structure is that two bodies of equal mass have equal numbers of protons and neutrons.

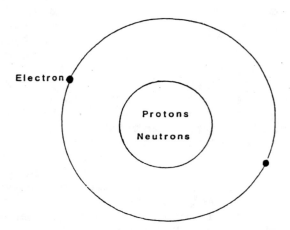

Figure 4-1. Atomic structure. Each atom is composed of three fundamental particles: protons, neutrons, and electrons. The positively charged protons and the massive neutral neutrons make up the very dense nucleus of each atom. The negatively charged electrons move in a much larger volume around the nucleus. The number of electrons equals the number of protons, hence, an atom is electrically neutral. The atomic number is the number of protons (or electrons).

Compounds can be decomposed by chemical change into their component elements, and every compound has each component element in definite amounts. The latter observation has resulted in the concept of the chemical formula of which H_2O is a familiar example. This formula tells us that water is composed of the elements hydrogen (H) and oxygen (O) with two atoms of H for each O atom. The unit H_2O is the smallest submicroscopic division of water and is a molecule of water. The atoms in a molecule are held together by chemical bonds, and a molecule is uniquely identified when the chemical formula (identity and number of atoms composing the molecule), chemical bonds (how atoms are linked together), and molecular structure (positions of atoms in space) are known. Covalent chemical bonds result from the sharing of electrons by two atoms and are represented by single, double, or triple lines between atoms. Figure 4-2 presents the chemical bonding for several examples.

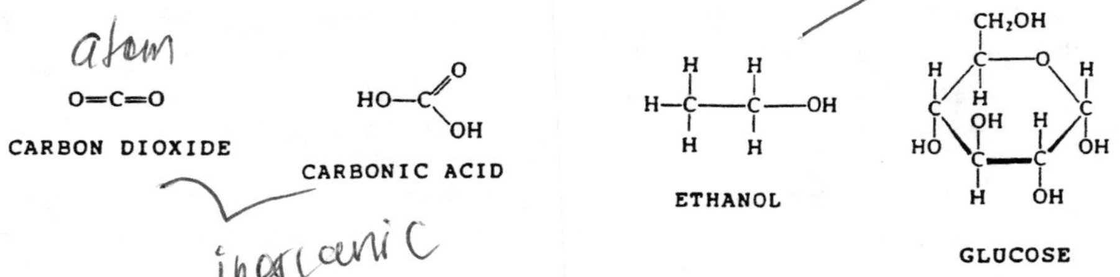

Figure 4-2. Elements, molecules, and compounds. An element is a kind of matter whose atoms all have the same atomic number. Two or more atoms may join together to form a molecule of a new substance. A compound is a substance formed by the chemical union of two or more elements. Carbon dioxide, for instance, is an inorganic compound formed from two elements--carbon and oxygen--always combined in the ratio of one carbon to two oxygen atoms. Two atoms of hydrogen, three one atoms of oxygen, and one carbon atom combine to form the inorganic compound carbonic acid. Ethanol, an alcohol, is an organic compound found in beer, wine, and liquor. Glucose is the main fuel that organisms burn to supply energy for their various vital functions.

Compounds can be grouped into two broad classes--organic and inorganic compounds. Organic compounds always have a C atom and at least one C--H or C--C bond while inorganic compounds do not satisfy this definition. For the molecules given in Figure 4-2, carbon dioxide and carbonic acid are inorganic compounds while ethanol and glucose are examples of organic compounds. In our environment, rocks and minerals are examples of inorganic compounds while petroleum and coal are organic compounds.

Nutrients is a term that includes any substance required by an organism for normal growth and maintenance. Nutrients required for the proper function of living systems are termed macronutrients if necessary in large quantities, and micronutrients if small amounts will suffice. For example, the human body requires four groups of macronutrients (water, proteins, lipids, and carbohydrates) and two groups of micronutrients (vitamins and minerals).

In this exercise we will take a closer look at the importance of inorganic and organic compounds. We shall determine the water content of some given substances. We will also examine some representative organic compounds, using simple techniques to identify them.

INORGANIC CHEMICALS

Many inorganic nutrients or minerals are as essential for good health as the organic nutrients, and they are required in the diet. Minerals needed include water and ions of sodium, chloride, calcium, phosphates, iron, and iodine. Most of them are obtained by humans directly from plants or from animals that have eaten the plants, or from drinking water (some minerals are dissolved in water). Various symptoms develop when minerals are lacking in the diet.

Water serves as a structural component of living systems, both as a solvent and a metabolite for biochemical reactions. Recall that water, in addition to light and carbon dioxide, is an essential requirement for photosynthesis. In our society water also serves many purposes in agriculture, industry, and the home. It is utilized for irrigation, as a cooling medium in many processes, and for domestic and personal needs. Thus, water is an extremely vital environmental factor.

Water is also utilized as a place to live or habitat. In fact, seventy-five percent of the earth's surface is covered by water. Life on earth is thought to have originated in water about 3 to 4 billion years ago, and even humans bear vestige of the primeval past in the gill they possess for a time as developing embryo. Since most organic compounds require water either as a base or as part of the compound itself, active organisms (as opposed to spores or dry seeds) are usually composed of about 70 percent water. In some organisms, such as jellyfish, water makes up as much as 95 percent of the organism's body. Even the average human body is 65 percent water.

The following experiment considers the water content of some given substances.

Materials needed: (Per Group)
    (1) Sandy soil, clay soil, milk, and a potato
    (2) Four ceramic crucibles, scale, wax pencil
    (3) Hot plate

Procedures:
    (A) Secure four crucibles and number them 1 through 4. Weigh them to the nearest 0.01 gram and record their weights in Table 4-1 (tare weight).

(B) Fill each crucible with the following substances:
    Crucible 1--Sandy soil (fill to the rim)
    Crucible 2--Clay soil (fill to the rim)
    Crucible 3--Chopped potato (fill to the rim)
    Crucible 4--Milk (one-third full only)
    (C) Weigh the crucibles plus the materials (gross wet weights) and enter results in Table 4-1. Calculate net wet weights (gross wet weights minus tare weights) for your samples. Record your results in Table 4-1.

Table 4-1. Water content of some substances.

	SANDY SOIL	CLAY SOIL	POTATO	MILK
TARE WEIGHT	19.5	19.7	19.1	18.6
GROSS WET WEIGHT	78.9	71.2	38.6	28.2
NET WET WEIGHT	59.4	51.5	19.5	10.4
GROSS DRY WEIGHT	65.3	57.7	33.6	19.5
NET DRY WEIGHT	45.8	38	19.5	0.9
PERCENT WATER	22.9%	26.52%	25.64	91.35

(D) Place the crucibles on a hot plate for one hour. Make sure that the hot plate is set on high. Note the odor produced. The odor produced is similar to that created when organic waste is burned in a dump or in an incinerator. Does this indicate that additional air pollutants are being added? (While waiting one hour, do the organic compound experiment.)
    (E) After one hour, reweigh the crucibles plus materials and enter data in Table 4-1 as gross dry weights.
    (F) Now compute net dry weights (gross dry weights minus tare weights) and percent water content of the substances (net wet weights minus net dry weights divided by net wet weights times 100). Enter results in Table 4-1. What is the percentage of water content present in the substances? Explain the differences observed between the substances in relation to their water content. Which substance had the most water? Which substance had the least? How does the type of soil (sandy versus clay) affect the frequency of fire in an ecosystem?
    (G) When your lab is complete, unplug your hot plate. After the crucibles have cooled, scrape out your crucibles into the trash--especially the milk and potato. (Warning: You may accidentally start a fire by placing burning materials in the trash!) Place the crucibles in the soapy solution on the front counter.

ORGANIC COMPOUNDS

In nature, organic compounds are produced only by living things, although many may now be synthesized by chemists. When living things die, some of their organic molecules end up in the environment as decaying detritus. The organic compounds mainly include carbohydrates, lipids, proteins, nucleic acid, and vitamins. The carbohydrates (sugars, starches, glycogen, cellulose) are a principal source of energy. Starchy vegetable foods, such as bread and potatoes, provide the most amounts of carbohydrates, but so do meats and seafood because they contain glycogen. Glycogen or animal starch serves as a food reserve in humans and other organisms (other animals, bacteria, and fungi); it can be broken down readily into glucose. Carbohydrates are also used as structural materials or as part of other molecules.

The lipids (fats, oils, waxes, steroids, carotenes) contain twice as much energy than carbohydrates. The lipids, in addition to serving as a source of energy, function as important components of cells, energy storers, and hormones. Food rich in lipids include butter, margarine, meat, eggs, milk, nuts, and a variety of vegetable oils.

Proteins provide the physical framework of the human body. For example, the cartilage that binds your bone joints together is composed of a protein (collagen). Other proteins serve to transport oxygen (hemoglobin). Others function as catalysts and regulate the speed at which chemical reactions occur in your body (enzymes), and still others function as hormones and chemical messengers. Proteins are present in meat, fish, poultry, cheese, nuts, milk, eggs, cereals, beans, and peas. Proteins are built of long chains of basic molecular units called amino acids. There are 20 different amino acids which, except for eight, your body has no difficulty in changing from one type to another. Those that cannot be changed or synthesized are called essential amino acids (they are lysine, tryptophan, threonine, methionine, phenylalanine, leucine, isoleucine, and valine) and must be provided in the diet.

Nucleic acids, such as deoxyribonucleic acid (DNA) and ribonucleic acid (RNA), are composed of nucleiotides. Nucleic acids are the carriers of genetic information. The nucleic acids are present in small amounts in foods.

Vitamins are essential organic compounds that the human body cannot synthesize for itself. They are required in small quantities in the diet or can be absorbed by the intestine after they have been produced by the bacteria living there. The vitamins are required by enzymes in order to function (as cofactors of enzymes). Thus, the absence of a particular vitamin may result in various diseases.

Materials needed: (Per Group)
(1) Four ml of Benedict's solution, several drops of iodine, several grains of Sudan red, and 1 ml of Biuret reagent.

(HANDLE THESE CHEMICALS VERY CAUTIOUSLY. IN CASE OF ACCIDENTAL CONTACT, FLOOD WITH WATER IMMEDIATELY.)

(2) Five test tubes, one test tube rack, and one test tube holder.

(3) Four labelled solutions of glucose, starch, olive oil, and protein

(4) One unknown solution

(5) Graduated cylinder (10 ml) & Erlenmeyer flask (250 ml)

(6) Hot plate, wax pencil, and eye dropper

Procedures:

(A) Pour approximately 75 ml of water into the flask. What is the function of the water bath? Place a test tube in the flask (Fig. 4-3). Place 4 ml of Benedict's solution into the test tube and add about 1 ml (about 20 drops) of glucose solution. Place the flask on a hot plate and let the water bath boil for three minutes. (CAUTION: DO NOT HAVE THE MOUTH OF THE TUBE FACING ANYONE. THE HOT SUBSTANCE MAY BOIL VIOLENTLY AND SHOOT OUT OF THE TUBE INTO SOMEONE'S FACE.) Remove the flask from the hot plate and allow to cool. Note what happens. The ultimate formation of reddish-orange precipitate is a test for the presence of simple sugar like glucose. Record your observation in Table 4-2.

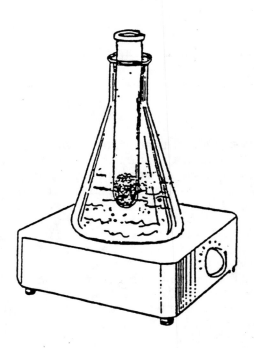

Figure 4-3. Place the flask and test tube on the hot plate.

(B) Place 4 ml of starch solution in a test tube and add a few drops of iodine solution. Observe the color change. Starch should show a blue or black color when iodine is added. Record observation in Table 4-2.

(C) Place 2 ml of water in a test tube and add several grains (or drops) of the stain Sudan red. Shake the test tube thoroughly. What happened? Next add 10 drops of olive oil and shake. Note what happens. In the presence of lipids, Sudan red exhibits a characteristic red color reaction. Record what you saw in Table 4-2. (Note: lipids are organic compounds that are insoluble in water.)

(D) Prepare a test tube containing 20 drops of protein (albumin) and add 20 drops of water and 20 drops of Biuret reagent. Record any color changes in Table 4-2. A pink or violet color indicates a positive test.

Table 4-2. Identification of organic compounds.

ORGANIC COMPOUNDS	TESTS (OBSERVATIONS)
SUGAR	orange on top
STARCH	black
OIL	red on top / clear on bottom
PROTEIN	blue
UNKNOWN	oil

(E) Now that you have validated the reagents against known organic compounds, perform these four tests on an unknown sample. To identify the unknown compound, you repeat Procedures A through D as described above. For example, to determine whether your unknown is glucose, repeat Procedure A. Briefly, place 4 ml of Benedict's solution into a test tube and add 20 drops of the unknown organic compound. Heat in a water bath for 3 minutes. If a reddish-orange precipitate is formed, your unknown is glucose. If not, then test whether your unknown is starch, lipid, or protein, as described in Procedures B through D above. Record your data in Table 4-2. What type of unknown do you think you had? Check your results with your instructor.

(F) Clean up your area and materials. Unplug your hot plate and wipe up any spills or soils.

Aquatic Environments

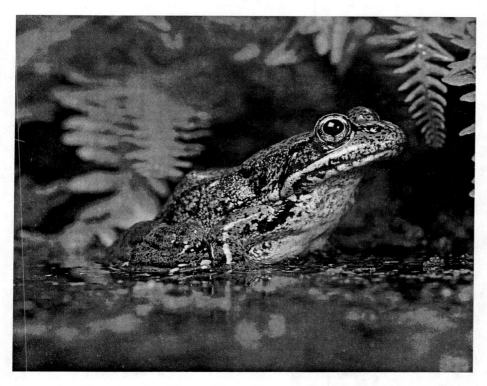

Figure 1   Threatened red-legged frogs (*Rana aurora draytonii*) depend on shrinking aquatic habitats, which have been reduced in quality and area in California.

INTRODUCTION

California red-legged frogs (*Rana aurora draytonii*) were once familiar aquatic animals in the Western United States (Figure 1). Mark Twain wrote about these frogs, and about the California gold miners who gambled on their leaping ability in "The Celebrated Jumping Frog of Calaveras County." Larger than any other native frog in the region, these amphibians were intensively harvested for food in the 1800s. Overharvesting, along with widespread diversion of surface water for irrigation, pollution of streams, and introduction of aggressive competitors such as the bullfrog, caused a steady decline in red-legged frog populations over the past century, according to the U.S. Fish and Wildlife Service (2001). Now listed as a threatened species, red-legged frogs are emblematic of our general concerns about aquatic ecosystem health.

Amphibians all over the world are declining, not for a single reason, but because their fragile wetland habitats, and the pure water they require, are impacted by so many different human activities. Synthetic hormones released as pollutants in wastewater, nutrients and sediments from agricultural runoff, draining of marshlands, exotic diseases, increased ultraviolet penetration of atmospheric ozone, and gradual changes in climate have all been suggested as possible contributing factors (Davidson *et al.*, 2001). Although rare species like the red-legged frog do eventually merit protection under the Endangered Species Act, recovery efforts are daunting after the species has been reduced to a few fragmented populations. The Endangered Species Act has been a valuable conservation tool, but its application usually involves damage control rather than prevention. Basing conservation policy solely on a species' endangered status is like waiting to see the dentist until you have only one tooth left in your mouth. Ecologists recognize that effective biodiversity protection for wetland and aquatic species depends on ecosystem-level understanding of our environment, and thoughtful management of entire watersheds. Mark Twain's miners may have bet on one frog at a time, but our task is to improve the odds for the aquatic community as a whole.

What are the most important environmental factors affecting life in aquatic systems? Dissolved oxygen is certainly critical, and this variable is always linked with temperature. Cold water is able to carry more oxygen than warm water. At one atmosphere of pressure, a liter of water near the freezing point can dissolve about 14 milligrams of oxygen. The same water heated to 30° C can dissolve only about 7 milligrams of oxygen. In other words, water in a temperate zone creek loses nearly half its ability to carry dissolved oxygen between January and July. Metabolic activity by bacteria or by aquatic organisms reduces oxygen levels below this maximum limit, so accelerated decomposition of organic matter in warm weather can make this difference even more extreme. Add to this the effects of water movement, with stream flow slower and more sluggish in summer, and faster with more aeration in winter, and the difference is greater still.

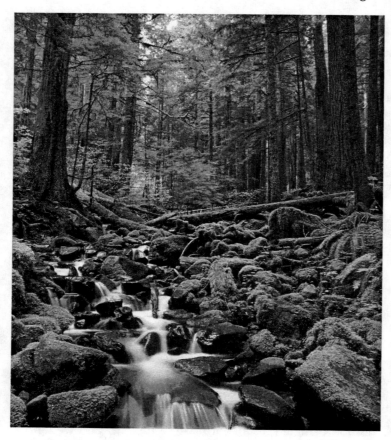

Figure 2 Trees reduce water temperature in shaded upper reaches of a stream.

Within a watershed, a stream tends to be more oxygenated in its upper reaches, where flow rates are greater and overarching trees shade the water (Figure 2). As a stream slows down and gets wider in its lower reaches, temperature increases and oxygen levels decline. A slower flow rate downstream provides less mixing, and this reduces oxygen levels as well. These changes in the physical environment affect life forms in the stream. Active fish with high oxygen demand are limited to cool streams with rapidly flowing water (Figure 3). Fish inhabiting warm stagnant waters tend to lower their metabolic demand for oxygen by

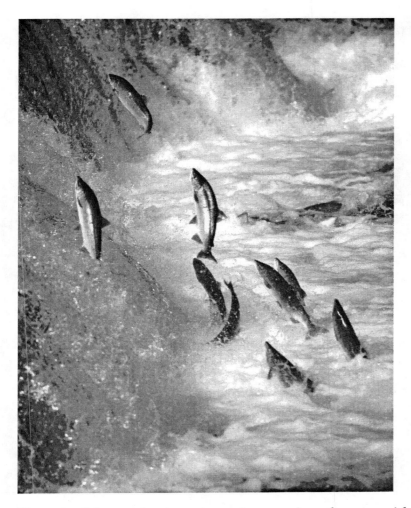

Figure 3   Salmon migrate upstream to spawn in cool, oxygen-rich waters.

moving slowly and spending much of their lives sitting still and waiting for prey to come to them (Figure 4). Human activities that increase water temperature, such as cutting shade trees away from stream banks or discharging heated water from power plants into rivers, significantly affect resident aquatic life.

Check your progress:

Aside from the obvious advantage of leaving more time for tadpole development, why might so many species of frogs in temperate zones shed their eggs very early in springtime?

Hint: Frog eggs need high levels of dissolved oxygen for development.

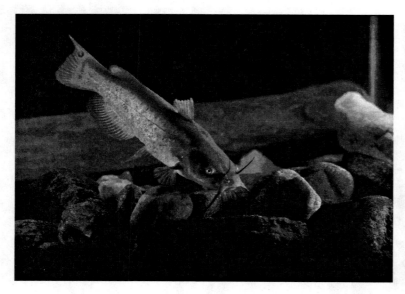

Figure 4   Brown bullhead catfish tolerates warm waters with low oxygen.

In a lake, warm water floats on top of cold water, so **stratification** of the water column occurs as the sun warms the surface (Figure 5). The warm upper layer, called the **epilimnion**, is the most biologically active. Since light penetrates only a few meters in most freshwater lakes and ponds, photosynthesis is limited to the epilimnion. The cooler, darker zone at the bottom is called the **hypolimnion**. Algae and other plankton "rain" down from the epilimnion above, to be decomposed by bacteria living in the mud at the bottom. There is little mixing of water between layers, so oxygen used up by these decomposers is not immediately replaced. Over the summer, the hypolimnion becomes richer in dissolved nutrients, but poorer in dissolved oxygen. Growth of algae near the surface slows down in midsummer, because their recycled nutrients are trapped in the hypolimnion.

Lake Stratification

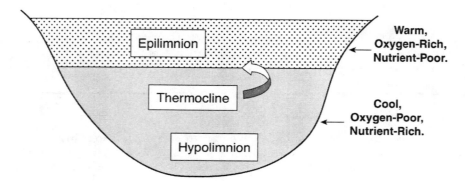

Figure 5   Temperature stratification in a freshwater lake.

On the interface between the warm epilimnion and the cold hypolimnion is a dividing line called the **thermocline**. This boundary layer can be found near the surface in early summer. If you have ever been swimming in a northern lake in June, you know the "toe test" may indicate warmth near the surface, but the near-freezing hypolimnion becomes all too apparent when you jump in. Through the summer, the thermocline drops lower and lower as solar heating expands the epilimnion. When fall comes, stratification is reversed.

Water exposed to cold air gets colder and heavier, so surface water sinks to the bottom. This mixes the upper and lower layers of the lake, a phenomenon known as "**fall turnover.**" The thermocline disappears as epilimnion and hypolimnion are blended together. Since water resists temperature changes, it can take a long time to cool the entire lake to 4° C, which is the temperature at which water is heaviest. Below that temperature, water molecules begin organizing themselves into the lattice of crystalline ice, becoming less dense than liquid water. By the time ice forms on the top of a lake, the entire water column has been cooled to 4° C, all the while mixing nutrient-rich waters from below with oxygen-rich waters from above. By the time of the spring thaw, surface waters can again support algae growth as the epilimnion begins to re-form in a new season.

Check your progress:

If a shallow lake and a deep lake both have the same surface area and the same average water temperature of 20° C, which will freeze over first when winter comes? Why?

Answer: Deep lakes take longer to freeze over because all the water must be cooled to 4° C before any of it turns to ice.

In addition to temperature and dissolved oxygen, light is a critical variable in aquatic systems. Aquatic food chains are built on productivity of microscopic algae, called **phytoplankton**, floating in the water. These algae tend to float near the surface because light intensity declines exponentially with depth. For example, if we measure red light of wavelength 620 nm at 100% intensity at the surface of a perfectly clear lake, its intensity declines to 10% at a depth of 9 m, 1% at 18 m, and 0.1% at 27 m. Not all wavelengths of light penetrate water equally well. Blue light, with wavelengths in the 400–500 nm range, is transmitted much more effectively than red light (600–700 nm). When sunlight composed of all colors enters water, the red wavelengths are preferentially absorbed, so light that has passed through water looks blue. Chlorophyll, the photosynthetic pigment for land plants and many algae, absorbs blue and red portions of the spectrum, so the rapid attenuation of red light near the surface significantly reduces energy available to phytoplankton. In deepwater marine habitats, some algae actually use a different photosynthetic pigment, which absorbs only the blue light available at that depth. Since their cells reflect red light rather than absorb it, they have a red appearance when brought up to the surface. They are appropriately called red algae.

Suspended particles and pigments interfere with light transmission in direct proportion to their concentration. This is the principle behind the spectrophotometer, which you may have used in chemistry laboratory to measure the concentration of a colored solution. Silt and clay soil washing into streams reduces photosynthesis by interfering with light transmission to algae and submerged plants. This reduction in clarity is called **turbidity.** It can be measured in an instrument similar to a spectrophotometer, called a turbidimeter. Standard units of turbidity, called nephalometric turbidity units, or N.T.U., are often included in water quality assessments of streams. A more traditional way to measure water transparency is with a Secchi disc (Figure 6). The Secchi disc is a round flat piece of metal or plastic, 20 cm in diameter, painted white and black in alternating quarters and weighted so that it will sink. A ring in the center is tied to a chain or rope which is marked off in meters, and the Secchi disc is lowered over the side of a boat. The observer lets out the line until the Secchi disc disappears from view. Then the observer pulls up the line until the Secchi disc is just visible, and a depth measurement is recorded. Ideally, Secchi disc readings are taken between 10:00 am and 2:00 pm, and observation is off the shady side of the boat for better visibility. The greater the depth a Secchi disc can be seen, the clearer the water.

Secchi Disk

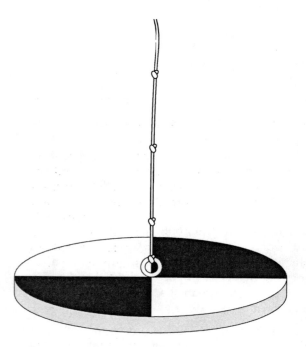

Figure 6   A Secchi disc is lowered into a body of water from a boat to measure turbidity of the water.

Finally, dissolved chemicals determine viability of aquatic life. Nutrients such as phosphates, nitrates, and potassium are needed in small amounts for biosynthesis, but can wreak havoc with aquatic communities if added in large amounts. A body of water receiving too much fertilizer is said to be **eutrophic**, which literally means "overfed." Algae grow exponentially in "blooms" or floating mats that block out all the light below the surface. Shaded algae die and decompose. Bacterial decomposition uses up dissolved oxygen, with predictable results for other aquatic organisms.

Some sources of pollution are easier to find than others. **Point sources**, such as industrial spills, pulp mill effluent, and insufficiently treated municipal wastewater, enter a body of water at an identifiable location. **Non-point sources**, which include runoff from lawns or farm fields, acid rain, manure from feed lots, silt from road construction, or leachates from mining operations, are more diffuse in their origin and thus harder to identify and control. Toxicity may be acute, resulting in dramatic fish kills, or chronic, causing gradually declining biodiversity in an affected waterway. The growing number of biologically active compounds entering streams from antibiotics in animal feed and from medicines incompletely metabolized by humans has more recently raised concerns about effects on animal fertility, reproduction, and development.

Chemical tests have been designed for many kinds of pollutants in water, but it is difficult to assess how much damage is being inflicted on stream biota in this way. A more direct approach is to test the water directly on organisms, monitoring their viability over time. So called **bioindicator** organisms are chosen for their short life spans and high sensitivity to pollutants. Two organisms used routinely for biomonitoring work are *Daphnia* (also called water fleas—Figure 7) and the small fish *Pimephales promelas* (also called fathead minnows—Figure 8). The premise of this biological approach is that water clean enough to support bioindicator organisms is probably safe for the aquatic ecosystem as a whole. Bioindicators are studied in two settings. Laboratory experiments expose a subject population to suspected toxins or suspect water sources in carefully controlled experiments. For example, a pesticide might be screened by making up a series of dilutions and exposing fathead minnows in aquaria to these dilutions over a period of time. A concentration of the pesticide just strong enough to kill half of the fish is called the lethal dose for 50%, or LD_{50} value. This critical concentration can then be compared with LD_{50} values for other pesticides to determine which has the lowest effect on fish if it runs off of fields into streams.

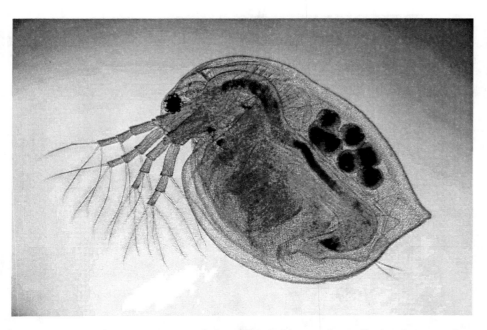

Figure 7   Daphnia are commonly used bioindicators for pollution in aquatic environments.

A second biomonitoring approach looks at organisms already living in a stream. A convenient group of bioindicators for on-site assessment are **benthic macroinvertebrates**. Benthic means living on the bottom, and macroinvertebrates are non-vertebrate animals large enough to be seen with the naked eye. This group includes strictly aquatic species, like amphipods and snails, that live all their lives in the water. It also includes the aquatic larvae of many insects, such as dragonflies, that live near aquatic habitats as adults and lay eggs in the water (Figure 9). Some of these macroinvertebrates, including the juvenile forms of mayflies, caddis flies, and stoneflies, are quite sensitive to pollution. If any toxins have entered the stream in the past few months, these organisms will be absent from the benthic community. Other macroinver-tebrates, including aquatic annelids and the larvae of midges, can tolerate a high pollution load. By comparing numbers of pollution-sensitive vs. pollution-tolerant species, ecologists can develop a water quality index that is more inclusive than a battery of chemical tests. In a sense, the bioindicator species have been monitoring pollution in the stream 24 hours a day, 365 days a year, for every pollutant that can harm organisms, right up to the time of your arrival.

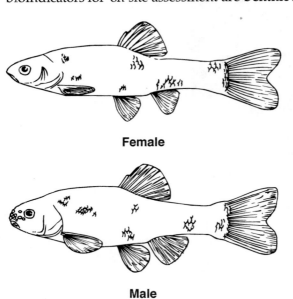

Female

Male

Figure 8   Fathead minnows (*Pimephales, promelas*) are commonly used as bioindicators for toxins affecting survival and development of vertebrate animals.

Check your progress:

To monitor non-point sources of pollution, what advantages would you see in a series of chemical tests, such as pH, ammonia nitrogen, and dissolved oxygen assays? What advantages would you see in using bioindicators instead?

Hint: One approach is more comprehensive, the other potentially yields a more specific diagnosis of the problem.

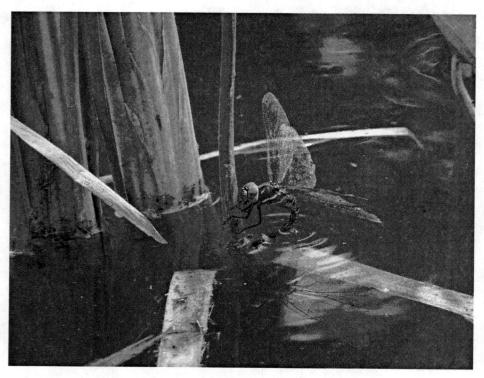

Figure 9   A dragonfly deposits eggs on aquatic vegetation.

METHOD A: DISSOLVED OXYGEN AND TEMPERATURE

[Laboratory/outdoor activity]

Research Question

How does temperature affect dissolved oxygen concentration?

Preparation

A series of five water baths at different temperatures between 0° C and 40° C will be needed for the laboratory portion of this experiment. If you do not have water baths that can be set at a range of temperatures, a fair substitution can be made with inexpensive fish tank heaters placed in 1000-ml beakers. Beakers can also be left overnight in an incubator or refrigerator. Make sure the water stays uncovered at temperature for several hours so that oxygen has a chance to equilibrate before testing.

Kits that include a chemical test for dissolved oxygen are inexpensive and widely available. These are adequate for the experiment if groups cooperate on testing and share data to save time. A portable meter with a dissolved oxygen probe is a better way for an individual to collect all needed data in a short time. For greater accuracy, groups can be instructed to pool their data, and to plot a standard curve through mean values for the class.

Outside water sources depend on your campus environment. Fish ponds, fountains, puddles, ditches, and adjacent streams are all possible sample sites. If outdoor sources do not exist, try measuring dissolved oxygen in aquaria as a model system.

Materials (per laboratory team)

Access to five water baths, of varying temperature

Access to at least one outdoor water source

Dissolved oxygen test kit or portable dissolved oxygen meter

Thermometer for assessing water temperature

Procedure

1. In each of the water baths, measure temperature and dissolved oxygen. Record your results in the Data Table for Method A.
2. Generate a graph on the Results for Method A page, showing the relationship between temperature (x-axis) and dissolved oxygen (y-axis). Draw a smooth curve through your points. This will be your standard curve.
3. Find a water source outdoors (or use an aquarium if necessary). Measure temperature and dissolved oxygen. Note water clarity, organic debris, flow rate, any organisms present, and other factors that may affect dissolved oxygen concentration. Repeat for more than one site if you can.
4. Draw circled points representing your field or aquarium data on the graph with your standard curve. Use your observations and measurements to answer Questions for Method A.

Data Table for Method A

PURE WATER SAMPLE NUMBER	TEMPERATURE °C	DISSOLVED OXYGEN (mg/l)
1		
2		
3		
4		
5		
FIELD SAMPLE(S) (Describe sites below.)	**TEMPERATURE** °C	**DISSOLVED OXYGEN** (mg/l)

Results for Method A:
Dissolved Oxygen as a Function of Water Temperature

DISSOLVED OXYGEN (mg/l)

WATER TEMPERATURE (°C)

Field Observations:

_____

_____

_____

_____

_____

_____

_____

Questions for Method A

1. Describe the shape of your standard curve. Is this relationship linear or curvilinear? Explain.

   _____

   _____

   _____

   _____

   _____

2. If oxygen is dissolved in cold water, what happens to the oxygen when the water warms up? Have you ever observed this phenomenon?

   _____

   _____

   _____

   _____

   _____

3. In your field (or aquarium) site, how did the data compare with your standard curve? Was the water at this site saturated with oxygen, based on its temperature, or not? Explain other factors that may have affected oxygen levels, based on your observations.

   _____

   _____

   _____

   _____

   _____

4. How might the relationship between temperature and dissolved oxygen explain the adaptive significance of symbiotic algae within the bodies of coral polyps on tropical reefs?

   _____

   _____

   _____

   _____

5. Trapping of infrared radiation by carbon dioxide in the atmosphere has the potential to warm the atmosphere a few degrees over the next century. This does not seem very significant to a terrestrial mammal like yourself, but how might this change affect tropical aquatic habitats?

   _____

   _____

   _____

   _____

METHOD B: SEDIMENT LOAD AND WATER CLARITY

[Laboratory/outdoor activity]

Research Question

How do suspended sediments affect water clarity?

Preparation

A simple turbidity meter can be made from a clear plastic tube, with inside diameter about 5 cm, and about a meter long (Figure 10). A 2-inch diameter plastic mailing tube 3 feet long will work, but extruded acrylic is sturdier. Next, you will need a black, one-hole rubber stopper to fit the bottom of your plastic tube. Use white waterproof paint to make a Secchi disc design on the inside surface (small end) of the stopper. (See Figure 6 for a standard Secchi pattern.) Insert a short piece of glass tubing into the hole in the outside surface (larger end) of the stopper. Slip a 2–3 foot length of surgical tubing over the glass tubing, making sure you have a tight fit. Place a pinchcock on the surgical tubing to control water flow. A meter stick can be used to measure depth of water in the tube. A funnel for adding water to the top of the tube and a bucket for catching water let out completes the apparatus.

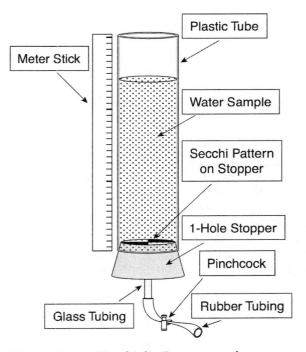

To create a standard, soil is suspended in water at a known g/l ratio. Clay or fine silt stays suspended much better than sandy soil. Silty soils may be obtained near rivers or stream banks. If stream water can be collected from your local watershed, you may wish to use soil from the campus itself. Since each soil is unique, try mixing 1 g soil per liter as a starting point. Put the soil into a 4-liter reagent bottle or plastic milk jug, add a liter of water, and shake well. Then add the rest of the water and shake again to suspend all the particles. Fill the tube to a depth of 20 cm, and take a turbidity reading as described below. If the disc is not visible, add more water. If it is very easily visible, add more soil. When you have a suspension that yields a Secchi disc reading of approximately 20 cm, make a 3-liter stock suspension at this soil/water ratio for each laboratory group.

Figure 10 A "Secchi disc" apparatus for measuring turbidity of water samples.

For the environmental water sample, collecting water from a campus lake, stream, or drainage ditch would be ideal. If not, you can collect samples or make up an unknown sample to simulate collected stream water. *Use caution when collecting water samples, especially from steep-sided channels and near fast moving water.* When filling a 4-liter bottle for a sample, be sure to avoid stirring up sediments from the bottom. If wading into the stream, stand downstream of the collecting point.

Materials (per laboratory team)

Local topographic map (or access to Web-based maps)

Turbidity apparatus (described above)

Meter stick

5-gallon plastic bucket for waste water

Large plastic funnel

1-liter graduated cylinder

4-liter reagent bottle or gallon plastic milk jug, for mixing

3-liter sample of stock soil suspension

1-liter sample of water from a local stream or lake

Access to tap water

Procedure

1. Obtain from your instructor the concentration of sediments in the stock suspension, expressed in grams of sediment per liter of suspension. Record this figure beside the label "Stock suspension concentration" in the Data Table for Method B.
2. Assemble the turbidity tube as shown in Figure 10, with the stopper securely in place and the pinchcock closed. Put the surgical tubing in the waste bucket to catch water drained from the tube, or conduct your trials outside.
3. Pick up the jug containing the stock suspension and shake it up well to suspend the sediments. Place a funnel in the top of the tube and fill it half full of the standard suspension.
4. Remove the funnel. Have one of the laboratory team hold the tube upright and look down through the water column while another operates the pinchcock. Open the pinchcock to let the water sample run slowly out. When the Secchi pattern on the stopper at the bottom of the tube is just visible, stop the water flow and measure the height of the water column from the Secchi disc pattern to the surface. If you overshoot the mark, pour in stock suspension until you cannot see the pattern, and try again. Record your turbidity measurement, in cm, in the data table beside the concentration figure you entered before.
5. In the empty jug, mix 500 ml of the stock solution with 500 ml of tap water. Call this "stock × 1/2." Divide the concentration of the stock solution by 2 and place this number (expressed in mg/l) in the second row of the data table. Shake the new suspension well, and rinse out your turbidity tube. Fill the turbidity tube about 2/3 full with the new mixture. Measure turbidity as described above. Record your turbidity measurement in the data table.
6. Empty your mixing jug into your waste bucket, and rinse it out with tap water. Then add 500 ml of stock solution to 1000 ml of tap water. Shake well. Call this suspension "stock × 1/3." Divide the concentration of the original stock solution by 3 and place this number in the third row of the data table. This time, fill your turbidity tube all the way to the top to begin your measurement. Measure and record turbidity as before.
7. Repeat step 5, but fill the rinsed mixing jug with 500 ml stock solution and 1500 ml tap water. Call this suspension "stock × 1/4." Record concentration and turbidity readings in the fourth row of the data table.
8. Repeat step 5, this time filling the mixing jug with 500 ml stock solution and 2000 ml tap water. Call this suspension "stock × 1/5." Record concentration and turbidity readings in the fifth row of the data table.
9. Complete the graph on the Results for Method B page by plotting sediment concentration (in milligrams of suspended material per liter of water) on the x-axis and turbidity tube reading (in cm) on the y-axis. Draw a smooth line through these points to produce a standard curve.
10. Collect water from at least one site on your campus, or use a water sample supplied by your instructor. Shake up the sample to ensure sediments are suspended, and then measure its turbidity.

11. Plot the turbidity readings as circled points on your graph. Based on the standard curve you have prepared, estimate sediment concentrations in your field sample or samples.
12. Consult a local topographic map, or on-line map of your region to find the streams that drain the sites you sampled. Interpret your results by answering Questions for Method B.

Data Table for Method B

SOIL SUSPENSION SERIES	SEDIMENT CONCENTRATION (mg / liter)	TURBIDITY TUBE READING (cm)
STOCK SUSPENSION		
STOCK × 1/2		
STOCK × 1/3		
STOCK × 1/4		
STOCK × 1/5		
FIELD SAMPLE(S) (Describe sites below.)	SEDIMENT CONCENTRATION (est. from standard curve)	TURBIDITY TUBE READING (cm)

Field Observations:

_____

_____

_____

_____

_____

_____

_____

Results for Method B:
Turbidity Tube Reading vs. Sediment Concentration

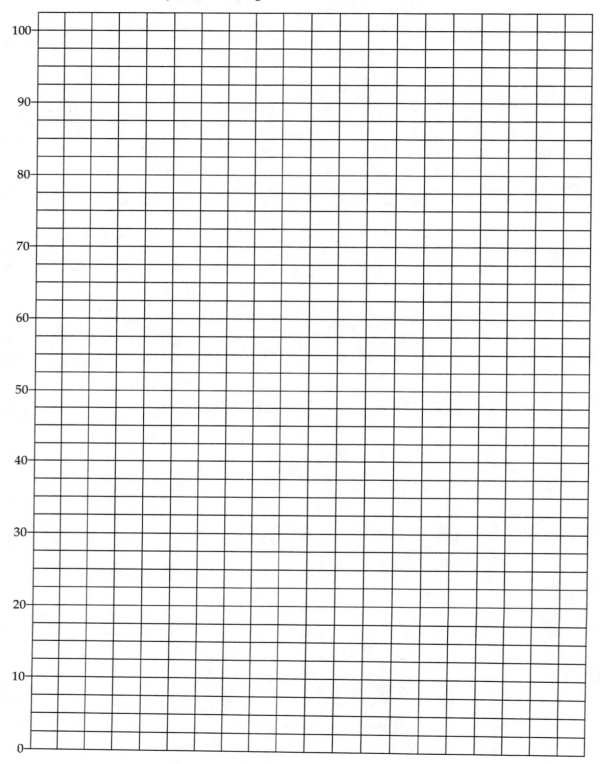

SEDIMENT CONCENTRATION (mg/l)

Questions for Method B

1. Describe the shape of your standard curve. Is this relationship linear or curvilinear? How did your data compare with solubility values mentioned in the Introduction?

   _____

   _____

   _____

   _____

   _____

2. How did your field sample(s) compare with your standard samples? Do you think turbidity at this site might be high enough to restrict photosynthesis?

   _____

   _____

   _____

   _____

   _____

3. Consult a topographic map to find the watershed in which your campus is situated. What streams or rivers drain the land you are on right now? What sources of sediment might be entering streams in this watershed?

   _____

   _____

   _____

   _____

   _____

4. Why is water clarity so important in aquatic ecosystems? What are the consequences of increased turbidity due to sediments washed into streams?

   _____

   _____

   _____

   _____

   _____

5. Suppose a lake received both suspended particles, such as silt, and dissolved particles, such as humic acids from leaf litter, after a heavy rain. Over time, will these two components of turbidity have similar or different impacts on the lake system? Explain.

   _____

   _____

   _____

   _____

   _____

METHOD C: LD$_{50}$ DETERMINATION FOR PESTICIDE
[Laboratory/outdoor activity]

Research Question
What concentrations of common pesticides are toxic to *Daphnia*?

Preparation
Daphnia cultures should be ordered close to the time they are to be used, since their culture in aquaria is sometimes difficult. *Daphnia pulex* is a good bioindicator, and somewhat easier to maintain than the larger *D. magma*. Chlorine in tap water is toxic to *Daphnia*, so water for dilutions and controls should be either spring water purchased for this purpose or aged tap water which has been left open to the air to allow chlorine to evaporate before use.

A 1% copper sulfate solution can be used as the pesticide. Under its common name of "bluestone," copper sulfate is commonly added to lakes and is even incorporated in swimming pool chemical systems to control algae. If desired, other home and garden pesticides such as carbamate insecticides or glyphosphate herbicides can be used for comparison by different laboratory groups. For the initial full-strength concentration, mix soluble pesticide according to package directions. *Make sure to follow warning labels on any pesticides used, and instruct the class to handle these chemicals carefully.*

Materials (per laboratory team)
Test tube rack

Nine 15-ml test tubes

100 ml spring water or chlorine-free water

Daphnia culture (at least 60 individuals)

Large-bore dropper for capturing *Daphnia*

1% solution of copper sulfate

10-ml pipette

8 disposable 1-ml pipettes

Pipette bulbs or pipette pumps

Vortex test tube mixer (optional)

Marking pen, for labeling test tubes

Dissecting microscope

Petri dish or depression slide

Procedure
1. Label your test tubes as shown in the top row of the following table. Take a minute to look at the pesticide concentrations that will be added to each tube. Note that each tube in the **dilution series** will hold a pesticide concentration 1/10 as concentrated as the one before. Also, note that we can express dilute concentrations as fractions of a gram per liter, or as parts of pesticide per parts of solution. One gram per liter is one part pesticide per thousand parts of the solution (or 1 **ppt**). Similarly, 0.001 gram per liter is equivalent to one part pesticide per million parts solution (1 **ppm**), and 0.000001 gram per liter is equivalent to one part pesticide per billion parts solution (1 **ppb**).

Tube Label	#1	#2	#3	#4	#5	#6	#7	#8	Control
Concentration (grams per liter)	10	1	0.1	0.01	0.001	0.0001	0.00001	0.000001	0
Concentration parts per thousand, parts per million, parts per billion	10 ppt	1 ppt	100 ppm	10 ppm	1 ppm	100 ppb	10 ppb	1 ppb	0

2. Line up your test tubes in the rack as shown in Figure 11. Using a 10-ml pipette, fill Tubes #2 through #8 with 9 ml clean water each. Add 9 ml to the control tube as well.

Serial Dilution of a Pesticide Solution for Bioassy

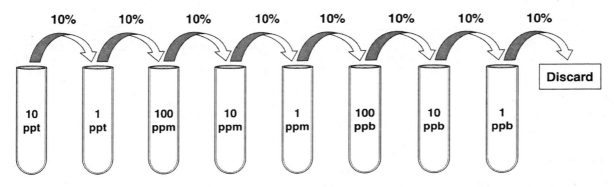

Figure 11 Serial dilution of a pesticide (copper sulfate) is accomplished by transferring 10% of each tube in the series into the next. A 1:10 dilution in each tube results in a pesticide concentration 1/10 as strong with each step.

3. Use the large pipette to measure 10 ml of 1% copper sulfate into Tube #1.
4. Using a 1-ml pipette with bulb or pipette pump, transfer 1 ml of the copper sulfate solution from Tube #1 into Tube #2. *Do not mouth-pipette chemical agents.* Mix tube #2 with a vortex or by placing the pipette into the tube and carefully stirring the solution. You have now completed a 1:10 dilution, so the concentration in Tube #2 is 1 ppt.
5. Using a new pipette, transfer 1 ml of solution from Tube #2 into Tube #3. Mix.
6. Repeat Step 5 for each tube in the dilution series, transferring 10% of each solution into the next tube to dilute by factors of 10, as shown in Figure 11. After mixing tube 8, take out and discard 1 ml so that all tubes will contain the same volume of 9 ml.
7. Using a large-bore dropper, transfer *Daphnia* into each of the eight solutions. Try to add six individuals to each tube. Note the time that *Daphnia* were exposed to the pesticide.
8. Save at least one individual *Daphnia* for observation under the microscope. Put several drops of water on a Petri dish, and place the *Daphnia* into the water. Observe under a dissecting scope. Make drawings and notes about *Daphnia* morphology and normal behavior.
9. After *Daphnia* have been exposed to copper sulfate for one hour, observe the tubes carefully. Any ill effects you notice after this brief time would be attributed to **acute toxicity**, meaning an immediate effect. Note changes in viability and behavior among the treatments.
10. If possible observe your *Daphnia* over 2–3 days to determine longer term effects of the toxin.
11. Record your results in the Data Table for Method C. Answer Questions for Method C.

Data Table for Method C

Tube Label	#1	#2	#3	#4	#5	#6	#7	#8	Control
Concentration	10 ppt	1 ppt	100 ppm	10 ppm	1 ppm	100 ppb	10 ppb	1 ppb	0
Number of viable *Daphnia* after 1–2 hours									
Number of viable *Daphnia* after 1–2 days									

Drawing of *Daphnia*

Notes on Behavior

Notes on *Daphnia* Response to Copper Sulfate:

Questions for Method C

1. What was the LD_{50} concentration for this pesticide? Does your answer depend on the time that has elapsed since exposure?

   _____

   _____

   _____

   _____

   _____

2. For routine testing of pesticides, what arguments would favor using *Daphnia* over fathead minnows? What arguments would favor fathead minnows over *Daphnia*?

   _____

   _____

   _____

   _____

   _____

3. This method determines the toxic threshold only to the nearest order of magnitude. How would you adapt this experiment to find an LD_{50} with greater accuracy?

   _____

   _____

   _____

   _____

   _____

4. *Daphnia* are representative of small aquatic invertebrates that float in freshwater lakes, eat phytoplankton, and in turn are prey for larger species. Based on your experiment, what would you say to fishing enthusiasts who propose to add copper sulfate to a lake to control aquatic "weeds"?

   _____

   _____

   _____

   _____

   _____

5. Suppose copper sulfate from an abandoned industrial site were leaking into a stream, and your tests of the effluent on live *Daphnia* show it to be in the toxic range. How might you test the hypothesis that dilution in the stream is reducing concentrations of the pollutant below threshold levels that would harm life in the stream?

   _____

   _____

   _____

   _____

   _____

FOR FURTHER INVESTIGATION

1. It does not take long to learn to identify families of macroinvertebrates and calculate your own biological index of water quality. State natural resource agencies may be able to help get you started. A few sample Web sites of water monitoring agencies who work with volunteers are included in the suggested readings.

2. Sample stream water for dissolved oxygen, temperature, and turbidity just after a rainstorm, and then repeat your sampling several times a day for two or three days afterward. How does the surge of stormwater through a stream affect water quality?

3. Use topographic maps or on-line geographic data to find the watershed you live in. How many hectares of land are drained by the river or stream nearest you? What land use is prevalent in your watershed? What might be done to improve water quality by improved watershed management?

FOR FURTHER READING

Davidson, Carlos, H. Bradley Shaffer, and Mark R. Jennings. 2001. Declines of the California Red-legged Frog: Climate, uv-B, Habitat and Pesticides Hypotheses. *Ecological Applications* 11(2): 464–479.

Ferrando, M. D., E. Andreu-Moliner, and A. Fernandez-Casalderrey. 1992. Relative Sensitivity of *Daphnia magna* and *Brachionus calyciflorus* to Five Pesticides. *Environ Science and Health Bulletin* 27(5):511–22.

National Science Foundation. 2004. "Water on the Web" http://www.waterontheweb.org/aboutus/index.html

University of Wisconsin Extension, Citizen Stream Monitoring Program. 2005. http://clean-water.uwex.edu/wav/monitoring/biotic/index.htm

U.S. Environmental Protection Agency. 2005. Biological Indicators of Ecosystem Health. http://www.epa.gov/bioindicators/html/benthosclean.html

U.S. Fish and Wildlife Service. 2001. http://www.fws.gov/endangered/features/rl_frog/rlfrog.html

Photosynthesis

*The human brain, so frail, so perishable, so full of inexhaustible
dreams and hungers, burns by the power of the leaf.*

Loren Eiseley, 1964

The flow of energy through living systems begins with plants, algae, and other chlorophyll-containing organisms that can make their own food. In other words, we depend on these organisms to live.

Autotrophic organisms make their own food. Heterotrophic organisms cannot make their own food and must get their energy from other sources.

In the process of **photosynthesis**, these autotrophic organisms capture solar energy and make glucose (Figure 1). These glucose molecules are then used both by autotrophic and heterotrophic organisms (including plants and animals) for cellular respiration.

In reality, glucose is only one product of photosynthesis. Most of the simple sugar resulting from photosynthesis is converted into starch (a glucose polymer) for storage, into sucrose for transport, or into structural components of plants [**Krogh section 8.5**].

The process of photosynthesis utilizes carbon dioxide, water, and light in the production of glucose. Oxygen is released as a by-product of this process. It is a very important by-product from the viewpoint of most organisms! You need to learn the balanced chemical equation for photosynthesis, given here. Does it look familiar? It is the opposite of aerobic cellular respiration.

$$6CO_2 + 6H_2O \xrightarrow{\text{light}} C_6H_{12}O_6 + 6O_2$$

The exercises in this chapter allow you to manipulate components of this equation. By manipulating

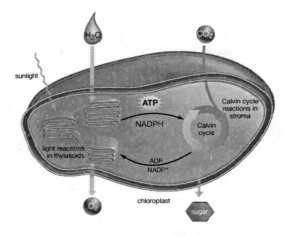

FIGURE 1   Summary of Photosynthesis in the Chloroplasts of Plant Cells.

the components, you can measure their effects on the rate of photosynthesis.

Exercise 1 EFFECTS OF CARBON DIOXIDE AND LIGHT ON PHOTOSYNTHESIS

On demonstration are four jars containing *Elodea* under different conditions, prepared in such a way that oxygen production by the plants can be measured. Two of the jars contain sodium bicarbonate (baking soda) as a source of carbon dioxide enrichment, and two of the jars contain tap water. One carbon dioxide–rich jar and one jar containing tap water were placed near a grow light. The two remaining jars were left in ambient light. Each jar is labeled with the start time of the experiment and the mass of the *Elodea* in that particular jar (Figure 2).

1. Answer Questions 1 through 5.
2. The size of the bubble is a direct measure in ml (cc) of oxygen production by the plants. When directed by your instructor, record the volume of oxygen trapped in each graduated cylinder. Record your results in Table 1.

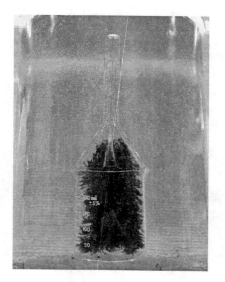

FIGURE 2   Setup for Exercise 1. If the jar is tall enough, use a 50-ml beaker to hold the *Elodea* sprigs upright. The sprigs release oxygen, which is trapped by the funnel and graduated cylinder.

3. To standardize the oxygen consumption in each jar, divide the cc of oxygen consumed by the weight of the *Elodea*, and divide again by the number of hours elapsed during the exercise. Compare these numbers in all four jars.

Questions

1. **Construct a hypothesis regarding this experiment.**

    Bubble in the light will be greatest.
    The ones in the sunlight will produce the most oxygen.

2. **State your prediction(s) regarding which *Elodea* sprigs will produce the greatest amount of oxygen.**

    the baking soda in the light will produce the most oxygen.

3. **What are the independent variables?**

    light and the amount of carbon available

4. **What is the dependent variable?**

    oxygen production

3:40

TABLE 1 OXYGEN PRODUCTION BY *ELODEA*				
Start time:				
Independent variables	**O_2 produced (cc)**	**Weight of *Elodea* (g)**	**Time elapsed (hour)**	**Standardized O_2 production (cc/g/hour)**
Water, grow light	0.442	0.9	1 hr	1.05
Water, ambient light	0	0.4	1 hr	0
Sodium bicarbonate, grow light	1.884	0.7	1 hr	2.69
Sodium bicarbonate, ambient light	0.314	0.5	1 hr	0.608

start / end
14.2 / 13.9
14.5 / 14.5 no change
14.1 / 13.5
13.5 / 13.4

5. What is the source of the bubbles?

The O_2 produced because its a byproduct of the glucose production

6. Which *Elodea* plants exhibited the greatest rate of oxygen production? Do the data support your hypothesis?

The sodium bicarbonate with light Not

7. According to your data, what has the greatest effect on the rate of photosynthesis—amount of carbon dioxide or amount of light? Explain.

The light had more effect.

8. Now consider what is lost when a tree is removed from an ecosystem (Figure 3). When plants are lost, a very important source of life-sustaining oxygen is lost. Deforestation (particularly of tropical forests) results not only in the loss of an oxygen source but also in the loss of one of the chief means by which CO_2 is removed from the atmosphere. Carbon dioxide is one of the most important of the greenhouse gases contributing to global warming [Krogh section 32.4]. To make matters worse, the burning of logging wastes releases excess CO_2 into the environment.

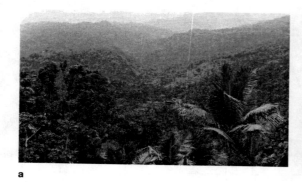 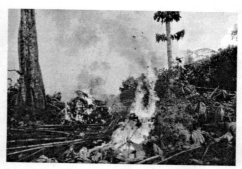

a   b

FIGURE 3   a. El Yunque Rainforest, Puerto Rico. It is the only tropical rainforest in the U.S. National Park System.
b. Destruction of Amazonian Rainforest.

Devise a way to estimate the amount of oxygen a tree can produce in a day.

9. **Assume that a resting adult human consumes about 1000 cc (ml) of oxygen per minute. At its current rate of photosynthesis, how long would it take the sprig of *Elodea* to produce enough oxygen to support a human for 1 minute? To support a human for 24 hours?**

Exercise 2 CARBON DIOXIDE CONSUMPTION BY *ELODEA*

When in an aqueous solution, carbon dioxide reacts with water to form carbonic acid.

$$CO_2 + H_2O \rightleftharpoons H_2CO_3$$

This results in lowering the solution's pH. As CO_2 is consumed by aquatic plants through photosynthesis, the level of carbonic acid in a solution will decrease, leading to an increase in pH. Thus, monitoring pH provides an indirect measure of the amount of CO_2 consumed in the photosynthesis. This experiment uses bromothymol blue (BTB), a pH indicator that turns yellow at pH < 6.0, green at pH 6.0–7.6, and blue at pH > 7.6.

1. Place 75 ml of BTB solution into a 100-ml beaker. Blow exhaled air through a straw into the BTB solution just until it changes from blue to greenish-yellow, then stop.

2. Fill four test tubes three-fourths full with CO_2-rich BTB solution.

3. Wrap two of the test tubes with aluminum foil, leaving only the top open.

4. Obtain two 2-cm sprigs of *Elodea*, and place one into a wrapped tube and one into an unwrapped tube. The other two tubes will have no *Elodea* in them—use these for comparison. Immediately finish covering the two tubes wrapped in aluminum foil.

5. Place the unwrapped test tubes directly in front of the grow light, and the wrapped ones on your lab bench.

6. Allow the tubes to "incubate" for 1 hour. Answer Questions 1 to 5 while you wait. In Table 2 record any color changes that have occurred by marking an *X* in the appropriate space.

Questions

1. **State your hypothesis regarding this experiment.**

2. **State your prediction(s).**

3. **Dependent variable:**

4. **Independent variable:**

TABLE 2 CARBON DIOXIDE CONSUMPTION IN *ELODEA*			
	Yellow: pH < 6.0	**Green: pH 6.0–7.6**	**Blue: pH > 7.6**
Elodea, light			
Elodea, dark			
No *Elodea*, light			
No *Elodea*, dark			

5. **Why did the BTB turn yellow as you blew through the straw?**

6. **What is responsible for the color change of the solutions containing *Elodea* in front of the grow light?**

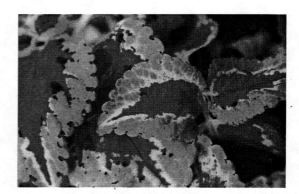

FIGURE 4   *Coleus* is a common houseplant. Use a *Coleus* plant with leaves that are red in the center, green on the margins, and white in between.

7. **Why might wrapped tubes with *Elodea* exhibit an increase in pH level?**

8. **Why might wrapped tubes with *Elodea* exhibit a decrease in pH level?**

Exercise 3   PHOTOSYNTHETIC PIGMENTS

Wear goggles. Be very careful with the boiling water and ethanol!

A variety of pigments found in plants provide the brilliant colors observed in the botanical world. In this exercise you will examine the pigments of the multicolored leaves of a common houseplant called *Coleus*, whose leaves are green and red

(Figure 4). As photosynthesis proceeds, glucose is produced, converted to starch, and then stored in the leaves. By looking at the distribution of starch in *Coleus* leaves, you can determine which pigments facilitate photosynthesis and which do not. The green color is a result of chlorophylls *a* and *b*, and pigments called *anthocyanins* impart the red color.

Anthocyanins may be extracted in boiling water, and chlorophyll may be extracted in boiling 95% ethanol. The distribution of starch may be determined by conducting an iodine test. Recall that starch reacts with iodine to produce a very dark blue or black color.

1. Obtain a leaf from each of the *Coleus* plants. One of the plants has been maintained under a grow light and the other has been kept in the dark for several days.

2. Sketch the leaves (see Question 1), indicating the distribution of the different colors.

3. Using tongs, place leaves from each plant into boiling water. After 1 to 2 minutes, remove the leaves and note their appearance.

4. Using tongs, place the leaves into boiling 95% ethanol.

Exercise great caution at this step. Ethanol is VERY FLAMMABLE!

After 1 to 2 minutes, remove the leaves and note their appearance. Remove the ethanol from the hot plate, using an oven mitt.

5. Place the leaves into petri dishes and cover them with iodine. After a reaction occurs, remove the leaves and note the distribution of starch.

Questions

1. **Sketch the color distribution in the leaves.**

   Green, red, white

2. **What happens to the water as the leaves are boiled in it?**

   Nothing happen.

3. **Describe or sketch the appearance of the leaves after boiling them in water.**

   the leaves start to lose their pinkey color

4. **What happens to the ethanol as the leaves are boiled in it?** *alcohol*

   It turns green

5. **Describe or sketch the appearance of the leaves after boiling them in ethanol.**

   It's almost all white. Like a lecture color

6. **In what manner is starch distributed throughout the leaves?**

   on the outside edges, where the green was, the starch is a black

7. **Are anthocyanins photosynthetic pigments? How do you know?**

   No, because there is no starch, so there's no photosynthesis

8. **How does the appearance of leaves from the plant kept in the dark differ from those kept in the light? What caused this difference?**

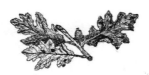

85

References and Suggested Readings

Hickman CP, Roberts LS, Hickman FM. 1984. Integrated principles of zoology, 7th ed. St. Louis, MO: Times Mirror/Mosby College Publishing. 1065 p.

Eiseley L. 1964. The hidden teacher. In: The Star Thrower (1978). New York: Times Books. pp. 82–93.

Mader SS. 2001. Biology, 7th ed. Boston: McGraw-Hill. 944 p.

Mathis ML. 1996. Biology 1400 laboratory manual, Fall 1996 edition: Biology for general education. Plymouth, MI: Hayden-McNeil Publishing, Inc. 102 p.

Perry JW, Morton D. 1995. Laboratory manual for Starr & Taggart's biology: The unity and diversity of life and Starr's biology: concepts and applications. Belmont, CA: Wadsworth Publishing Company. 515 p.

Credits

2 Dennis and Kristen Richardson
3a Dennis and Kristen Richardson
3b Jacques Jangoux/Peter Arnold, Inc.
4 Dennis and Kristen Richardson
end Barbara Nitchke

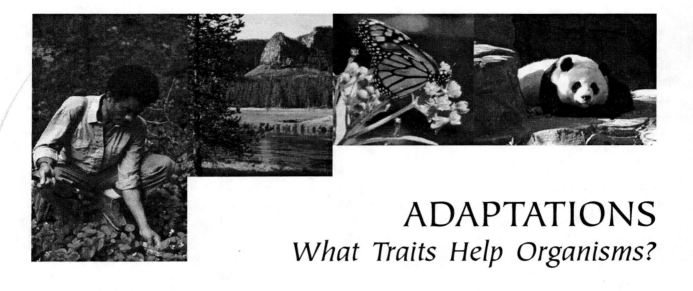

ADAPTATIONS
What Traits Help Organisms?

Objectives

In this laboratory exercise, you will test the function of a presumed adaptation by building a model butterfly or by manipulating the wing of a wind-dispersed seed. After completing this exercise, you will be able to:

- define adaptation
- discuss the importance of testing the adaptive value of organism traits
- devise an experimental question and design an experiment to answer that question
- collect and display data graphically
- interpret the data correctly
- suggest additional studies
- produce a report of your project, either in oral or poster form
- demonstrate improved skills in working with other people

Introduction

Organisms live in a physical environment—that is, in an environment that consists of certain temperatures, light environments, pH, wind conditions, etc. Many traits of organisms appear to enable organisms to survive specific physical conditions. For example, plants that live in dry environments may have thick waxy coatings on their leaves (to prevent water loss) or mammals that live in cold areas may have thick pelts (to prevent heat loss).

Many traits that appear to confer survival advantages have been tested experimentally and we have evidence that these traits actually do confer a survival advantage. For example, kangaroo rats have a variety of traits that allow them to survive the very dry environments of the western United States. These traits include appearing above ground only after dark when temperatures are lower and water loss through evaporation is lower, and having kidneys that produce very concentrated urine and colons that extract almost all the water from their feces. In that same environment, cacti have leaves reduced to thin spines to conserve moisture.

The match between organisms' traits and their physical environment results from the action of natural selection on previous generations of those organisms. Imagine a population of chickadees that varies genetically in the thickness of their feather coverings—those with more feathers will lose less heat in cold weather. Since chickadees can lose 10% of their body weight between dusk and dawn on a cold night, good insulation is important. Those chickadees with more insulation will lose less heat on a cold night and thus have a higher chance of survival than chickadees with less insulation. They may also have more energy reserves at the end of winter and then be able to put more energy into reproduction. During a cold winter, birds with less insulation will be more likely to die or less likely to reproduce in the following spring. Thus, the next generation will have more individuals with genes for thick insulation. This process, driven by natural selection (cold weather, in this case), can be called "adaptation" or "evolution." The trait that has evolved (thick insulation in this case) is called an "adaptation." (Note that the use of the word "adaptation" as both a process and as a trait can be confusing.)

But not all traits are adaptations. Some traits are by-products of other adaptations. For example, hemoglobin is a mammalian adaptation to transport oxygen in the blood. The fact that it is red in the presence of oxygen is a by-product of its chemical structure. Sickle-cell hemoglobin is an adaptation to the presence of malaria in the environment. People with one allele for sickle hemoglobin and one for normal hemoglobin are less at risk from malaria than are people with two normal hemoglobin alleles. Obviously, however, the health problems sometimes suffered by the homozygotes are not adaptations; they are by-products of the presence of sickle hemoglobin.

It is interesting to look at the traits of organisms and speculate about whether those traits confer a survival or reproductive advantage. It is even more interesting to test traits of organisms to see if they could confer a survival or reproductive advantage. The following two exercises will allow you to test either how physical traits of butterflies affect butterflies' abilities to regulate their body temperatures or how the characteristics of winged fruits affect the distance the fruits travel on the wind.

Exercise A: How Can Butterflies Get Hot Enough to Fly?

Butterflies, like many other animals but unlike mammals and birds, do not control their body temperatures internally. You, for example, will keep a constant body temperature (98.6°F = 37°C) in air that is 60°F (15.6°C) or 90°F (32.2°C)—your body produces its own heat and physiologically regulates itself to maintain a constant temperature. Butterflies do not have this same ability to produce heat internally and regulate their temperatures internally.

Butterflies can control their body temperatures—but not to the same degree as mammals. They take advantage of environmental conditions to regulate their temperatures. For example, on a cool morning, many butterflies "bask" in the sun by holding their wings flat and facing the sun. This behavior allows them to warm their flight muscles so they can fly. Most butterflies need a thoracic temperature between 75 and 112°F (25 and 44°C) for flight. When butterflies get too warm, they close their wings and turn toward the sun so they absorb less energy or move out of the sun.

Structural aspects of butterflies can also potentially affect the ability to regulate body temperature. Body color, wing color, wing size, thorax size, and presence of small hairs on the thorax can all affect a butterfly's ability to warm itself. Your job in this lab exercise is to study real butterfly specimens, note differences among species, and make model butterflies to test the importance of some aspect of body structure for heat gain in butterflies.

Light

"Visible light"—the light we can see—is emitted in large amounts from the sun. It is the part of the electromagnetic spectrum with wavelengths from 390 to 710 nanometers (nm). Each photon that arrives contains energy. The more photons there are in a light beam, the more energy in the beam and the greater the "irradiance"—a term that physicists use when common language would say "intensity." Irradiance is measured in watts/m². As light moves further away from its source, it tends to spread out and its irradiance (intensity) decreases (that is, the further you are from a light source, the fewer photons and the less energy there is in a given area).

When light photons hit an object, two things can happen—either the photon is reflected or the photon is absorbed. If the photon is reflected, the object does not gain or lose energy. If the photon is absorbed, the object gains the energy that was carried by the photon and its temperature will increase. (Some of that energy will be re-radiated to the environment as "heat.")

Visible light is composed of waves with different wavelengths. We detect these different wavelengths as different "colors." Shorter wavelengths have greater energy than do longer ones. "Violets" are the shortest wavelengths we can see. "Ultraviolets" are the wavelengths just shorter than violet. "Reds" are the longest wavelengths we can see. "Infrareds" are the wavelengths just longer than red.

Objects appear "colored" to us when they reflect particular wavelengths. Objects that are "white" reflect all wavelengths. Plants appear "green" because they absorb most wavelengths but reflect waves that are approximately 525–600 nm. Black objects absorb all wavelengths.

Heat and temperature

Atoms are constantly in motion. The more energy they have, the faster they move. We measure this motion as "temperature" and call it "heat." It is important to realize that all molecules have "heat"—there is "heat" in an ice cube because even water molecules in ice have a certain amount of movement.

If two objects with different temperatures are placed in contact with one another, the warmer one (the one with a higher temperature) will lose energy (heat) to the other object. If they are left in contact long enough, they will equilibrate to the same temperature. Two examples are what happens to a hot cup of coffee or a cold can of soda. The coffee cools and the soda warms. (Remember that there are molecules in the air that are gaining or losing energy to the liquids and their containers.)

Energy transfer occurs in three ways: direct contact and energy transfer between molecules (conduction); movement of a liquid or gas past an object (convection); and by transfer of photons (radiation).

Assignment

Your job in this lab exercise is to first study real butterfly specimens and note differences among species. Next you will hypothesize how some aspect of body structure affects heat gain by butterflies. You may choose to vary either morphology (and test heat gain in one environmental condition) or vary the environmental conditions (and test heat gain of one aspect of morphology). After planning your experiment, you will make model butterflies, conduct the experiment, and test your hypothesis. You will then prepare either an oral or poster presentation.

Methods

1. Inspect the butterfly specimens and/or pictures. Look for differences among species and think about how various aspects of butterfly structure might affect heat gain.

2. In your group, discuss the traits that differ among butterfly species and may be suitable for experimentation.

3. Examine the "butterfly" that has already been constructed (Fig. 1).

4. Plan your experiment (see the section "Hints for Designing Experiments" at the end of this lesson).

   - what characteristic of butterflies or the environment will you manipulate?
   - what effect do you predict your manipulation will have?
   - what will you measure? (The answer to this may seem obvious—temperature—but the answer may not be quite that simple. There are other variables you could measure. Even if you are measuring temperature, you need to think about when you will measure temperature—for example, after 1 minute or some other short time or after temperature is stabilized?)

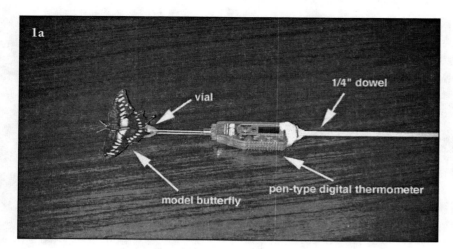

Fig. 1. The dorsal (a) and ventral (b) sides of a model butterfly. The vial contains water and the tip of the temperature probe; it is sealed with ear putty. The vial and temperature probe are taped to a 1/4'' dowel. A butterfly model is then attached to the vial with tape.

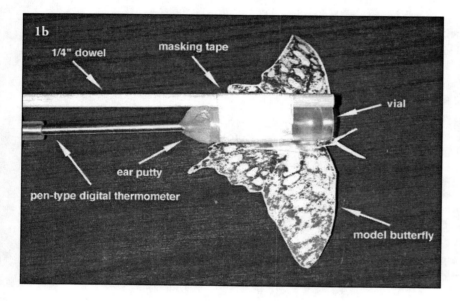

- what will be the experimental conditions (e.g., air temperature, light, distance from light, air speed)?
- how many replicates will you need?
- how will you graph your data?

5. Explain your experimental design to your instructor and modify it as necessary.

6. Conduct your experiment.

7. Graph and interpret your data (see the section "Hints for Graphing and Interpreting Your Data" at the end of this lesson). Was your prediction upheld?

8. Evaluate the results of your experiment in the light of the question "What is the likely adaptive trait of this characteristic with respect to butterflies' ability to regulate their body temperatures?" Include in your evaluation a quantitative assessment of the differences between groups (e.g., "After 5 min, the temperature of the experimental group was 10% higher than the control group.")

9. Prepare your oral presentation or poster on your project.

Making a butterfly

1. Use tape to attach a glass or plastic vial at the end a dowel, with the open end of the vial facing away from the end of the dowel.

2. Place the temperature probe in the vial, making sure the tip of the probe is in the center of the vial. Tape the probe to the dowel so that it will stay still.

3. Fill the vial with water and seal it with "ear putty."

4. Attach butterfly wings and thorax to the vial using a glue stick or hot glue.

5. If necessary, cover the top of the vial with petroleum jelly to help prevent leaks.

Exercise B: How Can Trees Disperse Their Seeds by Wind?

Unlike most animals, adult plants cannot move. Instead, they move their seeds. Why should plants move their seeds? Well, if the seeds just fell under the plant, there would be intense competition among siblings as the seeds germinated and grew. If, instead, the seeds are dispersed over a wider area, competition among siblings is reduced. Furthermore, the seeds differ genetically from the parent plant and dispersal may place them in a microhabitat that suits them better than the microhabitat of the parent.

Plants move their seeds in a variety of ways. Some have explosive fruits that, when dry, hurl the seeds away from the parent plant. Others depend on animals to move the seeds, either by attaching to the outside of the animal or by inducing the animal to swallow the fruits and seeds, digest the fruit, and defecate the seeds. Still other plants depend on wind to blow the fruits away from the parent tree.

Plants that depend on wind to disperse their fruits have some appendage to the seed that provides lift. Dandelions and milkweeds have fluffy white appendages that help the seed float on the wind. Other fruits have flat areas ("wings") that provide lift. Examples of winged fruits are ash (*Fraxinus*), maple (*Acer*), and tulip-poplar (*Liriodendron tulipifera*). If you look at different winged fruits, you will see that they vary in wing shape, wing area, placement of the seed in relation to the wing, and seed mass. These variables all affect how far a given fruit will travel in a wind of a given speed.

As are seen in many ecological and evolutionary situations, plants face trade-offs in producing fruits. Compared to small seeds, large seeds are more likely to produce a successful plant. However, these large seeds are 1) more energetically expensive to produce (and therefore fewer seeds can be produced), 2) potentially more attractive to seed predators (and therefore likely to experience a lower survival rate), and 3) likely to disperse shorter distances (and therefore be more likely to compete with siblings). Compared to fruits with small wings, large-winged seeds are likely to travel further. However, the larger the wing, the more energy that must be directed to tissue that does not directly lead to offspring production.

Wing loading is a measure that relates mass and area of a fruit. The lower the mass in relation to wing area, the lower the wing loading and the farther the fruit will move. Wing loading is calculated by dividing the mass of the fruit by its area.

Assignment

Your job in this lab exercise is to study fruits of wind-dispersed trees, note differences among species, and modify the fruits to determine how some aspect of the fruit affects the distance traveled.

In the first part of the exercise, you will calculate the wing loading of one species. Different groups might work with different species of plants.

In the second part of the exercise, you will manipulate some aspect of the fruit that will change the wing loading, predict how the alteration will affect the distance moved, measure how it affects dispersal distance, and evaluate the adaptive value of the trait you manipulated. You will need to find a way to drop the seeds from a point and then measure how far they travel.

Measuring and manipulating wing loading

You can measure wing loading by tracing the area of a fruit onto graph paper and then counting the number of boxes covered by the fruit. This process gives you the area of the fruit. Then weigh the same fruit. Calculate wing loading by dividing the fruit mass by the area. Then calculate the mean wing loading from at least 25 fruits.

You can easily manipulate wing loading by removing some wing area (cut it off with scissors), adding some wing area (glue on small pieces of copier paper, crepe paper, or other wings), adding mass (add small pieces of masking tape). You will need to decide what percentage change you would like to produce and then calculate how much change you need to make. For example, if you want to double the wing loading, you would need to either double the mass of the fruit or halve the area of the fruit (however, this is too big a change to try experimentally). Because it is too time-consuming to calculate wing loading for individual fruits, you can do the calculation on the mean wing loading for the species and then change all your fruits by the same amount (e.g., add the same mass, or remove the same area of wingspan).

For ease of identification of your fruits, lightly spray paint the fruits. Paint the altered and unaltered fruits different colors. This procedure will help you quickly identify the fruits after they are dispersed.

Methods

1. Collect winged fruits.

2. Measure the wing loading of a species.

3. If time allows, compare the wing loadings of different winged species. How different are they? This information can help you plan your experiment.

4. Plan your experiment (see the section "Hints for Designing Experiments" at the end of this lesson).

   - what characteristic of fruits will you manipulate?
   - what effect do you predict your manipulation will have?
   - what will you measure? (The answer to this may seem obvious—distance traveled—but make sure you know *exactly* what you will do.)
   - what will be the experimental conditions (e.g., place, height from which seeds are dropped, amount of wind)?
   - how will you drop the fruits?
   - how many fruits will you need to test?
   - how will you graph your data?

5. Explain your experimental design to your instructor and modify it as necessary.

6. Conduct your experiment.

7. Graph and interpret your data (see the section "Hints for Graphing and Interpreting Your Data" at the end of this lesson). Was your prediction upheld?

8. Evaluate the results of your experiment in the light of the question "What is the likely adaptive trait of this fruit characteristic with respect to dispersal or winged fruits?" Include in your evaluation a quantitative assessment of the differences between groups (e.g., "The mean distance dispersed decreased 10% when 5% more mass was added to fruits").

9. Prepare your oral presentation or poster on your project.

Hints for Designing Experiments

1. Make sure you vary only one factor.

2. Make sure everyone in the group knows what you are measuring/counting so that everyone will make the same measurement.

3. Make sure you have replication (how much is enough?—ideally you will have 10 or more trials per experimental or control group but you may have to decrease this number because of time, space, or material constraints). One trial in the butterfly adaptation experiment will be one test with an individual butterfly model. You can use each model several times, but you should make several models for each test group. One trial in the wind-dispersal experiment will be the release of a group of fruits (both experimental and control) at one time.

4. Ask one simple, small question, not a large complex one.

Hints for Graphing and Interpreting Your Data

Variability abounds in systems studied by biologists and this variability necessitates the use of replication in experiments, the graphing of data, and the use of statistics in data analysis. (If there were no variability, we could conduct one trial and know an answer.)

Graphs are a way for you to "see" your data. Visualizing data helps in choosing statistical tests and understanding your results.

In this laboratory exercise, you are most likely to use histograms, bar graphs, or line graphs to compare the data you generate. If these graphs don't seem to make sense with your data (which is a possibility), check with your laboratory instructor.

Histograms are most useful when you want to compare mean (or median) values for two groups and you want to see how the data are distributed. Histograms show the frequency of occurrence of data points. You will be able to see both the central tendency (mean or median) and the variability in the sample. With data of this sort, you would likely use a t-test to statistically analyze the data. Examine Fig. 2 for examples of histograms.

An alternative to the histogram is a bar graph (sometimes called a column graph by computer software programs). This type of graph (Fig. 3) is often convenient but you lose the ability to see the distribution of data points. You can give the viewer some indication of the variability in the data if you add "error bars" (variance, standard deviation, or standard error) onto the columns. I prefer histograms over bar graphs when you first inspect your data because it gives a better sense of variability in the data. However, bar graphs can be useful in presentations (but add error bars), especially if you have more than two columns.

Line graphs are useful when you have two measured variables. In this laboratory exercise, time might be an *x*-axis that is used frequently (Fig. 4). When you make a graph like this, plot each trial individually and connect the points. This procedure will allow you to see if the different trials overlap. Statistics can be rather complicated for this data set; a repeated-measures analysis of variance is often the best choice. Alternatively, a t-test on the model temperature after 10 minutes can be conducted.

Once you have plotted your data, you will need to ask yourself if there are differences between the groups. Ideally, you would conduct a statistical test, but time and material constraints might prevent you from generating a big enough sample size. Your instructor will tell you whether you will conduct statistical tests on your data. The availability of computers and statistical packages makes it very easy to conduct statistical tests (but care must be exercised to know which test to use).

The basic idea of statistics is actually easy to understand. The most important thing about using statistics is knowing how to interpret a result. Even if you don't conduct a statistical test, you should think about your data as if you were conducting a statistical test.

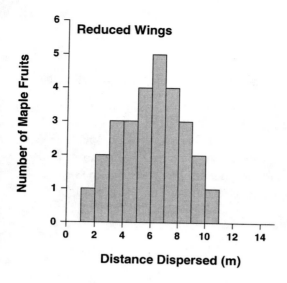

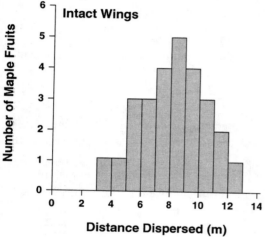

Fig. 2. Two histograms describing the distance that maple fruits dispersed. One group contained intact maple fruits while the other contained maple fruits whose wing area had been reduced by 10%. Each vertical bar represents the number of fruits that moved a given distance (for example, 5 of the intact fruits moved 8–9 m). Note that the lower graph (intact fruits) is shifted to the right relative to the upper graph—indicating that removal of wing area reduced the dispersal distance. If you were to conduct this experiment you would want to use a bigger sample size and disperse the fruits in several different trials. This type of graph can show if the effects of two treatments were different (the distribution of one group is shifted left or right of the other) or if the variability in the two groups was different (perhaps one of the distributions was quite narrow and the other was quite broad).

Fig. 3. The same data as shown in Fig. 2, but plotted as a bar graph. In this graph, the vertical bar represents the mean of a group (the mean distance traveled by reduced-wing fruits is 5.6 m). The vertical lines (error bars) show the standard deviation, a measure of variability. This graph is convenient for presentations but does not provide as much information on the distribution of data points as does a histogram.

Fig. 4. Comparison of heat gain by black vs. yellow butterfly models when placed 20 cm from a halogen light. Each line connects the temperature of a butterfly model at specific times after the models were place in front of the halogen light. Note that two trials for each model color are plotted and that the temperature appears to rise more quickly for the black models than for the yellow ones. If you were to conduct this experiment, you would want to conduct more trials.

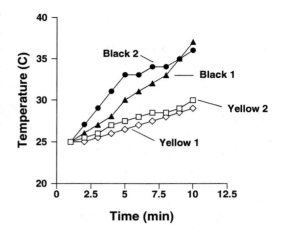

The easiest way, I find, to think about statistics is to ask yourself the following question, "What is the likelihood that differences between two groups are solely due to random variation in the system?" If differences are small, random variation may well account for them. If differences are big (and you have controlled your conditions appropriately), random variations probably can't account for the differences—the cause is likely to be your experimental variable!

Think about the two answers possible to your question:

1. "The likelihood that the difference between the two groups is solely due to random variation is high." This statement means that you will conclude that your experimental variable had little effect. Thus, differences between the two groups are not significant.

2. "The likelihood that the difference between the two groups is due to random variation is low." This statement means that you will conclude that your experimental variable caused the differences between the two groups. Thus, differences between the two groups are significant.

EXERCISE 14
ADAPTATIONS ASSOCIATED WITH FEEDING

Organisms exhibit many unusual and interesting adaptations associated with obtaining nutrients. Plants are extremely versatile in the synthesis of organic compounds. They capture the energy of sunlight and use it to build organic compounds from carbon dioxide and water. At the same time, they obtain other inorganic nutrients (nitrogen, phosphorus, potassium, etc.) from the physical environment and build them into amino acids, nucleotides, vitamins, and other vital compounds.

Different species of plants require, and have evolved to use, different quantities of nutrients. These species distribute themselves according to the availability of nutrients in the environment. Plants have undergone certain adaptations which permit them to maximize the uptake of nutrients. For example, leguminous plants, such as alfalfa, clover, peanut, and soybean are able to thrive in soil deficient in nitrogen. The roots of these plants are inhabited by nitrogen-fixing bacteria which are capable of taking nitrogen from the air in the soil and converting it into ammonia. The bacteria utilize the ammonia to build amino acids and the excess ammonia is utilized by the plants. Both organisms benefit from the process since the plants get needed ammonia and the bacteria get sugars and a place to live. This type of interaction is termed mutualism and is discussed in the next exercise.

From the standpoint of organic compound synthesis, animals are not as versatile as plants. Their energy requirements and principal sources of the carbon skeleton must be met through the principal types of food molecules; carbohydrates, lipids, protein and nucleic acids. Another group of essential organic nutrients, required by animals, are vitamins. As noted previously, these organic substances are not produced by the animal and are essential in minute amounts for normal growth and metabolism. Because they cannot be synthesized by a particular animal they must be obtained from its food or absorbed by the intestines after they have been produced by microorganisms residing there (see mutualism, Exercise 15). Thus animals rely directly or indirectly on plants as their sources of energy and matter.

In this laboratory exercise you will study some unusual and interesting adaptations associated with obtaining nutrients.

CARNIVOROUS, HERBIVOROUS, AND OMNIVOROUS MAMMALS

Heterotrophs, which cannot synthesize all of their necessary organic molecules, exhibit many unusual and interesting adaptations associated with obtaining these nutrients. A herbivore, like a cow, has teeth that are limited by the jaw margins. Like all mammals, the teeth are set in deep sockets and are differentiated into various types. Cows lack upper incisors and canines, and have a large gap (diastema) separating the cheek teeth (premolar and molars) from the cropping teeth (incisors). Cows do not have much force in the front of the mouth, thus dental battery is located in the back of the jaw. Hence the presence of the diastema. In the cow the cheek teeth are expanded into a grinding battery, and the cropping teeth work against a horny lip. The articulation of the jaw with the skull is made by a flattened facet which allows the jaws to move sideways to grind up vegetable matter.

The cow, like other herbivores, has other modifications that adapt it into an effective herbivore: a relatively large digestive tract, most of which is concerned with digesting cellulose matter from vegetation. Cellulose is a carbohydrate consisting of repeated glucose units. It is the main constituent of the cell walls of green plants. In addition, cows have microorganisms in their gut. These microorganisms aid in the digestion of cellulose while living in the intestines of their host. Like cows, most herbivores are unable to produce the cellulases (cellulose-digesting enzymes) needed to break cellulose into glucose. Exceptions include the little insects called silverfish, earthworms, and the wood-boring shipworm. Vertebrate herbivores have long legs and are fleet of foot to help them run away from carnivores.

A carnivore, like a cat, has on each side of the upper jaw three incisors at the anterior followed by one canine, three premolars, and one very small molar. The jaws articulate and the last premolar of the upper jaw and the lower molar intersect to form a specialized shearing mechanism. The cat uses the canines to catch and kill its prey, using the molars to cut it up. It does not have flattened, crowned crushing teeth. Each half of the lower jaw is hinged to the skull by a transverse roller that fits tightly into a trough on the underside of the skull which hampers rotary action of the jaw. Consequently, the jaws move mainly up and down to slice and tear meat. The cat has a short digestive system and the stomach is not complex. The stomach secrets enzymes that act primarily on meat which does not require much digestive action. The cat favors fish as food but eats birds and mammals readily. Since the prey of cats consists of other animals, composition of its food is very similar to that of their own bodies, with little of the waste that results from eating plants with their tough cell walls. In fact, predators, such as mountain lions, lions, tigers, and other wildcats receive so many usable nutrients from meat that they may not have to eat more than four or five times a week.

The cat can see with little or dim light. Its sense of smell is relatively poor. However, it can distinguish the odor of various foods. The cat's senses of hearing and touch are well

developed. The eyebrows, whiskers, hairs on the cheek, and fine
tufts of hair on the ears are all extremely sensitive to
vibratory stimulation. It also has a long tail that aids in the
maintenance of balance, and specialized claws that adapt it,
effectively, to a life of active hunting.

Materials needed: (Per Group)
    (1) Skull of a cat
    (2) Skull of a cow
    (3) Human skull

Procedures:
    (A) Examine the skull of a cat and note that the teeth are
limited to the jaw margins. Are the teeth set in deep sockets
and differentiated into various types? In each side of the upper
jaw there are normally three incisors at the anterior end,
followed by one canine, three premolars, and one very small
molar. How many teeth are in the lower jaw? Articulate the jaws
and note how the last premolar of the upper jaw and the lower
jaw molar intersect to form a specialized shearing mechanism.
Which teeth are used to catch and kill the prey? Do carnivorous
animals, such as cats and dogs, swallow their food without
chewing it? Note that each half of the lower jaw is hinged to
the skull by a transverse roller that fits tightly into a trough
on the underside of the skull. Does this aid or hamper grinding
movements? Cats have a short alimentary canal, a simple stomach,
a small cecum. Do most meat-eating animals usually empty their
stomach before eating again? Explain the adaptation of having a
short digestive tract?
    (B) Examine the skull of a cow--the cow is an herbivore.
Note that the cow's skull lacks upper incisors and canines, but
has a large gap (diastema) separating the cheek teeth (premolars
and molars) from the cropping teeth (incisors). What is the
benefit of a diastema? Do cows' teeth have a larger grinding
surface than cats' teeth? Why the difference? Note that the
articulation of the jaw with the skull is made by a flattened
facet. Does this articulation allow rotary action of the lower
jaw? Is the herbivorous diet easier for animals with ridged
teeth, long legs, and a long digestive tract? Why? Are cows
more gregarious and peaceful than cats? Explain.
    (C) Which spends most of their waking hour eating,
herbivores or carnivores? Which spends more energy in actually
obtaining their food, herbivores or carnivores? Which hardly
bothers to chew its food? Which has a relatively rich fecal
material containing undigested detritus?
    (D) Study the human skull. Do humans have large flattened
molars like that of cows? Do humans have the sharp pointed
canines exactly like those of cats? The digestive system of
humans is long but not as long as that of an herbivore. On the
other hand, the human digestive tract is more extensive than
that of a carnivore. Are humans herbivores, carnivores, or

omnivores? At what level of a food chain are humans?

PARASITES

A parasite is distinguished from a herbivore or carnivore in several ways. A parasite is usually much smaller than its prey and it usually does not kill its host. A parasite lives very much on the interest of its host, while a predator lives on the capital.

Endoparasites are internal parasites which feed within the host. The common tapeworm (Taenia) is a parasite that attaches itself to the intestinal wall of its host with the aid of suckers and sometimes hooks (Figure 14-1). The worms have no digestive system; they absorb molecular nutrients directly through their body surfaces. Tapeworms are composed of many sections, or proglottid, arranged in series to form a long ribbon. Each proglottid contains both male and female reproductive organs. Consequently, the animal is hermaphroditic. Specimens of tapeworms can be up to 50 feet long. The knoblike head or scolex is equipped with hooks and suckers for anchorage. The worms are very abundant as parasites in practically all mammals and many other vertebrates. Their adaptation includes a complex life cycle (Fig. 14-2). If the tapeworm eggs are accidentally eaten by a cow, hog, fish or some other vertebrate, the eggs are carried by the blood to the muscles, where they encyst. If a person eats insufficiently cooked meat of these infected animals, the eggs pass to the intestine, where they mature into adult tapeworms. They cause illness not only by encroaching on food supply of their host but also by producing wastes and by obstructing the intestinal tract.

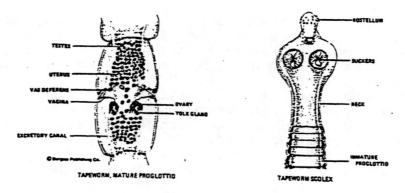

TAPEWORM, MATURE PROGLOTTID   TAPEWORM SCOLEX

Figure 14-1. Tapeworms are composed of many sections called proglottid, arranged in series to form a long ribbon. The knoblike head or scolex is equipped with hooks and suckers for anchorage.

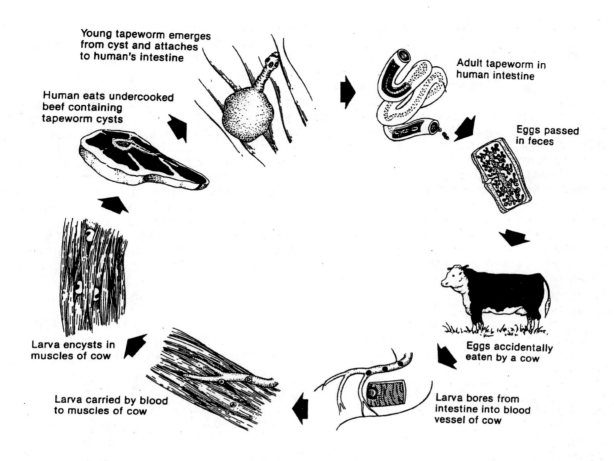

Figure 14-2. The infectious cycle of the endoparasitic tapeworm
(Taenia). If tapeworm eggs are accidentally eaten by a cow, hog,
fish or some other vertebrate, the eggs are carried by the blood
to the muscles, where they encyst. If a person eats
insufficiently cooked meat of these infected animals, the eggs
pass to the intestine, where they mature into adult tapeworms.

The dog tick (Dermacentor) is an ectoparasite of mammals
which feeds from the outside of the host (Fig. 14-3). The body
of an unengorged tick is oval, flattened dorso-ventrally and
indented on the anterior margin for reception of gnathosoma
which bears the mouth parts. Posterior to the gnathosoma is a
large region called idiosoma, which bears the walking legs and
other body parts. The tick pierces the skin with the chelicerae
and inserts the hypostome into the injury. The hypostome serves
to anchor the parasite to its host. The chelicerae and hypostome
have teeth. The sexes are separate with females being larger
than the males. This parasite requires three hosts. The larvae
first feed on host number one (rodents) and then drop from the
host to molt into nymphs. The nymphs attach themselves to host

number two (either the same or a different rodent) engorge and then drop off the host to molt to adults. The adults will later find a third host (any dog, fox, ungulate, or even people), feed, and drop off. Ticks generally feed from 2 to 11 days. Females are known to live more than one year without a blood meal, nymphs 300 days, and larvae for about a month. The ticks are a cosmopolitan group and they surpass all arthropods in the number and variety of diseases which they transmit to man and his domestic stock in temperate and tropical countries. Ticks can transmit to humans the causative agents of such diseases as the Japanese river fever, Tsutsugamushi disease, Colorado tick fever, Russian encephalatis, relapsing fever, and tick paralysis. Recently, spirochete bacteria has been found to cause Lyme disease. This particular bacteria are carried by deer ticks, which transmit them to humans by bites. Symptoms of Lyme disease are fevers, chills, sore muscles, arthritis, and general malaise. Some persons get a red skin rash within a month after a tick bite.

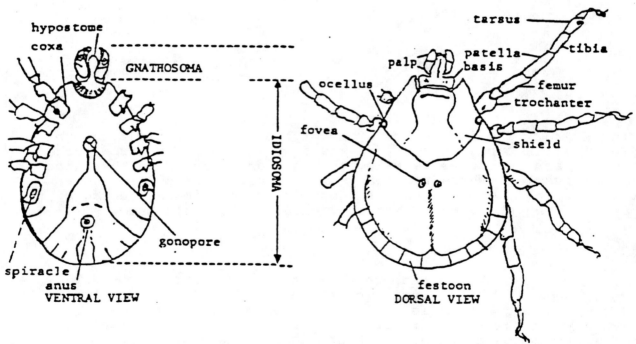

Figure 14-3. The tick (Dermacentor) is an ectoparasite attaching itself to its host for 3 to 27 days before dropping off. The ticks surpass all arthropods in the number and variety of diseases that they transmit to humans and livestock in temperate and tropical countries.

Materials needed: (Per Group)
    (1) Slides of tapeworm scolex & larvae encysted in
        muscle (Taenia)
    (2) Slides and specimen of the tick (Dermacentor)
    (3) Compound microscope

Procedures:
    (A) Study a prepared slide of the common tapeworm (Taenia)
under the scanning power of the microscope. Find the knoblike
head or scolex (Fig. 14-1). Note the series of sections (or
proglottids), which arise from the neck of the scolex. Each
proglottid contains both testis and ovaries (hermaphroditism).
What is the advantage of having both sexes in the same
individual? The tapeworm attaches itself to the intestinal wall
of its host with the aid of suckers and sometimes hooks
(rustellum). Can you see these structures? Does the parasite
have a digestive tract of its own? What kind of surface
structures would you expect the tapeworm to have to avoid being
digested by its host's digestive enzymes? Examine a prepared
slide of tapeworm larvae encysted in muscle. If a person eats
the raw or undercooked meat of the tapeworm's host, in what
stage is the tapeworm transmitted? Examine the preserved
specimens of the tapeworm which can be up to 50 feet long. Is
the tapeworm an endo- or ectoparasite? The infectious cycle of
the Taenia is demonstrated in Fig. 14-2.
    (B) Study specimens of the tick (Dermacentor) which is a
common parasite of mammals such as dogs, sheep, humans, etc.
Place the specimen on the stage of the microscope and examine it
under the scanning power. Note that the tick's body is divided
into only two regions: gnathosoma and idiosoma (Fig. 14-3).
Which region bears the mouth parts? Which regions bears the
legs? Look carefully at the gnathosoma and note the chelicerae
and snout-like hypostome. The tick pierces the skin with the
chelicerae and inserts the hypostome into the hole. The
hypostome serves to anchor the parasite to its host. Do the
chelicerae and hypostome have teeth? Is the tick hermaphroditic?
How long can the parasite survive without food? What is the
significance of this long survival period? Is the tick an endo-
or ectoparasite?

CARNIVOROUS PLANTS

    Some plants, such as the sundew, pitcher plant, and Venus's
flytrap, are also carnivorous. The sundew has gland-tipped hairs
with sticky, sweet fluid. Small insects are attracted to and
become stuck to a few of these hairs. The rest of the hairs then
bend over so that most of the hairs touch the insect's body.
Digestion is accomplished by secretion of enzymes onto the
trapped animal.
    The pitcher plant is another carnivorous plant. It

possesses pitcher-shaped leaves that collect small amounts of rainwater. The trapped water also has enzymes which digest proteins. Insects are attracted into the pitcher plant by the bright colors of nectar. Downward-pointing stiff hairs trap the prey. The insects eventually die and the soluble amino acids of the animals are then absorbed by the plant.

The leaves of Venus's flytrap are highly specialized, closing rapidly when "triggered" to catch insects. The mechanical trap is triggered by touching two or the three hairs in the center of a partially closed leaf lobe. Again, the leaf secretes protein-digesting enzymes, and absorbs nourishment for the plant from the dead insect.

None of the carnivorous plants are totally dependent on insects as a source of food, but in nature they grow larger and produce more flowers and seeds when animals are available to them. They use animals principally as a source of nitrogen and phosphorus. The plants are found in nature in bogs in which these elements are in short supply.

Materials needed: (Per Group)
(1) Specimens of the sundew (Drosera), pitcher plant (Sarracenia), and Venus flytrap (Dionera)
(2) Toothpicks, solution of carbohydrate, solution of protein, vestigial wings of the fruit fly, pH paper, slide and coverslip, and compound microscope

Procedures:
(A) Examine the carnivorous plant sundew. Add some vestigial wings of a fruit fly and attempt to observe their capture. Observe the sundew catch and enfold the wings. Gently touch the sundew's fine hairs with the three toothpicks, one soaked with protein, another with carbohydrate, and the other plain. What happens? How long does it take for the leaf involved to return to normal (hours or days)?
(B) The pitcher plant is another carnivorous plant. Look at the water in the pitcher plant. Dip a small piece (about 3 inches long) of pH paper into the water. After the paper is wet, remove it immediately. What is the pH of the water? In the water, you may find some small organisms which exist without getting digested. Make a wet-mount and study these microorganisms. How do these organisms aid the pitcher plant? How does the pitcher plant trap its prey?
(C) Observed the Venus flytrap.
(D) What color are the carnivorous plants? Are they totally dependent on animals as a source of food? What is the survival advantage of carnivorous behavior?
(E) If animal food is not available, do carnivorous plants suffer from malnutrition or undernourishment?
(F) Place microscope in the cabinet with lowest objective clicked in place. Return the prepared slides to proper box and in the proper sequence. Clean up your area.

Describing a Population

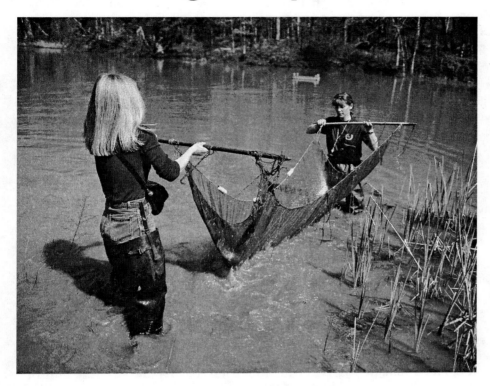

Figure 1   A fish population is sampled by seining.

INTRODUCTION

Ecology is the ambitious attempt to understand life on a grand scale. We know that the mechanics of the living world are too vast to see from a single vantage point, too gradual to observe in a single lifetime, and too complex to capture in a single narrative. This is why ecology has always been a quantitative discipline. Measurement empowers ecologists because our measuring instruments extend our senses, and numerical records extend our capacity for observation. With measurement data, we can compare the growth rates of trees across a continent, through a series of environmental conditions, or over a period of years. Imagine trying to compare from memory the water clarity of two streams located on different continents visited in separate years, and you can easily appreciate the value of measurement.

Numerical data extend our capacity for judgment too. Since a stream runs muddier after a rain and clearer in periods of drought, how could you possibly wade into two streams in different seasons and hope to develop a valid comparison? In a world characterized by change, data sets provide reliability unrealized by single observations. Quantitative concepts such as averages, ratios, variances, and probabilities reveal ecological patterns that would otherwise remain unseen and unknowable. Mathematics, more than any cleverly crafted lens or detector, has opened our window on the universe. It is not the intention of this text to showcase math for its own sake, but we will take measurements and make calculations because this is the simplest and most powerful way to examine populations, communities, and ecosystems.

Sampling

To demonstrate the power of quantitative description in ecology, you will use a series of measurements and calculations to characterize a **population**. In biology, a population is defined as a group of individuals of the same species living in the same place and time. Statisticians have a more general definition of a population, that is, all of the members of any group of people, organisms, or things under investigation. For the ecologist, the biological population is frequently the subject of investigation, so our biological population can be a statistical population as well.

Think about a population of red-ear sunfish in a freshwater lake. Since the population's members may vary in age, physical condition, or genetic characteristics, we must observe more than one representative before we can say much about the sunfish population as a group. When the population is too large to catch every fish in the lake, we must settle for a **sample** of individuals to represent the whole. This poses an interesting challenge for the ecologist: how many individuals must we observe to ensure that we have adequately addressed the variation that exists in the entire population? How can this sample be collected as a fair representation of the whole? Ecologists try to avoid **bias**, or sampling flaws that overrepresent individuals of one type and underrepresent others. If we caught our sample of sunfish with baited hooks, for example, we might selectively capture individuals large enough to take the bait, while leaving out smaller fish. Any estimates of size or age we made from this biased sample would poorly represent the population we are trying to study.

After collecting our sample, we can measure each individual and then use these measurements to develop an idea about the population. If we are interested in fish size, we could measure each of our captured sunfish from snout to tail (Figure 2). Reporting every single measurement in a data table would be truthful, but not very useful, because the human mind cannot easily take in long lists of numbers. A more fruitful approach is to take all the measurements of our fish and systematically construct a composite numerical description, or **statistic**, which conveys information about the population in a more concise form. The average length (also called the **mean** length) is a familiar way to represent the size of a typical individual. We might find, for instance, that the mean length of sunfish in this lake is 12.07 centimeters, based on a sample of 80 netted fish. The symbol μ is used for the mean of all fish in the population, which we are trying to estimate in our study. The symbol $\bar{x}$ is used for the mean of our sample, which we hope to be close to μ.

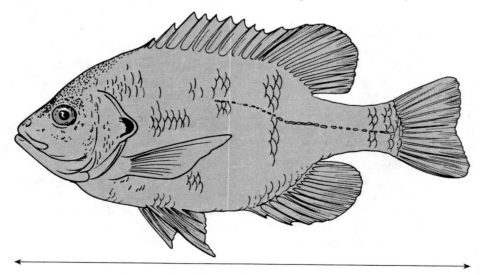

Figure 2   Measuring length of red-ear sunfish.

Means are useful, but they can be misleading. If a sunfish population were made up of small one-year-old fish and much larger two-year-old fish, the mean we calculate may fall somewhere between the large and small size classes—above any of the small fish, but below any of the large ones. A mean evokes a concept of the "typical" fish, but the "typical" fish may not actually exist in the population (Figure 3).

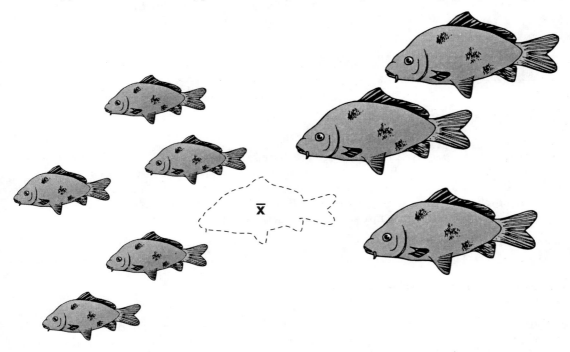

Figure 3   The calculated mean describes a "typical" fish that does not actually exist in a population composed of two size classes.

For this reason, it is often helpful to use more than one statistic in our description of the typical member of a population. One useful alternative is the **median**, which is the individual ranked at the 50th percentile when all data are arranged in numerical order. Another is the **mode**, which is the most commonly observed length of all fish in the sample.

Picturing Variation

After calculating statistics to represent the typical individual, it is still necessary to consider variation among members of the population. A **histogram** is a simple graphic representation of the way individuals in the population vary.

Check your progress:

If you wanted to determine the average height of students on your campus, how would you select a sample of students to measure?

Hint: Avoid statistical bias by making sure every student on campus has an equal chance of inclusion in the sample.

107

To produce a histogram:

1. Choose a measurement variable, such as length in our red-ear sunfish. Assume we have collected 80 sunfish and measured each fish to the nearest millimeter.
2. On a number line, mark the longest and shortest measurements taken from the population (Figure 4). The distance on the number line between these points, determined by subtracting the smallest from the largest, is called the **range**. In our example, the longest fish measures 15.7 cm, and the shortest fish measures 8.5 cm, so the range is 7.2 cm.

$$\text{Range} = 15.7 \text{ cm} \quad 8.5 \text{ cm} \ = \ 7.2 \text{ cm}$$

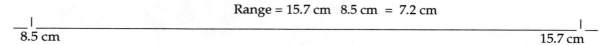

8.5 cm   15.7 cm

Figure 4   Number line indicating range.

3. Next, divide the range into evenly spaced divisions (Figure 5). In our example, each division of the number line represents a **size class**. It is customary to use between 10 and 20 size classes in a histogram. For our example, we will divide the range of sunfish sizes into 15 units of 0.5 cm each. The first size class includes fish of sizes 8.5 through 8.9 cm. The next size class includes fish of sizes 9.0 through 9.4 cm, and so forth to the last size class, which includes sizes 15.5–15.9.

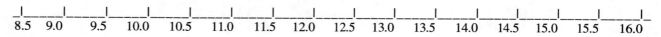

8.5   9.0   9.5   10.0   10.5   11.0   11.5   12.0   12.5   13.0   13.5   14.0   14.5   15.0   15.5   16.0

Figure 5   Number line divided into size classes of 0.5 cm.

4. Having established these size classes, it is possible to look back at our measurement data and count how many fish fall into each class. The number of individuals falling within a class is the **frequency** of that class in the population. By representing each measurement with an X, as shown in Figure 6, we can illustrate frequencies on the number line.
5. On the completed histogram illustrated in Figure 7, the stack of X-marks is filled in as a vertical bar. The height of each bar represents the proportion of the entire population that falls within a given size class.

Check your progress:

In the sample described by the histogram (Figure 7), how many fish measured between 10.0 and 10.4 cm?

Answer: 4

Figure 6 Counting frequencies.

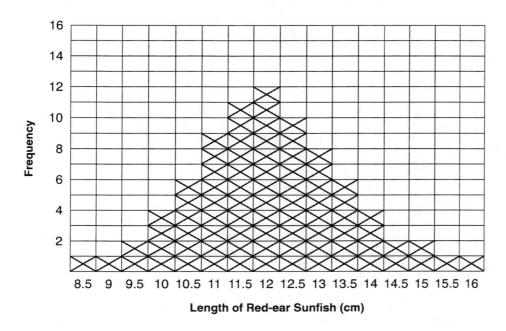

Length of Red-ear Sunfish (cm)

Figure 7 Histogram of fish lengths.

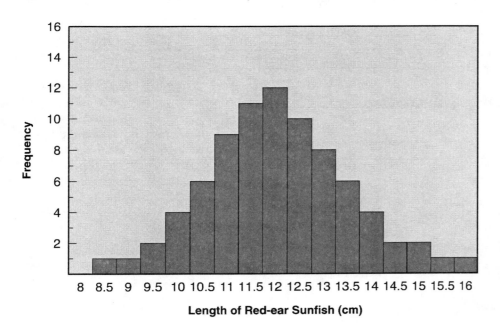

Length of Red-ear Sunfish (cm)

Describing the Pattern of Variation

Notice that in our sample histogram, the most common size classes are near the middle of the distribution (Figure 7). Extremely large and extremely small fish are rare, while intermediate sizes are more common. The "skyline" of the histogram fits under a bell-shaped curve that is symmetrical, and has characteristic rounded "shoulders" and "tails" that taper to the ends of the range in a predictable way. Statisticians call this shape a **normal distribution** (Figure 8).

Figure 8 Normally distributed data.

Length of Red-ear Sunfish (cm)

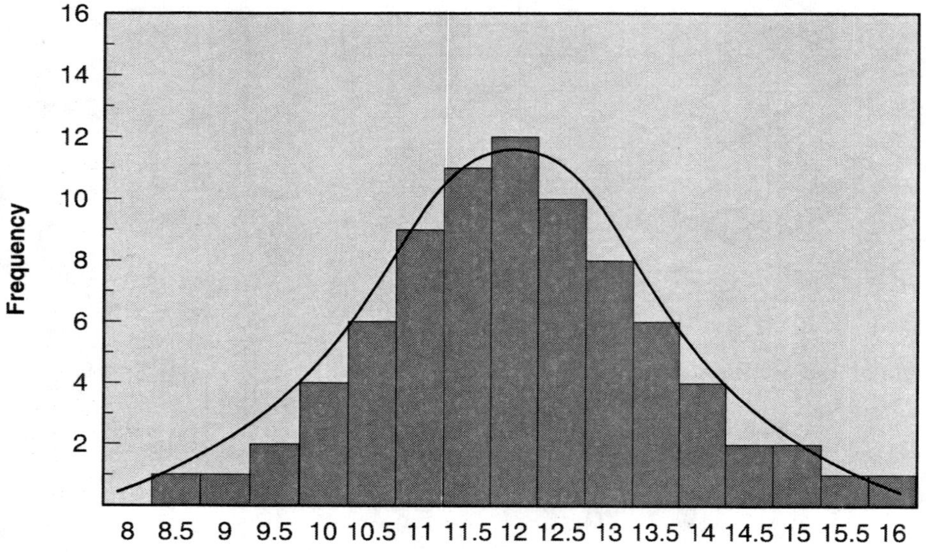

This pattern of variation is common in nature, and is encountered quite often when one effect is influenced by many independently acting causes. Since size in fish is influenced by temperature, diet, water purity, and

Figure 9a Normally distributed data.

Length of Red-ear Sunfish (cm)

many other factors, it would not be surprising to find that sizes of fish in a mixed-age population are normally distributed. Because the normal distribution is encountered so commonly, many of the statistical tools ecologists use to test hypotheses assume that variations in their data are distributed in this bell-shaped form. Models and tests based on this kind of distribution are called **parametric statistics**.

If the histogram of variation is lopsided, has more than one peak, or is too broad or too narrow, then parametric tests should not be used (Figure 9). **Non-parametric tests** have been developed for these kinds of data. Because the nature of variation in your measurements is critical to further analysis, it is always a good idea to draw a histogram and compare your data to a normal distribution before taking your analysis any farther.

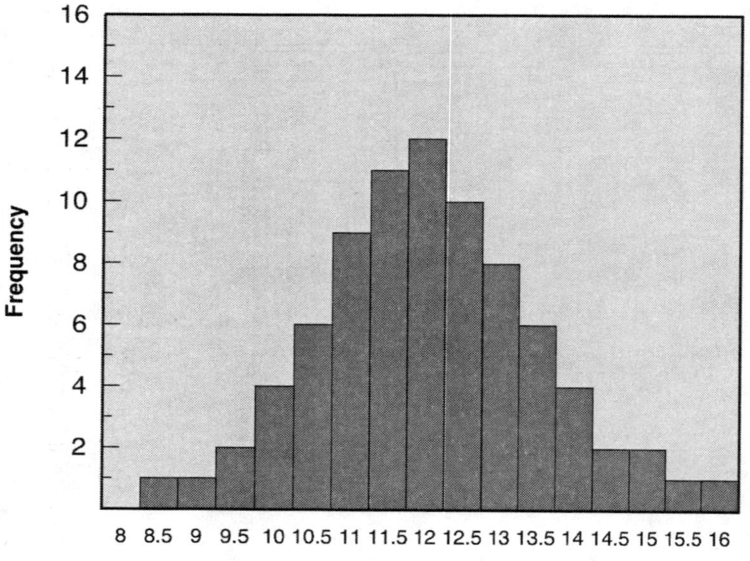

Measuring Variation

How trustworthy is the mean that we calculate from our sample of fish? Two factors come into play. First, the **sample size** is critical. If fish in the lake vary a lot in size, a mean calculated from a small sample (say 10 fish) might be significantly off the mark. By chance, the 10 fish you caught might be larger or smaller than the average population size you are trying to describe. If the sample is expanded to 1000, it is much more likely that your calculated mean will accurately reflect the population average. *A fundamental principle of data collection is that the sample size must be large enough to eliminate sampling errors due to chance departures from the population mean.* To keep our thoughts straight, we use **n = size of the sample**, and **N = size of the entire population**. N is usually unknown, but can be estimated in a number of ways.

Figure 9b Bimodally distributed data.

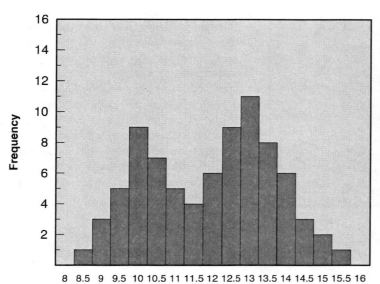

Length of Red-ear Sunfish (cm)

How large, then, must a sample be? This depends on the amount of variation in the population. Samples taken from a fish farm where all the fish are nearly the same size will give reliable estimates, even if the sample is small. In a natural population with a great range of sizes, the sample has to be expanded to ensure that the larger variation is accounted for. Thus, *the more variable the population, the larger the sample must be* to achieve the same level of reliability. It becomes obvious that we need a statistic to measure variation.

Figure 9c Skewed data.

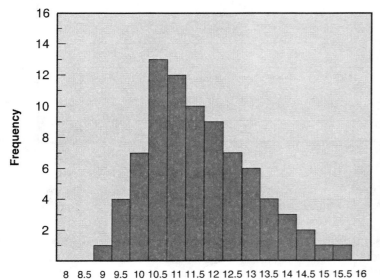

Length of Red-ear Sunfish (cm)

To measure the amount of variation around the mean, we use a statistic called the **standard deviation (abbreviated s.d.)**. To distinguish between our sample and the entire population, we define **s = the standard deviation of the sample**, and **σ = the standard deviation of the whole population**. The standard deviation is expressed in the same units as the original measurements, which would be cm in our hypothetical fish study. A standard deviation can thus be shown as a portion of the range on a number line. In normally distributed populations, 95% of all individuals fall within 1.96 standard deviations from the mean. This means that the X-axis of a histogram can be marked off in four standard deviation units (two above the mean, and two below), and roughly 95% of the observations will fall within that region (Figure 10).

Figure 10 Standard deviations.

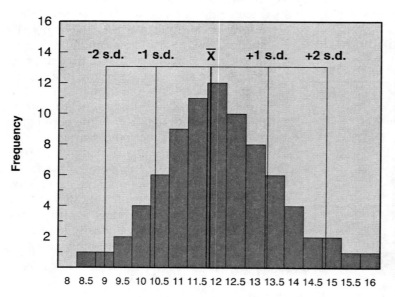

Length of Red-ear Sunfish (cm)

To calculate the size of a standard deviation, it is actually easier first to calculate a related statistic called the **variance**. The variance is the square of the standard deviation, so we use **s^2 = the sample variance**, and **σ^2 = the popula-tion variance.** Calculation of the variance is based on the difference between each observation and the mean. If all these differences are squared, and we calculate an average of the squared values, we have the variance. It is good to remember that the units on variance are the original measurement units squared. If we measure length in cm, then the sample variance is reported in cm^2. In calculating standard deviations, we take the square root of the variance, which returns us to our original measurement units, which is length in cm.

$$s = \sqrt{s^2} \quad \text{and} \quad \sigma = \sqrt{\sigma^2}$$

s = sample s.d. σ = population s.d.

s^2 = sample variance σ^2 = population variance

Check your progress:

If the standard deviation of a population is 9.5, what is the population variance?

Answer: 90.25

Confidence Intervals

There is one more statistic that you will find useful when characterizing the typical sunfish in your population with a mean. Incorporating sample size and variation, you can develop a measure of reliability of the mean called the **standard error (S.E.)**.

Assume there are 25 people in your ecology class. Each of you goes to the same pond sometime this week, nets a sample of sunfish in the same way, and measures 100 randomly selected individuals. Releasing the fish unharmed, you return to the lab and calculate a mean and standard deviation from your data.

Everyone else does the same. Would your 25 sample means be identical? No, but the variation in means would be considerably smaller than the total variation among the fish in the pond. Repeating a sampling program 25 times is usually impractical. Fortunately, statistics gives us a way to measure reliability when we have only one mean developed from one sample. The variation among all possible sample means can be predicted from the sample size and the variation in the pond's sunfish with the following formula:

Looking at the formula, you can see the relationship between error in our estimate, the variability of sunfish, and the sample size. The smaller the S.E. is, the more trustworthy your calculated mean. Note that the sample standard deviation is in the numerator of the calculation, so the more variable the size of the fish, the less accurate the estimate you made from a random sample. Sample size, on the other hand, is in the denominator. This implies that a large sample makes your mean more reliable. The formula shows that the more variable the population, the larger our sample must be to hold S.E. to an acceptably small margin of error.

$$\text{S.E.} = s/\sqrt{n}$$

S.E. = standard error of the mean

s = standard deviation of sample

n = sample size

Since standard errors tend to be normally distributed, it is a safe assumption that 95% of the variation in all possible means will fall within 1.96 S.E. of the actual mean. This fact can be used to calculate a 95% confidence interval as follows:

95% Confidence interval = $\bar{x} \pm 1.96$ S.E. $\bar{x}$ = **sample mean**

S.E. = standard error

Check your progress:

Calculate the 95% confidence interval for a mean of 14.3, derived from a sample of 25, where the standard deviation is 4.2. What are the upper and lower limits?

Answer: 12.65 to 15.95

To go back to our number line, the confidence intervals can be represented by brackets around the sample mean. A 95% confidence interval implies that the actual population mean (μ) will fall within the brackets you have placed around your estimate ($\bar{x}$) 95% of the time under these experimental conditions (Figure 11).

The importance of confidence limits cannot be overstated. Scientifically, it is dishonest to report a sample mean by itself. Without sharing with your readers the sampling methods, sample size, and the variability of the population, there is no way for them to know how accurately the sample mean represents the population. *Always report sample size with a mean, and add some measure of variation.* Any of the statistics representing variation (s, s², or S.E.) can be reported, since any one of these can be used to calculate the other two.

Figure 11 95% Confidence interval.

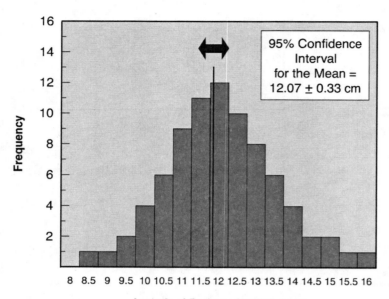

Length of Red-ear Sunfish (cm)

METHOD A: SEED WEIGHTS IN LEGUMES

[Laboratory activity]

Research Question
How does a population of bean seeds vary in weight around the typical individual?

Preparation
At a grocery or health food store, find uncooked dried beans of several types. Bags of approximately one pound are ideal. Lima beans, pinto beans, navy beans, and great northern beans are good varieties to choose from. If possible, buy unsorted beans; these best represent the population in the field.

Materials (per laboratory team)
1-pound bag of beans (Different teams can use different varieties.)

Analytical balance or electronic balance sensitive to 0.01 g (.001 g is preferable).

Plastic weighing tray, as large as the balance will accommodate.

Electronic calculator.

Procedure

1. *Recognize that each seed in your bag is a living organism*, harvested from a mature population of annual plants. If sprouted and allowed to mature, these seeds would produce a population of bean plants. Seed weight is of obvious interest in cultivated plants like beans, but is also biologically important in wild plants, because seed weight affects the distribution, growth rate, and survivorship of the seedling. (For example, see Rees, 1995.) Since the maternal plant must expend more resources to produce larger seeds, plants making larger seeds cannot produce as many. In most plant species, the tradeoff between larger seeds vs. more numerous seeds is influenced by genetics, subject to **natural selection**, and varying from one plant type to another. Identifying mean and variance for seed weights is therefore a biologically important description of **reproductive strategy** in a plant population.

2. *Develop a sampling plan*. Your sample size will be 80 beans. If you were to cut the bag open and take only the beans on top, would your "grab sample" represent the population fairly? If larger and smaller beans settled differently during shipment, this approach might result in a biased sample. Spreading beans out on a lab bench, mixing them to randomize your sample, and selecting a sample of 80 closest to your side of the bench is a much better way to ensure that your sample is random.

3. *Weigh and record observations*. Weigh each of the 80 beans in your sample. How accurate is your balance? To simplify your data analysis, record weights in milligrams. (For example, rather than 0.087 g, record 87 mg. If your balance measures only to two decimal places, record 0.09 g as 90 mg. Enter your measurements on the calculation page at the end of this chapter.

4. *Produce a histogram*. Following the example in the introduction, produce a histogram of seed weights.

5. *Calculate descriptive statistics*. Calculate a mean, standard deviation, standard error, and confidence limits for this population, following the directions in the introduction and appendices.

6. *Interpret your data*. What does the histogram show about the variation of seed weights in this species? Answer the Questions for Discussion that follow the calculation pages. Considering the way natural selection works, would you always expect symmetrical frequency distributions of seed weights?

7. *Check your accuracy*. Working with your lab partners, count every bean in the bag. Then weigh the whole population by weighing the beans in a plastic weighing tray and subtracting the weight of the tray. If your balance cannot accommodate all the beans at once, divide the population into parts, weigh each part, and then sum the separate measurements. Divide the weight of the whole population by the number of beans in the population to calculate the population mean. How does the population mean compare with the sample mean you calculated in step 3? Does the population mean fall within the 95% confidence intervals you calculated?

METHOD B: NEEDLE LENGTH IN CONIFERS

[Outdoor/indoor activity]

Research Question

How do pine needles vary in length, within and among individual trees?

Preparation

Locate several pine trees of the same species. Needles of other conifers may be used if they have needles long enough to be measured with a mm ruler. If students cannot collect needles themselves, pine branches can be collected elsewhere, or "pine straw" can be obtained from garden supply firms. Laboratory teams can be larger if greater effort is required to collect and measure 80 needles.

Materials (per laboratory team)

Metric ruler, marked in mm

Electronic calculator

Procedure

1. *Recognize that each needle is a plant organ, developing according to a genetic program influenced by local conditions.* A pine needle performs the critically important job of photosynthesis, producing chemical energy for the tree. A needle's length may affect how well it functions. If the needle is too short, it may lack sufficient photosynthetic tissue to produce an adequate supply of food. On the other hand, needles that are too long may fail to transport fluids adequately to the tip, or may accumulate too much ice and break limbs in the winter. Limits on size and shape affecting the performance of a biological trait are called **functional constraints**, and they help explain why many species' characteristics remain within predictable ranges.

   Although needles on the same tree might be expected to conform to a genetically determined size, differences in leaf age, sun or shade, exposure to wind, temperature, or moisture supplied through a particular branch could influence needle length. Within a tree, we can recognize many sources of variation. Among a population of trees, the variation is probably even larger because different trees have different genes, and probably experience a broader range of environmental conditions.

2. *Develop a sampling plan.* Your sample size will be 80 needles. If you have access to a grove or row of pine trees, spread out your needle collection to include roughly equal numbers of needles from each of the trees. A sampling plan that includes the same number of needles from each tree in your research area is a **stratified sample**. Decide whether you will pull a needle from a live branch, or pick a fallen needle from the ground. Since pine needles decay slowly, they can be collected long after they fall from the tree. If you collect live needles from the tree, will you always collect from a low branch, or will you try to collect equal numbers of needles from high, mid-height, and low branches?

   When collecting needles from pines (genus *Pinus*) you will discover that their needles come in bunches. The brown collar of tissue holding the bunch of needles together is actually a dwarf branch, called a fascicle. The number of needles in a bunch is fairly consistent, and is useful for identification. For instance, the Eastern White Pine (*Pinus strobus*) typically has five needles per fascicle, while Red Pine (*Pinus resinosa*) has two.

Make a decision about which needle in the bunch you will measure. The longest one? A randomly selected one? What will you do if you encounter a broken needle? Whatever your method, it would be best to measure only one needle per bunch, so that your data are not clustered into subgroups. Pull the needles apart carefully, so as not to introduce error by breaking the base, and measure one needle according to your predetermined sampling plan.

If the population of pines on campus is not that large, collect all your needles from the same tree. Recognize that this collection is not a population in the biological sense, since only one individual produced all the needles. However, your collection is a population in the statistical sense, because you are measuring a sample of a much larger number of needles. Different lab groups can sample different trees so that you can compare your results.

3. *Measure lengths and record observations.* Measure each of the 80 needles in your sample. How accurate is your ruler? Record needle lengths in mm on the data pages at the end of this chapter. Follow directions on the calculation page to produce a histogram of needle lengths and to calculate a mean, standard deviation, standard error, and confidence limits for this population.

4. *Interpret your data.* What does the histogram show about the variation of needle lengths in this species? Answer the Questions for Discussion that follow the calculation pages. Think about the functional constraints on evergreen needles, and try to explain the distribution of sizes in biological terms.

5. *Check your accuracy.* Compare your results with those of another lab group. Does the other group's calculated mean fall within the 95% confidence limits you calculated for your own mean? If not, how do you interpret the difference between the two estimates? If two groups sampled from the same tree, then significant differences in your calculated means might result from sampling bias, measurement error, or calculation mistakes. If two lab groups sampled different trees, then the data may reflect real biological differences between the two trees.

CALCULATIONS (METHOD A OR B)

1. *Enter your 80 measurements* (x_i) in the second column of the table, recording 20 measurements per page on each of the next four pages. You may wish to split up this task, with each member of your team completing a page.

2. *Sum the measured values* (seed weight or needle length) for each page, and then complete calculation of the mean ($\bar{x}$) in the calculation box at the end of the tables by adding totals from all four pages and dividing by the sample size (n = 80).

3. Subtract the mean from each of the 80 measurements to *obtain the deviation* above or below the average. (Deviation from mean for sample i = d_i.)

4. *Square each deviation* (d_i^2).

5. *Add up all the squared deviations* on each page, then sum the totals for the four pages to compute the sum of squared deviations (Σd^2).

6. Divide the sum of squared deviations by (sample size − 1) to *calculate the sample variance* (s^2).

7. Take the square root of the variance to *calculate the standard deviation* (s).

Describing a Population

Data (Methods A or B)—Page 1

Sample number (i)	Measurement for sample i (x_i)		Deviation (d_i)		Squared deviations (d_i^2)
1		$- (\bar{x}) =$		$^\wedge 2 =$	
2		$- (\bar{x}) =$		$^\wedge 2 =$	
3		$- (\bar{x}) =$		$^\wedge 2 =$	
4		$- (\bar{x}) =$		$^\wedge 2 =$	
5		$- (\bar{x}) =$		$^\wedge 2 =$	
6		$- (\bar{x}) =$		$^\wedge 2 =$	
7		$- (\bar{x}) =$		$^\wedge 2 =$	
8		$- (\bar{x}) =$		$^\wedge 2 =$	
9		$- (\bar{x}) =$		$^\wedge 2 =$	
10		$- (\bar{x}) =$		$^\wedge 2 =$	
11		$- (\bar{x}) =$		$^\wedge 2 =$	
12		$- (\bar{x}) =$		$^\wedge 2 =$	
13		$- (\bar{x}) =$		$^\wedge 2 =$	
14		$- (\bar{x}) =$		$^\wedge 2 =$	
15		$- (\bar{x}) =$		$^\wedge 2 =$	
16		$- (\bar{x}) =$		$^\wedge 2 =$	
17		$- (\bar{x}) =$		$^\wedge 2 =$	
18		$- (\bar{x}) =$		$^\wedge 2 =$	
19		$- (\bar{x}) =$		$^\wedge 2 =$	
20		$- (\bar{x}) =$		$^\wedge 2 =$	
Page 1 Sum $\Sigma(x_i) =$		**Page 1 Sum of Squared Deviations** $\Sigma(d_i^2) =$			

Data (Methods A or B)—Page 2

Sample number (i)	Measurement for sample i (x_i)		Deviation (d_i)		Squared deviations (d_i^2)
21		$- (\bar{x}) =$		$\wedge 2 =$	
22		$- (\bar{x}) =$		$\wedge 2 =$	
23		$- (\bar{x}) =$		$\wedge 2 =$	
24		$- (\bar{x}) =$		$\wedge 2 =$	
25		$- (\bar{x}) =$		$\wedge 2 =$	
26		$- (\bar{x}) =$		$\wedge 2 =$	
27		$- (\bar{x}) =$		$\wedge 2 =$	
28		$- (\bar{x}) =$		$\wedge 2 =$	
29		$- (\bar{x}) =$		$\wedge 2 =$	
30		$- (\bar{x}) =$		$\wedge 2 =$	
31		$- (\bar{x}) =$		$\wedge 2 =$	
32		$- (\bar{x}) =$		$\wedge 2 =$	
33		$- (\bar{x}) =$		$\wedge 2 =$	
34		$- (\bar{x}) =$		$\wedge 2 =$	
35		$- (\bar{x}) =$		$\wedge 2 =$	
36		$- (\bar{x}) =$		$\wedge 2 =$	
37		$- (\bar{x}) =$		$\wedge 2 =$	
38		$- (\bar{x}) =$		$\wedge 2 =$	
39		$- (\bar{x}) =$		$\wedge 2 =$	
40		$- (\bar{x}) =$		$\wedge 2 =$	
Page 2 Sum $\Sigma(x_i) =$		**Page 2 Sum of Squared Deviations**		$\Sigma(d_i^2) =$	

Data (Methods A or B)—Page 3

Sample number (i)	Measurement for sample i (x_i)		Deviation (d_i)		Squared deviations (d_i^2)
41		$- (\overline{x}) =$		$\wedge 2 =$	
42		$- (\overline{x}) =$		$\wedge 2 =$	
43		$- (\overline{x}) =$		$\wedge 2 =$	
44		$- (\overline{x}) =$		$\wedge 2 =$	
45		$- (\overline{x}) =$		$\wedge 2 =$	
46		$- (\overline{x}) =$		$\wedge 2 =$	
47		$- (\overline{x}) =$		$\wedge 2 =$	
48		$- (\overline{x}) =$		$\wedge 2 =$	
49		$- (\overline{x}) =$		$\wedge 2 =$	
50		$- (\overline{x}) =$		$\wedge 2 =$	
51		$- (\overline{x}) =$		$\wedge 2 =$	
52		$- (\overline{x}) =$		$\wedge 2 =$	
53		$- (\overline{x}) =$		$\wedge 2 =$	
54		$- (\overline{x}) =$		$\wedge 2 =$	
55		$- (\overline{x}) =$		$\wedge 2 =$	
56		$- (\overline{x}) =$		$\wedge 2 =$	
57		$- (\overline{x}) =$		$\wedge 2 =$	
58		$- (\overline{x}) =$		$\wedge 2 =$	
59		$- (\overline{x}) =$		$\wedge 2 =$	
60		$- (\overline{x}) =$		$\wedge 2 =$	
Page 3 Sum $\Sigma(x_i) =$		**Page 3 Sum of Squared Deviations** $\Sigma(d_i^2) =$			

Data (Methods A or B)—Page 4

Sample number (i)	Measurement for sample i (x_i)		Deviation (d_i)		Squared deviations (d_i^2)
61		$-(\bar{x})=$		$^2=$	
62		$-(\bar{x})=$		$^2=$	
63		$-(\bar{x})=$		$^2=$	
64		$-(\bar{x})=$		$^2=$	
65		$-(\bar{x})=$		$^2=$	
66		$-(\bar{x})=$		$^2=$	
67		$-(\bar{x})=$		$^2=$	
68		$-(\bar{x})=$		$^2=$	
69		$-(\bar{x})=$		$^2=$	
70		$-(\bar{x})=$		$^2=$	
71		$-(\bar{x})=$		$^2=$	
72		$-(\bar{x})=$		$^2=$	
73		$-(\bar{x})=$		$^2=$	
74		$-(\bar{x})=$		$^2=$	
75		$-(\bar{x})=$		$^2=$	
76		$-(\bar{x})=$		$^2=$	
77		$-(\bar{x})=$		$^2=$	
78		$-(\bar{x})=$		$^2=$	
79		$-(\bar{x})=$		$^2=$	
80		$-(\bar{x})=$		$^2=$	
Page 4 Sum $\Sigma(x_i)=$		**Page 4 Sum of Squared Deviations**		$\Sigma(d_i^2)=$	

Calculation of Variance and Standard Deviation

Page 1 Sum $\Sigma(x_i) =$		**Page 1 Sum of Squared Deviations** $\Rightarrow$ $\Sigma(d_i^2) =$	
Page 2 Sum $\Sigma(x_i) =$		**Page 2 Sum of Squared Deviations** $\Rightarrow$ $\Sigma(d_i^2) =$	
Page 3 Sum $\Sigma(x_i) =$		**Page 3 Sum of Squared Deviations** $\Rightarrow$ $\Sigma(d_i^2) =$	
Page 4 Sum $\Sigma(x_i) =$		**Page 4 Sum of Squared Deviations** $\Rightarrow$ $\Sigma(d_i^2) =$	
Grand Total $\Sigma(x_i) =$		**Grand Total Sum of Squared Deviations** $\Rightarrow$ $\Sigma(d_i^2) =$	
Mean $\Sigma(x_i) / n =$		**Sample Variance** $\Rightarrow$ $s^2 = \Sigma(d_i^2)/(n - 1) =$	
	Standard Deviation $\sqrt{s^2} =$		

(Methods A or B)

Summary of Results (Method A or B)

Sample Size (n) =   _____

Sample Mean ($\overline{x}$) =   _____

Sample Variance (s^2) =   _____

Standard Deviation (s) =   _____

Standard Error (S.E.) =   _____

95% Confidence Interval for Mean =   _____

Histogram of Group Data

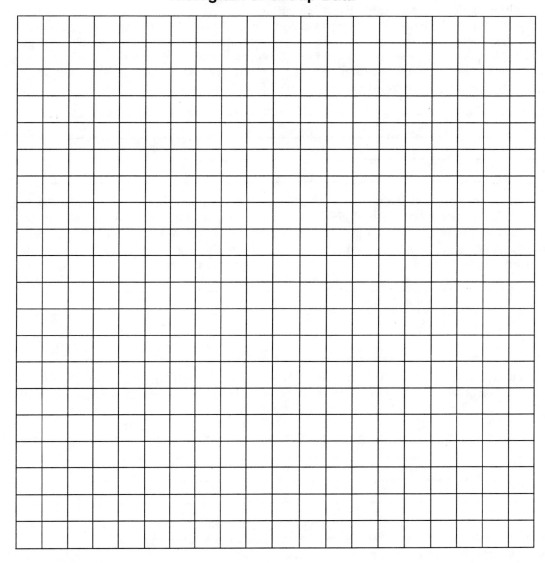

FREQUENCY

MEASUREMENT CLASSES

Questions (Method A or B)

1. In comparing your histogram to the description of a normal distribution, did you seem to get a fairly good fit to the bell-shaped curve, or did you notice a different pattern? Describe these differences: was the histogram bimodal? skewed? flattened or sharply peaked? If you performed statistical tests using these data, would you be comfortable using parametric statistics, or would you seek a non-parametric alternative? Do you think you made enough measurements to make a certain judgment on this question, or do you think more data may be needed?

   It was bimodal – two numbers are closed – bell shaped curve ∩ you use parametric statistics when you have a normal distribution

2. The mean, median, and mode are three different statistical approaches to describe the "typical" individual in a population. Recall that the median is the middle observation when all data are arranged in numerical order, and the mode is the most commonly observed measurement. Based on your data, does it matter very much which of these three statistics is used? Explain how this answer is related to your answer for the previous question.

   Sure, if you use the mode it will give you a better idea of the population. If you use the median, it would not be actual.

   mode   mode
   mean circled *this individual doesn't exist*

3. What do the variance, S.E., or standard deviation estimates tell you about your population that the mean does not tell you? Why is it important to report some measure of variation, along with the sample size, whenever you report a calculated mean?

   It tells you how the population varies. It helps your data be more accurate.

4. Variation among members of a population can lead to natural selection, but only if two conditions are met: First, the trait must be relevant to an individual's survival and/or reproductive rate. Second, variation in this trait must be **heritable**, that is, at least partly controlled by genes. How would you design experiments to determine the importance of this trait in determining survival and reproduction? How would you test the extent to which this trait is heritable?

FOR FURTHER INVESTIGATION

1. In a field guide to the trees in your region, identify the species of evergreen you sampled in this exercise. What does the book say about the needle length of this species? Does the description include a range of needle lengths, or just a mean length? If keys are included in the guide, is needle length used to distinguish this species from others? Based on your data, how often might a single measurement of a randomly selected needle lead to an incorrect species identification?
2. Are some varieties of beans inherently more variable than others? Calculate variances for different types of beans, or from the same variety purchased from different suppliers. Is genetic variety a good predictor of seed weight, or are other considerations such as growing conditions in a given crop year more significant?

FOR FURTHER READING

Howe, H.F. and J. Smallwood. 1982. Ecology of seed dispersal. *Annual Reviews of Ecology and Systematics* 13:201–228.

Preston, Richard J. Jr. 1989. *North American Trees.* Iowa State University Press, Ames.

Rees, Mark. 1995. Community structure in sand dune annuals: Is seed weight a key quantity? *The Journal of Ecology* 83(5):857–863.

Population Growth

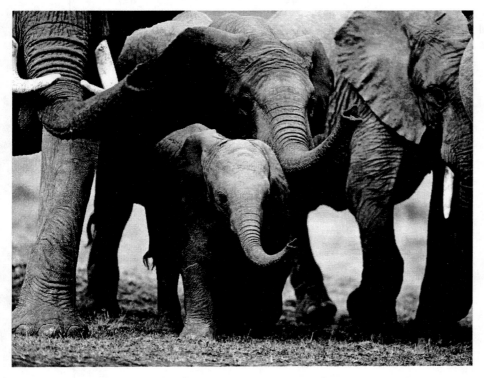

Figure 1 Elephants reproduce slowly, but have the potential to generate large populations.

INTRODUCTION

The great 19th century biologist **Charles Darwin** developed an important ecological idea while reading a book on population growth by **Thomas Malthus** (*An Essay on the Principle of Population*, 1798). Although Malthus was an economist concerned about an expanding human population with a limited food supply, Darwin saw in Malthus' thesis a more general ecological principle. He realized that populations of all species have the potential to grow, and if that growth continues unchecked, competition for resources will eventually limit the size of every population in nature. Darwin documented the staggering growth rate of rapidly breeding organisms such as insects and weedy plants in his *Origin of Species* (1859), but he most effectively illustrated the universal impact of population growth with an example at the opposite end of the life history spectrum: the long-lived and slowly reproducing elephant. In Darwin's own words, "The elephant is reckoned to be the slowest breeder of all known animals, and I have taken some pains to estimate its probable minimum rate of natural increase: it will be under the mark to assume that it breeds when thirty years old, and goes on breeding till ninety years old, bringing forth three pair of young in this interval; if this be so, at the end of the fifth century there would be alive fifteen million elephants, descended from the first pair" (*Origin of Species*, Ch. 3).

From *Ecology on Campus Laboratory Manual*, Robert W. Kingsolver. © Copyright 2006 by Pearson Education, Inc. Published by Benjamin Cummings, Inc. All rights reserved.

How did Darwin arrive at this amazing result? Let's try to duplicate his calculations. If an elephant begins breeding at age 30, then let's assume its generation length is close to 40 years of age. If a pair of elephants has an average family size of "three pair of young," then the population triples every generation. In other words, Darwin's elephants would have the capacity to tripl their numbers in approximately 40 years. To keep our model simple, we will ignore post-reproductive survival and mortality, simply counting each new generation as it replaces the old. With these simplifying assumptions, let's look at the projected growth for Charles Darwin's hypothetical population of elephants:

Year	Population Size
0	2
40	6
80	18
120	54
160	162
200	486
240	1,458
280	4,374
320	13,122
360	39,366
400	118,098
440	354,294
480	1,062,882
520	3,188,646
560	9,565,938

Indeed, before year 600, Darwin's elephants have passed the nine million mark! Darwin probably used a more complex population model, keeping track of surviving adult elephants and overlapping elephant generations, but even in our oversimplified calculation, the conclusion is clear. Any population can overrun its environment if parents continue to produce more offspring than are needed to replace themselves.

Exponential Growth

Let's look at our calculations of elephant growth in the form of a graph (Figure 2). The x-axis shows time in years, with year 0 marking the beginning of our calculations. The y-axis shows population numbers, in millions. Although the rate of growth is a constant, tripling every 40 years, the consequences begin to show dramatically after generation 12. This kind of increase is called **exponential population growth,** and a standard plot of its numbers always produces this kind of J-shaped curve. Although we would need different time scales to graph population growth for fruit flies or dandelions, their exponential growth curves would follow a similar pattern. Darwin's prolific pachyderms provide a good general model for population growth any time resources are in abundant supply and surviving offspring outnumber their parents.

Population Explosion of Darwin's Elephants

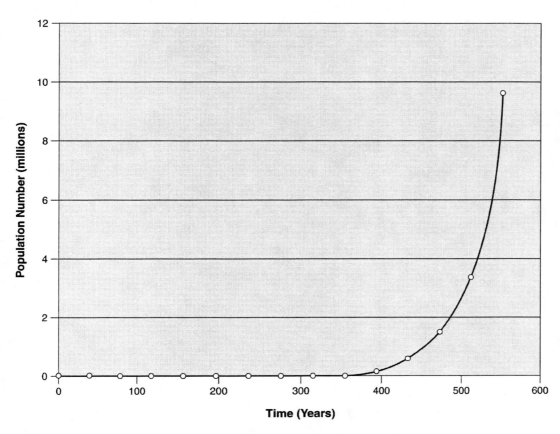

Figure 2   Projection of population size in Darwin's elephant example. The curve indicating population size bends upward in a J-shape, as is typical of exponential growth.

Why use the term *exponential growth?* Take a look at Figure 3. This graph shows exactly the same population growth numbers, and the x-axis is identical to Figure 2. You will notice, however, that they-axis shows numbers in powers of ten (1, 10, 100, 1,000, 10,000, etc.). Another way of writing this series is to use *exponents* of ten. The y-axis would then show 10^0, 10^1, 10^2, 10^3, 10^4, and so on. These *exponents* increase at a constant rate on the population growth line in Figure 2, so we say this population demonstrates *exponential* growth. Another name for a variable exponent attached to a constant base (base 10 in this example) is a *logarithm*. For this reason, graphs in the form of Figure 3 are called **logarithmic plots.** *Population ecologists find logarithmic graphs (or log plots for short) very handy, since they straighten out exponential curves, and display a broad range of data on a single axis.*

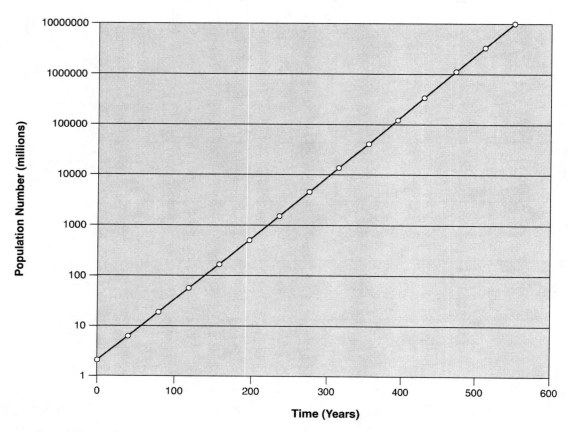

Figure 3 Logarithmic plot of Darwin's elephant example. Note that the y-axis shows numbers in a scale that increases by factors of ten. This changes the exponential growth curve to a straight line.

To describe the growth of an exponentially reproducing population accurately, we need a measure of its growth rate. The symbol used for this measure by ecologists is r, the **intrinsic rate of population increase**. One way to calculate r is to compare birth rates and death rates. The birth rate is simply the number of new individuals added to the population over a unit time period divided by the total population size. In the human population of a city, for example:

Birth rate = (newborns in the past year)/(total city population)

Similarly, the death rate is the number of deaths over a unit of time divided by the population size. For the city example:

Death rate = (deaths in the past year)/(total city population)

For humans, we chose a year as a convenient unit of time, but the appropriate time scale depends on the organism's life history. For fruit flies, we may want to calculate birth and death rate in days; for bacteria, the appropriate time scale may be minutes. Calculating r over a short time interval relative to the life of the organism is important, since r theoretically provides an instantaneous measure of the population's growth trajectory at a particular moment in its history.

Check your progress:

If the number of newborns in a city of 300,000 was 15,000 this year, and the number of deaths during the same period is 9000, what is the intrinsic rate of increase for the population?

Answer: r = 0.02

Since a population's growth depends on its birth rate in comparison to its death rate, we can define r for our city in these terms, assuming no net change due to people moving in or out of town:

r = population birth rate – population death rate

In exponential growth calculations, r is a constant, usually a small fraction near zero. The following table shows values of r for different biological situations:

r value	Population status
r < 0	Population is declining. Death rate exceeds birth rate.
r = 0	Population is stable. Birth rate equals death rate.
r > 0	Population is growing. Birth rate exceeds death rate.

Once you know the value of r, you can use a simple exponential equation to predict next year's population size:

To state this equation in words, we would say the population next year is equal to the population this year plus the new individuals added. The number of new individuals added equals the current population size times the intrinsic rate of growth. We will call this the "discrete form" of the equation, since it calculates growth in a series of discrete steps. To predict two years ahead, you must use the equation to generate N_1, and then plug that

Exponential Growth Equation (Discrete Form)

$$N_{t+1} = N_t + N_t(r)$$

N_{t+1} = population size at the next time interval
N_t = population size at the current time
r = intrinsic rate of population increase

number in as the new value of N_t and repeat the calculation to get N_2. For a hundred years of growth, you would have to repeat the calculation 100 times!

Check your progress:

If r = 0.02 for a city, and the current population is 300,000, then what will the population be next year?

Answer: N_{t+1} = 306,000

The discrete form of the exponential growth equation can be repeated as many times as you wish to make long-range projections, but this is a cumbersome method, and it tends to magnify small errors as you repeat the calculations. A form of the exponential growth equation that provides continuous tracking of population growth over time is as follows:

To demonstrate the power of this formula, let's return to the city example. For a population of 300,000 with r = 0.02, what is the projected population size 10 years in the future?

> ### Exponential Growth Equation (Continuous Form)
>
> $$N_t = N_0 (e^{r\,t})$$
>
> N_t = population size at any time in question
> N_0 = population size at the beginning
> e = base of natural logarithms $\cong$ 2.718
> r = intrinsic rate of population increase
> t = time

$$N_{10} = N_0 (e^{r\,t}) = 300{,}000\ (2.718)^{.02\ (10)}$$
$$= 300{,}000\ (2.718)^{.2}$$
$$= 300{,}000\ (1.22)$$
$$= 366{,}000$$

Note that the number of individuals added in ten years (66,000) is more than ten times the number added in one year (6,000). Like compound interest, the number of babies born each year increases as the number of parents increases, so additions to the population accelerate over time to produce a J-shaped curve.

There is one more form of the exponential growth equation you will find useful. By taking the natural logarithm of both sides of the equation, we can convert the J-shaped curve to a straight line, just as we saw in the log 10 plot of elephant numbers in Figure 3.

$$ln\ N_t = ln\ N_0 + r\,t$$

ln means "natural log of"
N_t = population size at time t
N_0 = population size at the beginning
r = intrinsic rate of population increase
t = time

Note that $ln\ N_0$ is a constant, as is r. The equation is therefore in the form of a straight line, y = a + bx. Furthermore, r represents the slope of that line. To calculate r from population numbers over time, simply take the natural logarithm of all population size data, and plot time on the x-axis vs. *ln* (population size) on the y-axis. Then calculate the slope of that line, which you may recall is the change in y divided by the change in x. The slope of the resulting line is a good estimate of the intrinsic rate of increase, r. (See Figure 4.)

Check your progress:

Use the formula to predict the number of individuals in a city of 300,000 with r = 0.02 after 20 years of exponential growth.

Answer: N_{20} = 447, 529

Calculating r from Darwin's Elephant Example

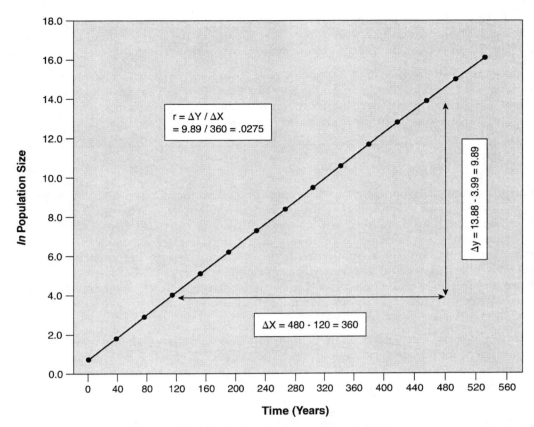

Figure 4   Calculating r from exponentially growing population numbers. If time in years is plotted against the natural log of population size, then r is the slope of the resulting straight line. To calculate the slope, pick two points on the line. Change in Y (denoted as ΔY) is simply the difference between the *ln* population sizes of the two points. Change in X (denoted as ΔX) is the difference between the years designated by the two points. To calculate the slope, divide $\Delta Y / \Delta X$, as shown in the figure. For Darwin's elephants, r is approximately 0.0275.

You may choose any two points on the line to calculate the slope; let's choose two points near the beginning and end of the elephant growth calculations as follows:

	x value (year)	y value (*ln* population size)
Point 1	120	3.99
Point 2	480	13.88

To calculate the slope,   r $= \Delta y / \Delta x$
$= (y_2 - y_1)/(x_2 - x_1)$
$= (13.88 - 3.99)/(480 - 120) = 0.0275$

Check your progress:

Use the formula $ln\ N_t = ln\ N_0 + r\ t$ to check the numbers in the elephant growth table at the beginning of this chapter. Since $N_0 = 2$ in Darwin's example, use $ln\ N_0 = ln\ 2 = 0.693$ in the formula. Plug in the calculated value of $r = 0.0275$, and you can project the population for any year you wish.

Remember that your calculation will yield the ln of population size, so you will have to find the inverse ln (or anti-log base e) button on your calculator or computer spreadsheet to convert your answer back to the number of elephants in the year you selected. Expect minor discrepancies due to rounding errors, but your answer should be fairly close to the number presented in the table.

Logistic Growth

The exponential growth equation is a good model for rapidly expanding populations, but as Darwin pointed out in the *Origin of Species*, it is ridiculous to assume growth can continue indefinitely. Whether made up of fruit flies or elephants, sooner or later, an increasing population will outstrip the natural resource base it needs to keep growing. Inevitably, the number of individuals in the population reaches the maximum number that the environment can sustain. This population level is called the **carrying capacity** of the environment. It is important to note that carrying capacity depends on the quality of the habitat, but also on the body size and resource requirements of the organism. Carrying capacity for elk in a meadow may be only one or two individuals, while carrying capacity for field mice in the same location may number in the hundreds.

If the population grows past carrying capacity, resources are being used faster than they are being regenerated, and the habitat becomes unsuitable for further survival and reproduction. Overpopulation by elephants may mean the woody plants they feed on are stripped from the savannah. Overpopulation by rabbits may mean a shortage of hiding places, and easy hunting for their predators. Overpopulation by oak trees may mean too much shade for seedlings to survive.

Some species tend to overshoot carrying capacity, and then crash to local extinction when they degrade their own habitat. These organisms tend to exhibit drastic fluctuations in population size, with "boom and bust" cycles throughout their range. Other species tend to slow their reproductive rate as they approach carrying capacity. Reproductive success in these organisms is **density-dependent**, that is, sensitive to the numbers of individuals per unit area. Population growth in these species is called **logistic growth**, because their rate of increase is adjusted as the population grows. As an example, many songbirds defend a territory large enough to rear a nest of young. If the population size grows too large, many birds fail to reproduce because all the nesting sites are taken. As a result, per-capita production of nestlings stabilizes as the population size approaches carrying capacity.

Ecologists use the symbol **K** to represent carrying capacity. If we can imagine a population occupying resource space in its habitat, then K represents the number of individuals that would completely fill that space. Recall that N represents the size of the population. The number of "empty spaces" in the environment could therefore be expressed as K – N. If we wanted to measure the *proportion* of habitat space still available for newcomers, we could divide empty spaces by total capacity, which would be:

Proportion of habitat space available $= \dfrac{K - N}{K}$ **K = carrying capacity**

N = population size

For example, if carrying capacity K = 100, and there are 80 animals in the population, then the proportion of the habitat still open for additions to the population would be (K – N)/K = 0.20, or 20%.

Check your progress:

If carrying capacity = 1500, and the population size is 600, what proportion of the resource base is still available?

Answer: 0.60 or 60%

To create an equation for population growth that takes available resources into account, we simply take the discrete form of the exponential growth equation, and multiply the growth term by our expression for available resources as follows:

The Logistic equation produces an S-shaped population growth curve, beginning with an accelerating increase in size, and ending with a gradual approach toward carrying capacity. To demonstrate with Darwin's elephants, if we presume the intrinsic rate of increase is still 0.0275, and that the beginning number of elephants is still 2, but the population occupies a grassland biome that can support a carrying capacity of

Logistic Growth Equation

$$N_{t+1} = N_t + \left(N_t \cdot r \cdot \frac{K - N}{K} \right)$$

N_t = population size at time t
N_0 = population size at the beginning
K = carrying capacity
r = intrinsic rate of population increase
t = time

no more than 500,000 individuals, then Figure 5 illustrates the resulting logistic population growth reaching a plateau at about 600 years. Compare Figures 2 and 5 to see the difference between exponential and logistic growth.

Check your progress:

If carrying capacity = 500,000, the intrinsic rate of increase is 0.0275, and the population size is 350,000 in time t, what does the logistic model predict for time t + 1?

Answer: N_{t+1} = 352,887.5

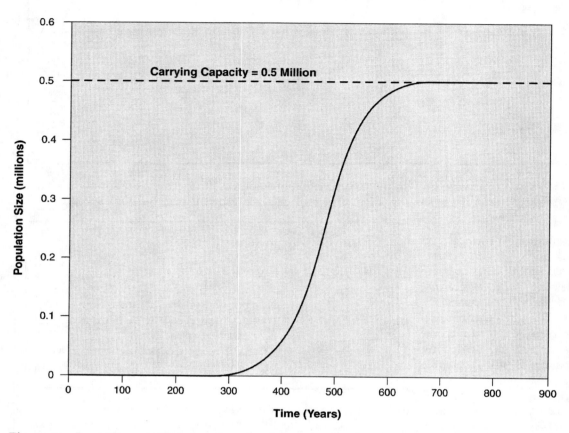

Logistic Growth of Darwin's Elephants

Figure 5 Logistic growth approaches carrying capacity as an S-shaped curve.

One final thought: in logistic growth models, K is treated as a constant. For general predictions of population behavior in relatively stable ecosystems, this is an appropriate assumption. We must realize, however, that carrying capacities in nature fluctuate with the weather, with changes in prey or predator numbers, and with many other kinds of environmental disturbance. Ecologists use growth models to understand basic patterns of population biology, but superimposed on these patterns we almost always see an overlay of random perturbation and continuous population adjustment. If a population fluctuates within definable limits, we say it is in **dynamic equilibrium**. The changing nature of carrying capacities does not negate the value of models such as the logistic growth equation, but variable upper limits to population size do need to be considered in applications to ecological problems such as wildlife management and biological pest control.

METHOD A: CALCULATING r FROM A PUBLISHED DATA SET

[Laboratory activity]

Research Question

How rapidly did populations of the Egyptian goose grow in the Netherlands?

Preparation

Students will need calculators with natural log functions or access to computers with spreadsheet software for this exercise. Extra graph paper may be useful for students attempting log plots.

Materials (per laboratory team)

Calculator or computer with spreadsheet software to calculate *ln* values

Ruler

Background

Figure 6 illustrates an Egyptian goose (*Alopochen aegyptiacus*), a species broadly distributed in Africa. Population biologist Rob Lensink documented exponential population growth of the Egyptian goose in the Netherlands in the years following its introduction to that country (Lensink, 1998). The following population numbers are cumulative census data from Lensink's observations along three rivers during the period 1985–1994. Each count included an entire winter's observations. For example, the population number for 1985 is the number observed during the winter of 1985–86.

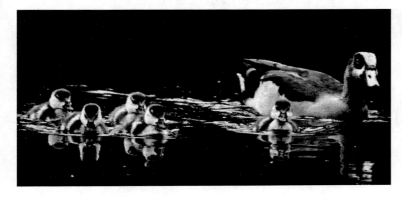

Figure 6 Egyptian goose.

Year	Population Size
1985	259
1986	277
1987	501
1988	626
1989	897
1990	1,324
1991	2,475
1992	2,955
1993	5,849
1994	7,259

Procedure

1. Enter the year and population size for each of the numbers above in the calculation page for *Method A*.
2. Calculate the log base e, also called *ln*, of each population number, and enter those data in the calculation page. This number is *ln* N.
3. Plot time in years (on the x-axis) vs. *ln* N (on the y-axis) on the graph following the calculation page.
4. Using a ruler, draw the best straight line you can through the points on the graph. If some points fall off the line, try to leave the same number of points above and below the line you draw.
5. Use the method explained in the Introduction to calculate the slope of the line. The slope is an estimate of r for Egyptian geese in the Netherlands during this period. Be sure to choose two points on your line for the calculations.
6. Use the population growth equation to project the numbers of geese in the winter of 2000, assuming continued exponential growth.

CALCULATIONS (METHOD A)

Year	Population Size	*ln* Population Size
1985	259	
1986	277	
1987	501	
1988	626	
1989	897	
1990	1,324	
1991	2,475	
1992	2,955	
1993	5,849	
1994	7,259	

Data Analysis: Calculating r from the Slope of a Log Plot

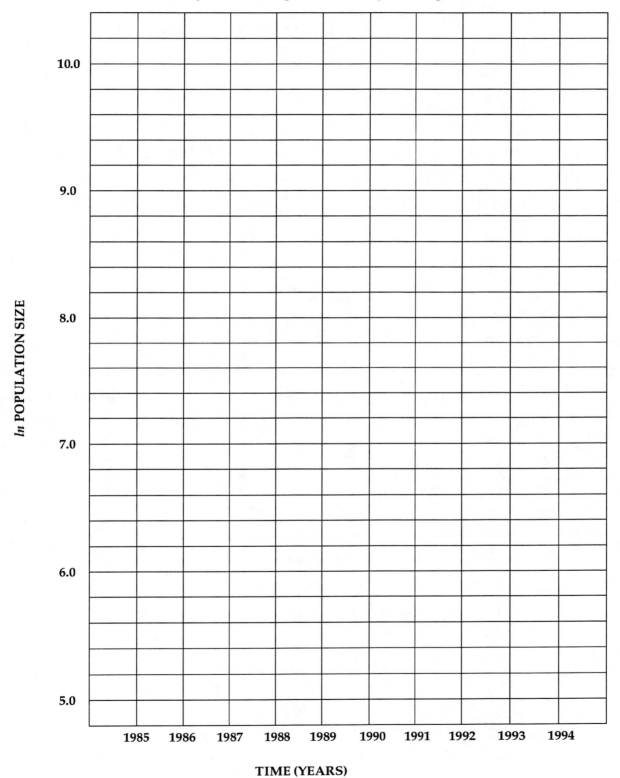

In POPULATION SIZE

TIME (YEARS)

Slope Calculation (From your graph of years vs. *In* population size)

	x value (year)	y value (*ln* population size)
Point 1		
Point 2		

To calculate the slope, $r = \Delta y / \Delta x$

$= (y_2 - y_1)/(x_2 - x_1)$

$$= \boxed{\qquad - \qquad} \; / \; \boxed{\qquad - \qquad}$$

change in *ln* N   divided by   change in time

$$r = \boxed{\qquad\qquad\qquad}$$

intrinsic rate of increase

Comment on the biological meaning of the r value you have calculated:

_____

_____

_____

_____

_____

_____

_____

_____

_____

_____

Questions (Method A)

1. In the exponential population growth equation, $N_t = N_0 (e^{rt})$, identify what each of the symbols stands for, and explain whether it is a variable or a constant for a given growing population.

_____

_____

_____

_____

2. In 1985, the number of Egyptian geese observed was 259. Starting with this as an initial population size, $N_0 = 259$, and using the value of r that you calculated in Method A, use the exponential growth equation to project numbers of geese in year 1994. Since that date is nine years later, use $t = 9$ in the equation. Does the calculated number approximate the number actually observed in 1994? Explain any discrepancies you encounter.

_____

_____

_____

_____

3. To calculate r, you plotted ln (population size) as a function of years, drew the best straight line through the points, and used two points on that line to determine a slope. Why is this method more reliable than simply choosing two points from the data table to determine $\Delta y / \Delta x$?

_____

_____

_____

_____

4. Why do you think Egyptian goose populations are increasing exponentially in the Netherlands, but not in Africa where they originated?

_____

_____

_____

_____

5. When species are introduced to a new continent, they often grow so quickly that they out-compete native species. It may be too soon to tell if this is the case for the Egyptian goose, but there are North American examples of introduced (exotic) species that have become an ecological problem. Can you name an example, and explain why this species is an ecological threat?

_____

_____

_____

_____

METHOD B: COMPARING EXPONENTIAL AND LOGISTIC GROWTH
[Computer activity]

Research Question
How do projections of the exponential and logistic growth models compare?

Preparation
Students will need a basic understanding of spreadsheet software such as Microsoft's Excel©. Corel's Quattro Pro© is also suitable, but the cell formulas in Quattro will require an opening parenthesis (rather than an equals sign =) as a first character. Graphing population data works best with the scatter-plot option in Excel.

Materials (per laboratory team)
One computer work station, equipped with spreadsheet software

Background
Wildlife biologists Anna Whitehouse and Anthony Hall-Martin studied growth of the elephant population of Addo National Elephant Park in South Africa over a 23-year time span. Hunting prior to 1950 had reduced elephants to low numbers, but the population recovered after Addo Park was established for their protection. The study generated the following population data (Whitehouse and Hall-Martin, 2000).

Year	Population Size		Year	Population size
1976	94		1988	160
1977	96		1989	170
1978	96		1990	181
1979	98		1991	189
1980	103		1992	199
1981	111		1993	205
1982	113		1994	220
1983	120		1995	232
1984	128		1996	249
1985	138		1997	261
1986	142		1998	284
1987	151			

Procedure
1. Using a spreadsheet program, set up a spreadsheet, labeled as shown in the following table.
2. Use the first row as column labels, "Year" in A1, "Observed Number" in B1, "Exponential Model" in C1, and "Logistic Model" in D1 as shown.
3. In column A, enter years 1976 through 1998 in cells A2 through A24. Make sure you enter all of the 23 years of data in your spreadsheet.
4. In column C, enter the beginning population size of 94 in cell C2. This number is N_t in the exponential population growth equation. Likewise, enter the beginning population size of 94 in cell D2 to supply a starting population number for the Logistic growth model.

	A	B	C	D
	Year	Observed Population Size	Exponential Model r = 0.0525	Logistic Model r = 0.0525 K = 500
1				
2	1976	94	94	94
3	1977	96	= C2 + (C2*0.0525)	= D2 + (D2*0.0525*(500−D2)/500)
4	1978	96	copy previous cell	copy previous cell
5	1979	98	copy previous cell	copy previous cell
6	1980	103	copy previous cell	copy previous cell
7	1981	111	copy previous cell	copy previous cell
8	etc.	etc.	etc.	etc.

5. Type the equation = **C2 + (C2*0.0525)** in cell C3. This is the spreadsheet version of the discrete form of the exponential growth equation $N_{t+1} = N_t + N_t(r)$ discussed in the Introduction. Compare the equation with the spreadsheet formula. We have already said that C2 is the number we have entered to represent N_t. The number **0.0525** is an estimate of this elephant population's value for **r**, calculated from these data estimated from the slope of a log plot, as demonstrated in Method A. Note that we are using the population size in cell C2, which stands for N_t, and placing the result in cell C3, which holds the value for N_{t+1}.

6. Now COPY the spreadsheet formula in cell C3, and PASTE it in every cell from C4 to C24. By dragging to highlight the entire area before you select PASTE, you can do this in one step. You have now commanded the spreadsheet to make a series of annual calculations, computing the population size for each year from the previous year's population size, located just above it in column C.

7. Type the equation = **D2 + (D2*0.0525*(500 − D2)/500)** in cell D3. This is the spreadsheet version of the discrete form of the logistic growth equation $N_{t+1} = N_t + [N_t \cdot r \cdot (K − N)/K]$ which was discussed in the Introduction. Note that the cell D2 holds the initial population size represented in the equation by N_t. We have used 0.0525 as our value for the intrinsic rate of increase **r**, and 500 as our value for the carrying capacity **K**. Note that we are basing our calculation on the population number in cell D2, which holds the value for N_t, and placing the result in cell D3, which holds the value for N_{t+1}.

8. Now COPY the spreadsheet formula in cell D3, and PASTE it in every cell from D4 to D24. By dragging to highlight the entire area before you select PASTE, you can do this in one step. You have now commanded the spreadsheet to make a series of annual calculations, computing the population size for each year from the previous year's population size, located just above it in column D.

9. Use your spreadsheet software to produce a graph. The x-axis should show time in years, the y-axis population numbers. To simplify the y-axis labels, you can display population numbers in millions, or billions if you choose. You should be able to produce three lines on the graph: the actual population growth over time, an exponential curve, and a logistic curve. Which model best projects the actual growth of this population?

10. Copy and paste the formulas in columns C and D through C49 and D49 to predict the fate of the Addo elephant population 25 years into the future. Repeat the graphing procedure in step 9 to show the fate of the elephants in Addo Park, as described by these two models of population growth. Remember that in column D you presumed the carrying capacity of the park was 500. This carrying capacity figure is NOT based on data from Whitehouse and Hall-Martin, so you may try substituting other values for K, and recopying the formulas in column D to produce alternative logistic projections if you wish.

11. Print out your graph and spreadsheet to attach to the Questions for Method B.

Questions (Method B)

1. Compare the tables for Addo Elephants in this exercise with the table at the beginning of the Introduction for Darwin's hypothetical elephants. Was Darwin as conservative in his calculations for elephant reproductive rates as he claimed to be?

_____

_____

_____

_____

2. If the Addo elephants do eventually reach carrying capacity, what factors might limit the further growth of the population? As a park manager trying to maintain biodiversity and ecosystem health, would you prefer to limit population growth at some point below carrying capacity? Explore some of the practical and ethical issues involved.

_____

_____

_____

_____

3. Since we really do not know what K is for Addo Elephant park, we presumed a carrying capacity of 500 for the purpose of this exercise. How might you determine a more realistic value for K in a field study of these animals?

_____

_____

_____

_____

4. Thomas Malthus was concerned that the global human population was growing exponentially, doubling every 50 years or less, and that we would eventually outgrow our food supply. What scientific advances since 1798 have altered r and increased K for human beings? Have these technologies actually solved the problem, or just postponed the famine Malthus was concerned about?

_____

_____

_____

_____

5. The global human population is over 6 billion and still climbing. What do you think the global carrying capacity might be for humans? Consider agricultural production as a possible limiting resource, but also fresh water, regeneration of oxygen by plants, energy, minerals, and cultural factors. How might our lifestyle choices and diet affect the maximum number of people the earth can sustain?

_____

_____

_____

_____

METHOD C: POPULATION GROWTH OF YEAST

[Laboratory activity]

Research Question

What kind of population growth do yeasts exhibit in laboratory cultures?

Preparation

Use potato dextrose broth in large (e.g., 20 mm × 150 mm) culture tubes to grow yeast cultures in advance. Make sure the tubes are sterilized and capped for aerobic culture of a yeast. From a stock culture of the common yeast *Saccharomyces cerevisiae*, transfer a small number of yeast cells to a sterilized culture tube using a flame-sterilized inoculation loop. For several days before this lab begins, set up a schedule to inoculate two yeast cultures a day, each day, until the lab begins. A five-day series would produce 10 cultures, which is certainly enough to count in one laboratory session. Be sure to label the hour of the day as well as the date on each yeast culture you inoculate. Cultures can be incubated at room temperature. In an incubator, a temperature of 21° C allows for population growth over a period of days. A higher setting of 28° C is recommended for rapid growth, but incubation at higher temperatures will require more frequent inoculation and observation to ensure that yeasts do not overgrow the cultures before the laboratory time.

Materials (per laboratory team)

Compound microscope with maximum magnification 400× or higher

Access to a series of yeast cultures of different ages

Pasteur pipettes for each culture in the series

Standard glass microscope slides and cover slips

Wax pencil or fine-point marker

Vortex test-tube mixer to suspend yeast cells (or lots of patience)

Background

Yeasts rarely if ever exhibit sexual reproduction. Instead, yeast cells produce asexual offspring by budding (Figure 7). A bud begins as a weak point in the cell wall. The cytoplasm then bulges out through the hole, forms a new cell, and builds its own cell wall as it grows. DNA is replicated and passed into the new cell before it separates from its parent, so that each cell retains a copy of the yeast genome. This process occurs frequently in the life of the cell, so yeasts have a prodigious reproductive rate. In some cases, the bud has another bud before it separates, so yeast cells often appear as short chains of cells producing smaller cells.

In this laboratory, you will work with a series of cultures of the common nonpathogenic yeast *Saccharomyces cerevisiae*. The cultures are of varying ages, so you can observe populations at different stages of growth. These yeasts do not normally cause disease, but you should always handle microbial cultures carefully. Keep test tubes upright, and keep pipettes oriented tip-down to avoid contamination. Wash your hands and clean up lab benches at the end of the laboratory.

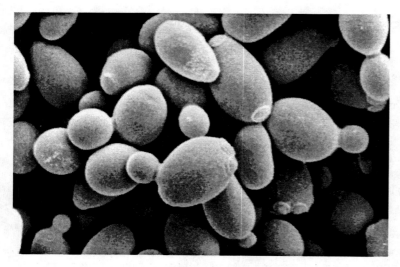

Figure 7 Yeasts reproduce by budding.

Procedure

1. Label a glass slide with a wax pencil or fine-point marker for each culture you will examine.
2. Obtain a culture tube, taking note of the time it was inoculated. Record the date and time this culture was started on the calculation page for *Method C*.
3. Using a vortex test-tube mixer, thoroughly suspend the contents of the yeast culture. Be careful not to set the mixer's speed too high; it is easy to spill your culture. Thorough mixing is important before obtaining your sample, since cells tend to settle in the bottom of the tube. If you do not have a vortex tube mixer, you can hold the tube near the top with one hand, and tap the contents repeatedly with the fingers of the other hand to suspend the cells. Try a drumming motion, as if you were drumming your fingers on the table top.
4. When cells are thoroughly mixed, have a lab partner hold the tube and remove the cap. Quickly insert a Pasteur pipette (with bulb attached) into the middle of the tube, about halfway down into the culture medium, and withdraw a small sample.
5. Without giving your cells too much time to settle, place the pipette over a clean slide and squeeze out exactly one drop onto the slide. A drop is 1/20 ml, so this method ensures you are counting cells in the same volume of culture from each sample.
6. Place the edge of a cover slip against the glass slide at the edge of your culture drop, and lower it gently over the drop, trying not to trap any air bubbles.
7. Under a compound microscope, find the cells under low power, then move to high power (400×). Compare the cells you see with Figure 7.
8. Sample 10 fields of view as follows: move the slide slightly, look in the eyepiece, and count the number of cells you see in this field of view. Move the slide again, and recount. After 10 counts, compute an average number of cells per field and record your result on the calculation page.
9. Repeat steps 2 through 8 for each yeast culture in the series. You may want to share the counting tasks with others in the lab to make sure all the counts are completed. If so, be sure everyone agrees on a convention for counting buds: do they count as a cell, and if so, how big should a bud be before it is counted?

10. Calculate the age of each yeast culture in hours. Add 24 hours for each day since the culture was inoculated, and then add hours if the culture was started earlier, or subtract hours if it was started later in the day than your lab time. Record age in hours for each culture on the calculation page.
11. Plot time (in hours) vs. cell density (mean number per field).
12. Convert your mean cell counts to a log scale by taking the natural log (base e) of each mean number of cells per field. Record these transformed cell density numbers in the calculation page.
13. Plot time in hours vs. *ln* (cell density).
14. If growth is exponential, calculate r from the slope, as shown on the calculation page.
15. Interpret your graphs, and answer Questions for Method C.

CALCULATIONS (METHOD C)

Culture Number	Date of culture inoculation (Date and time)	Age of culture (hours)	Mean number of yeast cells per field	*ln* (number of cells per field)
1				
2				
3				
4				
5				
6				
7				
8				
9				
10				

Results: Yeast Cell Density vs. Time

YEAST CELL DENSITY (mean number per field)

TIME (hours)

Results: *In* Yeast Cell Density vs. Time

LOG OF YEAST CELL DENSITY (*ln* mean number per field)

TIME (hours)

Slope Calculation (From your graph of hours vs. *In* population size)

	x value (year)	y value (*In* population size)
Point 1	27	r
Point 2	117	

To calculate the slope, $r = \Delta y / \Delta x$

$$= (y_2 - y_1)/(x_2 - x_1)$$

$r = $ [　　　 –　　　] / [　　　 – 27]

         change in *In* N   divided by   change in time

$= $ [　　　 0 　　　]

      intrinsic rate of increase

Questions (Method C)

1. Many rapidly growing organisms, including yeasts and bacteria, exploit temporary habitats such as a rotting apple. Compare advantages and disadvantages of asexual reproduction for organisms exploiting these kinds of resources.

   _____

   _____

   _____

   _____

2. Was the logistic or the exponential growth model best for describing your yeast population growth? Could the exponential model work for early stages of population growth, even if cell growth slows and stops as the population approaches carrying capacity?

   _____

   _____

   _____

   _____

3. In this experiment, you did not actually estimate population size, but only the number of cells per microscope field. Under carefully replicated conditions, are these two variables related? What errors in procedure could compromise the value of cell density per field as an index of population numbers?

   _____

   _____

   _____

   _____

4. Most microorganisms exhibit faster growth at higher temperatures, up to the point that their enzyme functions are compromised. If you incubated cultures at a higher temperature, how might the population growth curve be affected in your experiment?

   _____

   _____

   _____

   _____

5. Suppose an r value is calculated for yeast cells by plotting _ln_ population number vs. time in hours, and the same kind of calculation is performed for elephants, plotting _ln_ population number vs. time in years. Can the two r values be compared? Explain your answer.

   _____

   _____

   _____

   _____

FOR FURTHER INVESTIGATION

1. Try using exponential and logistic equations to model growth of the human population over the past 55 years, using the following data from the United Nations Population Division, World Population Prospects 2002 revision (http://esa.un.org/unpp/p2k0data.asp).

   After you have set up your spreadsheet, try projecting the human population 100 years into the future—a time span that will include lives of today's young adult generation and their children. How do your two models compare? What criteria did you choose to determine the global carrying capacity for human beings?

Year	Global Human Population
1950	2,518,629,000
1955	2,755,823,000
1960	3,021,475,000
1965	3,334,874,000
1970	3,692,492,000
1975	4,068,109,000
1980	4,434,682,000
1985	4,830,979,000
1990	5,263,593,000
1995	5,674,380,000
2000	6,070,581,000
2005	6,498,225,000

2. When yeast populations fill their test-tube habitat, their growth is eventually slowed by depletion of food such as sugars in the broth medium, but also by metabolic wastes (alcohols) that accumulate in the culture. To show logistic growth over a longer period of time, start your own series of yeast cultures, and sample them periodically over an extended time. Repeat your census of cells per field, calculating standard errors on your population estimates. Then try constructing a logistic growth model, with **r** derived from the "log phase" of fastest population growth as we did in Method C, but also with **K** calculated from the maximum number of cells per field you see at carrying capacity. If followed long enough, do yeast cultures exhibit logistic growth?

FOR FURTHER READING

Darwin, Charles R. 1859. The Origin of Species. In: *The Harvard Classics, Vol. XI.* New York, P. F. Collier & Son. On Line Edition: Bartleby.com, 2001. www.bartleby.com.

Lensink, Rob. 1998. Temporal and spatial expansion of the Egyptian goose *Alopochen aegyptiacus* in The Netherlands, 1967–94. *Journal of Biogeography* 25(2): 251–263.

Malthus, Thomas Robert. 1798. *An Essay on the Principle of Population.* J. Johnson. Library of Economics and Liberty. 31 December 2004. On Line Edition: www.econlib.org/library/Malthus/malPop1.

United Nations Population Division, *World Population Prospects, 2002 Revision.* http://esa.un.org/unpp/p2k0data.asp.

Whitehouse, Anna M. and Anthony J. Hall-Martin. 2000. Elephants in Addo Elephant National Park, South Africa: reconstruction of the population's history. *Oryx* 34(1): 46–55.

Estimating Population Size

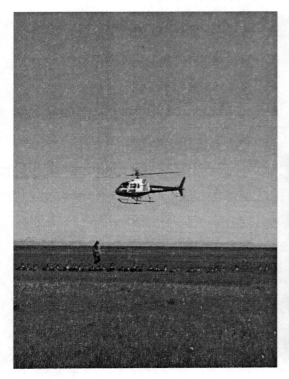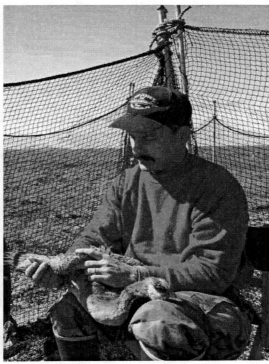

Figure 1   Banding Canada geese.

INTRODUCTION

One of the first questions an ecologist asks about a population is, "How many individuals are here?" This question is trickier than it appears. First, defining an individual is easier for some organisms than others. In the Canada geese shown in Figure 1, a "head count" of geese captured on the ground during their summer molt gives a clear indication of adult numbers, but should eggs be counted as members of the population or not? In plants, reproduction may occur sexually by seed, or asexually by offshoots that can remain connected to the parent plant. This reproductive strategy, called **clonal reproduction,** makes it difficult to say where one individual stops and the next one begins.

Consider the Kentucky bluegrass plant (Fig. 2), which is a common turf grass on college campuses. If it escapes mowing long enough, the plant can produce seed in the inflorescence depicted at the top of the drawing, but bluegrass also sends out vegetative shoots, called tillers, which run laterally just under the surface of the ground. Patches of bluegrass many feet in diameter may be interconnected parts of the same genetic individual. Botanists use the term **genet** to refer to the entire clonally produced patch of grass, and the term **ramet** for a standard unit of growth such as a bluegrass tiller.

Check your progress:

If you were asked to count the number of bluegrass plants in a quad area on your campus, which definition would you use? How would you go about it?

Hint: The purpose of your count determines the best methodology. Are you more concerned with area covered by this species or by the number of genetic individuals in the population?

Once the individual is defined, ecologists working with stationary organisms such as trees or corals can use spatial samples, called **quadrats**, to estimate the number of individuals in a larger area.

Mobile animals are usually simpler to define as individuals, but harder to count, because they tend to move around, mix together, and hide from ecologists. Quadrats are not a good approach with mobile animals because **immigration** and **emigration** in and out of the study site make it hard to know what area the entire population occupies. For largemouth bass in a farm pond, you could easily draw a line around a map of the population, but how would you define the edges of a population of house sparrows in your community? Although house sparrows tend to be more concentrated in towns and urban areas, they do not stop and turn back at the city limit sign. For zoologists, a fuzzy definition of the space occupied by the population often forces an arbitrary designation of the survey group, such as the "population" of robins nesting on your campus in the spring. Knowing the number of animals in a designated study area is interesting, but we must bear in mind that the **ecological population** is defined in terms of interactions among organisms of the same species, and not by the ecologist's convenience.

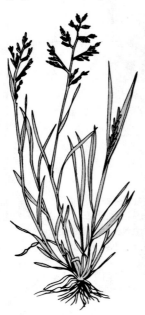

After defining the individual and establishing the limits of the population you wish to count, your next task is to choose a counting method. Arctic and prairie habitats such as the tundra in Figure 1 lend themselves to accurate survey by aerial reconnaissance. This approach works poorly in forests, at night, underwater, or in soil habitats. If animals can be collected or observed in a standard time or collecting effort, you can get an idea of relative abundance, but not absolute numbers. For example, the number of grasshoppers collected in 50 swings with an insect net through an old field community produces data that could be used to compare relative abundance in different fields, but would not tell you how many grasshoppers were in the population.

Figure 2 Kentucky bluegrass, *Poa pratensis*.

For estimates of absolute numbers, **mark-recapture methods** can be very effective. The first step is to capture and mark a sample of individuals. Marking methods depend on the species: birds can be banded with a small aluminum ankle bracelet, snails can be marked with waterproof paint on their shells, butterflies can have labels taped to their wings, large mammals can be fitted with collars, fish fins can be notched, and amphibians can have nontoxic dyes injected under the skin. Marked animals are immediately released as close as possible to the collection site. After giving the animals time to recover and to mix randomly with the whole population, the ecologist goes out on a second collecting trip and gathers a second sample of the organisms. The size of the population can then be estimated from the number of marked individuals recaptured on the second day.

The assumption behind mark-recapture methods is that the proportion of marked individuals recaptured in the second sample represents the proportion of marked individuals in the population as a whole. In algebraic terms,

$$\frac{R}{S} = \frac{M}{N}$$

M = **animals marked and released**

N = **population size**

R = **animals recaptured on a second day**

S = **size of the sample on the second day**

Let's consider an example. Suppose you want to know how many box turtles are in a wooded park. On the first day, you hunt through the woods and capture 24 turtles. You place a spot of paint on each turtle's shell and release all turtles back where you found them. A week later you return, and with an extraordinary effort, catch 60 turtles. Of these, 15 are marked and 45 are unmarked. Since you know how many turtles you marked, sampled, and recaptured, you can figure out the size of the whole population. By the definitions above, M = 24 marked and released, S = 60 in the second sample, and R = 15 recaptures. If the second sample is representative of the whole population, then:

$$\frac{15}{60} = \frac{24}{N} \quad \textbf{This can be rearranged to:} \quad N = \frac{(24)(60)}{15} = 96 \textbf{ turtles.}$$

This method is called the
Lincoln-Peterson Index of population size.
(See box at right.)

Lincoln-Peterson Index:

$$N = \frac{M \cdot S}{R}$$

N = population size estimate
M = marked individuals released
S = size of second sample
R = marked animals recaptured

In the rearranged version of the general formula, notice that *the smaller the number of recaptures, the larger the estimate of population size*. This makes good biological sense, because if the population is very large, the marked animals you release into the wild will be mixing with a greater number of unmarked animals, so you will recapture a lower percentage of them in your second sample.

Check your progress:

A biologist nets 45 largemouth bass from a farm pond, tags their fins, and releases them unharmed. A week later, she nets 58 bass from the pond, including 26 with tags. Based on the Lincoln-Peterson index, estimate the number of bass in the pond.

Answer: 100.4

Note that the estimate is carried out to one decimal place.

The Lincoln-Peterson method is fairly simple, and its calculations are straightforward, but it does depend on several assumptions. Violating the conditions of the Lincoln-Peterson model can seriously affect the accuracy of your estimate, so it is very important to bear these assumptions in mind as you interpret your results:

1. *Individuals with marks have the same probability of survival as other members of the population.* It is important to choose a marking method that does not harm your animal. If a predator used your paint marks to locate and capture marked turtles at a higher rate than other turtles, your number of recaptures would be lower, and the estimate would therefore be too high.

2. *Births and deaths do not occur in significant numbers between the time of release and the time of recapture.* If marked individuals die and are replaced with newborns, then you will recapture few or no marked individuals, and your estimate will be too high. This is not a large concern in studies of box turtles, but can significantly affect estimates for rapidly breeding organisms.

3. *Immigration and emigration do not occur in significant numbers between the time of release and the time of recapture.* If marked individuals leave the study area and new unmarked individuals come in to replace them, you will get fewer recaptures than the equilibrium population size would lead you to expect. To think about this another way, the real population covers a much larger area than the habitat you thought you were studying.

4. *Marked individuals mix randomly with the population at large.* If your marked turtles do not move among unmarked turtles, and you recapture them near the place you released them, then recaptured turtles may be overrepresented in your second sample, driving down your population estimate.

5. *Marked animals are neither easier, nor harder, to capture a second time.* If marking an animal frightens it so that it hides from you a second time, then recaptures will be underrepresented in a second sample. If animals become tame and are easier to recapture, then the opposite error is introduced.

6. *Marks do not come off of your marked organisms.* Invertebrates molt and shed marks, mammals can wriggle out of their collars, and many things can happen to obscure your marks. If this happens, recaptures will be undercounted, and your estimate will be too high.

7. *Recapture rates are high enough to support an accurate estimate.* The Lincoln-Peterson calculation tends to overestimate the population size, especially if the number of recaptures is small.

Assumption 7 is often violated, because it is difficult to generate sufficient recaptures in large populations. To correct for this source of error, ecologists often use a slightly modified form of the Lincoln-Peterson index, called the Bailey correction (Begon, 1979).

There are other mark-recapture methods designed to account for violations of several other assumptions of the Lincoln-Peterson method, but most of these require repeated sampling and day-specific marks. To begin simply, we will use the Lincoln-Peterson method with the Bailey correction to estimate the size of a population.

Bailey Correction for the Lincoln-Peterson Index:

$$N = \frac{M(S+1)}{R+1}$$

N = population size estimate
M = marked individuals released
S = size of second sample
R = marked animals recaptured

Check your progress:

Recalculate the number of bass in the pond in the last progress check, using M = 45, S = 58, and R = 26, but with the Bailey correction formula. Did the correction significantly change your estimate?

Answer: N = 98.3

After you calculate a value for N, you should use the following formula to calculate the 95% confidence intervals on your estimate of population size. Recall that confidence intervals give you an idea of the accuracy of your estimate. By adding a standard error term for the upper limit, and subtracting the same amount for a lower limit, you know with 95% confidence that the true population size falls within this range. In common language, we could say the true population size is our estimated value of N, "give or take" the confidence interval. With a 95% confidence limit we would be wrong only 5% of the time. The formula for 95% confidence intervals, using the Bailey method (Begon, p. 7) is shown in the box on this page.

Confidence Interval for population size estimate:

$$95\% \text{ Confidence Interval } = N \pm 1.96 \sqrt{\frac{M^2(S+1)(S-R)}{(R+1)^2(R+2)}}$$

N = population estimate
S = size of second sample
M = marked individuals
R = recaptured individuals

Check your progress:

Using the same data for bass mark-recaptures, estimate a 95% confidence limit for your population estimate. (Use the Bailey-corrected estimate of N.)

Answer: N = 98.3 ± 26.8

In summary, to estimate the size of a population: 1) define what you mean by an individual, 2) determine the area you will study, 3) decide on a counting method, and then 4) calculate your estimate and confidence intervals.

METHOD A: MARK-RECAPTURE SIMULATION

[Laboratory activity]

Research Question

How can mark-recapture methods be used to estimate the number of beans in a container?

Preparation

At a grocery or health food store, purchase dried white beans. Navy or Great Northern varieties in bags of approximately one pound are ideal.

Materials (per laboratory team)

1-pound bag of dried white beans

1-liter beaker, jar, or wide-mouthed flask

Felt-tip marker

Calculator

Procedure

1. Partially fill the container with beans, making sure there is room to shake and mix them. This jar of beans represents your population in the wild.
2. Remove a sample of 100 individuals from your population. Mark each bean on both sides with a felt-tip marker so that the marked beans are always easy to see. Return the beans to the jar. Shake well to simulate release and mixing of animals in the wild. Enter the number you marked (number = M) on the calculation page at the end of the chapter.
3. Take a second sample by shaking about 200 beans out of the jar onto a table or lab bench. After you have shaken your sample out, count the total number sampled (this number = S in the index formula) and the number of marked beans in your sample (this number representing recaptures = R in the formula). If you do not have at least 10 recaptures, shake out some more beans and recount. Enter the size of the second sample (S) and the number of recaptures (R) in the calculation page at the end of this chapter.
4. Calculate N and 95% confidence intervals on your estimate of population size, as explained in the Introduction.
5. Count all the beans in the jar, dividing up the task with your lab partners. How close was your estimate? Was the actual population size within the confidence intervals you calculated? Compare your results with others in the class to interpret your results.

Questions (Method A)

1. Why was it important to shake beans out onto the table in your second sample, rather than picking them out of the jar by hand? Can you imagine similar sampling issues arising with the box turtle example from the Introduction?

   random sampling to get accurate results.

   _____ where they usually live._

2. If you did not shake up the beans very well after returning them to the jar, how would that have affected your estimate of population size? Can you imagine a comparable problem arising in a field study?

   If we didn't shake it well, our results would be throw

   off, your estimate population would decrease.

3. Looking at the formula for confidence intervals, how would you expect the 95% interval to be affected by increasing the size of the second sample? How would it be affected by marking a larger number of individuals?

   _S =_
   sample
   size

   It would be bigger because you increase the numerator

   which would increase the population interval.

4. Suppose one of your classmates simulated a predator by removing some of the beans from the jar between the release of your marked individuals and your second sample. Would your estimate of population size be too high or too low? Explain why.

   It would be too low because the chance of recapture

   would be inaccurated.

   The problem is removing marked individuals.

5. Suppose one of your lab partners simulated **emigration** and **immigration** between the release of your marked individuals and your second sample. Your partner removed a third of the population and replaced it with an equal number of new beans from the grocery store. Would your estimate of population size be too high or too low? How would your error compare with the previous example?

   _____

   _____

   _____

   _____

METHOD B: MARK-RECAPTURE ESTIMATE OF A STUDENT POPULATION

[Campus activity]

Research Question

How can mark-recapture methods be used to estimate the number of students on campus?

Preparation

This exercise uses human subjects, but in a nominal and nonintrusive way. However, if this method is adapted for use in a study leading to a student talk or publication, be sure to follow protocols for research on human subjects established for your institution. For best results, at least 5% of the student body should be "marked." If the number of participating students is much less than 5% of the population as a whole, estimates will vary substantially.

Materials (per student)

Colored yarn cut to 30-cm (12-inch) length

Procedure

1. During a lecture session before lab, ask all volunteers for this experiment to tie a piece of yarn on her/his left wrist, (not too tight) and to leave it on for 24 hours. The wristband can be removed at night, but should be displayed whenever students are out on campus. Get a count of the "marked" students in your class, and enter this number as (M) on the calculation page. If there are multiple sections of your class participating in this experiment, ask your professor to sum all the sections for a grand total of marked participants.

2. After marked students are "released" from class, allow them time to go their separate ways and mix with the population as a whole. Then take a second sample. Your second sample should be in a place where you can observe a large number of students without counting the same person twice. The library, a cafeteria, another class, or a sporting event might be reasonable choices. To take your sample, observe the left wrist of every student you encounter. Count both the total number of students in your sampling effort and the number who have a wristband. Enter the total number in your sample as (S) on the calculation page at the end of this chapter. Also record the number of students with wristbands as "recaptured" individuals (R).

3. Use the Lincoln-Peterson Index to calculate the population size of students on your campus. Also calculate confidence intervals on your estimate.

Questions (Method B)

1. When students left the classroom after being "marked," did they really mix randomly with the entire student body? How do the daily routines of ecology students differ from the average student on your campus? How does this difference in behavior potentially affect your estimate?

    _____

    _____

    _____

    _____

2. When you selected your sample site, was it a good place for observing a random sample of the student body, or were some categories of students overrepresented or underrepresented? Was the likelihood of a "recapture" higher or lower than the likelihood of encountering a nonparticipating student? How do these considerations compare with ecologists' concerns about biased sampling in a field study?

    _____

    _____

    _____

    _____

3. If several students in your class became irritated with the wristband and took them off too soon, how would your estimate of population size be affected? How does this concern compare with the field ecologist's concerns about marking methods for animals in the wild?

    _____

    _____

    _____

    _____

4. If some "marked" commuter students leave campus after class and other commuter students arrive before your sampling effort, how will this affect your estimate? How does this source of error compare with the field ecologist's concerns about emigration and immigration of animals?

    _____

    _____

    _____

    _____

5. This method has actually been used, with personal identification data rather than wristbands, to estimate numbers of transient and homeless persons in urban areas. (See Peterson, 1999, and Fisher *et al.*, 1994.) Based on what you have learned in this study, do you think this method could help develop a more accurate census of the city's population? What sources of error would you anticipate?

    _____

    _____

    _____

    _____

METHOD C: MARK-RECAPTURE ESTIMATE OF MEALWORM POPULATION

[Laboratory activity]

Research Question

How can mark-recapture methods be used to estimate the number of insects in a mealworm culture?

Preparation

Mealworm cultures must be started well in advance, preferably several months before students do the exercise. Mealworms (actually larvae of the beetle *Tenebrio molitor* L.) are easily cultured in plastic shoe-boxes or sweater boxes half-filled with wheat bran. An apple or potato cut up and layered in the bran provides all the moisture needed by the mealworms. Larvae are most useful for the experiment. These can be purchased from biological supply companies, or reared from a starting population of adults if you allow sufficient time for egg laying and maturation.

Plan two short laboratory periods for this exercise: one to mark the larvae, and a second day for recapturing them and calculating results. This could easily be combined with Method B.

Materials (per laboratory team)

Mealworm culture, with large numbers of larvae

Screen sieve, #5, with 4-mm openings

Acrylic paint, in several colors

Small paintbrush

A sheet of newspaper

Procedure

1. Observe the life cycle of *Tenebrio molitor*, the mealworm or darkling beetle, in Figure 3. You may be able to find adults, pupae, and larvae of various sizes in a well-established mealworm culture. If you have adults, you probably also have eggs, but they are about the size of the period at the end of this sentence, and so are difficult to see. The purpose of this exercise is to count numbers of larvae, but you may also decide to include other life stages.

2. With your #5 sieve, scoop out a sample of the mealworm culture. Shake the sieve carefully over the box, allowing the bran meal to fall back into the culture. Remove bits of potato, bread, or apple by hand if they are included in your culture. Do you see any mealworms in the sieve?

3. Use water-based acrylic paint to mark the insects in your first sample. (Volatile solvents in oil-based paints are more likely to penetrate the cuticle and harm the mealworms.) Place the captured mealworms on a sheet of newspaper on the laboratory bench. Use a small paintbrush and acrylic paint to put a small mark on each insect. (See Figure 4.) Leave the insects on the newspaper while the paint dries. Make sure the paint is dry to the touch before releasing the mealworms back into their culture.

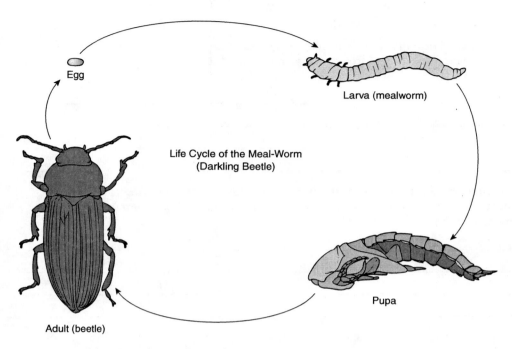

Figure 3 Mealworm life cycle, *Tenebrio molitor*.

4. Record the number marked (M) in the calculation page, and let the cultures sit overnight.

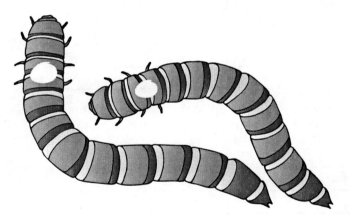

5. A day or two later, repeat the sampling procedure by sieving about half of the mealworm culture. As you collect mealworms, place them on the newspaper or in the shoebox lid. Count and record on the calculation page how many mealworms are included in your second sample (S), and how many of these are marked individuals that you recaptured (R).

6. Use the Bailey correction of the Lincoln-Peterson Index to calculate the population size of mealworms in the culture. Also calculate confidence intervals on your estimate.

Figure 4 Marked mealworm larvae.

Questions (Method C)

1. Are all life stages represented equally in the sampling procedure used in this experiment? How might life history complicate mark-recapture estimates in field studies of birds, reptiles, fish, or mammals?

   _____

   _____

   _____

   _____

2. Like all animals with an exoskeleton, larval mealworms must shed their skin periodically as they grow in size. This is called molting. If some of the larval mealworms molted between your first and second sample, how would this affect your estimate?

   _____

   _____

   _____

   _____

3. You could have estimated the size of the mealworm culture by measuring the volume of bran in your first sample, and simply calculating numbers of mealworms per unit volume of bran. If you measured the volume of the culture box, you could then come up with an estimate by multiplication, without using mark-recapture methods. What assumptions would you have to make in a volumetric calculation? Which method do you think would be more accurate?

   _____

   _____

   _____

   _____

4. Were mealworms equally distributed throughout the medium, or did you notice that concentrations varied with depth or proximity to the edge of the culture box? How might a clumped distribution of insects affect your results?

   _____

   _____

   _____

   _____

5. Although larvae and adult mealworms are mobile, the pupae do not move through the culture. If you marked a large number of pupae, and sampled in the same part of the culture on your second sampling effort, how would your estimate of population size be affected? How could you avoid this source of error?

   _____

   _____

   _____

   _____

CALCULATIONS (METHODS A, B, OR C)

M = Total number marked and released =

S = Total number in second sample =

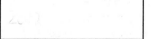

R = Number marked individuals recaptured =

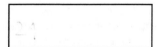

Using the Bailey correction for the Lincoln-Peterson formula, estimate N.
(Show calculations.)

$$N = \frac{M(S+1)}{R+1}$$

N =

$$\text{95\% Confidence Interval} = N \pm 1.96 \sqrt{\frac{M^2(S+1)(S-R)}{(R+1)^2(R+2)}}$$

(Show calculations.)

$$= N \pm 1.96$$

In other words, we can say with 95% confidence that the true population lies between:

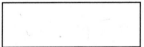   and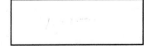

High end of estimate   Low end of estimate.

If available, the **actual count** of the population size =

Does this fall within the 95% confidence interval? _____

FOR FURTHER INVESTIGATION

1. Use "Mark-recapture" and "Lincoln-Peterson" as keywords in a literature search to find field studies that used this method to estimate population size. Did the authors use the Bailey correction, or not? Based on what you have learned in this exercise, did the authors mark enough individuals? Did the number of recaptures merit their conclusions? Try to calculate confidence intervals to compare with any published in the study.

2. From the college web site or catalog, find the total number of students attending your college or university. How does this compare with your estimate from Method B? Is the "student population" published by the institution really the same as the number of people on campus at any given time? How many definitions of the term "student population" could be applied to your institution?

3. In early autumn before the first frost, most campus environments are home to adult insects which could be sampled and counted in a mark-recapture experiment. Moths can be collected around security lights at night. Beetles can be collected by burying a sample jar up to its rim to make a pit trap. (You would need to find an undisturbed location, behind a fence or beneath shrubs, for this method.) Hopping insects can be collected with sweep nets if there is tall grass anywhere on your campus, and many small invertebrates can be collected beneath leaf litter. Try marking adult insects of the most abundant species with acrylic paint as you did in Method C, releasing them, and estimating population size by the Lincoln-Peterson method.

FOR FURTHER READING

Begon, M. 1979. *Investigating animal abundance: capture-recapture for biologists.* Edward Arnold, London.

Fisher, N., S. Turner, R. Pugh, and C. Taylor. 1994. Estimating the number of homeless and homeless mentally ill people in north east Westminster by using capture-recapture analysis. *British Medical Journal* 308: 27–30.

Litzgus, J. D. and T. A. Mousseau. 2004. Demography of a southern population of the spotted turtle (*Clemmys guttata*). *Southeastern Naturalist* 3(3): 391–400.

Peterson, I. 1999. Census sampling confusion. *Science News* 155(10): 152–154.

Spatial Pattern

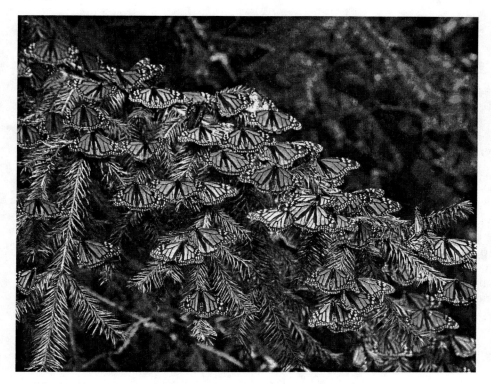

Figure 1   Monarch butterflies congregate during their fall migration.

INTRODUCTION

Members of a population constantly interact with physical features of their environment, one another, and other species in the community. Distinctive **spatial patterns**, describing the distribution of individuals within their habitat, result from these interactions. Movements, family groupings, and differential survival create spatial patterns that vary from one population to another. A population can also change the way it is scattered through space as seasons or conditions change. As an example, monarch butterflies spread out to feed and reproduce during the summer, but congregate in dense assemblies during fall migration and winter dormancy (Figure 1). The physical arrangement of organisms is of interest to ecologists because it provides evidence of interactions that have occurred in the past, and because it can significantly affect the population's fate in the future. Analyzing spatial distributions can reveal a lot more about the organism's natural history than we could ever know from estimates of population size alone.

Since it is often impossible to map the location of every individual, ecologists measure features of spatial pattern that are of particular biological interest. One such feature is the dispersion of the population. **Dispersion** refers to the evenness of the population's distribution through space. (Dispersion should not be confused with **dispersal**, which describes movement rather than pattern.) A completely uniform distribution has maximal dispersion, a randomly scattered population has intermediate dispersion, and an aggregated population with clumps of individuals surrounded by empty space has minimal dispersion (Figure 2).

From *Ecology on Campus Laboratory Manual*, Robert W. Kingsolver. © Copyright 2006 by Pearson Education, Inc. Published by Benjamin Cummings, Inc. All rights reserved.

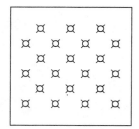
Uniform distribution
High dispersion

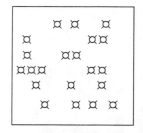
Random distribution
Intermediate dispersion

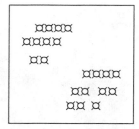
Aggregated distribution
Low dispersion

Figure 2   Three types of spatial distribution. Individuals spread evenly through the environment are highly dispersed, individuals clumped together exhibit low dispersion.

How can we measure dispersion in populations? A typical approach involves **quadrat** sampling. Quadrats are small plots, of uniform shape and size, placed in randomly selected sites for sampling purposes. By counting the number of individuals within each sampling plot, we can see how the density of individuals changes from one part of the habitat to another. The word "quadrat" implies a rectangular shape, like a "quad" bounded by four campus buildings. Any shape will work, however, as long as quadrats are all alike and sized appropriately for the species under investigation. For creatures as small as barnacles, an ecologist may construct a sampling frame a few centimeters across, and simply drop it repeatedly along the rocky shore, counting numbers of individuals within the quadrat frame each time. For larger organisms such as trees, global positioning equipment and survey stakes may be needed to create quadrats of appropriate scale.

The number of individuals counted within each quadrat is recorded and averaged. The mean of all those quadrat counts (symbolized as $\bar{x}$) yields the **population density**, expressed in numbers of individuals per quadrat area (barnacles per square meter, for example, or pine trees per hectare). An alternative approach is to measure **ecological density**, expressed in numbers of individuals per resource unit (numbers of deer ticks per host, for example, or numbers of apple maggots per fruit). To get a measure of dispersion in our population, we need to know how much variation exists among the samples. In other words, how much do the numbers of individuals per sampling unit vary from one sample to the next? The **sample variance** (symbolized as s^2) gives us a good measure of the evenness of our distribution. (For an introduction to the variance, see Appendix 1—Variance.) Consider our three hypothetical populations, now sampled with randomly placed quadrats (Figure 3).

Notice that the more aggregated the distribution, the greater the variance among quadrat counts. To standardize our measurements for different populations, we can divide the variance by the mean number of individuals per quadrat. This gives us a reliable way to measure aggregation. Statisticians have demonstrated that the **variance/mean ratio**, symbolized as $s^2/\bar{x}$ yields a value close to 1 in a randomly dispersed population, because in samples from a random distribution the variance is equal to the mean. Any ratio significantly greater than 1 indicates aggregation, and a ratio less than 1 indicates a trend toward uniformity. We could therefore call the variance/mean ratio an index of aggregation, because it is positively related to the "clumping" of individuals in the population. The variance/mean ratio is also called an **index of dispersion**, even though dispersion is inversely related to $s^2/\bar{x}$. It is good to remember: a high value of $s^2/\bar{x}$ means high aggregation, but low dispersion.

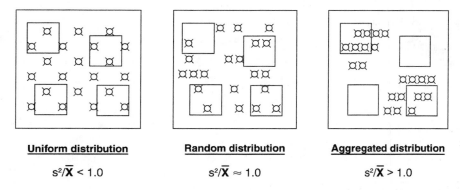

Uniform distribution   **Random distribution**   **Aggregated distribution**

$$s^2/\overline{X} < 1.0 \qquad\qquad s^2/\overline{X} \approx 1.0 \qquad\qquad s^2/\overline{X} > 1.0$$

Figure 3   Quadrat sampling allows measurement of dispersion by counting numbers of individuals within each sampling frame, and then comparing the variance to the mean. Note that the mean number per frame is the same for all three patterns, but variance increases with aggregation.

Bear in mind that the size of the sampling frame can significantly influence the results of this kind of analysis. A population may be clumped at one scale of measurement, but uniform at another. For example, ant colonies represent dense aggregations of insects, but the colonies themselves can be uniformly distributed in space. Whether we consider the distribution of ants to be patchy or uniform depends on the scale of our investigation. Figure 4 illustrates a population that would be considered uniformly distributed if sampled with large quadrats, but aggregated if sampled with smaller quadrats. For organisms distributed in clusters, the $s^2/\overline{x}$ ratio will be maximized when the size of the sampling frame is equal to the size of the clusters.

Check your progress:

If densities are equal, which would yield a higher variance in numbers of individuals per quadrat: a highly aggregated population or a highly dispersed population?

Answer: High variance in relation to the mean results from highly aggregated spatial pattern.

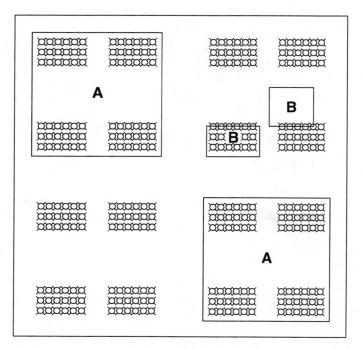

Figure 4   The calculated index of dispersion depends on the size of the quadrats used to sample the population. This hypothetical spatial pattern would exhibit a uniform dispersion index if sampled with large quadrats (A), but a clumped dispersion index if sampled with small quadrats (B).

The significance of aggregation or dispersion of populations has been demonstrated in many kinds of animal and plant populations. **Intraspecific competition**, for example, tends to separate individuals and create higher dispersion. Territorial animals, such as male robins on campus lawns in the spring, provide an excellent example. As each male defends a plot of lawn large enough to secure food for his nestlings, spaces between competitors increase, and the population becomes less aggregated. Competition can also create uniform plant distributions. In arid habitats, trees and shrubs become uniformly distributed if competition for soil moisture eliminates plants growing too close together (Figure 5).

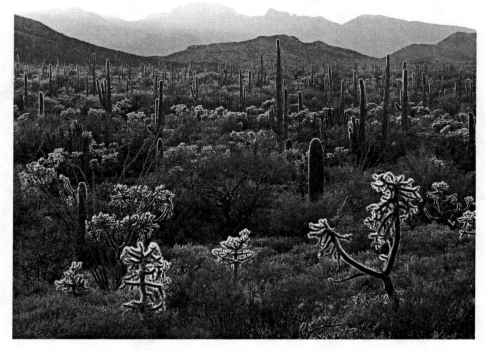

Figure 5   Saguaro and cholla cactus exhibit highly dispersed spatial patterns because of intense competition for water in a desert ecosystem.

If organisms are attracted to one another, their population shows increased aggregation. Schooling fish may limit the chance that any individual within the group is attacked by a predator. Bats in temperate climates conserve energy by roosting in tightly packed groups (Figure 6). Cloning plants and animals with large litter sizes create aggregation as they reproduce clusters of offspring. For example, the Eastern wildflower called mayapple generates large clusters of shoots topped by characteristic umbrella-like leaves as it spreads vegetatively across the forest floor (Figure 7). By setting up quadrats, and calculating the variance/mean ratio of the quadrat counts, you can gain significant insights about the biology of your organism.

Check your progress:

Give an animal example of high dispersion; of low dispersion.
Give a plant example of high aggregation; of low aggregation.

Hint: Dispersion is the opposite of aggregation.

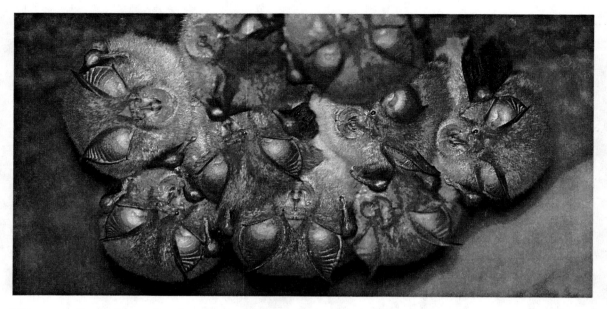

Figure 6   Lesser horseshoe bats roost in clusters to conserve body heat.

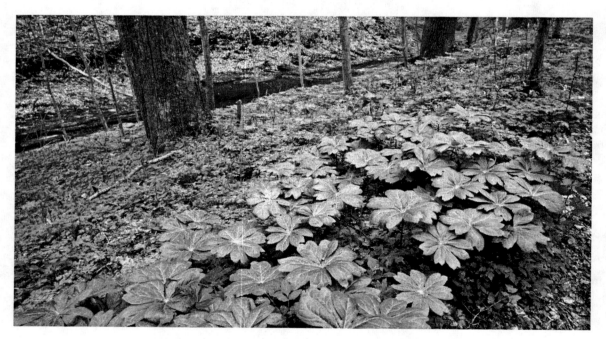

Figure 7   Mayapple (*Podophyllum peltatum*) forms highly aggregated stands through asexual reproduction.

METHOD A: DISPERSION OF PLANTS IN A LAWN COMMUNITY

[Outdoors, spring, summer, or fall]

Research Question

What can we infer about the natural history of lawn species from their spatial distribution?

Preparation

Before laboratory, carefully examine lawns on campus. Regardless of maintenance efforts, few lawns are actually monocultures. Almost all lawn communities include some broad-leaved plants such as dandelions, plantain, or clover growing among the turf grasses (Figure 8).

Check with your facilities management department to ensure that pesticides have not been applied to campus lawns within a few days prior to this laboratory.

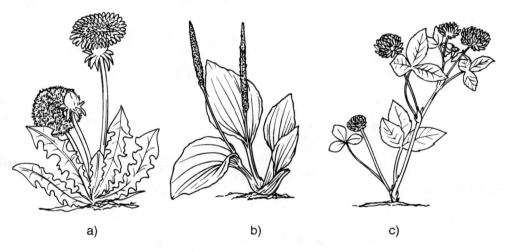

a)   b)   c)

Figure 8   Three common broad-leaved lawn weeds: (A) dandelion (*Taraxicum*), (B) Plantain (*Plantago*), and (C) clover (*Trifolium*).

Materials (per laboratory team)

   1 large nail (#16 galvanized or aluminum gutter nail)

   1 meter stick

   1 piece of nylon string, about 1-1/2 m long

Procedure

1.   Make quadrat sampler by tying one end of the string around the nail, tightly enough to stay on, but loosely enough to swivel around the head (Figure 9). Then using the meter stick, mark a point on the string 56 cm from the nail by tying an overhand knot at that position. Repeat the procedure to make a second knot 80 cm from the nail, then a third knot 98 cm from the nail, and a fourth knot 113 cm from the nail. The distance from the nail to each knot will become the radius of a circle in your sampling plots. Distance to the first knot represents the radius of a circle of area 1 m². (Try verifying this calculation, using the formula Area = π r² for a radius of 0.56 m.) The knots farther along the string will be used to sample circles of areas 2 m², 3 m², and 4 m², respectively. Take your sampler with you to a lawn area.

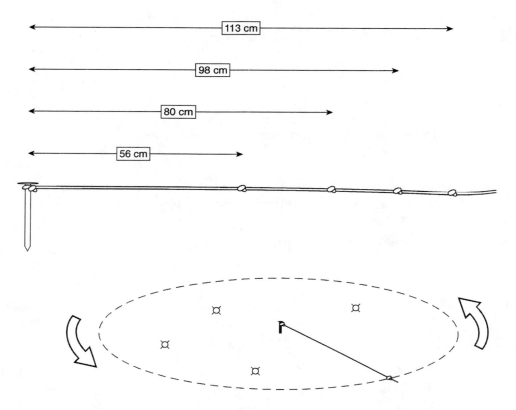

Figure 9 A string tied to a large nail, with knots tied at specified distances, can be used to sample a fixed area of lawn. Put the nail in the ground and pull the string taut. Moving the knot around the nail, count how many of your organisms fall within the circle.

2. Choose one lawn species exhibiting an interesting spatial pattern and common enough to find some specimens growing less than a meter apart. Decide what vegetative unit of this plant you will designate as an individual for the purpose of counting plots. For non-cloning plants such as dandelions, one rosette of leaves constitutes one individual. For cloning plants such as violets, choose a unit of plant growth, such as a shoot, as an arbitrary unit of population size.

3. Choose an area of lawn for sampling in which this species is relatively common. Before taking any samples, observe physical features of the habitat such as shade, soils, or small dips or mounds affecting water runoff that might help you interpret the pattern you see. Develop hypotheses relating the reproductive history of your species and habitat features with the distribution you are measuring.

4. Next, you must select sites for quadrat samples within your study area. You can obtain a fairly unbiased sample by tossing the nail within the sample area without aiming for any particular spot, and then pushing it into the soil wherever it lands. Hold the string at the first knot and stretch it out taut from the nail.

5. Now move the string in a circle (Figure 9). The length marked by your closest knot becomes a radius of a circular quadrat with area 1 m². If this circle is too small to include several individuals, move out to the second knot for a 2-m² quadrat, the third knot for a 3-m² quadrat, or the fourth knot for a 4-m² quadrat, as needed. After you decide on the appropriate scale, use the same size quadrat for all your samples.

6. As you move the string in a circle, count how many individuals fall within this quadrat. When the circle is complete, record this number in the Data Table for Methods A, B, and C. On the third column of the table, make notes of any landscape features that may affect your plant. Pull out the nail, make another toss to relocate your circular plot, and repeat for a total of 20 samples. Your sampling is complete when you have recorded 20 quadrat counts.

7. Analyze results on the Calculations for Methods A, B, and C page following the data table. By comparing the variance of your 20 quadrat counts with the mean, you will determine whether the plants you sampled are aggregated, random, or uniformly dispersed.

METHOD B: DISPERSION OF HERBIVORES ON PLANT RESOURCE UNITS

[Indoors/outdoors, employs biological collections, year-round]

In this exercise, we make use of plant parts serving as resource units for herbivorous animals. Leaves are resource units for plant-eating insects. Seeds and fruits, such as acorns or crab apples, serve as resource units for seed predators and fruit-eaters. An even-aged stand of campus trees can be considered a series of resource units for foraging birds or nesting squirrels.

Rather than constructing quadrats to count individuals per unit of space (absolute density), we will count the number of animals per resource unit (ecological density). By counting animals or animal signs in each plant part in a collected sample, we can calculate a variance as well as a mean, and get a determination of the aggregation or dispersion of animals among their resource units. As seen with quadrat counts in the Introduction, analysis of pattern among resource units can yield interesting insights into the population biology of the species.

Research Question

When animals choose resources, or insects choose egg-laying sites, do they randomly disperse themselves (or their offspring) among resource units?

Preparation

Campus landscapes provide many options for collecting plant parts bearing evidence of associated animal species (Figure 10). Leaves of almost all temperate deciduous trees are riddled with leaf miner tunnels and insect galls in late summer. Close examination of nuts or acorns almost always reveals small, round emergence holes made by seed-eating weevils or bruchid beetles, which have matured inside the seed and escaped through the seed coat. Seeds are easy to preserve, so the instructor can make a large collection (on or off campus) to use repeatedly for this exercise. Leaf samples can be preserved in a plant press, and maintained as a permanent collection, provided the brittle specimens are handled carefully. (It is best not to use leaves from existing herbarium pages, since these tend to be biased toward perfect specimens without visible insect damage.)

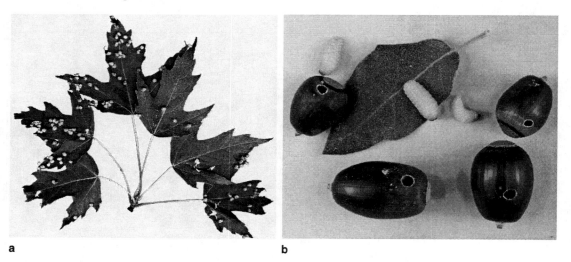

a   b

Figure 10   Ecological density is measured as numbers of individuals per resource unit. Insects on plant parts provide good study organisms: (A) Galls on maple leaves, (B) Acorn weevil larvae.

Alternatively, students may venture out onto the campus to collect their own specimens as part of this laboratory. Fall is best for collecting leaves, but seeds can be found throughout the year. In temperate locations, winter is the best time to find squirrel nests, which look like balls of leaves, in the bare branches of large deciduous trees. Empty bird nests are also apparent in winter and early spring, and provide a good index of ecological density if enough of them can be found. In spring, the class may find aphids or scale insects, which can be counted under a dissecting microscope. Once the collection is brought back to the laboratory, this exercise requires little time for data collection.

Materials (per laboratory team)

Collection of 20 resource units, or data from 20 resource units collected outside

Dissecting microscope or hand lens for small organisms

Procedure

1. If making your own collection, observe or collect 20 plant parts of equivalent size. Decide on a sampling plan in advance, so that the specimens are chosen with minimal bias. If using a laboratory collection such as a box of acorns, select 20 plant parts in a random sampling plan.
2. Count animals, or evidence of animal activity, on each plant part. Observe any life history observations you can, to help interpret intraspecific interactions that result in a pattern of dispersion among resource units.
3. Record numbers of animals for each of the 20 resource units as a data column in the Data Table for Methods A, B, and C at the end of this chapter. Bear in mind that one plant resource unit is a sampling unit in your study. Complete the Calculations section following the table, and answer the questions to discuss your results.

METHOD C: DISPERSION OF ISOPODS IN AN ARTIFICIAL HABITAT

[Laboratory, year-round]

Research Question

Do terrestrial isopods seek out conspecifics when selecting a habitat, or do they disperse to partition resources more evenly by avoiding habitat spaces occupied by others?

Preparation

Terrestrial isopods (Figure 11) include "pill bugs" (genus *Armadillium*), which roll into a ball when threatened, and the flatter and less flexible "sow bugs" (genus *Oniscus*). These arthropods are widely distributed, and are easily collected from leaf litter, under rocks and logs, or in lumber piles around buildings in most of North America. They can also be obtained from laboratory supply companies. Isopods feed on decaying organic material and are not difficult to handle or maintain in the laboratory. Use a covered container with some air exchange, such as a terrarium, plastic food container with perforated lid, or plastic shoe box. You might find a spoon and a small paintbrush handy to "sweep" them up and transport them from one place to another. It is very important to keep damp leaf mold or moistened paper toweling in their habitat at all times, because isopods use gills for respiration, and require high humidity.

If you are turning over logs, rocks, or lumber piles in search of isopods, remember that more aggressive animals, such as scorpions and venomous snakes, frequently hide in the same places. It is always wise to lift the side of a rock farthest from you first, and to be careful where you place your hands. When you are finished searching in a natural setting, replace rocks and logs where you found them.

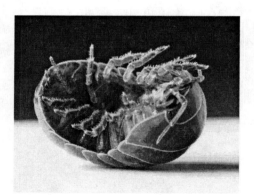

Figure 11 Terrestrial isopods, also called "pill bugs" (genus *Armadillium*), roll into a ball when threatened.

Materials (per laboratory team)

Plastic sweater box or other box-shaped container with a flat bottom, about 30 × 50 cm

5 medium potatoes

3–4 inch paring knife

60 map pins (with round heads, about 5 mm diameter)

20–30 live terrestrial isopods

Cutting board or cutting surface on lab bench

Procedure

1. Prepare "resource islands" from potatoes. First, cross-section a potato with parallel cuts evenly spaced 1 cm apart. You should get four or five round sections from each potato. Discard the ends, and cut more potatoes until you have 20 sections of approximately equal size and thickness. Then insert three map pins in a triangle formation on the bottom of each potato slice, so that the potato slice will stand on the map pins like a three-legged stool (Figure 12). The pins should leave about ½ cm of space for the isopods to crawl underneath.

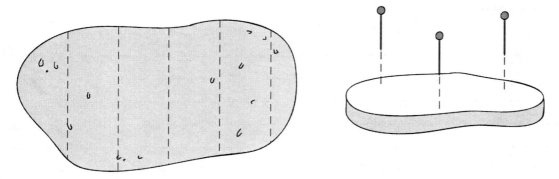

Figure 12   Slice potatoes and insert pins to make isopod shelters.

2. Arrange the 20 potato slices, pinheads down, in the bottom of the sweater box. Distribute the potato slices uniformly, with space separating each one. You now have an artificial habitat with 20 resource islands suitable for isopod colonization.
3. Release 20–30 isopods into the box. Take a few minutes to observe their behavior. How do they react to the box edges? to the potato "islands"? to one another?
4. Leave the isopods overnight. The underside of the potato slice islands provide a dark, humid microclimate that is preferred by isopods. They also feed on the potatoes. If lights are left on in the room, all isopods should select one of the potato slices to hide under.
5. After the isopods have had time to adjust to their habitat (12–48 hrs), count the number of isopods underneath each potato slice. You will need to pick up each "habitat island," because the isopods often invert themselves and cling to the potato. Record 0 if there are none in that sample. The 20 numbers you record should sum to the number of isopods you released into the box.
6. Complete the Data Table and calculation page at the end of this chapter. The mean number of isopods per potato slice ($\bar{x}$) is the ecological density, and the variance/mean ratio provides an index of aggregation for the captive isopod population.
7. Interpret your results by answering Questions for Methods A, B, and C.

Data Table for Methods A, B, and C

Sampling Unit	No. of individuals in the sample	Note any habitat features associated with this sample.
1	3	
2	2	
3	9	
4	1	
5	1	
6	1	
7	1	
8		
9		
10		
11		
12		
13		
14		
15		
16		
17		
18		
19		
20		

−2
dead

CALCULATIONS FOR METHODS A, B, AND C

1. Enter your 20 counts of organisms per sampling unit (x_i) in the second column of the table below.
2. Calculate a mean ($\overline{x}$) by summing all the counts and dividing by the sample size ($n = 20$).
3. Subtract the mean from each data value to obtain the deviation from the average (d_i).
4. Square each deviation ($d^2)_i$. (Note that this step takes care of the negative signs.)
5. Add up all the squared deviations (Σd^2).
6. Divide the sum of d^2 values by (sample size − 1) to calculate the sample variance (s^2).
7. Finally, divide the variance by the mean ($\overline{x}$) to compute the variance/mean ratio ($s^2/\overline{x}$).
8. Refer to the Introduction, and to the methods section you used, to interpret this ratio.

Sample number (i)	No. of organisms in sample i (x_i)	0.7	Deviations (d_i)		Squared deviations (d^2)$_i$
1	3	$- \bar{x} =$	2.3	$^2 =$	5.29
2	2	$- \bar{x} =$	1.3	$^2 =$	1.69
3	9	$- \bar{x} =$	8.3	$^2 =$	68.89
4		$- \bar{x} =$		$^2 =$	
5		$- \bar{x} =$		$^2 =$	
6		$- \bar{x} =$		$^2 =$	
7		$- \bar{x} =$		$^2 =$	
8		$- \bar{x} =$		$^2 =$	
9		$- \bar{x} =$		$^2 =$	
10		$- \bar{x} =$		$^2 =$	
11		$- \bar{x} =$		$^2 =$	
12		$- \bar{x} =$		$^2 =$	
13		$- \bar{x} =$		$^2 =$	
14		$- \bar{x} =$		$^2 =$	
15		$- \bar{x} =$		$^2 =$	
16		$- \bar{x} =$		$^2 =$	
17		$- \bar{x} =$		$^2 =$	
18		$- \bar{x} =$		$^2 =$	
19		$- \bar{x} =$		$^2 =$	
n = 20		$- \bar{x} =$		$^2 =$	
Total # organisms $\Sigma (x_i) =$	14	Sum of Squared Deviations $\Sigma (d^2)_i =$			75.87
Mean $\Sigma (x_i)/n =$	0.7	Sample Variance $s^2 = \Sigma (d^2)_i/(n-1) =$			$\frac{75.87}{19} \approx 4$
	Variance/Mean $(s^2 / \bar{x}) =$	5.71			

greater then 1   aggregated distribution

Questions for Methods A, B, and C

1. Based on the variance/mean ratio, what can you conclude about the spatial pattern of your population? How might you explain this pattern, given observations you made as you were sampling?

   aggergated distrubution

2. Random sampling is very important if the data you collected are meant to represent a larger population. In retrospect, do you have any questions or concerns about the validity of the sampling method? If bias exists, how might you alter your method to randomize your samples?

   The larger the potato preces would incoease the size of the specieres on Ito the avalrable space hus peenlty of space for them.

3. An index of aggregation is maximized in patchy distributions if the size of the quadrat is the same as the size of the organism's aggregations. Might a larger or smaller sampling unit (or a different sized resource unit) have affected your results?

   Yes, the avalrable spece will moese.

4. Would you expect another organism from the same biological community to exhibit a similar index of dispersion? Is spatial pattern a property of the organism, or of its habitat?

5. Lesser horseshoe bats (Figure 6) and many other bat species are increasingly rare. How does a highly aggregated distribution, for at least part of the life cycle, influence the status of endangered species?

FOR FURTHER INVESTIGATION

1. In Method A, does spatial pattern vary among species of lawn plants, or in different parts of the campus? What does spatial pattern tell you about community interactions?
2. In Method B, how would you expect population density to affect the pattern of resource use by your herbivore? It might be possible to compare collections from different years or from different sites to address this question.
3. In Method C, how might the addition of predators such as centipedes affect patterns of settlement by an isopod population in the laboratory? If the same population is sampled repeatedly over a period of time, does its pattern of dispersion change? What environmental factors influence these changes?

FOR FURTHER READING

Eliason, E. A. and D. A. Potter. 2001. Spatial distribution and parasitism of leaf galls induced by *Callirhytis cornigera* (Hymenoptera: Cynipidae) on Pin Oak. *Environmental Entomology* 30 (2): 280–287.

Krebs, C. J. 1998. *Ecological Methods* (2nd edition). Menlo Park (Benjamin Cummings).

Competition

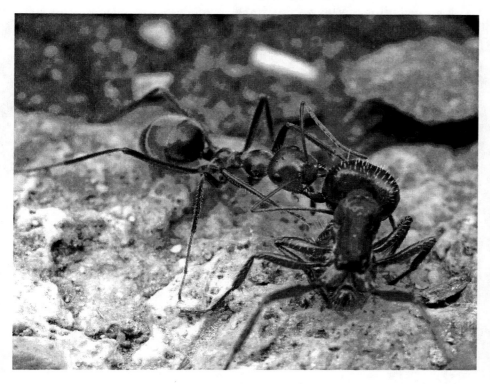

Figure 1   Honeypot ant (left) and harvester ant (right) compete for resources in the Chiricahua Mountains of Arizona.

INTRODUCTION

Harvester ants (Figure 1, right) are ecologically important members of desert communities. These ants range far and wide to collect small seeds for food, hoarding their substantial harvest in huge underground nests. Honeypot ants (Figure 1, left) often feed on nectar, so they have a somewhat different **niche**. However, honeypot ants do compete with harvester ants for dead insects and other scavenged food. In fact, honeypot ants frequently attack harvester ants to rob the larger ants of food they are carrying. This kind of negative community interaction is called **interference competition**, because one species actively interferes with the success of the other. Interference can be behavioral, as seen in warring ants, or it can be chemical, as seen in plants and fungi. A *Penicillium* fungus growing through rotting fruit produces antibiotics that interfere with the growth of its bacterial competitors.

Creosote bush (Figure 2) releases chemical herbicides that interfere with the growth of grasses and other plants. This sort of chemical warfare against competitors, called **allelopathy**, has been proposed as an explanation for creosote's dominance in dry scrub environments across the American southwest. Although allelopathy can be clearly demonstrated in controlled laboratory experiments, field researchers have identified many complicating factors, including herbivory by small mammals, drought, fire, and soil microorganisms, all potentially influencing the way plant chemicals affect the outcome of competition in nature (Halsey, 2005).

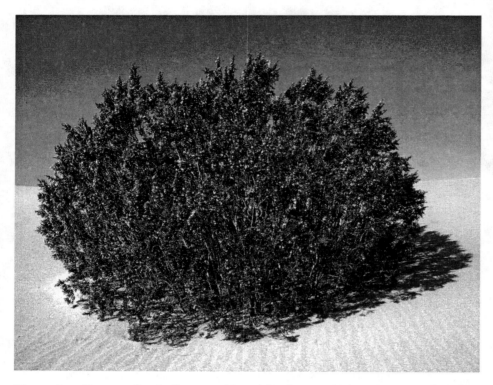

Figure 2   Creosote bush (*Larrea tridentata*) releases allelopathic chemicals that can retard the growth of competing plants around its root zone.

Competitors do not always face off in head-to-head contests. Hawks and owls hunting for the same rodents in a meadow may not hunt at the same time, but the presence of one predator reduces food for the other. Two tree species in a forest, though in physical proximity, compete primarily by extracting nutrients, water, and sunshine from their habitat to the exclusion of other trees, and not necessarily through active interference. These more passive forms of mutually detrimental interaction are called **exploitative competition**.

It is important to recognize that individuals pursuing limited resources are generally faced with two sources of competition. Competitive interaction among members of the same species is called **intraspecific competition**. Competitive interaction among members of different species is called **interspecific competition**. (Similar prefixes are used to distinguish intramural sports, among members of your own school, from intermural sports, between rival schools.)

Laboratory Studies

Key insights into the nature of competition came from the microbiology laboratory of Georgyi Frantsevitch Gause, who worked in Russia during the 1930s. Gause understood that the complexity of ecological systems makes identification of cause and effect very difficult, so he used his training in microbiology to develop the simplest model ecosystem he possibly could. Gause cultured *Paramecium*, a genus of ciliated protozoans, in small culture tubes on a diet of the rod-shaped bacterium *Bacillus subtilis*. To eliminate bacterial population growth as a confounding variable, Gause cultured the bacteria separately on solid media, scraped mature colonies off the culture plates, and resuspended the cells in a nutrient-free solution of physiological salts. Paramecia could then be introduced to feed on bacteria in these suspensions, but the bacteria could not reproduce. Every day, Gause put his protozoan cultures in a centrifuge at low speed to push all Paramecia to the bottom without killing them. He then used a pipette to remove the old fluid on top, and replaced it with a fresh bacterial suspension. He then gently stirred the Paramecia up from the bottom. This method guaranteed a constant food supply and constant waste removal for the ciliate. With bacterial food supply and the chemical environment held constant, growth of Paramecia was the only variable Gause needed to monitor in his experiments.

Gause's most famous experiment involved two closely related species: *Paramecium caudatum*, which is the larger, and *Paramecium aurelia*, which is the smaller of the two organisms illustrated in Figure 3. Species in the same genus, which are called **congeners**, were a wise choice for Gause's competition studies, because taxonomically related species would be expected to use similar resources in similar ways. To determine growth characteristics of each species, Gause first cultured each species separately. These isolated populations followed **logistic growth** curves, reaching similar **carrying capacities** when cell volume was taken into account. When Gause introduced both *Paramecium* species into the same culture tube, *P. aurelia* always persisted, and *P. caudatum* always died out. Although smaller, *P. aurelia* was consistently the stronger competitor (Figure 4).

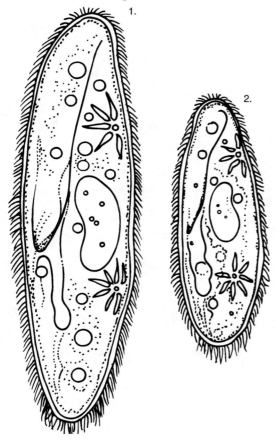

Figure 3 *Paramecium caudatum* (1) and *Parame-cium aurelia* (2), from Gause's classic publication on competition.

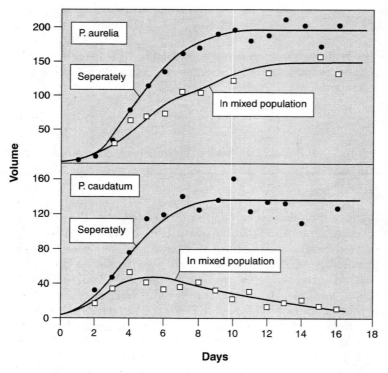

Further experiments with other pairs of protozoans produced similar results; when grown in mixed culture, even slight advantages in efficiency or stress tolerance allowed one species to survive and grow while the other species declined to extinction. The only way Gause was able to keep two species alive for any length of time was to create a more complex environment, such as a culture tube with glass wool in the bottom, which allowed each species to dominate in a different microhabitat. These observations led to Gause's **competitive exclusion principle**. Stated simply, Gause (1934) determined that *competing species cannot coexist within the same ecological niche.*

Figure 4   Gause's results for *Paramecium aurelia* (top graph) and *Paramecium caudatum* (bottom graph). Each species was grown separately (solid data points) and then in mixed population (open data points). Results show total biomass accumulation (numbers of individuals multiplied by cell size) over a 16-day period. Under competitive pressure in mixed cultures, *P. aurelia* growth is only slowed down, but *P. caudatum* is driven to extinction.

Check your progress:

If the competitive exclusion principle applies to all of nature, how can we account for so many species still existing in the world?

Hint: Natural ecosystems contain a great variety of niches.

Intraspecific vs. Interspecific Competion in Plants

In plants, the number of individuals is an indicator of the success of a population, but size of individuals is important as well. Large individuals tend to consume more resources and produce more offspring than small ones. For example, if sagebrush and bunchgrass are competing in a Great Basin habitat, counting individuals may not be the best way to determine which species is more successful, since individual size at maturity varies so much in plants of this type (Figure 5). A better measure of competitive outcomes in plants is **biomass** accumulation over time. To measure biomass, ecologists harvest all plants from a sampled area, separate the harvest by species, dry the plant material, and weigh the samples to determine which species has amassed more grams of tissue per unit area over the time of the study.

Dutch biologist C. T. de Wit developed a method for comparing the effects of intraspecific and interspecific competition in plants. His experimental design, called a **replacement series,** begins with seeds of two species planted in a series of pots. Let's call these plants Species A and Species B. An equal number of seeds are started in each pot. However, the proportions of the two species vary from all Species A to combinations of A and B, to all Species B (Figure 6). This is called a replacement series because Species B individuals are gradually replaced by Species A individuals, illustrated in the figure from left to right. If interspecific competition is less severe than competition within the species, results resemble Figure 7A. The two bottom curves on the graph show dry weights of Species A and Species B, separately, for each combination of planting frequencies. The top curved line shows the biomass of both species summed together. The straight line connecting the 100% A biomass and the 100% B biomass represents a null hypothesis: that the total yield at each frequency along the replacement series is predicted by the proportions of A and B planted in that pot. This is what we would expect if competition between species is exactly as intense as competition within the species. For example, for a mixed planting begun with 50% species A seeds and 50% species B seeds, the null hypothesis projects total biomass exactly halfway between the maxima for Species A and Species B.

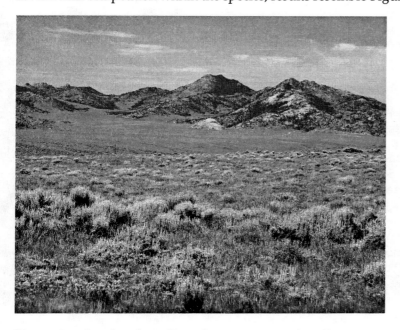

Figure 5   Sagebrush and bunchgrass compete in a Great Basin habitat.

Seedlings Planted in a Replacement Series

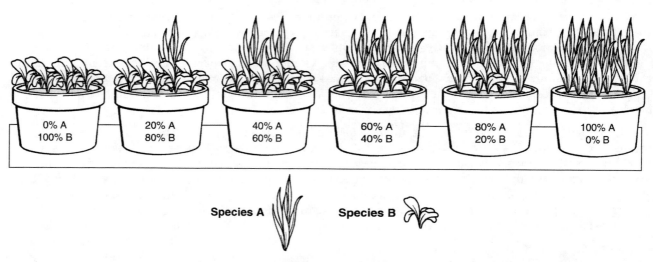

Figure 6 Replacement series of two-species plantings for de Wit competition experiment. Each pot in this example has five plants, but frequency of the narrow-leaved species A ranges from 0% at the left to 100% at the right.

The actual biomass totals can be compared with the null model to determine whether interspecific competition compares with intraspecific competition. If the two plants produce a higher combined biomass in mixed planting than in pure stands, then the total biomass line curves above the straight line predicted by the null model. This would be expected if the two plants are extracting different nutrients from the soil, or are in other ways exploiting different niches. Sometimes the de Wit experiment indicates high interspecific competition (Figure 7B). If one species interferes with growth of the other, as expected in allelopathic plants, then the combined biomass line sags below the straight line of the null model. Agricultural scientists conduct this kind of experiment to find out whether mixed species plantings could improve productivity of cropland or rangeland. For ecologists, the de Wit method can give insights into the extent of **niche overlap** between two competing plant species. The more closely two species compete in the same niche, the more likely combined yield in mixed plantings will be depressed below null expectations.

Check your progress:

What is the expected shape of the total yield curve in a de Wit diagram if interspecific competition is equivalent to intraspecific competition?

Answer: A straight line connecting the two 100% points

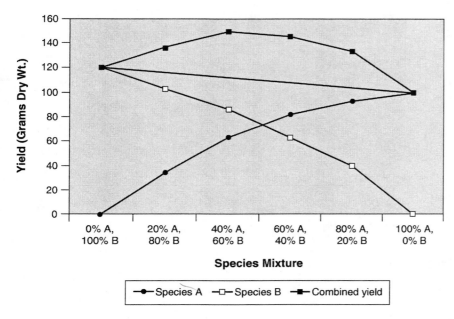

**de Wit Diagram
Low Interspecific Competition**

Yield (Grams Dry Wt.)

Species Mixture

— ● — Species A — □ — Species B — ■ — Combined yield

Figure 7A   de Wit diagram showing competition between species less severe than competition within species. The combined yield (top curved line) is above null expectations based on averaging individual species yields (straight line).

Modeling Competition

Although the de Wit diagram is a good way to describe the results of competition among plants, it does not forecast the outcome of competition in population terms. The challenge of predicting population growth in the presence of competitors was taken up by two researchers on different continents at the beginning of the 20th century. American biophysicist Alfred Lotka and Italian mathematician Vito Volterra independently discovered that well-known population growth equations could be modified to incorporate the effects of competition. Their simple mathematical models, called the **Lotka-Volterra competition equations**, have generated many useful questions and experimental investigations of competition in nature. (Lotka and Volterra also followed parallel approaches to the study of predator-prey relationships.)

Lotka and Volterra's model of competition begins with the assumption that two species are competing for the same resources, and that their rates of population growth are described by the **logistic growth** equation. To demonstrate how this model works, let's name our two competitors Species 1 and Species 2. To keep track of the numbers of both species, we will identify their population sizes as N_1 and N_2. We can assume each species has a maximum **intrinsic rate of reproduction** (**r**), so we can designate the population growth rates of the two species r_1 and r_2. Since resources are finite, each species has a **carrying capacity** (**K**) within the shared environment. Even if both species are limited by the same resource, their carrying capacities may not be the same. For example, if Species 1 is a bison and Species 2 is a prairie dog, we would not expect a patch of grassland to support equal numbers of bison or prairie dogs! We therefore need to designate K_1 as the

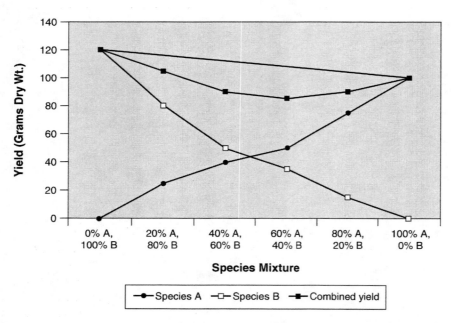

**de Wit Diagram
High Interspecific Competition**

Figure 7B de Wit diagram showing competition between species greater than competition within species. The combined yield (concave curve) lies below null expectations based on averaging individual species yields (straight line).

carrying capacity for Species 1, and K_2 as the carrying capacity for Species 2. Finally, we will need symbols to show the negative impact of these two species on each other. The impacts are not always equal. To go back to our bison and prairie dog example, we would expect a single bison to have a greater negative influence on the colony of prairie dogs than a single prairie dog would have on a herd of bison. We will therefore define α as the per-capita effect of Species 2 on Species 1, and β as the per-capita effect of Species 1 on Species 2. The constants α and β are called **competition coefficients**.

Check your progress:

Identify each of these symbols from the Lotka-Volterra equations.

$N_1 =$ $K_1 =$

$N_2 =$ $K_2 =$

$r_1 =$ $\alpha =$

$r_2 =$ $\beta =$

Hint: Remember that each species must have a population size, a growth rate, a carrying capacity, and a competitive effect on the other.

To begin as simply as possible, let's imagine that Species 1 is enjoying population growth by itself in the absence of any competitors. Its numbers are predicted by the logistic model:

Look at the fraction at the end of the equation. The numerator of this fraction is the carrying capacity of the environment (measured in numbers of individuals the environment can hold) minus the number of individuals already there. In other words, the numerator shows the number of "empty slots" available for colonization. Since this number of openings is divided by total carrying capacity, $(K_1 - N_1)/K_1$ represents the proportion of the environment that remains unfilled.

Growth Equation for Species 1 in isolation:

$$\Delta N_1 = (r_1)(N_1)\frac{K_1 - N_1}{K_1}$$

ΔN_1 = change in population size from one time interval to the next

r_1 = population growth rate of Species 1

N_1 = population size of Species 1

K_1 = carrying capacity of Species 1

Now considering the whole equation, this mathematical statement says the change in the number of individuals of Species 1 is equal to Species 1's intrinsic rate of increase multiplied by the current population, multiplied by the portion of the environment that is still open for colonization. If numbers of Species 1 are low, then N_1 is near 0, and $(K_1 - N_1)/K_1$ approximates (K_1/K_1), which would be equivalent to multiplying by 1. This means that the third term in the equation has little impact on population growth as long as population size is low. However, as N_1 approaches K_1, the third term approaches zero, and multiplying by zero results in no change in the population. In other words, as the environment fills up, the population approaches zero population growth so that numbers are stabilized at carrying capacity. This is the meaning of logistic growth.

Check your progress:

How does the size of N_1 relative to K_1 determine the growth rate of species 1 in the absence of competition? Explain what $(K_1 - N_1)/K_1$ means, in biological terms.

Hint: Consider the effects of multiplying by the third term in the growth equation when $N_1 = 0$. Compare this answer to your result if $N_1 = K_1$.

Next, we will assume that Species 2 enters the habitat. As Species 2 occupies space and consumes resources, the number of "empty slots" for growth of Species 1 in the environment will decline. How much will they decline? We can show carrying capacity being consumed by both species as follows:

Number of "empty slots" for Species 1 = $K_1 - N_1 - \alpha N_2$

From the total carrying capacity for Species 1, we subtract the number of Species 1 individuals, and we also subtract the number of Species 2 individuals multiplied by the competition coefficient α. Think of α as a conversion factor that transforms each individual of Species 2 to an equivalent number of Species 1, for the purpose of calculating resource consumption. For example, α would be quite large if we were converting bison to an equivalent number of prairie dogs, but quite small if we were converting prairie dogs to an equivalent number of bison.

Having incorporated both species into the model, we can now calculate the growth rate of Species 1 in the presence of its competitor as follows:

Note that this is just the logistic growth equation, with Species 2 thrown into the numerator of the third term. As long as the carrying capacity K_1 exceeds the total numbers of Species 1 and Species 2 (converted by α to Species 1 equivalents), then populations of Species 1 will grow. The actual rate of growth depends on the numbers already present (N_1) and the population growth rate (r_1). Population growth is indicated by a positive value of ΔN_1, stable population size is indicated by a zero value of ΔN_1, and population decline is indicated by a negative value of ΔN_1.

Competition Equation for Species 1:

$$\Delta N_1 = (r_1)\,(N_1)\,\frac{K_1 - N_1 - \alpha N_2}{K_1}$$

ΔN_1 = change in population size from one time interval to the next

r_1 = population growth rate of Species 1

N_1 = population size of Species 1

N_2 = population size of Species 2

α = per-capita effect of Species 2 on Species 1

K_1 = carrying capacity of Species 1

Check your progress:

Use the competition equation to calculate the number of new individuals expected in the population if $N_1 = 43$, $N_2 = 86$, $\alpha = 0.4$, $r_1 = 0.75$, and $K_1 = 110$.

Answer: 9.6 new individuals added, so we project a total of 52.6 individuals of Species 1 in the next time period.

To simplify interpretations of the model, it is useful to ask, under what conditions does the population have zero population growth? Examine the competition equation for Species 1. There are three terms multiplied together in the equation. If any of these terms is zero, then ΔN_1 will be zero. However, the first two terms give trivial solutions. In the case of the first term, population growth is obviously zero if N_1 is zero, because the species cannot grow if it is already extinct. In the case of the second term, the population cannot grow if $r_1 = 0$, because that would indicate a zero intrinsic rate of increase, with no biological capacity for reproduction beyond population replacement. The third term is therefore the interesting case. As we saw in our earlier discussions, ΔN_1 will be zero whenever $K_1 - N_1 - \alpha N_2 = 0$. In biological terms, the population stops growing whenever the two species fill up the carrying capacity of the environment. Solving this equality for N_1 gives us the following zero-growth equation conditions for Species 1:

Zero-growth Equation for Species 1:

$\Delta N_1 = 0$ whenever:

$$K_1 - N_1 - \alpha N_2 = 0$$

or:

$$N_1 = K_1 - \alpha N_2$$

$\Delta N_1 =$ change in population size from one time interval to the next
$N_1 =$ population size of Species 1
$N_2 =$ population size of Species 2
$\alpha =$ per-capita effect of Species 2 on Species 1
$K_1 =$ carrying capacity of Species 1

Note that the zero-growth equation is in the form of a straight line with a slope equal to $-\alpha$. The best way to illustrate the conditions for zero growth is with a **joint abundance graph** (Figure 8). This graph shows numbers of Species 1 on the x-axis and numbers of Species 2 on the y-axis. A point on this kind of graph shows both population sizes simultaneously. Changes in the joint abundance of the two populations can be shown by moving this point around within the graph space. The figure shows the zero growth equation for Species 1 plotted as a line on the graph. This line is called the **zero growth isocline** for Species 1. Remember that the zero growth isocline represents the combined numbers of Species 1 and Species 2 that equal the carrying capacity for Species 1. Anywhere below this line (closer to the graph's origin) is a set of conditions allowing growth of Species 1. Anywhere above and to the right of this line represents an overloaded carrying capacity, which will result in decline of Species 1. Arrows on the graph show the direction the joint population point will move, depending on its position relative to the isocline.

Check your progress:

Beginning with the zero-growth equation for Species 1,

$$N_1 = K_1 - \alpha N_2$$

Solve for N_1 when $N_2 = 0$

Then solve for N_2 when $N_1 = 0$

Answer: Look at the isocline on the graph.
When $N_2 = 0$, the line intersects the x-axis. What value of N_1 do you see at this point?
When $N_1 = 0$, the line intersects the y-axis. What value of N_2 do you see at this point?

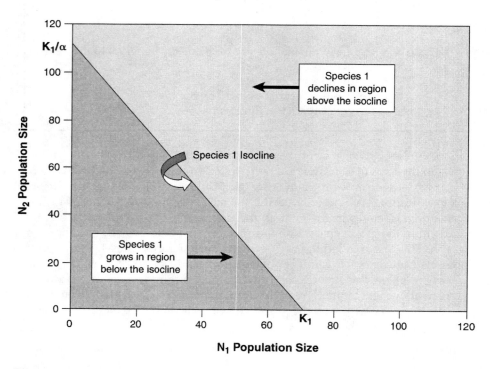

Lotka-Volterra Competition Model
Species 1 Isocline

Figure 8   Joint abundance graph showing the Species 1 zero-growth isocline. The N_1 population, shown on the horizontal axis, grows whenever the joint abundance lies in the region to the left of the isocline (shaded) and declines whenever the joint abundance lies in the region to the right of the isocline (unshaded).

Now we need to consider Species 2. By the same arguments we used for Species 1, we can generate the following complementary equations:

Competition Equation for Species 2:

$$\Delta N_2 = (r_2)(N_2)\frac{K_2 - N_2 - \beta N_1}{K_2}$$

ΔN_2 = change in population size from one time interval to the next
r_2 = population growth rate of Species 2
N_2 = population size of Species 2
N_1 = population size of Species 1
β = per-capita effect of Species 1 on Species 2
K_2 = carrying capacity of Species 2

And by similar logic, the following equation can be used to draw a zero growth isocline for Species 2 (Figure 9).

Zero-growth equation for Species 2:

$\Delta N_2 = 0$ whenever:

$$N_2 = K_2 - \beta N_1$$

ΔN_2 = change in Species 2 population size from one time interval to the next
K_2 = carrying capacity of Species 2
N_1 = population size of Species 1
β = per-capita effect of Species 1 on Species 2

Lotka-Volterra Competition Model
Species 2 Isocline

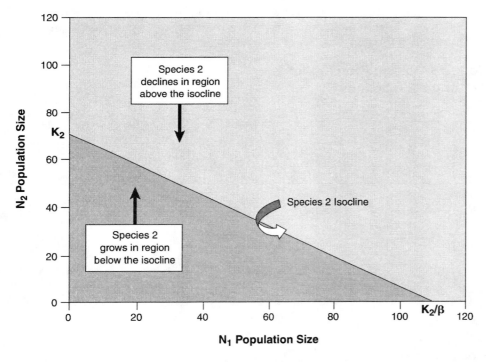

Figure 9   Species 2 isocline. The N_2 population, shown on the vertical axis, grows whenever the joint abundance lies in the region below the isocline (shaded) and declines whenever the joint abundance lies in the region above the isocline (unshaded).

Note that numbers of Species 2 are represented vertically on the graph, so the labels on the isocline are inverted relative to the isocline for Species 1.

Check your progress:

By inspecting the zero-growth isocline for Species 2 in Figure 9, can you estimate the value of K_2 in this example? Can you estimate the value of β?

Answer: $K_2 = 70$
$\beta = 0.64$

The Lotka-Volterra model gets interesting when both species isoclines are shown on the same graph (Figure 10). Since the isoclines cross in the illustrated example, the graph space is divided into four regions. Near the origin is a region below both isoclines, so both species can grow. The black arrow in the figure shows the direction of change on the joint abundance graph within this region. Above and to the left is a region below the Species 1 isocline, but above the Species 2 isocline. Species 1 can continue to grow below its isocline, so the joint abundance moves toward the right, but Species 2 is declining so the joint abundance moves down. The arrow is a vector summing both of these trends, indicating a change down and toward the right. At the lower right is a region above the Species 1 isocline but below the Species 2 isocline, so the joint abundance moves up and to the left as Species 1 declines and Species 2 grows. Finally, at the upper right is a region above both isoclines, so the joint abundance declines down and to the left in this region.

Lotka-Volterra Competition Model
N1 and N2 Isoclines

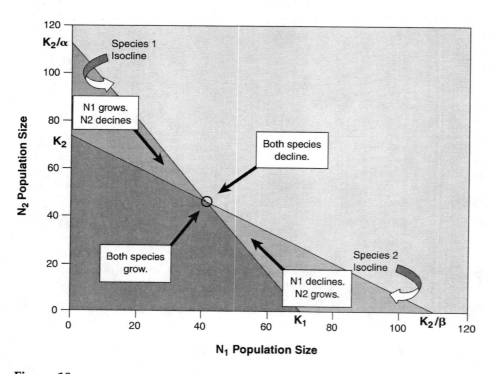

Figure 10

Note that wherever the two populations begin, their joint abundance moves toward the point of intersection of the two isoclines. This point, indicated by a circled dot on the graph, is a point of equilibrium because it is the only place on the graph in which ΔN_1 and ΔN_2 both equal zero. The model predicts coexistence of Species 1 and Species 2, with stable populations determined by the intersection of the isoclines. If environmental perturbations move the joint equilibrium off this stable equilibrium point, the system returns to equilibrium. You can think of this model like a round-bottomed bowl holding a marble: whatever happens to move the marble away from equilibrium, it tends to return to the same point.

The particular outcome predicted in Figure 10 occurs only when $K_2/\beta > K_1$ and $K_1/\alpha > K_2$. This tends to happen when the competition coefficients are low, making K_2/β and K_1/α large in relation to carrying capacity. Biologically, this makes sense. Coexistence between competitors would be expected if their competitive effects on one another are small. As α and β become larger, the value of the fractions decreases, and it is less likely the isoclines will cross in this direction.

Figure 11 shows four possible outcomes for Lotka-Volterra competition, depending on the orientation of the two zero-growth isoclines. Graph A predicts coexistence, as you have already seen. In Graph B, the isoclines cross in the opposite direction, with $K_2/\beta < K_1$ and $K_1/\alpha < K_2$. There is still an equilibrium point at the intersection, but note the direction of the vectors of change pointing away from the center of the graph. Any small perturbation moving the point away from the center will result in one species or the other driving its competitor to extinction. You can think of this condition as an upside-down bowl with a hemispherical bottom and a marble balanced carefully on top. A slight push destroys the unstable equilibrium, and the marble falls to rest at a more stable equilibrium point. This model predicts either one species or the other will win, but the outcome depends on initial conditions.

Graphs C and D in Figure 11 show what happens when the isoclines do not cross. In these cases, the species whose isocline lies farthest from the origin will continue to grow when its competitor is above capacity, so the same species always drives the other to extinction. A marble on an inclined plane is a good way to visualize these graphs.

There is no question that the Lotka-Volterra competition models are oversimplified, and fail to incorporate all the factors influencing competition in nature. However, we should remember that models are supposed to be simplifications of a complex reality. The key to a good model is retaining a few key elements of the system so that we can better grasp how it works. For nearly a century, the Lotka-Volterra competition equations have helped ecologists to explain community interaction, and to generate more interesting questions for their studies of competition.

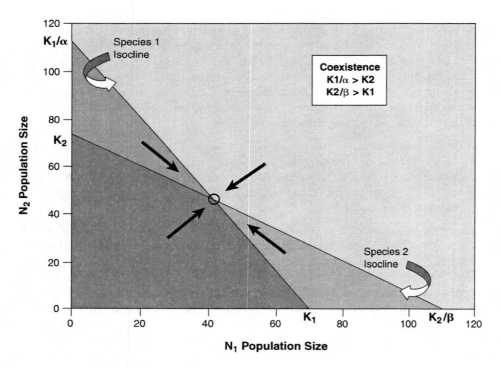

Figure 11A

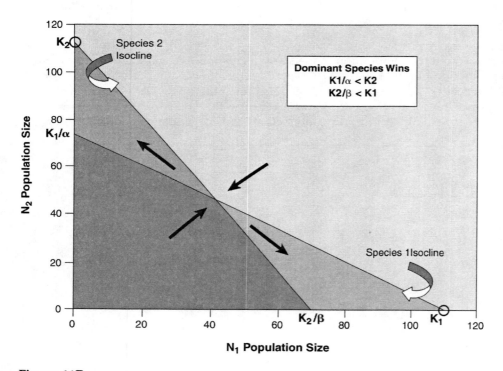

Figure 11B

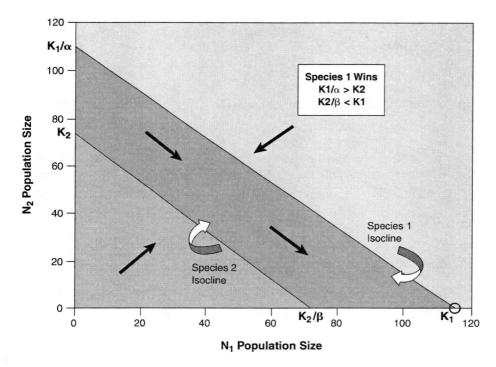

Figure 11C

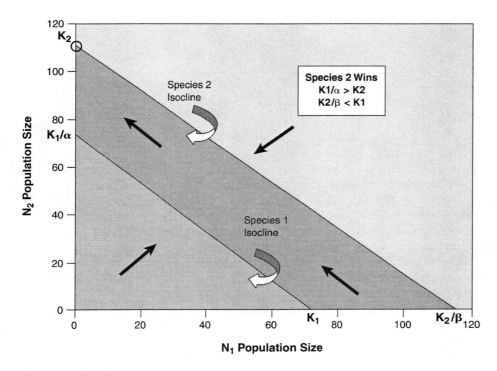

Figure 11D

STOP

METHOD A: ALLELOPATHY

[Laboratory activity, spring, summer, or fall]

Research Question

Is lettuce sensitive to allelopathic compounds found in black walnut leaves?

Preparation

Seeds can be obtained at garden supply stores, but plant parts as a source of allelopathic compounds are seasonal. The exercise calls for black walnut leaves, but radish leaves, sweet potato plants grown from cuttings, or alfalfa sprouts can be substituted.

Materials (per laboratory team)

3 Petri dishes, 10 cm diameter

9 sheets of round filter paper, 9 cm diameter

Grease pencil or marker to label glassware

Lettuce seeds (packet of 75 or more seeds)

Lettuce leaves, 100 g

Black walnut leaves, 100 g

Distilled water (1 liter)

Blender

2 large funnels

3 flasks, 500-ml each

Paper toweling or cheesecloth

Access to refrigerator

Procedure

1. Weigh out 50 grams of lettuce leaves and 50 grams of walnut leaves.
2. Place 50 g lettuce leaves in blender with 300 ml distilled water. Blend long enough to disrupt cells.
3. Push the center of a paper towel (or piece of cheesecloth) into a large funnel. Place the funnel in a large flask. Pour your leaf extract through the funnel, filtering out leaf fragments to get a clear solution of plant compounds. Collect about 250 ml of lettuce leaf extract, then label the flask and place it in a refrigerator.
4. Wash the blender thoroughly with soap, and rinse several times.
5. Repeat steps 2 and 3 with black walnut leaves to make a walnut leaf extract.
6. Place three sheets of filter paper in each of the three Petri dishes. Add 5 ml of lettuce extract, or enough to saturate the filter paper, to one of the dishes. Add an equal amount of walnut extract to the paper in a second dish, and an equal volume of distilled water to the third dish.
7. Place 25 lettuce seeds on top of the wet filter paper in each of the dishes. Cover the dishes, and label them on the sides of the lids so that the tops transmit light. Place both under constant light from a growth lamp or fluorescent light. Incubate at room temperature.
8. Check dishes every couple of days to ensure that the filter paper stays moist. Add equal amounts of distilled water to all dishes as needed to keep paper moist. Seedlings should be fully developed within a week.
9. Compare germination success and seedling size in the three dishes. If you wish, use a Chi-square contingency test to test the null hypothesis that germination is equal in the three treatments. If seedlings do emerge, measure the length of the root and calculate a mean and variance for each treatment group. Answer the following questions to analyze your data:

Questions (Method A)

1. Do black walnut leaves seem to have an allelopathic effect on germination of lettuce seedlings? on growth rates after germination?

_____

_____

_____

_____

_____

2. Why was lettuce extract used in one of the treatments? Why was plain water used in the third treatment? Were there any differences between lettuce extract and plain water treatments? Why do you think this might be so?

_____

_____

_____

_____

_____

3. What does this experiment imply about the way black walnut might compete with other plants? How might you test this hypothesis in a field setting?

_____

_____

_____

_____

_____

4. If other trees react in the same way as lettuce to black walnut compounds, how would results of a replacement series involving black walnut appear in a de Wit diagram? Draw and label a sketch to indicate your conclusion.

_____

_____

_____

_____

_____

5. With reference to the Lotka-Volterra models, what sort of competition coefficient would you expect for the effects of black walnut on a broad-leaved competitor?

_____

_____

_____

_____

_____

METHOD B: COMPETITION WITHIN AND BETWEEN SPECIES

[Laboratory activity, spring, summer, or fall]

Research Question

How do intra- and interspecific competition compare among legumes and grains?

Preparation

This experiment requires bench space in a greenhouse, growth chamber, or extensive growth lights in a laboratory. Small peat pots of the type that expand when wet work well for this experiment. Mung beans and wheat seeds can be ordered from supply houses, but are also available from health food stores.

Materials (per laboratory team)

6 seed-starting pots (2–3" diameter) in trays, with potting soil

Mung bean seeds

Wheat seeds

Tap water, aged in a watering can or large flask for watering

Electronic balance, accurate to 0.01

12 large plastic weighing dishes

Procedure

1. Use label tape to identify each pot as shown in the first row of the following table. Fill pots with potting soil. Place the pots in a tray to catch excess water and water all pots liberally. To plant seeds, push a pencil point into the wet soil to make a hole and push in the seed until it is just below the soil surface. Plant *initial numbers of seeds* as shown in the second and fourth rows of the following table:

Label	0% B 100% W	20% B 80% W	40% B 60% W	60% B 40% W	80% B 20% W	100% B 0% W
Initial # bean seeds	0	4	6	8	10	12
Final # bean seeds	0	2	4	6	8	10
Initial # wheat seeds	12	10	8	6	4	0
Final # wheat seeds	10	8	6	4	2	0

2. Note that two extra seeds of each species are placed in each pot to account for any failures in germination. After seeds germinate, pull out excess seedlings to achieve the final number of seeds in each pot, as shown in the second and fourth rows of the table.
3. Place all pots in a randomized pattern under growth lights or on a greenhouse bench. Grow at room temperature (20–25° C) for 3–4 weeks. Check plants frequently and add water to the underlying tray to ensure all pots are equally moist.
4. After 3–4 weeks, cut all plants off flush with the soil, and separate plants from each pot into two weighing dishes; one for wheat and one for beans. You should have 10 weighing dishes for six pots, because the 100% pots contain only one species and the others have two. Expose all your harvested plant material to the air in a fairly dry place for a week.

5. Weigh the dried plant material in their weighing dishes, then dump out the plant material and reweigh the dish itself. Subtract the weights to determine the dry weight of beans (or wheat) in that pot. Enter data in the following data table.
6. Calculate class means for each species in each pot, and use the class averages to complete a de Wit diagram for this experiment. Answer the questions for Method B to interpret your results.

Results for Method B
Yields from Plant Competition Replacement Series
(Dry Weight in Grams)

TREATMENT GROUP:	0% B 100% W	20% B 80% W	40% B 60% W	60% B 40% W	80% B 20% W	100% B 0% W
Bean weight (Individual data)	X					
Wheat dry wt. (Individual data)						X
Bean weight (Group average)	X					
Wheat weight (Group average)						X

de Wit Diagram for Group Data

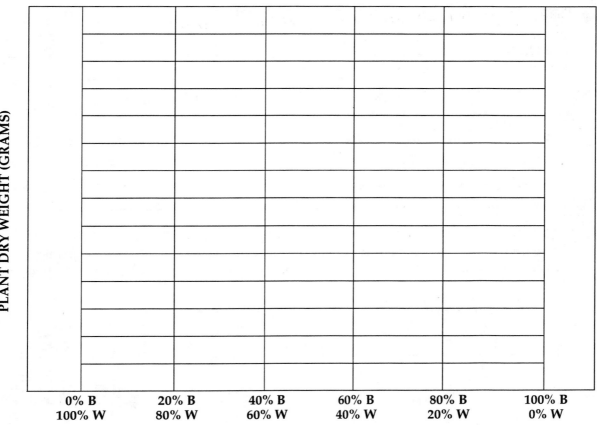

PLANT DRY WEIGHT (GRAMS)

| 0% B 100% W | 20% B 80% W | 40% B 60% W | 60% B 40% W | 80% B 20% W | 100% B 0% W |

Questions (Method B)

1. Explain the null hypothesis in this experiment. What is the value of a null hypothesis?

    _____

    _____

    _____

    _____

    _____

2. For mung beans growing with wheat, is interspecific competition stronger or weaker than intraspecific competition? Is the same true of wheat?

    _____

    _____

    _____

    _____

    _____

3. Do mung beans and wheat seem to have substantial niche overlap, or do they occupy distinct niches? How can you tell from the de Wit diagram?

    _____

    _____

    _____

    _____

    _____

4. Would beans and grain be good candidates for mixed plantings in the same field to increase agricultural yields, or not? Explain.

    _____

    _____

    _____

    _____

    _____

5. Referencing the Lotka-Volterra model of competition, would you suspect the two competition coefficients α and β to be large or small in this system? Are they likely to be equal or unequal in size? Explain.

    _____

    _____

    _____

    _____

    _____

METHOD C: COMPETITION PROBLEMS

[Classroom or homework activity]

1. Observe the population dynamics of the two *Paramecium* species illustrated in Figure 4. Assume the carrying capacities of each species (in volumetric units as shown on the graphs) are indicated by the maximum size of the populations when cultured in isolation. Draw a joint abundance graph, with Lotka-Volterra isoclines consistent with the results of competition in this experiment. (Consult Figure 11 for possible arrangements of the isoclines. You will not have values for α and β, so the important consideration is the relative positions of the isoclines.)

2. Assume the maximum density of harvester ants in a desert region is eight colonies per hectare in the absence of honeypot ants. Five colonies of honeypot ants move into the area, and as a result of interference competition, the number of harvester ant colonies falls to six colonies per hectare. If α is a competition coefficient representing the effect of honeypot colonies on harvester colonies, what is the value of α?

3. Assume a prairie reserve in Kansas has sufficient grassland to maintain a herd of up to 180 bison. Both bison and elk are introduced to the reserve. From past experience, assume that α, the effect of elk on bison, is 0.3 and that β, the effect of bison on elk, is 0.45. Carrying capacity for elk is 230. Use the Lotka-Volterra equations to predict the equilibrium population sizes of these two competing species. Draw a joint abundance graph with isoclines to illustrate your answer.

4. In the Kansas preserve described in problem 3, if the bison herd is culled every year and maintained at a constant number of 50 individuals by the park staff, predict the equilibrium number of elk. Explain your answer by referencing isoclines on the joint abundance graph.

5. Assume that Species 1 (cattails) and Species 2 (rushes) compete for space around a pond in such a way that $K_1 = 80$ shoots per m^2 and $K_2 = 115$ shoots per m^2. Competition coefficients are $\alpha = 0.8$ and $\beta = 1.6$, indicating a high level of niche overlap. Draw a joint abundance graph with isoclines, adding arrows to indicate the direction of change within each area of your graph. In theory, if the populations were at the point of intersection of the two isoclines in your drawing, both cattails and rushes would demonstrate zero growth, and the system would be in equilibrium. Is the population likely to remain at this point? What biological factors might determine the actual outcome for this pond?

FOR FURTHER INVESTIGATION

1. Locate ant colonies on your campus. Sidewalks and paving stones often shelter nests. Map colony sites, measuring distances between colonies. Use small dabs of acrylic paint to mark individual ant workers, and follow them as they forage. Do ants forage near other colony sites, or do the colonies seem to have territorial boundaries?

2. Many weed species, such as crabgrass and ragweed, have been shown to release biologically active compounds. Try collecting weeds of different types from your campus or weedy lots or fields to extend the allelopathy investigation outlined in Method A.

3. Try the replacement series experiment for seeds collected from wild plants or trees in your area. Does the de Wit diagram you produce explain distribution patterns of these species?

4. Use a spreadsheet program to model the Lotka-Volterra equations. Because the growth equations are in the discrete form, you can use the solution from one year as the population size input for the next. Plot results on a joint abundance graph to see what happens as populations approach the zero-growth isoclines.

FOR FURTHER READING

de Wit, C. T. 1961. Space relationship within populations of one or more species. *Society of Experimental Biology Symposium* 15:314–329.

Gause, G. F. 1934. *The Struggle for Existence.* Accessible at: http://www.ggause.com/Contgau.htm

Halsey, Richard W. 2005. In search of allelopathy: an eco-historical view of the investigation of chemical inhibition in California coastal sage scrub and chamise chaparral. *Journal of the Torrey Botanical Society* 131:343–367.

Holldobler, Bert. 1986. Food robbing in ants: a form of interference competition. *Oecologia* 69(1):12–15.

Predators and Prey

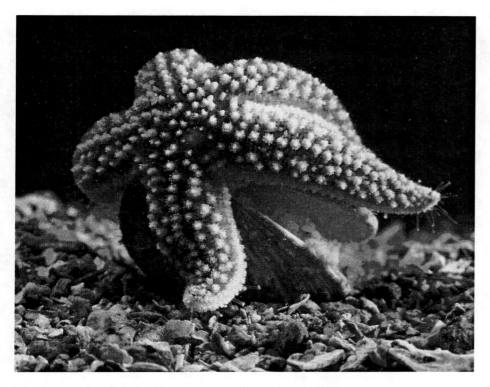

Figure 1   Starfish are important predators in marine ecosystems.

INTRODUCTION

The sea star *Asterias* may seem slow and benign to human observers, but it is a formidable predator on mollusks (Figure 1). Moving on flexible arms and hundreds of tiny tube feet, the sea star actively seeks its prey on the sea floor. When it encounters a clam or mussel, the sea star grasps the bivalve, pries open the shell, and everts its stomach into the opening to digest the soft body of the mollusk inside. Although the bivalve's shell seems impenetrable, the sea star has evolved a body plan and predatory behavior that circumvents the prey's defenses. This kind of evolutionary arms race is typical of predators and prey; each adaptation of the prey leads to **co-adaptation** by its predators.

On an ecological time scale, studies of sea stars have taught ecologists a lot about the influence of predators on natural communities. In a classic field experiment, Robert T. Paine (1966) artificially removed sea stars from tide pools and monitored the resulting changes in diversity of invertebrate animals in a rocky intertidal environment. Released from predation, mollusk populations grew and competition among species increased. As a result, some species drove others to extinction, and overall **biodiversity** decreased. The so-called "**top-down control**" of ecological community structure by predators has been demonstrated in many kinds of biological communities. If a single species at the top of the food chain seems especially crucial to maintaining the character of a biological community, the top carnivore is called a **keystone** predator. The term "keystone" is borrowed from architecture, and refers to a structural element that holds an entire system together (Figure 2). The supposition is that the entire structure collapses if the keystone is removed. Prey can function as keystone species as well. Population dynamics of plankton in freshwater lakes, for example, can significantly impact kinds and numbers of fish in the community. This is called "**bottom-up control.**"

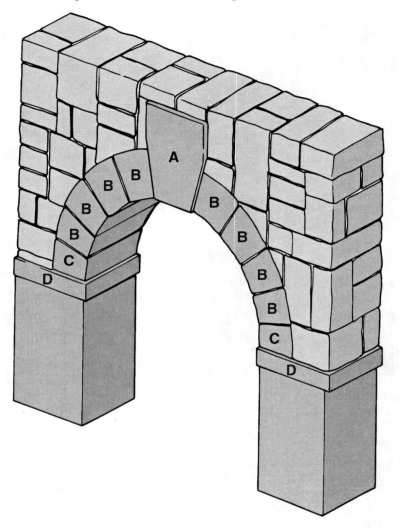

Figure 2   The keystone (A) holds other parts of an arch in place. By analogy, a keystone species is essential to maintaining community structure. Removal of the keystone (or extinction of a keystone species) results in drastic community change.

Not all types of sea stars enhance biodiversity. In Pacific waters from Australia to the South American coast, a spiny sea star called the crown of thorns "starfish" has increased both its distribution and its numbers, inflicting terrible damage to coral reefs throughout its range (Figure 3). Hard corals may seem unlikely food for a predator without teeth, but the crown of thorns feeds by extruding its stomach over the thin layer of living polyps that cover a coral's calcareous skeleton. As it moves across the reef, the crown of thorns leaves behind a white swath of dead coral. Without its living foundation, the reef deteriorates and many other species of fish and invertebrates are lost. Why are crown of thorns sea stars increasing in numbers? One widely accepted theory is that population growth of the sea star is linked to a decline in largepredatory marine snails called tritons. In a reverse of the *Asterias*/clam relationship, the triton is a

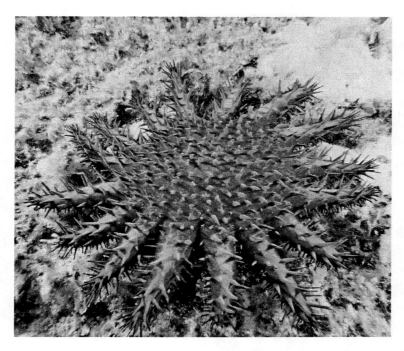

Figure 3   Crown of thorns starfish feeding on corals off the coast of Hawaii.

mollusk that feeds on crown of thorns sea stars (Figure 4). Unfortunately, the triton shell is highly sought by collectors, and its populations have been depleted by divers taking living tritons from reefs throughout the Pacific. Released from predation by the increasingly rare triton, populations of the crown of thorns sea star have grown exponentially, with predictable consequences for reefs. Whether sea stars eat mollusks or mollusks eat sea stars, the importance of predator-prey relationships in maintaining a stable community structure emerges as a common ecological theme. To understand why some predator/prey systems are more stable than others, we need a more quantitative understanding of predator and prey populations.

Check your progress:

Based on the two predator/prey cases listed above, what ecological consequences would you expect from overfishing large predatory fishes from the world's oceans?

Answer: Removal of top predators often causes loss of species diversity due to competitive interactions among smaller species released from top-down control.

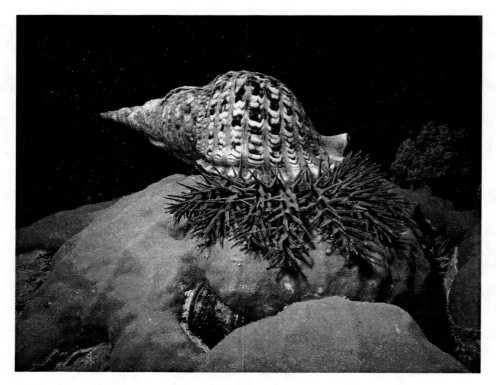

Figure 4   A giant triton snail attacks a crown of thorns sea star.

When ecologists speak of stability in biological communities, we should not imagine a static environment with no year-to-year changes. Populations of predators and prey rise and fall, often demonstrating cyclic changes in numbers over many generations. An instructive example of fluctuations in mammalian predator/prey populations is found on Isle Royale, a large forested island 24 km off the north shore of Lake Superior. Here moose and wolf populations have existed together for over 50 years, but many smaller mammals otherwise expected in woodland habitats at this latitude are absent because of the great distance across very cold water to the mainland. Hunting is prohibited, as the entire island has been preserved as a national park. Movement of animals on or off the island is practically nonexistent. Isle Royale wolves have few other prey than moose, and moose have no other predators. For ecologists, this kind of simplified natural system provides an opportunity to study interactions between one predator and one prey without the confounding variables encountered in more complex communities. Results of 50 years of population census data are shown in Figure 5. Note that wolves and moose are shown on separate scales; it is typical for prey to exist in much larger numbers than their predators. Like many systems dominated by one predator and one prey species, these populations fluctuate in cycles. Although longer monitoring will test the generality of the trend, a period of roughly 20 years between peak numbers seems to characterize both populations, with the predator peak lagging several years behind the prey peak. Our understanding of this process involves mutual feedback as follows: 1) If prey and predator populations are both low, prey numbers increase exponentially. 2) When predators have more food, their survival and reproductive success increases, and their population growth follows that of their prey. 3) As predator populations increase, the death rate for prey exceeds the birth rate, and prey populations decline. 4) After prey numbers decline, predators deprived of food face population collapse. 5) The cycle begins again with low numbers of both species.

Wolf and Moose Populations on Isle Royale

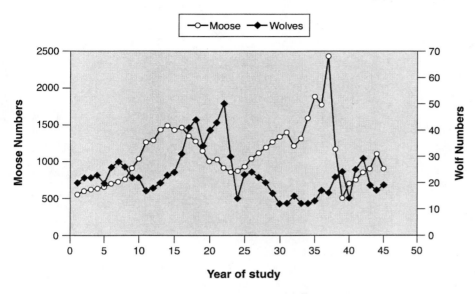

Figure 5 Population cycles of wolf and moose on Isle Royale. (Data from John Vucetich, 2005, "The Wolves and Moose of Isle Royale." http://www.isleroyalewolf.org/)

This is a common scenario in two-species systems, though the period of predator-prey cycles depends on the life spans and reproductive rates of the organisms. For predatory mites feeding on herbivorous mites in laboratory experiments, population peaks occur every three months. Snowshoe hare and Canada lynx cycles, documented over 200 years through fir trading records, show a predictable pattern of peaks every nine years (Figure 6). Clearly, any model we develop to explain predator-prey interactions must incorporate predator and prey population cycles.

Check your progress:

When predator and prey populations are plotted over several generations, why do predator population peaks usually lag behind prey population peaks?

Hint: Predators usually have longer lives and slower reproduction than their prey.

Ecology on Campus

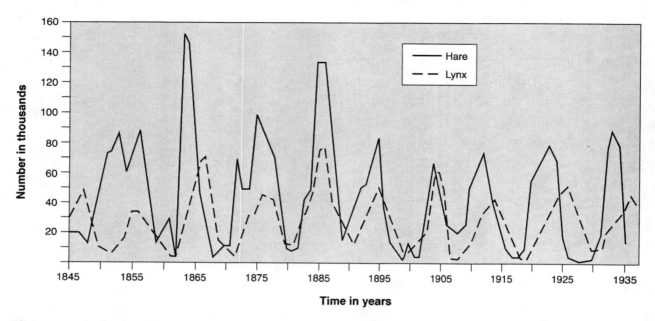

Figure 6 Snowshoe hare and Canada lynx populations rise and fall on a 9-year cycle. (After Bolen, E. G. and W. L. Robinson. 1999. *Wildlife ecology and management*. Prentice Hall, N. J.)

Modeling Predator and Prey Populations

Alfred Lotka, in the United States, and Vito Volterra, in Italy, independently modeled not only mathematical descriptions of competition but also developed equations that describe the cyclic patterns of change in predator and prey numbers. To follow their reasoning, let's first define some terms. Let **P** be our symbol for the numbers of predators in our system, and let **H** stand for the numbers of prey (herbivores). Prey grow exponentially in this model with an intrinsic rate of growth equal to **r**. We also need to quantify the rate of capture when predators encounter prey; let's call this the predation constant **p**.

As for predators, Lotka and Volterra assumed a constant death rate **d**. Since predator birth rate depends in part on prey consumed, they used the constant *a* as the predator birth constant. Think of *a* as the rate at which a predator converts food into offspring.

Check your progress:

Identify each of these symbols from the Lotka-Volterra predator-prey equations.

P =   d =
H =   p =
r =   *a* =

Hint: P, d, and *a* describe the predators.
H and r describe the prey.
The value of p affects both.

To model prey populations, we assume that changes in population size result from births minus deaths. Births are assumed to follow an exponential curve, with changes in prey numbers equal to the prey population size times the intrinsic rate of increase, or $r \cdot H$. Death rate of prey is assumed to be due to predation, which is modeled as the predation constant times the number of prey times the number of predators. In other words, negative change in population numbers due to predators killing prey is equal to $p \cdot H \cdot P$. Note that by multiplying the prey and predator populations together, we get a number proportional to the probability that a predator meets its prey during a given time interval. If both populations are high, the product of their numbers is very high. If one or both populations are low, the product of their numbers is low, and therefore the frequency of predation is low. Multiplying by p simply tells us how often an encounter becomes a successful kill for the predator. The population size for prey can therefore be stated as follows:

Growth Equation for Prey:

Change in prey numbers   Births   Deaths

$$\Delta H = r\,H - p\,H\,P$$

ΔH = change in prey numbers per unit time p = predation constant
H = population size of prey P = population size of predators
R = prey population growth rate

Any time the constants are known and census data indicate predators and prey numbers, we can use this equation to project the number of prey added to or subtracted from the population. In other words, $H + \Delta H$ = the herbivore population for the next time period.

Check your progress:

For a population of sea stars feeding on clams in the shallows around a small island, assume that $H = 1200$, $p = 0.004$, $r = 0.7$, and $P = 130$. What is the projected population size for clams?

Answer: 216 new clams added, so the prey population will grow to 1416.

To examine conditions critical to prey survival, it is instructive to ask, under what conditions can prey populations maintain a stable population size? If the population is not growing under these conditions, then $\Delta H = 0$. The equation can be simplified as follows:

Zero-Growth Condition for Prey:

$$0 = r\,H - p\,H\,P$$

Adding pHP to both sides: $$p\,H\,P = r\,H$$

Dividing both sides by **H**,
this simplifies to: **P = r/p**

H = population size of prey   p = predation constant
  r = prey population growth rate   P = population size of predators

Since both **r** and **p** are constants, the value **r/p** represents a constant number of predators needed to hold prey populations in check. Let's look at the biological meaning of the fraction on the right side of the equation. When **r**, the growth rate of the prey, is large, the number of predators needed to control the prey will be large. It also makes sense that the predation constant **p** is in the denominator, because if the predator is highly efficient at capturing prey, **p** will be large and thus the number of predators needed to control the prey will be relatively small.

Think of r/p as a threshold number of predators. Whenever P is lower than the threshold number, prey populations grow. Whenever P is higher than the threshold number, prey populations decline. A joint abundance graph (Figure 7) is a good way to illustrate both populations at the same time. Prey numbers (H) are shown on the horizontal axis of the graph, and predator numbers (P) are shown on the vertical axis. A point on this kind of graph represents both populations at the same time. Movement of this point within the graph space shows how both populations change over time.

Zero-growth conditions for the prey are represented by the line at the top of the shaded area, representing the number of predators (r/p) that would create zero-growth conditions for prey. On a graph, we call this an **isocline**. It is a graphic representation of the equation for zero-growth conditions for prey explained above. Note that the joint abundance point will move to the right (indicating prey growth) in the area under the isocline, and to the left (indicating prey decline) in the area above the isocline.

Check your progress:

For the predator-prey system illustrated in Figure 7, assume the predation constant is 0.004. Estimate the reproductive rate of the prey.

Answer: estimating r/p = 12.5 yields r = 0.05

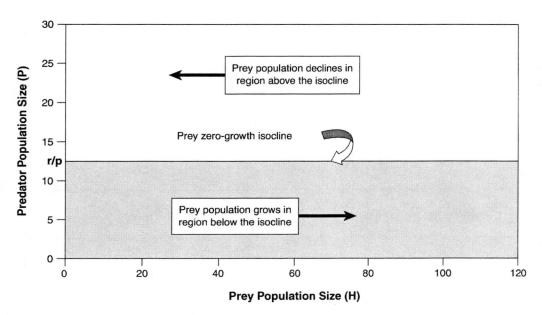

Lotka-Volterra Predation Model
Prey Isocline

Figure 7   Zero-growth isocline for prey. The position of the isocline is determined by the number of predators (r/p) required to keep prey numbers in check. Lower predator numbers allow prey population growth; higher predator numbers cause prey population decline.

Next we need to look at an equation to model predator population growth. Lotka and Volterra assumed that predators suffer a constant death rate (**d**), and that their growth was based on the amount of prey they are able to capture (**p**) multiplied by the reproductive rate per captured prey (**a**). As we saw for prey, changes in predator populations are equal to births minus deaths, as shown in the following equation:

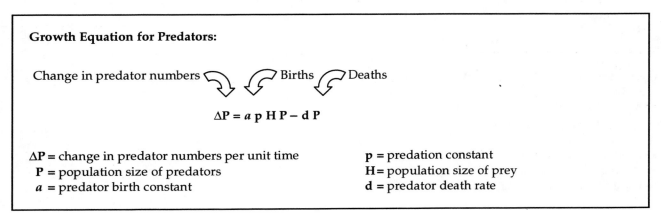

Growth Equation for Predators:

Change in predator numbers   Births   Deaths

$$\Delta P = a\ \mathrm{p}\ \mathrm{H}\ \mathrm{P} - \mathrm{d}\ \mathrm{P}$$

ΔP = change in predator numbers per unit time   **p** = predation constant
 P = population size of predators   **H** = population size of prey
 a = predator birth constant   **d** = predator death rate

It is interesting to note that the three terms determining numbers of prey captured by predators once again appear as **p H P**, which is the capture rate multiplied by the two population sizes. However, number of captures determines deaths of prey, whereas it contributes to births of predators.

Check your progress:

To return to our sea star/clam example, assume that **H** = 1200, **p** = 0.004, *a* = 0.025, **d** = 0.12, and **P** = 130. What is the projected population size for sea stars?

Answer: **ΔP = 0,** so the sea star population retains its current size of 130.

To calculate a zero-growth condition for predators, we again set ΔP = 0, as shown below:

Zero-Growth Condition for Predators:

$$0 = a\,p\,H\,P - d\,P$$

Adding dP to both sides: $\quad d\,P = a\,p\,H\,P$

Dividing both sides by P and rearranging, the equation simplifies to: $\quad H = d\,/\,(ap)$

a = predator birth constant
p = predation constant
H = population size of prey

P = population size of predators
d = predator death rate

What does this equation say biologically? Predator growth will be zero whenever the number of prey is equal to a value determined by **d / (ap)**. This is the threshold number of prey needed to maintain the predator population. The **d** in the numerator makes sense, because the higher the death rate of the predator, the more births (fueled by prey) it will take to replace those dying each generation. It also makes good biological sense for the predation constant (**p**) and the predator birth rate (*a*) to occupy the denominator, since these two terms measure the effectiveness of the predator at catching prey and converting them to offspring. The more offspring the predator can produce out of each prey encountered, the fewer prey are needed to maintain the predator population.

On a joint abundance graph, we can show this threshold number of prey as a zero-growth isocline for predators (Figure 8). This time the position of the isocline depends on a number of prey on the H axis, so the line runs vertically. Everywhere to the right of this line, the predators have sufficient food for population growth, so the joint abundance point moves upward. Everywhere to the left of this line, the predators are starving, so the joint abundance moves downward.

Check your progress:

From inspection of Figure 8, what is the minimum number of prey needed to maintain a population of predators in this system?

Answer: at least 50

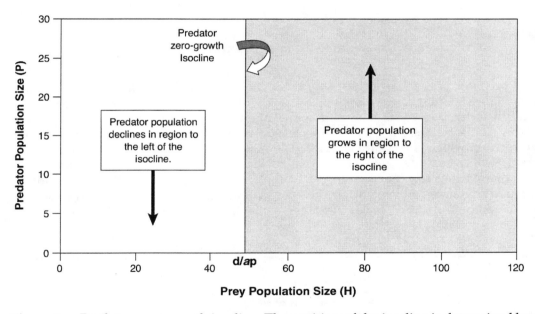

Lotka-Volterra Predation Model
Predator Isocline

Figure 8 Predator zero-growth isocline. The position of the isocline is determined by the number of prey (d/ap) needed to maintain the predator population. Larger numbers of prey allow predator population growth; smaller numbers of prey cause predator population decline.

To see how the Lotka-Volterra predation model generates population cycles, let's look at both isoclines on the same graph (Figure 9). The isocline for zero prey growth intersects the isocline for zero predator growth near the center of the graph. If the two species were introduced to an environment at precisely this joint abundance, the model predicts equilibrium. At the intersection, predators are just sufficient to keep prey in check, and prey are just sufficient to feed the predators. If the joint abundance begins a bit off center, the populations will enter a cycle, as shown by the curved arrows in the graph. With two simple equations, Lotka and Volterra provide a quantitative theory for the periodic fluctuations often observed in predator and prey abundance.

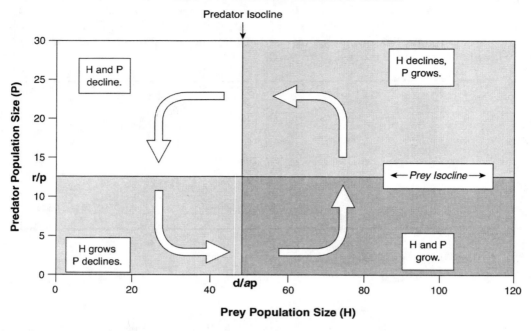

Figure 9   Predator/prey joint abundance cycles around the intersection of the zero-growth isocline.

Though common, not all predator-prey cycles persist over time. The joint abundance plot may produce a closed circle as shown in Figure 8, but it often forms a spiral. If the joint abundance plot spirals in toward the center, ecologists call it a damped cycle, because the oscillations get smaller and smaller until the populations come to rest at the intersection of the isoclines. The intersection of the isoclines thus represents a **stable equilibrium** which is resistant to small environmental disturbances. Alternatively, the two populations may spiral outward in an exploding cycle, oscillating at greater and greater extremes until one species or the other crashes to extinction. In this example, the isoclines intersect at an **unstable equilibrium** point, because any small movement off this joint abundance results in major irreversible changes in the system. To compare damped cycles, repeating (or limit) cycles, and exploding cycles, see Figure 10.

Check your progress:

In which kind(s) of cycle on Figure 10 would the intersection of the zero-growth isoclines be considered a stable equilibrium point? In which kind(s) would it be considered an unstable equilibrium point?

Hint: When disturbed, a system quickly returns to a stable equilibrium point. A disturbed system rarely returns to an unstable equilibrium point.

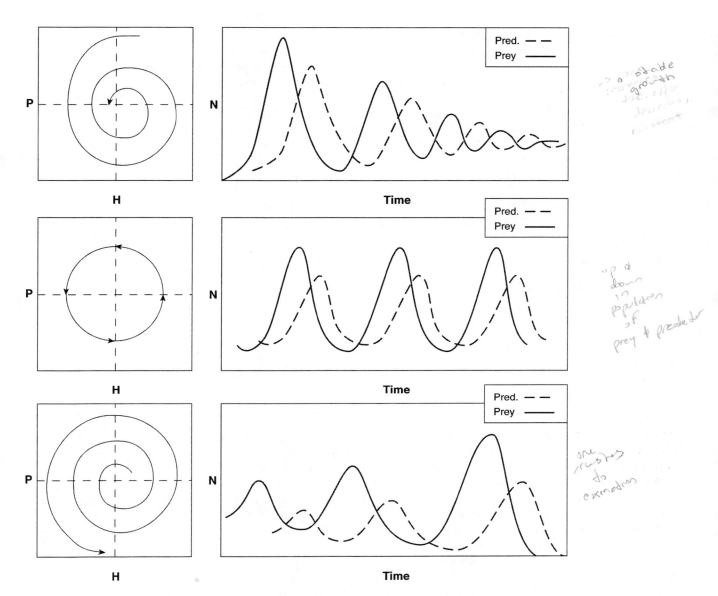

Figure 10 Predator-prey dynamics can produce damped cycles (top), limit cycles (middle), or exploding cycles (bottom). On the left are joint abundance graphs (see Figure 9). On the right, numbers (N) of predators and prey are plotted against time.

Functional Responses of Predators

The simple Lotka-Volterra equations assume that the rate at which predators capture prey (**p**) is a constant, so numbers of captures each predator makes per unit time is directly proportional to prey density. This is sometimes called a **type 1 functional response**. Can we assume predators always take prey in direct proportion to their numbers? An ecologist named C. S. Holling (1959) studying small mammals feeding on sawfly cocoons observed that predation is a two-step process: first the prey must be found, then it must be "handled." **Handling time** includes all activities required before the next capture, including removal of inedible parts, carrying the prey back to a nest, or eating and digesting the food item. If handling time is long in comparison to searching time, then it can become a limiting factor for a predator's consumption rate as prey density increases. When plotted against prey density, capture rate levels off in the type 2 response (Figure 11). Holling's disk equation, so-called because he did simulations in the laboratory involving sandpaper disks, recognizes that predators spend most of their time hunting for food when prey are scarce, but a greater proportion of their time handling food when prey become more abundant. The equation for the type 2 functional response is as follows:

Holling's Disk Equation:

$$C = A\,N/(1 + T_h\,A\,N)$$

C = number of prey captured
T_h = handling time
A = attack rate of predators
N = population density of prey

For vertebrate predators capable of learning from experience, the most abundant prey may be selected at an even higher frequency than their prevalence in the environment. The rarest prey may be ignored altogether. Vertebrate predators often develop a **search image** for prey with which they have experience. (This is not unlike a phenomenon you may observe in a university cafeteria. If unusual looking food items are presented on a buffet line, they are selected at a lower frequency than food items more familiar to students.) If predators form a search image, the functional response curve is S-shaped, due to disproportionately low predation of rare prey. This is called a **type 3 functional response** (Figure 11). At intermediate prey density, the rate of capture increases rapidly with enhanced predator experience, and then handling time slows the capture rate at very high density. Invertebrate predators such as hunting wasps are less likely to illustrate the S-shaped functional response curve, because most of their predatory behavior is genetically programmed, and not dependent on learning.

In conclusion, predators adjust to their prey over three time scales: 1) Over evolutionary time, predators develop adaptations in morphology and behavior to help them capture their prey. 2) Over generations, predator populations fluctuate up and down in response to prey numbers. 3) Over the lifetime of a single predator, handling time and learning affect rates of capture.

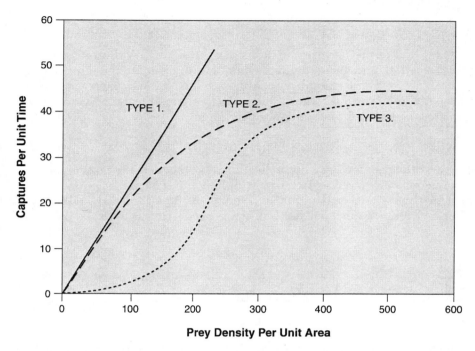

Functional Responses of Predators

Figure 11 Functional Response Curves. Type 1 (solid line) assumes prey consumption is directly proportional to availability. Type 2 (dashed line) levels off at high prey density as the capture rate becomes increasingly limited by "handling time" required to process and digest prey. Type 3 (dotted line) is seen in vertebrate predators developing a "search image" for the most common prey. In this model, rare prey are underrepresented in predator diets in comparison to their frequency, and common prey are overrepresented.

METHOD A: PREDATOR-PREY SIMULATION

[Computer activity]

Research Question

How do the Lotka-Volterra predator-prey equations generate population cycles?

Preparation

Because the Lotka-Volterra equations are built on ideas about population growth, it is highly recommended that students complete other readings and exercises before attempting exercises in this chapter. Instructions for this simulation are appropriate for Microsoft Excel software. If you use other spreadsheet software, instructions for writing cell formulas given in this procedure may require modification.

Materials (per laboratory team)

A computer station, with spreadsheet software

Background

This exercise simulates growth of prey and of predator populations using the Lotka-Volterra equations. The purpose of the exercise is to demonstrate how the equations work, and to examine the sensitivity of predator-prey systems to small changes in initial conditions. Although the Lotka-Volterra model is simplistic, and omits many factors operating in natural communities, it help us understand how even two-species interactions can generate interesting patterns of abundance over time.

Procedure

1. Set up a computer spreadsheet with the following column headings. Numbers in the first column (Column A) indicate the year in our simulation, so each row will show the state of the populations in another year as we go down the page. The second and third columns (B and C) will show numbers of prey and of predators. The next four columns will hold constants needed to calculate the Lotka-Volterra equations.

	A	B	C	D	E	F	G
1	Year	Prey	Predators	r	p	A	d
2							

2. The first entry in cell A2, under "year," should be 0, the starting point of our simulation. Go on down this column, numbering years 1, 2, 3, 4, etc. If you do not want to type all those numbers in, just enter 0 in cell A2, and then in cell A3 type the formula = **A2+1**. If you copy and paste this formula down the column to the one hundred fifty second row, you will get a series of numbered years from 0 through 150. Format all the cells below the first row in columns 1, 2, and 3 to display integer values, with no decimal places. The top of your spreadsheet should now look like this:

	A	B	C	D	E	F	G
1	Year	Prey	Predators	r	p	A	d
2	0						
3	1						
4	2						
5	3						
6	4						

3. Then you will need to enter starting numbers of prey and predators, along with values for the four Lotka-Volterra constants. To start off, try entering 100 prey and 15 predators. For the four constants, try the following values: Intrinsic rate of increase of the prey (r) = 0.1; the predation constant (p) = 0.01; the predator's birth constant (a) = 0.3; and the predator death rate (d) = 0.3. The top of your spreadsheet should now look like this:

	A	B	C	D	E	F	G
1	Year	Prey	Predators	r	p	*A*	d
2	0	100	15	0.1	0.01	0.3	0.3
3	1						
4	2						
5	3						
6	4						

4. Now you are ready to enter the Lotka-Volterra population growth equations for prey. In cell B3, which is the first empty cell under the Prey column, type the following formula:

$$=B2+(\$D\$2*B2)-(\$E\$2*B2*C2)$$

This formula calculates the number of prey in year 1 by starting with the number that were present in the previous year, then adding births and subtracting deaths. (This corresponds to the $\Delta H = r\,H - p\,H\,P$ equation from the Introduction.) Note that cell references in the formula include dollar signs in front of the letter and number of the cell address. This transfers the value within the cell, and not the position of the cell, which is necessary for constants. COPY cell B3 and then PASTE the formula into cells B4 through B152. Don't worry if you get an error message in the target cells at this point.

5. Next, you need to enter the Lotka-Volterra population growth equation for predators. In cell C3, in the first empty cell under the Predators column, type the following formula:

$$=C2+(\$F\$2*\$E\$2*B2*C2)-(\$G\$2*C2)$$

This formula calculates the number of predators in year 1 by starting with the number that were present in the previous year, then adding births and subtracting deaths. (This corresponds to the $\Delta P = a\,p\,H\,P - d\,P$ equation from the Introduction.) COPY cell C3 and then PASTE the formula into cells C4 through C152. You should see a cascade of numbers go down the page as the spreadsheet calculates numbers of predators and prey for each year of the simulation. The top of your spreadsheet should now look like this:

	A	B	C	D	E	F	G
1	Year	Prey	Predators	r	p	*A*	d
2	0	100	15	0.1	0.01	0.3	0.3
3	1	95	15				
4	2	90	15				
5	3	86	14				
6	4	82	14				

6. If your spreadsheet can display graphs, try highlighting the first three columns, including the headings, all the way down to row 152. Then click on the graph option on the menu bar, and select a scatter plot for your data display. You should be able to produce a graph with Year as the x-axis and Prey and Predator numbers as Series 1 and Series 2 on the y-axis. With the simulation parameters you have set by following these instructions, you should see an exploding cycle, with prey and predator populations cresting in three peaks of increasing size during the 150-year simulation. Ideally, you can display the graph within the spreadsheet just under the constants on the right, so that you can change initial

simulation conditions and observe results as the graph changes. You can also produce a joint abundance graph by highlighting columns 2 and 3, and using the same graphing options. For simulation conditions given above, your graphs should resemble those in Figure 12.

7. Try to stabilize the exploding cycles by adjusting the numbers of prey and predators you entered in Year 0. Small changes in initial numbers can make large differences in the simulation.
8. Adjust the four constants, one at a time, by replacing the numerical values under r, p, a, and d by numbers just a little larger or smaller. After each adjustment, look at the numbers output from the spreadsheet and the graphs. Take notes on your findings.
9. Produce large plots, both of numbers vs. time, and of joint abundance, of the most stable cycles you were able to produce in the simulation. If you cannot get computer printouts to show the graphs, draw them by plotting points by hand on graph paper. On the joint abundance plot, use the input parameters for the simulation to calculate the positions of the isoclines, and draw them in, as seen in Figure 9.
10. Use your experience with the model and your graphs to answer the Questions for Method A.

Predator-Prey Simulation Results

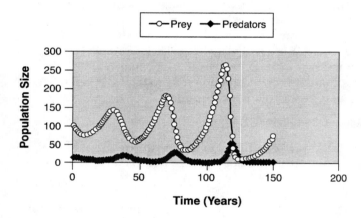

Joint Abundance Plot

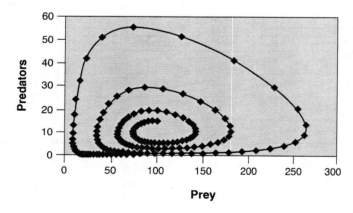

Figure 12   Sample output from predator-prey spreadsheet simulation.

Questions for Method A

1. On your joint abundance graph, use the values of the constants to calculate the positions of the isoclines (as shown in Figure 9) and draw the isoclines with a pencil and ruler on top of your population curve. Does the curve seem to spiral around the point of intersection? Explain.

   _____

   _____

   _____

   _____

2. On a joint abundance plot of cycles near the stable limit condition, are the circles symmetrical around the intersection of isoclines, as diagrammed in Figure 10, or not? Describe the shape of the cycles on the joint abundance graph, and reflect on why the increasing and decreasing parts of each cycle might be asymmetrical. (Hint: what controls predator births? deaths?)

   _____

   _____

   _____

   _____

3. During the 1920s, U.S. government policy encouraged extermination of predators such as wolves, mountain lions, and coyotes from large areas in the American West in order to maintain more abundant deer and antelope populations for hunters. Based on your model, what outcome would you expect from this effort to maintain prey in the absence of predators?

   _____

   _____

   _____

   _____

4. If you adjust each of the four constants, one at a time, by 10%, which seems to have the greatest impact on the simulation output? Examine the Lotka-Volterra equations to explain why this constant makes such a big difference in the predator-prey system. (Hint: This constant affects both the birth rate of predators and the death rate of prey.)

   _____

   _____

   _____

   _____

5. Predator-prey systems are difficult to balance when there is only one predator and only one prey. Would you expect a system with multiple prey species to be more stable? Why?

   _____

   _____

   _____

   _____

METHOD B: PREDATION BY *DAPHNIA* ON *EUGLENA*
[Laboratory activity]

Research Question
Do *Daphnia* feeding on *Euglena* experience population cycles?

Preparation
This laboratory works best if students are able to come in and check on their cultures frequently between laboratory periods. If student access to the lab is limited to weekly class meetings, it is very hard to monitor rapid changes in the populations. *Daphnia pulex* and *Euglena gracilis* are available from supply houses. Order large, mixed-age *Daphnia* cultures if possible. Make sure your *Euglena gracilis* strain has chloroplasts. Water quality is essential for culturing both *Daphnia* and protozoans. Traces of chlorine or detergent will kill protozoans and *Daphnia*, so all glassware should be carefully rinsed and water must be aged to let chlorine evaporate. Avoid deionized or distilled water, as it does not have sufficient trace minerals to support *Euglena*. Spring water can be purchased, but rainwater or tap water can be used if it is filtered or boiled for 15 minutes to remove contaminating algae. If boiled, cover container of water loosely with aluminum foil and allow to reoxygenate for several days before using it in cultures.

Euglena are photosynthetic, so they can grow without added food. *Daphnia* are notoriously difficult to culture for long periods, but most cultures go through at least one full cycle before they crash. While students are beginning their cultures with *Euglena*, keep *Daphnia* in the dark, and feed them a few drops of Baker's yeast suspended in water to avoid introducing algae along with the *Daphnia*. After inoculation with algae, cultures should be kept under fluorescent lights or grow lights at room temperature to support *Euglena* growth.

Materials (per laboratory team)
Access to stock cultures of *Daphnia pulex* and *Euglena gracilis*

Water for *Daphnia* culture

Glass culture dish, 4½" diameter × 3" high

Glass plate (or extra stacking dish) to cover culture dish

Plastic dropper, 6" (one-piece plastic pipette with tapered tip)

Scissors

Pasteur pipette

Glass slides

Cover slips

Compound microscope

Dissecting microscope (optional)

Background
Daphnia are very small crustaceans that swim in the water column and feed on *Euglena* and many other kinds of plankton in freshwater lakes and ponds. *Daphnia* are able to reproduce by **parthenogenesis** (a form of asexual reproduction), which allows rapid population growth when food is abundant. Because *Daphnia* have a short life span, their populations can also decline quickly when prey are scarce. Since *Euglena* also have rapid growth rates and very short life spans, predator-prey cycles in *Daphnia*/*Euglena* populations occur quickly, over a few days or weeks.

Procedure

1. Fill culture dish ¾ full of culture water. With a Pasteur pipette, transfer one or two drops of *Euglena gracilis* stock culture to your dish. Cover your dish with another dish or glass plate, and place it under a light source. About three feet below a fluorescent lamp is enough light. Incubate at room temperature (20° to 23° C) for one week.

2. After one week, stir the culture well with the end of a pipette and then draw up a sample. Put one drop on a glass slide, cover with a cover slip, and examine the culture under a compound microscope, using the 10 × objective (100 × total magnification). You should see green, cigar-shaped *Euglena* cells swimming through the water. After you have learned what they look like, census the population as follows: move the slide slightly to a new location. Look through the eyepiece and count the number of *Euglena* cells you see in this field of view. If you see no *Euglena*, record zero as the number in this field. Repeat ten times. Take an average of the number of cells per field, and record in the calculation page for Method B.

3. When you have established a *Euglena* culture, it is time to add *Daphnia*. First look at the tip of your large plastic pipette. If the hole in the end is smaller than 2 mm in diameter, use scissors or a sharp blade to trim some of the end off the pipette so that *Daphnia* can pass through unharmed. Use your modified pipette to capture *Daphnia* from the stock culture. Transfer three large and three smaller *Daphnia* into your culture dish.

4. Record the date, the mean number of *Euglena* per field, and the number of *Daphnia* you placed in your culture on the first line of the Method B Data Table. Every few days, count the number of *Daphnia* by placing your culture dish on a black surface under a bright light. If numbers are hard to count, estimate by counting a wedge-shaped part of the culture dish and multiplying by the number of parts in the whole. Count the number of *Euglena* as described in step 2. Record the date, the age of the culture (as number of days elapsed since Day 0), the number of *Daphnia* per culture, and the number of *Euglena* per field in the next line of the data table.

5. Continue monitoring your *Daphnia/Euglena* system for several weeks. You should be able to see the two populations peak and then decline for at least one cycle. Plot the data on a joint abundance graph, with *Euglena* per field on the x-axis and *Daphnia* per culture on the y-axis. Answer the Questions for Method B.

Data Table (Method B)

DATE	AGE OF CULTURE No. days since beginning	DAPHNIA Number per culture	EUGLENA Mean number per field
	0	6	

Joint Abundance Plot of Results (Method B)

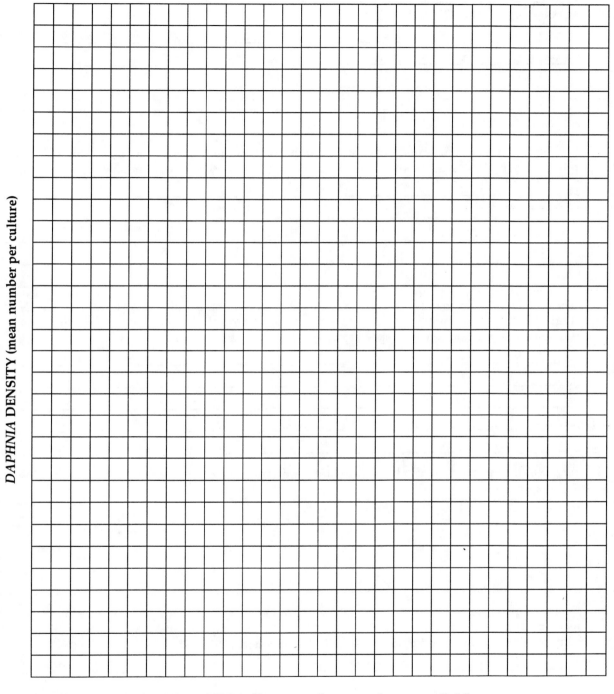

DAPHNIA DENSITY (mean number per culture)

EUGLENA DENSITY (mean number per microscope field)

Questions for Method B

1. How do population fluctuations of *Daphnia* and *Euglena* compare with the predictions of the Lotka-Volterra model?

   _____

   _____

   _____

   _____

   _____

2. When plotted on a joint abundance graph, did the joint abundance move in a counterclockwise direction? If so, how does the shape of the curve compare with the simulation output in Figure 11?

   _____

   _____

   _____

   _____

   _____

3. Based on your experiment, would you say this two-species community is very stable, or fairly fragile? What lessons might we apply to agricultural systems that replace natural communities with one or a few domesticated species occupying a very large landmass?

   _____

   _____

   _____

   _____

   _____

4. Why was it important to introduce some large and some small *Daphnia* in your initial population?

   _____

   _____

   _____

   _____

5. *Daphnia* reproduce asexually as long as the environment is favorable to population growth, but when conditions become less favorable, they produce male offspring and begin sexual reproduction. Why would asexual reproduction be linked to favorable conditions?

   _____

   _____

   _____

   _____

METHOD C: SIMULATING FUNCTIONAL RESPONSE OF A PREDATOR

[Laboratory activity]

Research Question
How does the functional response of a predator depend on handling time?

Preparation
Bolts and nuts used to represent organisms can be purchased at a hardware store. A 3/8" diameter is suggested, but other sizes are fine. Threads should go all the way to the head of the bolt, because a key variable is the number of turns necessary to remove a bolt—this represents handling time in the simulation.

Materials (per laboratory team)
25 2½" bolts, with nuts

1 sheet poster board (22" × 28" or larger)

Stopwatch or laboratory timer

Background
In this simulation, a student with eyes closed represents a predator searching for prey. A piece of poster board lying flat on a table or lab bench represents the habitat. Bolts represent prey, and nuts represent inedible parts of the prey (such as a clam shell or insect wings) that must be removed before the prey can be consumed. Time spent removing the nut from the bolt therefore serves as handling time in this experiment. The "predator" must search the board with only one finger, pointing straight down, moving across the "habitat" of the board. When a prey item is encountered, it is picked up and "handled" by removing the bolt. Bolt and nut are placed off the board and the search resumes, all without looking at the board. Other students in the lab group will time the simulations, count the number of prey "consumed," and replace the bolts with nuts reattached on the board to maintain a stable prey density.

Procedure
1. Designate one student in your group as the "predator." With eyes closed, hand the "predator" a bolt with the nut screwed all the way up to the head. Ask the student to remove the bolt from the nut (without spinning the nut around the bolt). After allowing once or twice for practice, conduct a time trial and measure the number of seconds it takes to remove the nut. Then divide the number of seconds by 60 to calculate handling time in minutes. Record this number, to the nearest hundredth of a minute, in the Data Table for Method C.
2. Lay the poster board flat on a table or lab bench. While the "predator's" eyes are still closed, scatter five "prey" (nut and bolt assemblies) onto the poster-board habitat. Your task is to determine how many prey can be captured and handled in a three-minute period. The "predator" searches for prey with one finger touching the board. The "predator" should try to move at a steady pace, and be careful not to touch prey with the whole hand. When a prey item is found, the "predator" picks up the prey, removes the nut from the bolt, places the "eaten" parts off the board, and then continues searching. Student observers should screw the nut back onto the bolt and quietly replace the "prey" item back on the board so that the prey density does not change during the experiment. Record the number of prey taken within a three-minute period. If a prey item has been found but not fully processed when time is up, count that bolt as an additional ½ prey consumed.

3. Calculate the "predator's" attack rate as follows:
   a) multiply the handling time per prey (in minutes) by the number of prey consumed during the three-minute interval. This is total handling time.
   b) subtract total handling time (in minutes) from the total predation time (three minutes) to determine total searching time (T_s). For example, if total handling time is 1.2 minutes, then T_s = 3 minutes – 1.2 minutes = 1.8 minutes.
   c) Use the following equation to calculate the attack rate for the "predator" in the first trial, which used five prey on the board. The total search time in the denominator is multiplied by 5 because that is the initial prey density.

Attack rate = (# prey consumed)/(5 T_s)

   d) Record the attack rate (A) for this "predator" in the data table.

4. Repeat step 2 with the same predator, but with 10 bolts on the board. Then repeat with densities 15, 20, and 25. Record results for each prey density in the Data Table for Method C.
5. Allow a second lab group member to take a turn as predator. Measure handling time, record the number of bolts the "predator" is able to "consume" in three minutes at densities 5, 10, 15, 20, and 25. Calculate the attack rate after the first trial, and record all data for the second predator in the second row of the data table. If time allows, allow every member of the laboratory group to take a turn as "predator." If you do not have time for five predators, simply leave the bottom of the table blank, and compute column means based on the number of predators who were able to do the simulation.
6. Calculate average numbers of bolts "eaten" at each of the five densities for your group, and write the means in the data table. Also calculate a mean handling time, in minutes, for the entire group, and record that grand mean as well.
7. Plot results on the Graph for Method C. Assume 0 prey will be caught when prey density is 0. For densities 5–25, plot your mean number of captures per three-minute trial as points on the graph, and connect your points to make a curve. Compare your curve to the Functional Response curves in Figure 11.
8. Use the following equation to calculate an expected number of captures for trials at each of the five prey densities. Draw a dotted line (or use a different color) to show the expected functional response on the Graph for Method C.

Holling's Disk Equation:

$$C = A\,N/(1 + T_h\,A\,N)$$

C = number of prey captured per trial
T_h = handling time
A = attack rate of predators
N = population density of prey

---

9. Refer to the data table and the graph when answering Questions for Method C.

Data Table for Method C

PREDATOR #	PREY DENSITY 5	PREY DENSITY 10	PREY DENSITY 15	PREY DENSITY 20	PREY DENSITY 25	HANDLING TIME	ATTACK RATE
1	C = 13	C = 16	C = 18	C = 17	C = 18	$T_h = 0,18$	A =
2	C = 9	C = 13	C = 19	C = 99	C = 21	$T_h =$	A =
3	C = 7	C =	C =	C = 2	C =	$T_h =$	A =
4	C = 12	C = 14	C = 17	C =	C =	$T_h =$	A =
5	C =	C =	C =	C =	C =	$T_h =$	A =
Mean Observed values:	10:05	14.3	18	18	19.5	20.	
Expected values:							

11 seconds - handling time
3:00 minutes
9½ preys

9

3 - 11 seconds

Functional Response of Predators to Prey Abundance

NUMBERS OF PREY CONSUMED (per three-minute simulation)

15
14
13
12
11
10
9
8
7
6
5
4
3
2
1
0

0   5   10   15   20   25

PREY DENSITY

Questions for Method C

1. Which of the three types of functional response curves shown in Figure 11 does your data plot most resemble? Does this make sense, given the rules of the simulation?

2. How did your expected functional response curve match the graph of your observations? Propose hypotheses to explain any discrepancies between the two.

3. If two nuts were placed on each bolt to simulate a prey harder to process and consume, how would you expect the functional response curve to change? Illustrate your answer with a small drawing.

4. Outline a method for an experiment with real predators (such as preying mantises fed with crickets) to test Holling's model for predator functional responses.

5. Why does a strong search image produce an S-shaped functional response curve? If one predator were feeding on many prey species, would this kind of functional response tend to increase or decrease biodiversity? Explain.

FOR FURTHER INVESTIGATION

1. Use the spreadsheet model you developed in Method A to simulate the predator/prey dynamics you observed in Method B. Values of r and d for *Daphnia* are reported in the literature. The positions of the isoclines crossing at the center of observed predator/prey cycles may then allow estimation of *a* and p. How valuable are the Lotka-Volterra equations for describing *Daphnia/Euglena* population dynamics?

2. Try culturing *Daphnia* on more than one species of algae. Does a more complex food web lend greater stability to the system?

3. In late spring or summer, observe songbirds nesting on your campus. During their nesting season, birds such as American robins tend to spend most of the day searching for food or feeding young. Since robins tend to patrol territories on lawns, searching time can be measured as you observe a robin hopping across the grass looking for prey. Time spent flying to and from the nest, or in feeding young, can be considered handling time. With binoculars and a stopwatch, you can measure search time and handling time for nesting birds. Although prey density may be hard to measure, you can compare the proportions of time spent in searching and handling food in different kinds of habitat.

FOR FURTHER READING

Holling, C. S. 1959. Some characteristics of simple types of predation and parasitism. *Canadian Entomologist* 91:385–398.

Lubchenco, Jane and Bruce A. Menge. 1978. Community development and persistence in a low rocky intertidal zone. *Ecological Monographs* 48(1):67–94.

Lubchenco web site: http://lucile.science.oregonstate.edu/?q=node/view/131

Paine, Robert T. 1966. Food web complexity and biodiversity. *American Naturalist* 100: 6575.

Peterson, Ralph O. and John A. Vucetich. 2005. Ecological Studies of Wolves 2004–05 Annual Report. School of Forest Resources and Environmental Science. Michigan Technological University, Houghton, Michigan, USA, 49931–1295 http://www.isleroyalewolf.org/

Mutualism

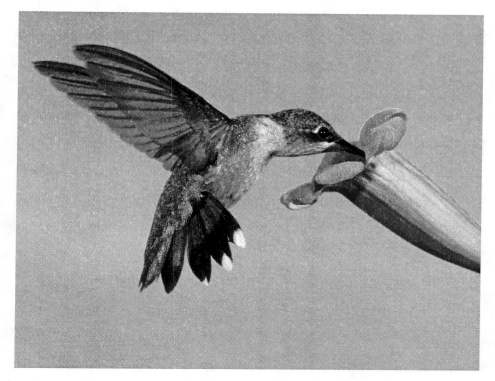

Figure 1   A ruby-throated hummingbird pollinates the red tubular flower of a trumpet creeper vine.

INTRODUCTION

The evolution of flowering plants over 100 million years ago was one of the greatest revolutions in the history of life. Flowers gave plants the capacity for faster gene exchange over longer distances, which in turn generated the variety of botanical forms that dominate our world today. Flowering plants owe much of their success to partnerships with pollinators. Early flowering plants may have been wind-pollinated, with insects visiting flowers primarily to feed on the energy-rich pollen, but plant/insect interactions quickly evolved as mutually beneficial relationships. Insects are still the most ecologically significant pollinators, but birds, bats, and even nonflying mammals are known to pollinate flowers. By attracting pollinators with strong scents, showy petals, and sugary nectar, flowers exploit the power of animal locomotion to overcome the disadvantages of a rooted existence. In return for a meal, the pollinator carries pollen cells clinging to its body to other flowers of the same species, facilitating sexual reproduction. This kind of relationship is called **mutualism** because the two organisms mutually benefit from their interactions.

Because pollen carried to a flower of the wrong species is of no value to the pollen donor or receiver, pollination is more efficient when the flower attracts a limited number of pollinators specializing in a single flower type. Flower color is an effective way to narrow the field of potential pollinators. Because insect vision is sensitive to ultraviolet wavelengths, but not to red light, a red flower is more likely to attract birds birds than insects. With the further adaptation of a trumpet-shaped flower more easily probed by a hummingbird's beak than a bee's tongue, the trumpet creeper eliminates many pollinators while powerfully signaling its preferred hummingbird pollinator (Figure 1). Hummingbirds in turn have an incentive to visit trumpet creeper, since its nectar resources are not likely to have been taken by insects prior to the bird's arrival.

Some mutualisms are so highly coevolved that the partners can no longer survive alone. *Yucca glauca*, a showy perennial flower of the Great Plains, has intrigued ecologists ever since its unique life history was first described over a century ago. Its pollination by the yucca moth *Tegeticula yuccasella* (Figure 2) presents a classic case of **obligate mutualism**. The relationship is obligate because the moth gets its only food from the seeds of the plant, and the plant has no other pollinator. As often seen in cases of obligate mutualism, each species has developed adaptive strategies to maximize its benefits from close association with the other organism.

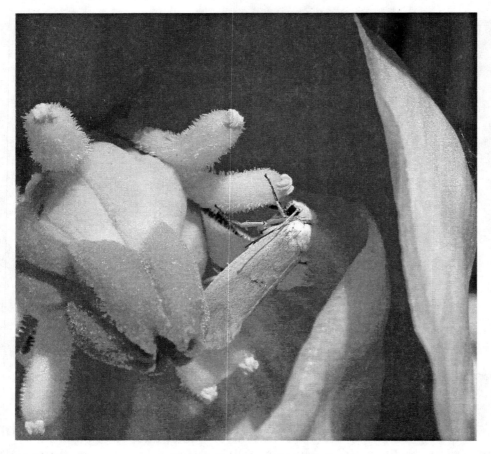

Figure 2   A yucca moth (*Tegeticula yuccasella*) pollinates a *Yucca* flower. The plant and moth are obligate mutualists; the plant has no other pollinator and the insect has no other food source.

Adult yucca moths normally live only a day or two, because their mouthparts are not adapted for feeding. Instead, the insect's specialized oral appendages are adapted for a totally different task. The female moth uses these mouthparts to gather sticky yucca pollen into a ball, which she carries under her chin. At sunset, the moth flies to another plant with her pollen load, settling on a fresh yucca flower. Stabbing into the base of the flower with a sharp abdominal appendage, she injects an egg into a seed chamber within the flower's ovary. Then, exhibiting behavior that looks quite intentional to human observers, the moth climbs to the receptive tip of the flower and rubs her pollen ball up and down on the stigma, ensuring pollination of the flower. Her eggs hatch inside the developing yucca fruit, and the young caterpillars chew their way through a row of immature seeds. Since there are generally more seeds in the chamber than one larva needs to complete its development, some of the seeds survive to propagate the yucca plant. Although nineteenth-century biologists credited the "wise little moth" with restraint and foresight in preserving the reproduction of her ally in this relationship, contemporary ecologists recognize that the plant's evolutionary adjustment of seed capsule size and of flower numbers contribute to a more biologically coherent explanation for the plant's reproductive success.

Check your progress:

Why have so many flowering plants evolved shapes and colors that limit, rather than expand, the number of pollinator species visiting their flowers?

Hint: Generalist pollinators are less likely to visit the same floral species twice in a row.

Not all mutualistic relationships are as completely codependent as *Yucca* and its moth. **Facultative mutualists** can survive on their own, but grow faster or produce more offspring in the presence of a coevolved species. Plants in the **legume** family, which includes peas and beans, exhibit facultative mutualism with bacteria of the genus *Rhizobium*. The bacterium has the rare ability to convert N_2 gas from the atmosphere into organic nitrogen (NH_4^+), which provides raw material for protein synthesis in both bacteria and plants. *Rhizobium* can grow alone in the soil, but when it encounters a legume root, the bacterium stimulates the growth of root nodules, in which the microbe takes up residence (Figure 3). Oxygen levels, which must be kept low to facilitate nitrogen fixation, are controlled inside the nodules by a layer of proteins similar to blood hemoglobin. Energy needed to drive the nitrogen-fixing reactions also comes from nutrients supplied by the plant. Legumes can grow without *Rhizobium*, but in unfertile soils, the plants have better access to growth-enhancing organic nitrogen with the help of their microbial **symbionts**.

Mutualistic associations frequently involve organisms from different kingdoms. Since mutualistic interactions are most likely to develop when the capabilities or by-products of one organism complement the needs of the other, this observation makes biological sense. Tree roots develop beneficial relationships with soil fungi, large-fruited plants rely on birds and mammals that eat their fruits to disperse seeds, cnidarian animals such as corals maintain living algae within their tissues for photosynthesis, and many herbivores rely on microbes in their guts to facilitate digestion. In the last example, mutualism is necessary because cellulose, a polymer of sugar, is the primary structural molecule in plant fibers. Although cellulose contains as

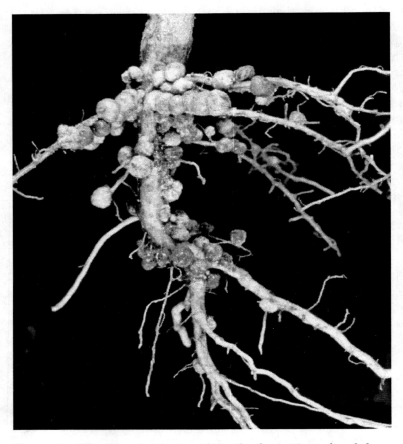

much chemical energy as starch, this food energy is unavailable to most mammals, including humans, because we do not have the enzyme required to cleave the sugar units from the polymer. This enzyme, called cellulase, is synthesized by a number of soil fungi, bacteria, and some protists. How can a cow, feeding on vegetation rich in plant fibers, derive energy from cellulose? The cow's rumen, a sac off the alimentary canal anterior to the stomach, is full of microorganisms that make the digestive enzyme for the cow, and in turn receive a warm, dark environment ideal for microbial growth. Termites (Figure 4), feeding almost exclusively on the cellulose in wood, have pockets off the hind gut that house a diverse community of cellulase-secreting microorganisms. One of these is a multi-flagellated protist called *Trichonympha* (Figure 5), an obligate symbiont that maintains its own mutualistic relationships with other microbes in the termite gut community.

Figure 3 *Rhizobium* bacteria induce the formation of nodules on the roots of legumes, which provide a hospitable environment for the microorganism. In return, *Rhizobium* fixes nitrogen in a chemical form useful to the plant.

Another two-kingdom partnership of great ecological significance is the lichen association. Lichens result from a partnership between algae (or in some cases, blue-green bacteria) and fungi. There are many lichen forms; some produce crusty splotches on rocks or tree bark, some develop leaf-like sheets, and others form spongy mats (Figure 6). The lichen body, called a thallus, is constructed like a sandwich. It has a thin layer of fungus on top, a layer of algae in the middle, and a thicker and looser layer of fungus filaments on the bottom (Figure 7). Laboratory studies of lichen reproduction suggest that the balance of power in this relationship is not equal. The fungus seems to control the growth and reproduction of its algal symbionts to such an extent that some lichenologists have questioned whether this association should be compared to a partnership or a kidnapping.

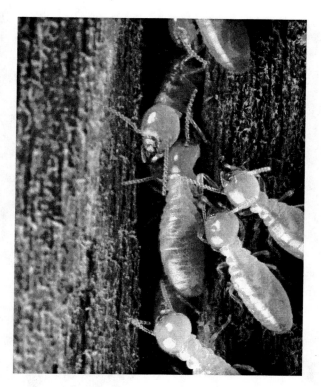

Figure 4   Termites digest cellulose in wood with the help of microbial symbionts.

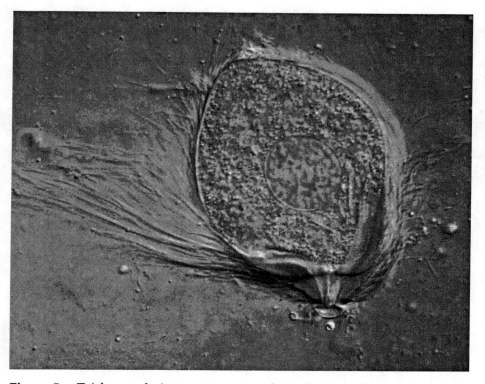

Figure 5   *Trichonympha* is a protozoan symbiont living in the gut of termites. The enzyme cellulase, provided by *Trichonympha*, breaks cellulose down into its component sugars and allows the termite to eat wood it could not otherwise digest.

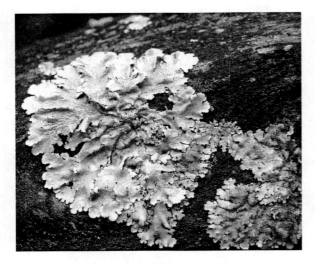

Figure 6A Crustose lichen (adheres tightly to substrate in a single layer).

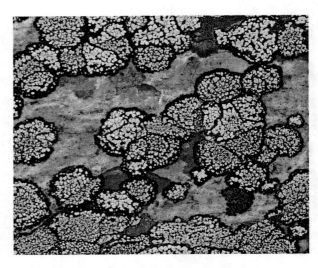

Figure 6B Foliose lichen (leafy growth form).

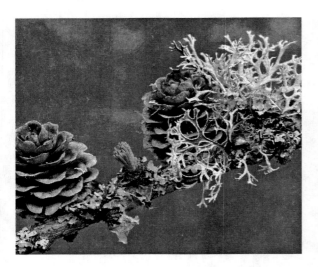

Figure 6C Fruticose lichen (bushy growth form).

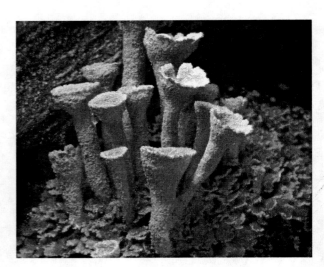

Figure 6D Squamulose lichen (with scale-like parts).

However controlled, a typical lichen association can tolerate drought and nutrient-poor conditions that would kill either component species. Algae inside the lichen produce food by photosynthesis, and the fungal layers protect the algae from drying out. The fungus can secrete acids to extract minerals from a rock substrate, so many lichens play an important role in soil formation in the early stages of ecological **succession**. The fungal elements of lichens also extract ions and organic molecules from water moving across their surfaces, so they help trap nutrients that would otherwise escape the ecosystem after a rain. This tendency to extract chemicals from the environment also makes lichens very susceptible to air pollution. Pollutants picked up by raindrops from the atmosphere are concentrated in lichens, and tend to kill them before other forms of life show ill effects. Where air quality is poor, lichens become less common, and some may disappear completely (Figure 8). Lichens are therefore useful as **bioindicators**, demonstrating long-term trends in air quality through changes in their diversity and distribution.

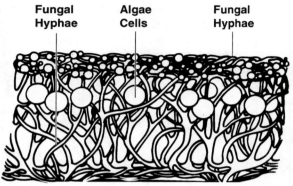

Fungal Hyphae **Algae Cells** **Fungal Hyphae**

Figure 7   A lichen thallus is made up of fungal hyphae, with a layer of algae cells embedded near the upper surface.

Check your progress:

Name the mutualist associated with each of these organisms, and explain what each partner receives from the association.

cow - enzyme
legume
yucca - yucca flower
lichen-forming fungi ~ algae

Hint: Mutualism tends to involve species from different kingdoms.

245

Although these and many other cases of mutually beneficial interactions among species have been studied by generations of biologists, only recently have we realized the full significance of mutualism in the natural world. Microbial ecologist Lynn Margulis (1999) has expanded our understanding of mutualism's importance with her work on the **endosymbiotic theory** of cell origins. This idea, since corroborated with genetic and biochemical evidence, is that mitochondria and chloroplasts originated as free-living prokaryotes that infected, and subsequently became obligate mutualists with, a larger cell. This explains why chloroplasts and mitochondria have circular DNA, binary division, and ribosomal and cell membrane characteristics similar to those of prokaryotes. Probing further into our general understanding of life, Margulis proposes that much of the genetic variation driving biological evolution may come from DNA exchanges among cooperating symbionts. Although competition and predation inspired nineteenth-century biologists to describe a natural world "red in tooth and claw," an appreciation for the essential role of mutualism gives us a more sophisticated understanding of community relationships and the history of life.

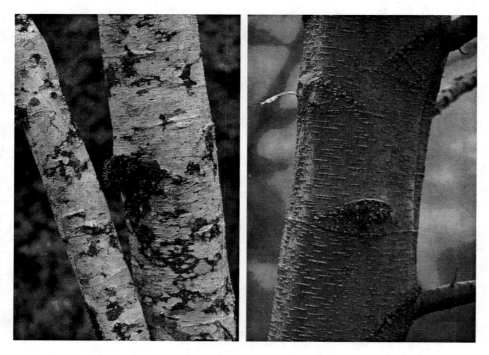

Figure 8   Lichens indicate air quality. The Red Alder tree on the left is in a clean air environment, and is covered with gray lichens. The Red Alder on the right, impacted by air pollution from a pulp mill, is devoid of lichens.

METHOD A: EFFECTS OF *RHIZOBIUM* ON LEGUMES

[Laboratory activity]

Research Question

Does association with *Rhizobium* affect the morphology and growth of legumes?

Preparation

Plan at least four weeks between planting and harvest of pea plants for this experiment. If previously exposed to soil, plastic pots for pea culture should be washed in 15% chlorine bleach solution and allowed to dry before use. Vermiculite, garden pea seeds, and the symbiont, *Rhizobium leguminosarum*, can be purchased in garden stores or through biological suppliers. Seeds should be untreated. *Rhizobium* is available as an inoculant designed for application to soil in granular form. Make sure package directions specify its use on peas, or list *R. leguminosarum* as the bacterial species.

Nitrogen-free or low-nitrogen fertilizer is sold under the names "Bloom Booster" or "Mor Bloom." Look for a fertilizer formulation with zero as the first number, such as 0-12-12, or 0-10-10. (The second and third numbers signify available phosphorus and potassium.) Apply according to package directions. If you wish to make up your own nitrogen-free fertilizer, mix the following reagents with four liters of water. Tap water is adequate, but let it stand to allow chlorine to evaporate before use.

Nitrogen-free fertilizer, per 4 liters of water:

   3.2 g potassium monohydrogen phosphate

   0.8 g magnesium sulfate

   0.8 g dihydrogen phosphate

   0.4 g calcium sulfate

   0.04 g ferric sulfate

Soak peas overnight in lukewarm water the night before the laboratory begins.

Materials (per laboratory team)

   For the Planting Lab:

   8 plastic flower pots, 4" diam.

   Labeling tape

   Paper towels

   2 trays (or plastic shoebox lids), one for treated pots and one for untreated

   Vermiculite potting medium, enough to fill pots

   Small amount of pea inoculant (a packet can be shared with other groups)

   40 garden pea seeds (previously soaked)

For the Harvesting Lab:

Metric ruler

Glass slides

Single-edge razor blade or scalpel

Dissecting microscope

Calculator or computer for computation of t-test

Procedure

Planting Lab:

1. Label four flower pots "*Rhizobium* treated," and four pots "Control." Fill all eight flower pots to within 1" of the rim with clean vermiculite potting medium. Water pots thoroughly, and allow to drain.
2. Press five previously soaked pea seeds onto the vermiculite in each of the eight pots, but do not bury the seeds.
3. In the "*Rhizobium* treated" pots, introduce the bacterium by sprinkling a very small amount of granular inoculant over the peas, making sure a few grains are touching each of the seeds. Be very careful not to contaminate the control pots with the bacterium. Washing hands before handling control pots is a good precaution.
4. Sprinkle a thin layer of Vermiculite over the peas in both treatment and control pots, covering them to a depth of 1/2". Cut a circle out of paper toweling 4" in diameter, and cover the surface of the planting medium in each pot with a layer of paper. Water the peas once more through the toweling to ensure the top layer is damp.
5. Place pots in a growth chamber at 70–75° F, with 16 hr light per day, or in a cool greenhouse, maintaining the treated and control pots in different trays. The entire class can randomize and rotate tray positions as the seedlings mature to control for any position effects on plant growth. Check for sprouts within a few days, and remove the paper toweling as soon as shoots emerge.
6. Let peas mature for 4–5 weeks before harvesting the plants. Once a week, water the pots with a low-nitrogen fertilizer solution. Add water to trays between fertilizer treatments as needed to keep vermiculite moist, making sure treated and untreated plants receive the same watering and fertilizer regime.

Harvesting Lab:

1. Ideal harvest time is when flower buds appear. First carefully unwind pea plants from each other and measure the height of each pea from the surface of the potting medium to the highest shoot tip, recording your results in the Data Table for Method A. Record any observations you can about the plants' condition, color, leaf size, and other details. Sample size could be as high as 20 for the treatment group and 20 for the control group, but may be less if some of the seeds failed to germinate.
2. After measuring heights of control peas and *Rhizobium*-treated peas, carefully invert the pots and remove the plants from the vermiculite. Shake and rinse off plant roots, keeping treated and untreated plants separated. Count the number of nodules on the roots of each plant, recording your numbers and noting sizes of nodules.
3. Remove one of the root nodules and place it on a glass slide. Use a single-edged razor blade or sharp scalpel to cross-section the nodule. Look for a rust-colored layer near the outside of the nodule. Make a drawing to record your observations.
4. Use a t-test to test the null hypothesis that *Rhizobium*-treated plants grow to the same mean height as controls. Complete the calculations in the box below the data table to determine significance for the difference between the two means.
5. Use your data and observations to answer Questions for Method A.

Data Table for Method A

RHIZOBIUM-TREATED SEEDLINGS				CONTROL SEEDLINGS		
Plant #	Height (cm)	# Nodules		Plant #	Height (cm)	# Nodules
1				1		
2				2		
3				3		
4				4		
5				5		
6				6		
7				7		
8				8		
9				9		
10				10		
11				11		
12				12		
13				13		
14				14		
15				15		
16				16		
17				17		
18				18		
19				19		
20				20		
Group Mean	$\bar{X}_1 =$			Group Mean	$\bar{X}_2 =$	
Standard Deviation	$S_1 =$			Standard Deviation	$S_2 =$	

t-TEST FOR PLANT HEIGHT DATA:

Null hypothesis: mean height of *Rhizobium*-treated plants is equal to that of controls.

t = test variable associated with data significance — d.f. = degrees of freedom
$\bar{X}_1$ = mean height of treated plants — $\bar{X}_2$ = mean height of control plants
n_1 = sample size of treated plants — n_2 = sample size of control plants
S_1 = standard deviation, treatment — S_2 = standard deviation, control

$$t = \frac{(\bar{X}_1 - \bar{X}_2)}{\sqrt{(S_1^2/n_1) + (S_2^2/n_2)}} = \boxed{}$$ d.f. = $n_1 + n_2 - 2 =$ ☐

From t-table, the t value equivalent to a significance level of p = 0.05 = ☐

Conclusion: ☐

Questions (Method A)

1. Compare the appearance of the plants treated with *Rhizobium* and the control plants. Did you notice any differences in vegetation? color? root growth?

    _____

    _____

    _____

    _____

2. Did your t-test produce the expected result, based on information in the Introduction? Explain.

    _____

    _____

    _____

    _____

3. If you had added nitrogen fertilizer to all pots, how would you expect the outcome to have been different? Would categorization of this mutualism as facultative or obligate depend on the environment? Explain.

    _____

    _____

    _____

    _____

4. Why do vegetarian diets rely heavily on foods made from legumes such as peanut butter, beans, and tofu? Why can't other kinds of plants produce storage compounds in their seeds equivalent to the dietary value of legumes?

    _____

    _____

    _____

    _____

5. Describe what you saw inside the root nodule. What makes the nodule a good site for nitrogen fixation?

    _____

    _____

    _____

    _____

METHOD B: MICROBIAL SYMBIONTS IN TERMITE GUT AND LICHEN THALLUS

[Laboratory activity]

Research Question

Do termites have symbiotic microorganisms?

Preparation

Termites can be ordered from biological supply houses, but a USDA permit is required for shipping to Arizona and Maine. The genus *Zootermopsis* is desirable for observing protists; some genera in the family Termitidae rely on bacteria rather than protozoans for cellulose digestion.

Termites can also be collected from rotting wood or old lumber piles. (Always exercise caution when turning over rocks, logs, or lumber—snakes and scorpions also occupy these sites.) Most termites are fairly easy to maintain in the laboratory. A battery jar or large glass container with air holes in the lid, half-filled with sandy soil, and a piece of wet sponge to maintain humidity provide good culture conditions for termites. Unlike ants, worker termites function well in the absence of a queen. Feed termites on brown paper, bark, or pieces of rotten wood dropped onto the surface of the soil. Avoid using pieces of treated lumber, as it contains chemicals toxic to termites.

A 0.7% saline solution will protect protozoa from osmotic shock. Add 0.7 grams NaCl or iodine-free table salt to 100 ml deionized water, and dispense into dropper bottles for each laboratory team. Termites can be distributed in Petri dishes, but put a small piece of damp paper towel in the dish if termites are to be kept this way for more than an hour or two.

For lichen observations, local lichens can be collected. Prepared slides of the lichen thallus in cross section are readily available.

Materials (per laboratory team)

Compound microscope, magnification to 400×

1 small Syracuse watch glass

Fine forceps

2 dissecting needles

Dropper bottle of 0.7% saline solution

Glass slides

Cover slips

Petri dish containing live termites

Lichen specimens

Prepared slide of lichen thallus cross section

Procedure 1 (Termite Symbionts)

1. Place a termite in the watch glass. With forceps and a dissecting needle, remove the head of the termite.
2. Cover the termite abdomen with about 10 drops of 0.7% saline. It is important to free protists from the gut under saline, because these microorganisms are anaerobes, and air is toxic to them. Tease the termite abdomen apart with dissecting needles. When the gut is opened, the saline should become milky.
3. With a Pasteur pipette, remove a few drops of fluid and place on a glass slide. Cover with a cover slip and observe with the compound microscope, first under medium power, and then on high.
4. Make observations of protozoans in the suspension, make drawings, and answer Questions for Method B.

Results for Method B: Drawings of Organisms Found in Termite Gut

Draw, label, and describe locomotion of organisms you found.

Questions for Method B on Termite Symbionts

1. Did you find *Trichonympha* in the termite gut (see Figure 5)? Describe these and any other types of protists you found in the termite gut community.

_____

_____

_____

_____

2. *Trichonympha* and other microbes supply cellulase, the enzyme needed to break down cellulose, which is the primary chemical constituent of wood and other fibrous plant parts. What ecological consequences would ensue if we did not have *Trichonympha* and other organisms producing this enzyme?

_____

_____

_____

_____

3. Young termites engage in proctodeal feeding, which involves ingesting secretions from the anus of older termites. Do your observations help to explain this behavior?

_____

_____

_____

_____

4. How could antibiotics designed to stop narrowly defined categories of infectious microbes be used to discover which organisms are mutualists and which are **parasites** or **commensals** in the termite gut?

_____

_____

_____

_____

5. Human beings carry a diverse community of bacterial species in their large intestine, including *Eschericia coli* strains that rarely cause disease in healthy people. The normal bacterial flora outcompete any foreign bacterial species passing through the system. Based on these facts, is it understandable that antibiotics taken for a sore throat might cause intestinal discomfort?

_____

_____

_____

_____

Procedure 2 (Lichen Symbionts)

1. Search for lichens on your campus. Examine sides of buildings, monuments, and tree trunks. Are lichens found in shady or sunny areas? Note color, texture, spore-forming "fruiting bodies," and shape. Count numbers of types that you find in each of the categories in Figure 6. Draw some of the lichen types in the space below:

2. Use a compound microscope to examine a prepared slide of the lichen thallus in cross section. Find layers illustrated in Figure 7. Note details in your specimen that differ from the illustration. Draw your specimen in the space below:

Questions for Method B on Lichen Symbionts

1. What, if any, kinds of lichens have you found on campus? What does lichen diversity tell you about air quality where you are?

   _____

   _____

   _____

   _____

   _____

2. From your observations of lichens and from Figure 6, which kinds of lichens have the lowest surface area per unit volume of tissue? Which have the most? How would you expect the form of a lichen to affect its nutrient retention ability? Its vulnerability to air pollution?

   _____

   _____

   _____

   _____

3. Lichen-forming fungi are generally capable of reproducing by the production of **ascospores**: single-celled reproductive units small enough to be carried away on the air. What questions does this fact pose about the obligate/facultative nature of this mutualism?

   _____

   _____

   _____

   _____

   _____

4. The blue-green bacteria (also called cyanobacteria) in some lichens are capable of nitrogen fixation. Why would this be especially advantageous in early stages of ecological succession?

   _____

   _____

   _____

   _____

   _____

5. Does the biological species concept apply to lichens? Should lichens be given species names? On what criteria should two similar-looking lichens be classified as different species?

   _____

   _____

   _____

   _____

   _____

255

METHOD C: FLOWER/POLLINATOR MUTUALISM

[Outdoor activity, spring]

Research Question
Do flowers on campus attract specialist or generalist pollinators?

Preparation
Most campus landscaping includes flowering trees and shrubs, as well as beds of annuals or perennials. Depending on your latitude, flowers may be blooming in fall or winter months, but in northerly locations spring is the best time to observe pollination. Two or more flowering plants must be available for student observations at the same time.

Some experience in identifying insects, particularly Diptera and Hymenoptera, is useful prior to the exercise, but not essential. Field identification of insect pollinators as butterflies, honeybees, beetles, etc., is adequate for preliminary analysis, but you may wish to collect and preserve voucher specimens for more accurate identification. Denatured ethanol (80% aqueous solution) and isopropyl alcohol are good preservatives for most kinds of insects.

Although observers near flowers are at low risk of bee stings, students should be asked about allergies to bee stings before participating in this laboratory.

Materials (per laboratory team)
Guide to insect identification

Insect net (optional)

Collecting vial with alcohol (optional)

Watch or timer

Procedure
1. Choose a flowering tree, shrub, or flowers of one species in a flower bed that are attracting insects. Set up a chair or something to sit on, and remain still during your observations. Insects will generally ignore you as they fly in to the flowers.
2. For a period of 30 minutes, record numbers and kinds of insects coming to the flower species you have selected. If you do not know the name of the insect, describe it as accurately as you can. As each new insect species arrives, give it a descriptive name and add it to the Preliminary Data Table for Method C. After that, make tally marks for each additional visit by the same species on the line next to the name. If too many insects are moving through your study area to observe individually, confine your observations to a smaller group of flowers. If the same individual insect moves from one flower to another within the patch of flowers you are observing, you do not need to record its presence more than once. At the end of your observation period, you may wish to collect specimens of the most common pollinators for more detailed taxonomic identification.
3. Move to a different site with a different flower species in bloom. Observe a patch of flowers approximately equal in size to the first site. Again record numbers and kinds of insects coming to the flowers for a period of 30 minutes. You may wish to collect specimens if new species are observed in this site.
4. From the data table for both sites, select the three most common pollinators overall. Fill in the Chi-square Table for Method C with numbers of these three species in each of the two sites. If a species was present at one site but not the other, then enter a 0 for the frequency at that site. Complete a Chi-square contingency test on your data. The null hypothesis for this test will be that pollinators visit the two floral species in equivalent frequencies. This means that the proportions of bees, butterflies, beetles, etc., would be the same for both flower types.

If you get a significant Chi-square value from the test, a fair conclusion is that the insects are exhibiting preferences, and that the flowers are attracting subsets of the total array of pollinator species flying at this time.

5. Use your field observations, any collections you have made, and your frequency data to answer the Questions for Method C.

Preliminary Data Table (Method C)

INSECT POLLINATOR (Name or briefly describe each species observed.)	FLORAL SPECIES A Name_____	FLORAL SPECIES B Name_____
1.		
2.		
3.		
4.		
5.		
6.		
7.		
8.		
9.		
10.		

Chi-square Contingency Table (Method C)

	FLOWER SPECIES A	FLOWER SPECIES B	Row Totals
Insect Species 1 observed:			
(expected):	( )	( )	
Insect Species 2 observed:			
(expected):	( )	( )	
Insect Species 3 observed:			
(expected):	( )	( )	
Column Totals:			
			⇑ GRAND TOTAL

1) For this analysis, you will need records for three insect species most common in the data set as a whole. Write the name of the first species in the box labeled "Species 1," the name of the second in the box labeled "Species 2," and the third in the "Species 3" box.
2) Inside the boxes marked "Flower Species A" and "Flower Species B," write plant names or descriptions of the two kinds of flowers you observed.
3) For Species 1, record the number of times you observed this species on Flower Species A inside the cell at the top left corner of the graph, *above the parentheses*. Going across the top row, enter the number of times you saw this insect on Flower Species B as well. Then enter observations for Species 2 in the second row, and Species 3 in the third row.
4) After entering your observations, add the two numbers in the top row and record the sum in the column labeled "Row Totals" at the right. Repeat for the other species, summing the total number of observations for each species as a row total.
5) Then add all the observations in the first column to determine the total number of insects you saw visiting Flower Species A. Enter the column total at the bottom of the Flower Species A numbers. Calculate column totals for Flower Species B in the same way.
6) Sum up all the row totals and enter the result in the cell labeled "Grand Total" at the bottom-right corner of the table. To check your math, sum the two column totals, and you should get the same result.

7) You should now have the table filled out as below. Three insect species are observed in this example.

	Flower Species A	Flower Species B	Row Totals
Insect Species 1	A_1	B_1	Row Total 1
Insect Species 2	A_2	B_2	Row Total 2
Insect Species 3	A_3	B_3	Row Total 3
Column Totals:	Column Total A	Column Total B	**GRAND TOTAL**

Expected values will be calculated from the **null hypothesis** that insects visit flowers randomly. Using the laws of probability we can calculate how many insects we would expect to observe on each type of flower, based on species abundance and total numbers of visits. If a pattern in the data does not conform to these expectations, we can reject the null hypothesis and follow the alternative reasoning that insects select flowers in nonrandom patterns.

For each cell in the table, you will need to calculate expected values using a simple formula: (Expected value) = (Column Total)(Row Total)/(Grand Total). For example, the expected number of observations for Insect Species 1 visiting Flower Species A would be calculated as follows:

$$\text{Expected number (A1)} = \frac{\text{(Column Total A)(Row Total 1)}}{\text{GRAND TOTAL}}$$

8) Perform this calculation, and *enter the expected number for Insect 1 on Flower A within the parentheses* in the top-left cell of the data table.

9) For each of the other cells, multiply the cell's row and column totals, divided by the grand total, to get an expected number. Enter the expected value within the parentheses at the bottom of each cell in the contingency table.

10) For a Chi-square test, you will need to calculate the number of independently varying cells in the table. This is called **degrees of freedom**, abbreviated as **d.f.** For a contingency test, degrees of freedom (d.f.) is calculated using the formula below. Calculate d.f. for your contingency table, and write the result in the box below.

The table has spaces for three insect species and two flower species, so d.f. should be $(3 − 1)(2 − 1) = 2$.

d.f. = (# insect species − 1)(# flower species − 1) = [ ]

11) Now calculate Chi-square by completing the table that follows. As you fill in the table, you will be calculating a Chi-square value for your data using the following formula:

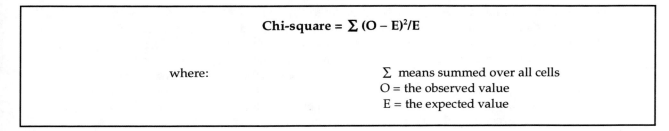

Chi-square = $\sum (O − E)^2/E$

where:

$\sum$ means summed over all cells
O = the observed value
E = the expected value

Chi-square Calculation Table

CELL LABEL Flower letter, Insect number	OBSERVED NUMBER (O)	EXPECTED NUMBER (E)	(O – E)	(O – E)^2	(O – E)^2/E
A1					
A2					
A3					
B1					
B2					
B3					
				Chi-square value =	

12) Enter a cell label for each cell you completed in your earlier table. For example, label the data for Flower B and Insect 2 as "B2." Note that each cell in the earlier table gets its own row in this one.

13) From your entries in the first table, copy all observed and expected values in the columns labeled "O" and "E."

14) Calculate the amount of deviation by subtracting the expected value from the observed value in each row. Enter the difference, with sign, in the column labeled "(O – E)." As a test of your math, check to make sure this (O – E) column sums to zero.

15) Square each deviation. Note that positive and negative signs disappear when you square these values. Enter the squared value in the column labeled "(O – E)^2."

16) Divide each squared deviation by the original expected value. Enter the result in the last column, which is labeled "(O – E)^2/E."

17) Finally, add up all the (O – E)^2/E values, and record the sum at the bottom-right corner of the calculation page. This is the **Chi-square** value for your data set. Because it is calculated from deviations of observed values from expected values, the greater the departure from null hypothesis expectations, the higher the value of Chi-square. If we observed no differences between observed and expected values, the value of Chi-square would be calculated as 0, meaning that insects are selecting flowers exactly as your null hypothesis predicted. Even if insects were selecting flowers at random, some degree of pattern could be expected due to sampling error, so we could anticipate a small Chi-square value most of the time, just due to chance.

As deviations from random expectations grow larger, Chi-square grows too. At some breaking point, called the **critical value** of Chi-square, we can no longer accept the null hypothesis as an explanation for data patterns generating these large deviations. At this point, we say an alternative, nonrandom explanation is warranted. By convention, scientists agree that the critical value of Chi-square has been reached if the odds of generating deviations of this magnitude by random sampling error alone are less than 5%. This 5% probability, written as **p = 0.05** by statisticians, means that our results can be considered **"statistically significant."** This does not mean the alternative explanation we pose is always right, but it does mean we have eliminated the null hypothesis with 95% confidence. An even higher value of Chi-square, corresponding to a p value of 0.01, is the threshold customarily designated as a "highly significant" departure from random expectations. In this case, our conclusion is the same, but our confidence in rejecting the null hypothesis has risen to 99%.

In summary, think of p as the error rate we can expect if we reject the null hypothesis based on a given Chi-square value. *A high value of Chi-square corresponds to a high level of statistical significance, which in turn corresponds to a low p value.*

18) Equating a Chi-square value (along with the degrees of freedom in your experimental design) with its corresponding p value is easily accomplished using a Chi-square table. A simplified Chi-square table is included below, for your convenience. First, find the row equivalent to the **degrees of freedom** you calculated for this data set. Remember this is (#Flowers − 1)(# Insects − 1) so your degrees of freedom should be 2 if you observed 3 insect species and 2 flower species. Next, compare your Chi-square value with the two Chi-square numbers in the table.

Under the heading "p = 0.05" and in the row corresponding to your degrees of freedom, you will find a critical value of Chi-square. *If your calculation of Chi-square yielded a number larger than the critical value, then your results can be considered significantly nonrandom.* In the context of your experiment, this supports the hypothesis that your insect species are partitioning themselves among flowers in a nonrandom fashion.

Under the heading "p = 0.01," you will find a Chi-square value indicating a higher level of significance. If your calculation of Chi-square yielded a number larger than this, you can have even greater confidence that your data show a nonrandom pattern. The conclusion is the same as for p = 0.05, but your evidence is stronger in this case.

A Chi-square value lower than the number in the p = 0.05 column could have come from observations of insects randomly selecting flowers. This may or may not be the case, but low Chi-square values mean you do not have sufficient evidence to reject the null hypothesis of random flower visitation.

Simplified Chi-square Table of Critical Values*

DEGREES OF FREEDOM	CHI SQUARE GREATER THAN THIS VALUE INDICATES SIGNIFICANCE p = 0.05	CHI SQUARE GREATER THAN THIS VALUE INDICATES HIGHER SIGNIFICANCE p = 0.01
2	5.99	9.21

*Critical values from Rohlf, F. J. and R. R. Sokal. 1995. *Statistical Tables*, 3rd ed. W. H. Freeman, San Francisco.

Questions (Method C)

1. Did you confirm any differences in pollinator preference between the two plant species? Do you think these plants have evolved mechanisms to limit mutualistic interactions to one or a few pollinator species, or are they acting as generalists?

   _____

   _____

   _____

   _____

2. What did you notice about flower color, scent, shape, or orientation that might affect attractiveness to different kinds of pollinators? Does flower structure explain any patterns in insect preference you observed?

   _____

   _____

   _____

   _____

3. How were the flowers you observed shaped to maximize pollen transfer? Were the insects forced to brush against the male parts of the flower (called anthers) in order to enter the flower or in order to access the nectar? How do you think pollen might be transferred to the receptive surface (called the stigma) of the female floral parts?

   _____

   _____

   _____

   _____

4. An insect's resource-seeking behavior is called a **foraging strategy**. What factors other than flower characteristics might influence the foraging strategies of the insects you observed? Is it possible that wind or sun exposure, proximity to shelter, humidity, or other site characteristics are in part responsible for differences in pollination frequency?

   _____

   _____

   _____

   _____

5. In natural plant communities, different species often open their flowers at different times of day or at different times of year. Why might this be advantageous to all members of the community?

   _____

   _____

   _____

   _____

FOR FURTHER INVESTIGATION

1. Try the pea and *Rhizobium* experiment with different varieties of peas. Are some pea varieties better able to accommodate the symbiont than others?
2. Observe and classify lichens on your campus. When you compare the lichens growing on trees on campus with lichens on trees in a less populated area nearby, do you see evidence of air quality differences between the sites?
3. Compare results of your pollinator foraging study at different times during the spring. Do some pollinators shift their preferences as different kinds of flowers become available?

FOR FURTHER READING

Borror, D. J. and R. E. White. 1998. *A Field Guide to Insects.* Houghton Mifflin.

Margulis, Lynn. 1999. *Symbiotic Planet: A New View of Evolution.* Basic Books, New York.

Ramsay, Marylee and John Richard Schrock. 1995. The yucca plant and the yucca moth. *The Kansas School Naturalist.* Emporia State University, Emporia KS. 41(2). http://www.emporia.edu/ksn/v41n2-june1995/KSNVOL41-2.htm

Richardson, D. H. S. 1992. Pollution monitoring with lichens. *Naturalists' Handbook No. 19*, Richmond Publishing Co. Ltd.

Biodiversity

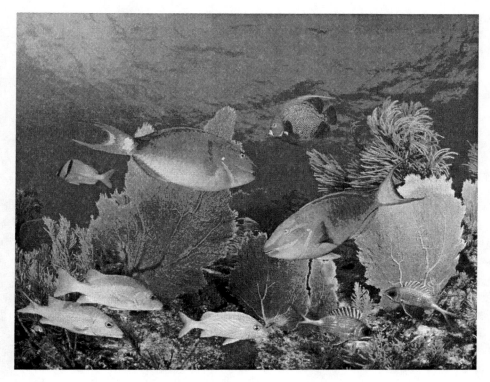

Figure 1   A coral reef off Key Largo in Florida. Tropical coral reefs are among the earth's most diverse systems.

INTRODUCTION

Biologists have always been awed and challenged by the diversity of life on earth. At the conclusion of "The Origin of Species," Charles Darwin contemplates with astonishment a riverbank covered in a tangled growth of vines, shrubs, fungi, birds, mammals, worms, insects, and scores of other living things. After hundreds of pages of carefully marshaled evidence supporting his concept of speciation as a natural and ongoing process, the methodical Victorian naturalist finds the outcome of biological evolution too amazing for words. **Biodiversity**, which Darwin described as "endless forms most beautiful and most wonderful," remains an object of scientific curiosity and passion. A contemporary biology student, snorkeling over a coral reef for the first time (Figure 1), is likely to share Darwin's wonderment at the "grandeur" of life. Coral reefs are incredibly species-rich communities. Surrounded by hard and soft corals, echinoderms, annelids, molluscs, arthropods, and fishes of all sizes, shapes, patterns, and colors, it is hard to fathom how so many different species can coexist in one place.

How many species are there? This question is easier to ask than to answer, because we have discovered and described only a fraction of the earth's biota. Most large terrestrial organisms, such as birds and mammals, are so well inventoried that discovery of a new species in these taxonomic groups is a newsworthy event. At the other extreme are soil bacteria, often impossible to culture in standard media, and so poorly studied that there are probably a number of undescribed species thriving beneath your campus grounds. In his influential book *The Diversity of Life*, ecologist E. O. Wilson (1999) reports an estimate of 1.4 million described species, based on interviews with taxonomists specializing in a wide variety of organisms, and comprehensive reviews of databases and museum records. As for the numbers of living species not yet known to science, estimates range from 5 million to 100 million. As ecologists discover new taxonomic categories and new microhabitats, they are constantly revising their estimates as previously unknown groups of organisms are discovered (e.g., Ellwood and Foster, 2004). Wilson's argument for more attention to taxonomic questions in biology is compelling, since intelligent management decisions for global species protection begin with some idea of the number of species we have to protect.

How can we improve our appraisal of biodiversity yet to be discovered? One practical approach is based on repeated sampling of a type of organism in a particular place, using the growing database to develop a **species accumulation curve**. To show how this works, let's visit La Selva, Costa Rica's national rainforest preserve. Here entomologists John T. Longino and Robert Colwell have been collecting ants from the leaf litter of the forest floor in an extended survey of the insect fauna of the park. One of their methods for trapping specimens is the Berlese apparatus (Figure 2). Leaf litter collected from the forest floor is returned to a lab and placed in a funnel lined with screening. A lightbulb placed over the top of the funnel heats up the leaf litter, and all the tiny invertebrates from that sample go down through the screening and into the funnel. The bottom of the funnel leads to a jar of preservative, so the species in this sample can be counted and identified (Figure 3).

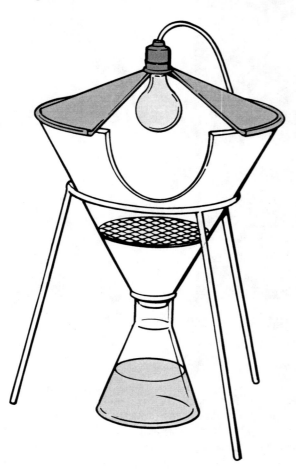

Figure 2 Berlese funnel apparatus for collecting arthropods from leaf litter.

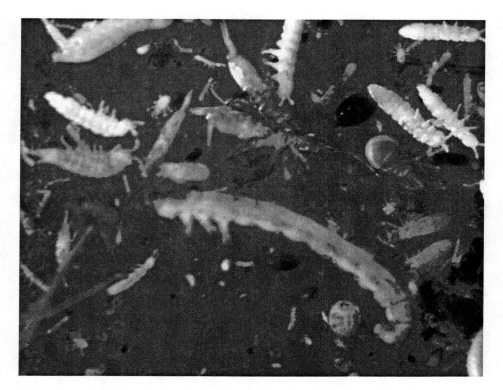

Figure 3   Arthropods sampled with a Berlese apparatus.

Longino and Colwell's Berlese results for La Selva are shown in Figure 4. The x-axis shows the number of samples analyzed, and the y-axis shows cumulative numbers of ant species found in all the samples up to that point. The curve rises steeply at first, because new species are discovered in nearly every sample at the beginning of the study. As more and more samples are examined, it becomes harder and harder to find species not already counted, so the slope of the curve gets less and less steep as the sampling effort continues. From a quick examination of the figure, you could predict that biologists could find more ant species if the study were continued, but you could also place an upper limit on the expected number, based on the decreasing slope of the curve. Species accumulation curves have been developed for many kinds of organisms in many kinds of habitats. The shape of the curve varies somewhat, depending on habitat patchiness and the relative frequency of rare species, but declining rates of return on sampling effort are common to all. At some arbitrary stopping point, say less than one new species per 1000 samples, we can conclude for all practical purposes that the fauna in this locale have been adequately described.

Check your progress:

Estimates of the total numbers of species on earth vary by orders of magnitude. How can we find out which estimates are correct?

Answer: More study of poorly investigated taxonomic groups and species-accumulation analysis in species-rich systems could lead to better global estimates.

Although we are not sure how many species exist in the world, we do know that ecosystems vary significantly in biodiversity. In general, numbers of species per unit area are highest in tropical systems, declining as you travel from the equator toward the north or south pole. A tropical forest may have as many as 300 tree species in a randomly selected hectare of land (Figure 5), but in a similar area of boreal forest in interior Alaska, you are likely to find only one or two species of spruce trees (Figure 6). Why does biodiversity per unit area decline with increasing latitude? One explanation is that **primary productivity**, which is the rate of biomass accumulation per unit area via photosynthesis, is highest in the tropics where the growing season lasts longer and high temperatures speed up biochemical reactions. If we assume the total **biomass** of an ecosystem can only be divided into a finite number of species, then higher productivity gives an ecosystem the capacity to support more kinds of organisms. This explanation presumes ecosystems are subject to **bottom-up control** by the plants at the base of the food chain. Better growing conditions, in this way of thinking, lead to greater biodiversity.

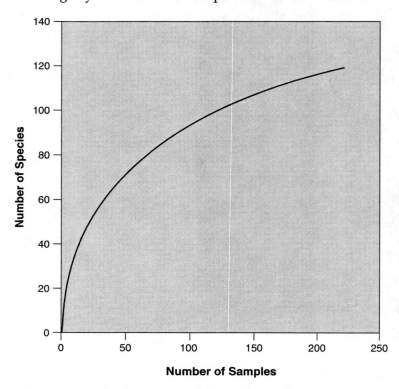

Figure 4   Accumulation curve for ants collected with Berlese trapping in La Selva Biological Station in Costa Rica. (After John T. Longino, http://www.evergreen.edu/ants/alascollns/2001.expeditions/reports/formicidae/home.html#fig1)

An alternative explanation recognizes the longer geologic history of tropical ecosystems. Since arctic and north-temperate communities were disrupted in the relatively recent past by glaciation, evolution has had a longer undisturbed period to produce species in the tropics. A third possibility is that stable climate in the tropics means organisms migrate less, so tropical populations remain more isolated within valleys or on mountains. Since speciation is thought to occur more quickly when populations are geographically separated, we might expect higher rates of speciation in the tropics as a result of greater climatic stability. All of these explanations may be true in part. As is so often the case in ecology, the trend we observe may have more than one contributing cause.

Check your progress:

Name two of the earth's most species-rich ecosystems. Why are they so diverse?

Hint: Tropical ecosystems have the most species. These include tropical forests and coral reefs.

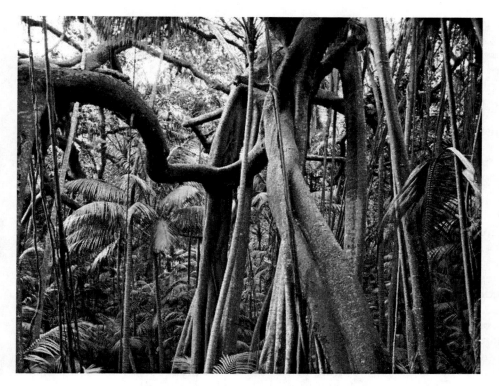

Figure 5 A tropical forest exhibits high biodiversity, with hundreds of species of trees in a single community.

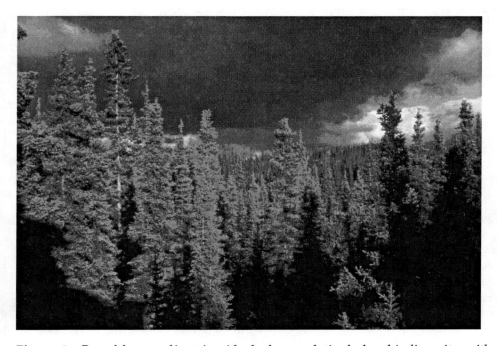

Figure 6 Boreal forests of interior Alaska have relatively low biodiversity, with a community dominated by two species of spruce trees.

We also know that biodiversity is unequally distributed among taxonomic groups. As impressed as we may be by the number of living mammals (4000 described, according to E. O. Wilson), there are more than 10 times as many mollusks as mammals (over 50,000 species). That is certainly a lot of snails and clams, but there are twice that number of butterflies and moths (Order Lepidoptera 112,000), and six times that many beetles (Order Coleoptera 290,000). Broad-leaved flowering plants make up 2/3 of the plant kingdom, and more than half of all animal species are insects. Why have some taxonomic groups been so successful at generating new species? Given our understanding of competitive exclusion, we understand that each species in a community must exploit a unique ecological niche. Small body size would therefore seem conducive to rapid speciation. It is reasonable to assume creatures as small as mites or beetles could find more ways to divide up an environment into distinct microhabitats or unique feeding niches than could a moose-sized animal occupying the same habitat.

Another factor made clear from the fossil record is that numbers of species in an emerging taxonomic group can expand rapidly when the normally slow evolution of organismal forms crosses a threshold into a truly novel body plan. The first winged insects, for example, were suddenly presented opportunities for hunting, grazing, escaping predators, and finding mates that were unprecedented in the history of arthropod life. In the absence of any serious competition save one another, these novel organisms spread across continents, adapting to newfound modes of existence like homesteaders in a land rush. Natural selection to local environments and unprecedented access to far-flung resources generated genetic differences among geographically distinct populations and pushed the process of speciation into overdrive. The result, which we see reflected in patterns of biodiversity in the present day, is a diverse array of related species, each applying the group's common evolutionary advantage as individual variations on the common morphological theme. Evolutionary biologists call this phenomenon **adaptive radiation.** In addition to the insects, the rapid development of flowering plants in the Cretaceous period (over 100 million years ago) presents a noteworthy example. A "breakthrough" to reproduction through flowers and fruits made plants much more successful in terms of species numbers than the older established lines of ferns and conifers. Emerging insect families, adapting to new niches as pollinators, seed predators, and herbivores, rode the tide of floral diversity to become the most species-rich animal group on planet Earth.

Check your progress:

Why are there so many kinds of beetles?

Answer: Beetles are small, and as a consequence of adaptive radiation, exploit a variety of niches.

In addition to species richness, we need to recognize that biodiversity exists in a hierarchy of variation. Genetic diversity within the species is an important consideration in understanding the history and predicting the future of a population. Above the species level, diversity of higher taxa such as orders or families is also of paramount importance to conservation efforts. Biologists first want to save taxonomic groups represented by one or a few species, because these "end of the line" species have a significant number of unique genetic traits. For example, the mammalian order Proboscidea includes many fossil species of mammoths and mastodons, but only two surviving species: the Asian elephant and the African elephant. In contrast, the Order Rodentia has approximately 2000 living species, so extinction of a rare species of vole or squirrel would not have the same impact on global animal diversity as losing a species of elephant.

Below the species level, biodiversity exists in subspecies and varieties. Florida panthers (*Puma concolor coryi*) were once broadly distributed through the American Southeast, but are now reduced to a few individuals in the Everglades. Although they are considered the same species as more abundant cougars (also known as mountain lions) in Western states, sufficient genetic differences exist among populations to merit separate protection for Florida panthers. At the bottom of the hierarchy of diversity is genetic variation within a population. Maintaining critical levels of genetic variation within populations is important too, because species reduced below a critical threshold lack the genetic variation needed to avoid inbreeding depression. This term refers to genetically related failures in vitality and reproduction due to mating of genetically similar individuals. This becomes a problem in many species when the breeding population drops below 100 or so.

Documenting and managing biodiversity is especially important in the twenty-first century because species extinction represents an increasing problem across the globe. Expanding human populations and an exponentially growing demand for primary resources such as coal, water, cropland, and timber take habitats away from more native species every year. In the oceans, pollution and changes in average sea temperature are stressing coral reefs and all their associated life forms. The vanishing rainforest is well publicized, but biologists are currently voicing serious concerns about the extent of habitat loss within the United States as well. For example, a particularly destructive form of mining in the Appalachians removes entire tops of mountains to expose seams of coal (Figure 7). The overburden of rock layers above the seam is dumped into surrounding creek valleys, so mountaintop removal affects water quality downstream as well as the obvious impact on high-altitude habitat for species not found at lower elevations. Although mining companies usually plant grass on the flattened peaks after the coal is removed, the resulting "reclaimed" land cannot support the same biological community that was destroyed.

Check your progress:

Given the rising extinction rates around the world, and the limited funding available for conservation, in what types of habitats should we focus our preservation efforts?

Hint: Consider species richness, unique taxa, and the economic status of the nations involved.

Making sound decisions about biodiversity management and protection begins with accurate data, so measuring diversity is important. Species lists are a good start, but relative numbers of individuals of each species in a community should also be considered. The number of species in a sample is called species **richness**. The degree to which total organism number is distributed equally among these species is called species **evenness**. Both richness and evenness need to be incorporated in a biodiversity index.

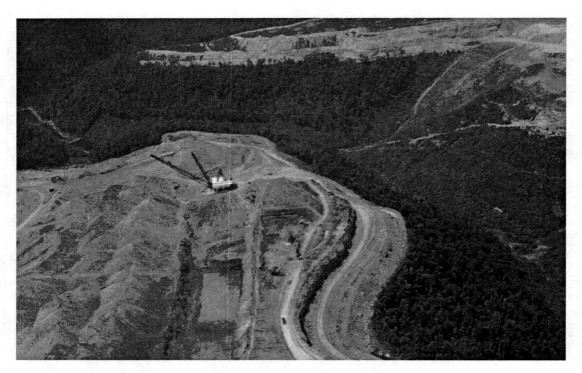

Figure 7   Mountaintop removal threatens biodiversity in the Appalachians.

To illustrate with an example, suppose ecology students at two hypothetical colleges held a contest to see which had the most biologically diverse bird community (or avifauna) on their campus. College A students spent a Saturday morning walking the campus, counting numbers of each species they encountered. Students at College B engaged in a similar sampling routine. Assume that both colleges had the same species richness (five species) and the same sample size of 100 birds, but that numbers of each kind of bird were distributed differently. (For a visual representation of the two campus data sets, see Figure 8.)

Number of Birds of Listed Species Identified on Campus

TYPE OF BIRD	CAMPUS A	CAMPUS B
Pigeon	96	20
Robin	1	20
Starling	1	20
Purple grackle	1	20
House sparrow	1	20

Campus A - Dominated by One Species

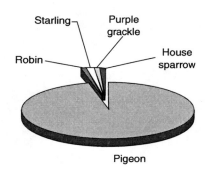

Campus B - Even Species Distribution

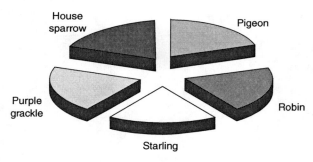

Figure 8 Species distribution contributes to biodiversity. Campus A, dominated by one bird species, is less biologically diverse than Campus B, even though both sites have 5 species.

Which school has the more diverse avifauna? Clearly, four of the birds on Campus A's species list make little contribution to the bird community. Campus B's sample, illustrating maximum evenness, demonstrates greater biodiversity. On Campus B, interactions between different species are much more frequent because the community has no single dominant type. Another way of thinking about this as an observer is to ask, what is the probability of encountering the same species twice in a row? On Campus A, the probability is very high, but on Campus B it is much lower.

This probability of change in encounters was used along with species richness to design a way to measure biodiversity that takes both numbers of species and their proportions into account. Called a **Shannon diversity index**, this methodology was originally derived for calculating variations in electronic signals. This index is also known as the Shannon-Wiener Index and as the Shannon-Weaver Index, because its author Claude Shannon collaborated both with Norbert Wiener and with Warren Weaver (Perkin, 1982). In any case, the index measures the likelihood of repetition in adjoining samples. The diversity index is calculated as follows:

Shannon Diversity Index:

$$H = \sum_{i=1}^{S} -(P_i \cdot ln\, P_i)$$

where:

H = the Shannon diversity index
P_i = fraction of entire population made up of species i
S = numbers of species encountered
Σ indicates the sum from species 1 to species S

To calculate the index, first divide the number of individuals of species #1 you found in your sample by the total number of individuals of all species. This is P_1, which should be expressed as a decimal value between 0 and 1. Then multiply this fraction times its own natural logarithm. This gives you the quantity $(P_1 \cdot ln\, P_1)$. Since the natural log of a fraction yields a negative number, a minus sign is placed in front of the parentheses in the equation to convert the negative product back to a positive number. Next, plug in species # 2 numbers to calculate $-(P_2 \cdot ln\, P_2)$. Repeat for all species through the last on your species list, which is species number **S**. Finally, sum the $-(P_i \cdot ln\, P_i)$ products for all species to get the value of the index, **H**.

The following table demonstrates calculations of the diversity indices for the bird data on Campus A and Campus B.

CAMPUS A BIRDS	N_i	P_i	$ln\ P_i$	$-(P_i \cdot ln\ P_i)$
Pigeon	96	0.96	−0.041	0.039
Robin	1	0.01	−4.61	0.046
Starling	1	0.01	−4.61	0.046
Purple grackle	1	0.01	−4.61	0.046
House sparrow	1	0.01	−4.61	0.046
TOTAL	100			H = 0.223

CAMPUS B BIRDS	N_i	P_i	$ln\ P_i$	$-(P_i \cdot ln\ P_i)$
Pigeon	20	0.20	−1.61	0.322
Robin	20	0.20	−1.61	0.322
Starling	20	0.20	−1.61	0.322
Purple grackle	20	0.20	−1.61	0.322
House sparrow	20	0.20	−1.61	0.322
TOTAL	100			H = 1.610

High values of H represent more diverse communities. A community of only one species would have an H value of 0, since P_i would equal 1.0, and it would be multiplied by ln (1.0) = 0. Campus A's H value is small, because its community is dominated by one species. If all species are equal in numbers, the equation yields a maximum H value equal to the natural logarithm of the number of species in the sample. For example, Campus B has five species. The H value of 1.61 = ln (5), so Campus B is as diverse as a five-species community can possibly be.

Check your progress:

What added information about biodiversity does the Shannon index convey that could not be derived from a simple species count?

Hint: The distribution of species abundance contributes to biological diversity.

METHOD A: MEASURING BIODIVERSITY OF CAMPUS BIRDS

[Outdoor activity, any time of year]

Research Question

How diverse is the community of bird species on campus?

Preparation

Birds can be censused almost any time of year. Early morning is best, especially in breeding season. A walk across a campus landscaped with trees and shrubs should allow observation of sufficient numbers of species to calculate a diversity index. If available to you, local parks, cemeteries, and residential areas are generally good habitats for songbirds as well. In northern states, migratory songbirds are present only in summer, but the birds that stay all winter are actually easier to see when the leaves are off the deciduous trees. If a bird feeder has been established for observation of feeding niches, you can collect data by counting birds visiting the feeder during a specified length of time.

Good field guides are available for identification of local birds, but a knowledgeable mentor is the best way to master bird identification. Local Audubon societies are a great source of expertise. You may want to participate as a class in the annual winter bird count that many local organizations hold, and use these data for biodiversity analysis.

This method can be used to accumulate species counts for a species accumulation curve if multiple laboratory sections standardize their observation time. Treat each class observation as a sample, and plot the cumulative number of species found vs. number of samples analyzed. In small institutions, you can accumulate data from multiple years for the same purpose, although changing habitat conditions could become a factor over a period of years.

Materials (per laboratory team)

Binoculars (One for every person is ideal, but binoculars can be shared.)

Field guide to local birds

Data from previous surveys, if available

Procedure

1. Establish a time (e.g., one hour) for your census of campus birds. Designate at least one observer and one recorder for your group. As you walk a survey route or watch a bird feeding station, all members of the class can look for birds and relay information to the recorder. The recorder should write the name of each bird on the Data Sheet for Methods A, B, or C. Each time this species is encountered, record numbers of individuals in the second column of the Data Sheet. If you see a flock of birds, have everyone in the group estimate numbers, and then choose the middle (median) estimate as your group record.
2. When your observation time is complete, sum the number of individuals of each species, and include these totals in the right-hand column of the data sheet.
3. Transfer these totals to the Shannon Calculation Page for Methods A, B, and C. Calculate H, the diversity index for this sample, following the example from the Introduction. Record your estimated value of H.
4. If multiple samples are available, either from your instructor for past classes or from multiple sections of your class, arrange the data in chronological order and fill out the Species Accumulation Data Sheet for Methods A, B, and C.
5. Plot numbers of species as a function of number of samples to create a species accumulation curve for these data sets on the graph paper provided at the end of the chapter.
6. Answer Questions for Methods A, B, and C to interpret your results.

METHOD B: MEASURING INVERTEBRATE BIODIVERSITY

[Outdoor or laboratory, two class meetings required]

Research Question

How diverse is the detritus invertebrate community?

Preparation

Small invertebrates are surprisingly common in decaying leaf litter, but organic landscaping such as shredded bark mulch works very well too. Look for last year's landscaping mulch or leaf litter around the bases of trees or shrubs. Partially decayed organic material in contact with damp soil is best. Samples should be collected using a standardized methodology. A 1-pound coffee can or large empty tin can will work fairly well for taking a standard core sample.

A Berlese apparatus can be made with a ring stand and a large funnel. Drywall joint tape is readily available in hardware and home supply stores, but cheesecloth can be substituted if necessary. A goosenecked lamp with a metal shade and a 60-watt incandescent bulb works quite well for the heat source. If your lab benches do not have an elevated middle section, use a box or overturned bucket to elevate the lamp above the funnel. *Although the lamp bulb should be positioned 10–15 cm above the mulch, maintain enough space to avoid fire hazard, making sure the bulb is not leaning against the funnel or touching the organic material.*

A wide-mouth glass specimen jar, containing 85% denatured ethanol, can be positioned under the funnel to collect specimens. Driving specimens out of the mulch requires several hours, so this is a two-period procedure. If someone can come by after several hours and turn off the lamps and put tops on the jars, counting the specimens can be completed at a later time.

If multiple samples are scored by different lab groups, the class can complete steps 10 and 11 in the Procedure to develop a species accumulation curve. The class will have to share species lists from 8–10 groups to make this meaningful. Previous years' data can be pooled for this purpose as well.

Most introductory entomology texts have illustrations of noninsect arthropods suitable for identification in this exercise. If species identification is not possible, higher-level taxonomy (such as identification of the family) is adequate, as long as all analyses used in the species accumulation data are conducted in a consistent way. If students find an organism they cannot identify, it can still be used as a species in the analysis.

Materials (per laboratory team)

Large sealable plastic bag

Empty tin can

Hand trowel or spade

Ring stand

Large polypropylene funnel, with top diameter 15–20 cm

Drywall joint tape: two pieces, 15 cm long

Wide-mouthed specimen jar

Goosenecked desk lamp

Dissecting microscope

Guide to invertebrate identification

Data from previous surveys, if available

PROCEDURE

1. Locate an area where decaying mulch or leaf litter is in contact with soil. Push the open end of the can through the litter layer down to the soil. Tip the can sideways, and use your hand trowel to scoop all the loosened material into the can. Empty the contents into a large sealable plastic bag and return to the laboratory.
2. Set up the ring stand so that the funnel can be positioned just above the specimen jar as shown in Figure 2.
3. Cut two pieces of drywall joint tape about 15 cm long. Cross them, sticky side down, as shown in Figure 9. Push the crossed tape into the bottom of the funnel, with the adhesive side down, to create a screened mesh over the bottom of the funnel, as shown in the figure. This will keep leaf litter from falling into your specimen jar.

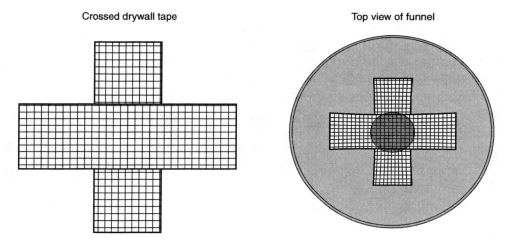

Crossed drywall tape   Top view of funnel

Figure 9   Procedure for lining funnel for Berlese apparatus. Cross two pieces of drywall joint tape about 15 cm long, sticky sides down, as shown at left. Then stick the crossed tape onto the bottom of the funnel to cover the hole, as shown at right.

4. Put a sample of leaf litter or mulch into the top of the funnel. Pour alcohol into the sample jar to a depth of 2 cm, and position it under the neck of the funnel.
5. Position the lamp a few inches above the funnel so that the bulb can warm and dry the sample. *Avoid direct contact between the lightbulb and the leaf litter*. Leave several hours or overnight. You should be able to see tiny organisms that have fallen in the jar as the Berlese trap begins to separate invertebrates from the decaying plant material.
6. Pour out your sample into a Petri dish or specimen dish, and examine under a dissecting microscope.
7. Identify or briefly describe species of organisms in your sample. Carefully count the numbers of individuals of each different species you see. Record each species on a separate line in the Data Sheet for Methods A, B, and C.
8. Sum the number of individuals of each species, and include these totals in the right-hand column of the data sheet.
9. Transfer these totals to the Shannon Calculation Page for Methods A, B, and C. Calculate H, the diversity index for this sample, following the example from the Introduction. Record your estimated value of H.
10. (Instructor's option) If multiple samples are available, either from your instructor for past classes or from multiple sections of your class, assign a recording student's name to each group, arrange group data in alphabetical order according to the student names, and use the samples in this order to fill out the *Species* Accumulation Data Sheet for Methods A, B, and C.
11. (Instructor's option) Plot numbers of species as a function of number of samples to create a species accumulation curve for these data sets on the graph paper provided at the end of the chapter.
12. Answer Questions for Methods A, B, and C to interpret your results.

METHOD C: MEASURING BIODIVERSITY IN SWEEP NET SAMPLES

[Outdoor or laboratory activity, late spring, summer, or fall]

Research Question

How diverse is the insect community in a field habitat?

Preparation

This method requires that students go to a weedy or grassy area not closely mown. Afternoon times are better than mornings for sweep samples, if nights are cool enough to restrict insect activity. The advantage over Method B is that collections can be made in minutes rather than hours.

Killing jars can be made inexpensively from any kind of large specimen jar or recycled jelly jar with a tight-sealing lid. Pour a layer of plaster of Paris, about 3 cm deep, in the bottom of the jar. (Alternatively, cut and layer paper toweling to fill the bottom fourth of the jar.) After the plaster of Paris has hardened, saturate it with ethyl acetate. This is a good killing agent for insects, but not as harmful to humans as other chemical alternatives. Ethyl acetate is the primary ingredient in many kinds of fingernail polish remover, which can be purchased in drugstores and works as well as reagent grade.

If multiple samples are collected by different lab groups, the class can complete steps 7 and 8 in the Procedure to develop a species accumulation curve. The class will have to share species lists from 8–10 groups to make this meaningful. Previous years' data can be pooled for this purpose as well.

Materials (per laboratory team)

Sweep net

Insect killing jar (one per sample)

Sealable plastic bags

Dissecting microscope

Insect identification guide

Procedure

1. Charge your killing jar by pouring 5–10 ml of ethyl acetate onto the absorbent material at the bottom of the jar. All the ethyl acetate should be absorbed; you should not have any pooled in the jar. Screw the lid on tightly and take it with your sweep net to a sample area.
2. In a field of high grass or weeds, collect insects with an insect net by "sweeping." This means to swing the net through the grass with a side to side stroke in front of you, so that insects are knocked off the grass and into the net. Take 30 swings as you walk through the field so that you sweep a new area of grass with each swing of the net. If you do not catch a variety of insects in 30 swings, increase the number of swings per sample, and standardize all further sampling at this number.
3. After you have collected a sample, shake all the insects down into the bottom of the net. Hold the netting closed with one hand to make a "pocket" containing the insects, and place the open mouth of the killing jar into the net adjacent to the pocket. Invert the "pocket" into your killing jar. Quickly slide the lid over the insects and screw it on tight. Insects should be held in the killing jar for at least 15 minutes before you examine them.
4. Examine your insect sample under a dissecting microscope. Identify or briefly describe each species of insect or other invertebrate in the sample. Carefully count the numbers of individuals of each species. Record each species on a separate line in the Data Sheet for Methods A, B, and C. Count the number of each species in your sample, and record those counts as tally marks in the second column of the data sheet.

5. Sum the number of individuals of each species, and include these totals in the right-hand column of the data sheet.
6. Transfer these totals to the Shannon Calculation Page for Methods A, B, and C. Calculate H, the diversity index for this sample, following the example from the Introduction. If you do not need all the rows in the table, leave the bottom rows blank. Record your estimated value of H in the indicated box at the bottom.
7. (Instructor's option) If multiple samples are available, either from past classes or from multiple sections of your class, assign a recording student's name to each group, arrange group data in alphabetical order according to the student names, and use the samples in this order to fill out the *Species* Accumulation Data Sheet for Methods A, B, and C.
8. (Instructor's option) Plot numbers of species as a function of number of samples to create a species accumulation curve for these data sets on the graph paper provided at the end of the chapter.
9. Answer Questions for Methods A, B, and C to interpret your results.

Data Table for Methods A, B, and C

SPECIES IDENTIFIED	TALLY MARKS (Numbers of individuals)	TOTAL # OF INDIVIDUALS
1.		
2.		
3.		
4.		
5.		
6.		
7.		
8.		
9.		
10.		
11.		
12.		
13.		
14.		
15.		
16.		
17.		
18.		
19.		
20.		
TOTAL # → Individuals in the sample		

Shannon Calculation Page for Methods A, B, and C

SPECIES FOUND IN SAMPLE	N_i	P_i	$ln\ P_i$	$-(P_i \cdot ln\ P_i)$
1.				
2.				
3.				
4.				
5.				
6.				
7.				
8.				
9.				
10.				
11.				
12.				
13.				
14.				
15.				
16.				
17.				
18.				
19.				
20.				
TOTAL			H =	

Species Accumulation Data for Methods A, B, and C

SAMPLE #	CUMULATIVE SPECIES NUMBER	SAMPLE #	CUMULATIVE SPECIES NUMBER
1.		11.	
2.		12.	
3.		13.	
4.		14.	
5.		15.	
6.		16.	
7.		17.	
8.		18.	
9.		19.	
10.		20.	

Species Accumulation Curve for Methods A, B, and C

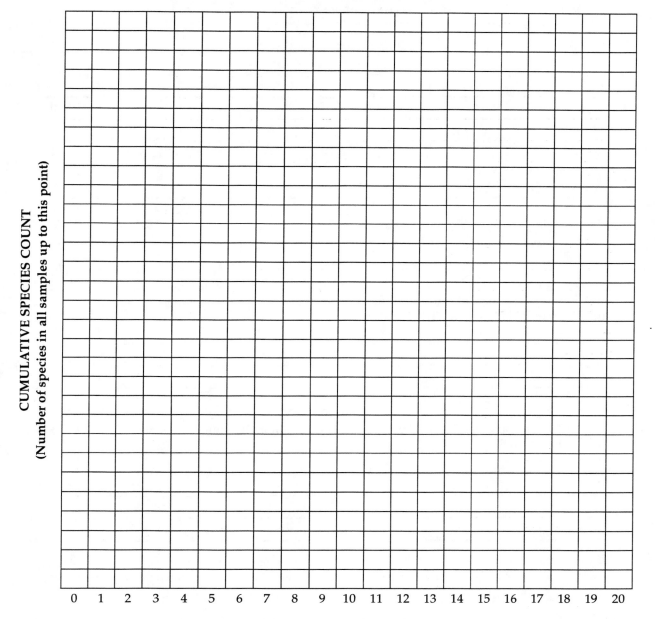

CUMULATIVE SPECIES COUNT
(Number of species in all samples up to this point)

SAMPLE NUMBER

Questions (Methods A, B, and C)

1. Describe the animal life you observed during your sampling process. Did you see species you had never seen before?

_____

_____

_____

_____

2. For any given sample, the highest possible value of H is equal to the natural logarithm of the number of species in the sample. For your sample, how does H compare with its theoretical upper limit? Explain what this means.

_____

_____

_____

_____

3. If the Shannon index were used to calculate a value of H for mammals in a multiuse national forest, would this be a good indicator of wildlife management practices? What management practices might increase H? Decrease H?

_____

_____

_____

_____

4. Which would you expect to yield the highest H value among the methods explained in this chapter: Method A or Method C? Why?

_____

_____

_____

_____

5. If you were able to draw a species accumulation curve, what conclusions can you draw about species richness at your site? Do you think your collection of samples includes more than half of all species present, or not? Explain.

_____

_____

_____

_____

FOR FURTHER INVESTIGATION

1. National Audubon Society members have been conducting bird surveys called "Christmas bird counts" for over 100 years. Data for your state and region can be accessed at http://cbc.audubon. org/cbccurrent/current_table.html. Use the census data from a survey conducted near your campus to develop a diversity index. You may also compare counts from a series of locations or a series of years to develop a species accumulation curve for birds in your state.
2. Longino and Colwell suggest the best mathematical description of their species accumulation curve is a logarithmic function of the following form:

Species Accumulation Curve:

$$S_T = \frac{ln(1 + Z A T)}{Z}$$

where:

S_T = cumulative numbers of species discovered up to and including sample T
T = numbers of samples taken
A is a constant (= 6.818 for ants at La Selva)
Z is a constant (= 0.013 for ants at La Selva)

    Using any of the methods in this chapter, generate a series of samples and produce a species accumulation curve. If you use A and Z values similar to those found empirically by Longino and Colwell, does the theoretical curve match your data? Can you find A and Z values more appropriate for your organism to fit your data to the theoretical curve?
3. Repeat one of these methods of species sampling in a natural area off campus, and compare results. How much difference can you document in the biodiversity of the two sites?
4. Devise a method for calculating a diversity index for plants. Compare animal diversity and plant diversity for a series of sites.

FOR FURTHER READING

Ellwood, Martin D. F. and William A. Foster. 2004. Doubling the estimate of invertebrate biomass in a rainforest canopy. *Nature* 429:549.

Longino, J. T. and R. K. Colwell. 1997. Biodiversity assessment using structured inventory: Capturing the ant fauna of a tropical rain forest. *Ecological Applications* 7, 1263–77.

Perkin, J. L. 1982. Shannon-Weaver or Shannon-Weiner? *Journal of Water and Pollution Contribution* 54: 1049–1050.

University of Arizona College of Agriculture and Life Sciences and The University of Arizona Library. 2005. *The Tree of Life Web Project.* http://tolweb.org/tree/phylogeny.html

University of California Berkeley Museum of Paleontology. 2005. http://www.ucmp.berkeley.edu/historyoflife/histoflife.html

Wilson, Edward O. 1999. *The Diversity of Life.* Norton, N.Y.

EXERCISE 23
ECOLOGICAL SUCCESSION

While organisms carry out their living processes, they live
in and interact with an environment. They obtain nutrients from
the environment and they also respond to different environmental
stimuli. All the preceding functions guarantee the survival of
the species in space and time. Living organisms as they interact
with their environment cause environmental changes.

The term "community" refers to a varied assemblage of
interacting species in a particular environment, such as a
forest or pond. Communities are not static, and the populations
of animals and plants vary widely from season to season and from
year to year. Many organisms have the ability to sense time in
an orientation related to circadian, annual rhythms or both.
Many organisms respond to seasonal changes in the relative
length of day and night. For example, deciduous trees lose their
leaves, some animals migrate and most animals hibernate or go to
sleep in anticipation of the winter. Changes also occur when a
tree or animal dies. The decaying organisms provide a substrate
on which bacteria and fungi live, succeed each other, and
eventually disappears becoming in the final stages a part of its
surrounding. Decomposition is characterized by early dominance
of decomposers and their consumers and because of this, some
ecologists termed it heterotrophic succession. This
microcommunity, however, cannot perpetuate itself through time.
After the stored energy is exhausted, heterotrophic succession
ends. The sequence of species that feed on decaying plants and
animals or animal waste demonstrates a detritus food chain.

Population cycles, biological rhythms, and decomposition,
illustrate the dynamic changes in community but do not, in
themselves, alter the overall characteristics of a community.
During the preceding phenomena, ecological succession or
community change does not occur. The community tends to return
to the same condition. The structure (e.g. species composition)
and function (e.g. material cycling and energy flow) of the
community remains relatively the same.

Ecological succession is the natural change which occurs in
the entire community. There is an orderly and sequential series
of changes in the community over a period of time. To a
considerable extent this flora and fauna change is predictable.
When succession is caused by factors outside the living part of
the ecosystem, it is termed an allogenic factor. When the
weather gets colder, for instance, deciduous trees (oak, maple,
hickory, etc.), are replaced by evergreens (spruce, fir, etc.).
When succession is caused by organisms within the ecosystem, it
is termed an autogenic factor. Some species of trees create
heavy shade under their canopies and thus make the area cooler

and more conducive to the growth of different plants like shade-tolerant species. In the following paragraphs, we will concern ourselves with discussion of succession that occurs on land.

Xerarch succession, by definition, is succession that begins on land surfaces (Fig. 23-1). Newly exposed rock or sand surfaces are first invaded by pioneer species. These species tend to live under uncrowded conditions and thus competition between members of the same species is rarely important. Lichens, bacteria, small plants such as mosses, annual grasses and herbs (annual plants that seed the first year and then die) are all examples of pioneer species. They grow from spores and seeds that have been swept in by wind and rain from nearby areas. These sun-adapted plants can grow in many exposed areas where sunlight is intense and the land is nutrient-poor. Pioneer species must be able to stand temperature extremes and severe drying.

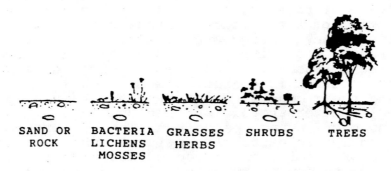

SAND OR   BACTERIA   GRASSES   SHRUBS   TREES
ROCK   LICHENS   HERBS
       MOSSES

Figure 23-1. Ecological succession is a natural change that occurs in the entire community. For example, if there are no disturbances made by outside factors (e.g. humans, climate), newly exposed sand or rock will be invaded by organisms in a predictable sequence. The changes which drive a bare piece of land to develop into a mature forest may require hundreds of years.

The pioneer species also tend to be "r-strategists." r-Strategists (r-Selection) are species with reproductive pattern typical of organisms that produce many small offspring which develop rapidly. Such species tend to increase in numbers at a rate close to the organism's intrinsic rate of increase (r).

During xerarch succession, the soil is formed by the weathering of rocks or sand surfaces together with activities of pioneer organisms that use the soil as a habitat. Thus, xerarch is caused by allogenic and autogenic factors. In this succession, organisms act on and interact with an environment which was previously uninhabited by flora or fauna. This interaction produces a change that will permit new and different species to survive in the same area. Some pioneer organisms such as lichens and bacteria, corrode rock and make the substrate suitable for plants like mosses. The mosses further trap dust and debris which permit grasses and herbs to survive. The pioneer organisms die and their remains are added to the soil. The soil layer becomes thicker and nutrients are available. Finally, the shrubs and trees invade the area and establish themselves as dominant species. Some species of trees create heavy shade under the canopies and thus make the area under the tree cooler and more conducive to the growth of shade-adapted plants like ferns. The shrubs and trees make up the climax community because they do not significantly change the environment any further. The conditions continue to be suitable for all members of the community. Such a climax community can maintain itself for a long time (Figure 23-1).

In contrast to pioneer species, climax species are "K-strategists." K-Strategists (K-Adaptation) are species with reproductive patterns typical of organisms that produce few large offspring which develop slowly. These species are usually large and long-lived, especially when they grow in stable climates. K-strategists are so-called because such organisms tend to maintain a population size close to their environment's carrying capacity (K).

The climax community is also characterized largely by the ability of its species to reproduce within the narrow range of environmental conditions. Many have highly specialized functional or habitat requirements. They live under carrying capacity conditions, and since they live under crowded conditions, competition between members of the same species is generally important. They also tend to utilize the resources of the environment to the maximum.

The term sere refers to the whole series of communities from the pioneer to intermediates to the climax communities. Each developmental stage in the sequence is called a seral stage. Therefore, the first seral stage is the pioneer stage and the final state of a sere is the climax stage. Xerarch succession tends to be gradual (it requires hundreds of years) because no soil was previously present and each step in the successional sequence depends on the changes in the environment brought about by the previous species.

At the beginning of the twentieth century, the American ecologist F.E. Clements (1916) formulated what he called the climatic theory. This principle states that in an unchanging physical environment, succession is a directional change. The ecosystem develops gradually from the pioneer stage to the final climax stage which is relatively stable.

As the change occurs, there are general internal changes in the ecosystem (illustrated in Fig. 23-2). There is a tendency for a greater biomass or total quantity of living organisms at any given time as the ecosystem gets older. (Trees weigh more than shrubs, shrubs weigh more than grass.) A greater variety of habitats for animals is created. This leads to more diversity of species at the preclimax stage, as well as a tendency for more interactions between species at the climax stage. Besides an increase in the number of terrestrial species, there is also an increase in the variety of soil organisms.

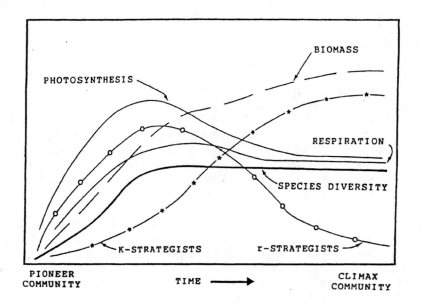

Figure 23-2. Expected pattern of biomass, species diversity, opportunistic species (r-strategists), equilibrial species (K-strategists), photosynthesis, and respiration in a hypothetical ecosystem.

Finally, as the climax stage is reached or approached, the photosynthesis/respiration ratio approaches one. This is due to the fact that in the pioneer state, the photosynthetic rate is greater than the respiratory rate. The pioneer stage contains fairly simple food webs comprised mostly of producers. However, as the community gets older, more animals colonize the region and the ecosystem's resources are mainly consumed by respiration. Matter and energy go primarily into maintaining the existing food webs. The more complex the ecosystem, the more efficiently it can use the available solar energy. The successional interactions in natural ecosystems have evolved over millions of years by natural selection to create an incidental "balance of nature."

As mentioned, ecological succession is a gradual sequential change in the composition of a community. The sequence in which one species after another succeeds to invade a habitat can be easily demonstrated in a milk culture containing several types of bacteria. The milk provides a substrate on which species of bacteria live, succeed each other, and eventually disappear, becoming in the final stages a part of the surrounding environment. On the front bench of the lab, there are a series of milk cultures which were established at different intervals so that you can witness in a laboratory period the microsuccession that would normally take weeks.

Materials needed: (Per Group)
    (1) On the front bench:
            fresh milk (labelled "O")
            one week old milk (labelled 1)
            two week old milk (labelled 2)
            three week old milk (labelled 3)
    (2) Xylene (Xylol) in a dropping bottle
    (3) 95% ethyl alcohol in a dropping bottle
    (4) Methylene blue stain
    (5) Four slides
    (6) Dissecting needle
    (7) Wax pencil and bibulous paper
    (8) Two compound microscopes
    (9) pH paper or pH meter

Procedures:
    (A) Secure four slides and using a wax pencil label them O, 1, 2, and 3, respectively. Transfer a drop of milk to the corresponding slide. Gently, with the dissecting needle, evenly spread the milk over the slides. Wait a few minutes and allow the milk to air dry.
    (B) Add two drops of xylene to each dried preparation. (<u>Caution</u>: xylene is caustic and toxic, handle it with care.) Gently, with the dissecting needle, evenly spread the xylene over the milk. Wait one minute and then pour off the xylene and again allow the four slides to dry. (Xylene is used as a fat solvent to remove lipid material from the milk which can interfere with the staining later on.)
    (C) Place four drops of alcohol on each slide. Wait about one minute, and then allow the alcohol to run off. Let the preparations air dry. (The alcohol removes the remaining xylol from the preparations. This facilitates staining later on.)
    (D) Cover the dried preparations with methylene blue stain. After stain has set for 5 minutes, gently wash off with soft stream of tap water. Blot dry (use bibulous paper).
    (E) Examine microscopically. After locating the bacteria under low power, rotate the high power objective into position and focus on the cells. You will need to use reduced

illumination and extreme care in focusing, in order to locate the bacteria. Bacteria appear to be tiny dots or spots. You should be able to determine the shapes of the individual bacteria. Identify as many of the bacteria as you can and record their number in Table 23-1. Graph data in Fig. 23-3.

(F) Is this microsuccession primary, secondary, or tertiary? Is this succession caused by allogenic or autogenic factors? Is this succession heterotrophic or autotrophic?

(G) During autotrophic succession, do biomass or species diversity increase? Does the photosynthesis/respiration ratio approach unity? As autotrophic succession ensues, do r or K-strategists increase?

(H) Clean up your lab area. Place the slides and coverslips in the "Glass Disposal Container." The microscope are placed in their numbered slots with the lowest objective in place.

Table 23-1. Bacteria in milk. Bacteria are different morphologically. Use Figure 7-2 (page 45) to help you identify the various shapes.

	AGE OF MILK			
TYPE OF BACTERIA	O	ONE	TWO	THREE
BACILLI				
COCCI				
SPIRAL				
DIPLOCOCCI				
STREPTOCOCCI				
STAPHYLOCOCCI				
pH				
OTHER				

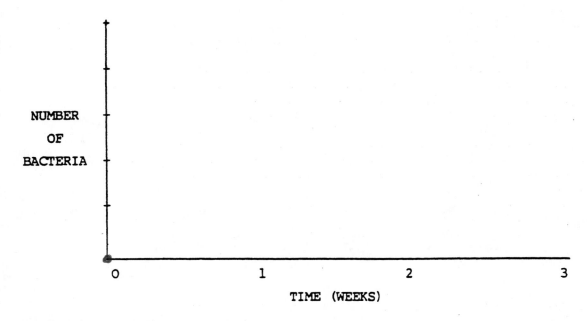

Figure 23-3. Plot of microsuccession in milk.

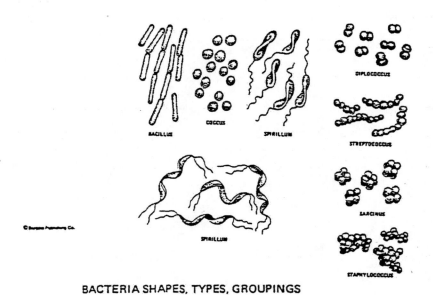

BACTERIA SHAPES, TYPES, GROUPINGS

Figure 23-4. Most bacteria can be divided into three major groups according to their particular shape.

Energy Flow

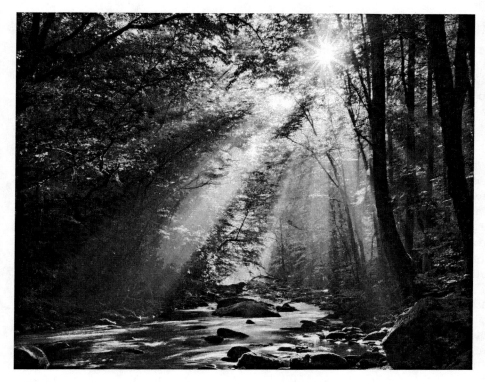

Figure 1   Sunshine powers life in the Great Smokey Mountains.

INTRODUCTION

Every day, a square meter of land at the equator receives about 3000 kilocalories of energy from the sun. A kilocalorie is the amount of energy needed to raise one kg of water 1° C. This means that a pool of water 3 meters deep could be warmed one degree per day of exposure to the tropical sun, provided none of the energy it received was reflected or radiated back into the atmosphere. Solar input declines with latitude, but even as far north as Anchorage, Alaska, solar energy input averages fully half as much as at the equator. What happens to all this energy? A third of it reflects off clouds or snow fields and bounces back into space. Another third warms the land and sea, and about a fourth is absorbed in the process of evaporation, driving the water cycle. A small fraction of the daily solar input is used by plants for photosynthesis; typically 1% to 2% of light striking a forest is captured as chemical energy in plant cells (Figure 1). Though little more than a footnote in the solar energy budget, photosynthesis is immensely important to life on earth. Kilocalories converted from sunlight to chemical bond energy by green plants provide the life force that flows through food chains to power the entire biotic community.

From *Ecology on Campus Laboratory Manual*, Robert W. Kingsolver. © Copyright 2006 by Pearson Education, Inc. Published by Benjamin Cummings, Inc. All rights reserved.

Although chemical constituents are cycled from one ecosystem component to another without being used up, energy flows through the ecosystem on a linear path, according to the laws of thermodynamics. The **first law of thermodynamics**, also known as the energy conservation rule, is that matter and energy are neither created nor destroyed. Although matter can be converted to energy in nuclear reactions, this does not happen in normal ecosystem processes. For the biologist, it is safe to assume energy flowing out of a system will ultimately balance energy flowing in. For example, our hypothetical three-meter pool in the tropics will absorb energy until it becomes as warm as the surrounding air. After that, the sum of energy radiating out of the water and energy used in evaporating the water will equal the radiant energy absorbed by the pool each day. Energy in ecosystems follows the same conservation rule. The chemical bond energy captured by photosynthesis is converted to heat when sugars and other biomolecules are metabolized by plants or the animals that eat them, ultimately warming the environment and radiating energy back into space. To put it simply, life on Earth depends on continuous solar radiation because living systems cannot make new energy, nor can they reuse what they expend.

The **second law of thermodynamics**, also called the **entropy** rule, recognizes that energy comes in many forms, which can be converted from one to another. A green plant transforms light energy to chemical energy. A thundercloud transforms mechanical energy to electrical energy. A muscle cell transforms chemical energy to mechanical energy. Energy conversion is a ubiquitous part of nature, but it is never 100% efficient. A portion of the transformed energy is always lost in the form of heat. Since heat is the least useful form of energy, the second law says that useful energy is always lost in energy conversions. As an example, think about the energy stored by plants in the Carboniferous period of our geologic past. Some of this energy has been lying under the ground, trapped in the chemical bonds of fossil fuels for millions of years. Then humans pumped the oil out of the ground and separated its chemical ingredients, saving the shorter, more volatile hydrocarbon chains to make gasoline. If you drive a gasoline-powered car, that fuel is burned in a series of small explosions within the cylinders of your engine. As chemical energy is converted to mechanical energy, the engine turns the wheels and you move down the road. If your engine and drive train were able to translate every kilocalorie of the energy in gasoline into forward motion, your car would be 100% efficient. The second law says this is impossible. Inevitably, much of the energy in auto fuel is converted to heat, which radiates from the engine, warms your tires as they rub against the road, and blows out your exhaust pipe with all the waste products of combustion. A typical gasoline engine is only 30% efficient, and if it is attached to a heavy vehicle that accelerates quickly, brakes often, and pushes tons of air out of its way at high speeds, the efficiency of the vehicle as a whole is significantly less. Thanks to the second law, as much as 4/5 of the energy you purchase at the gas station is used to heat up the atmosphere, and only 1/5 is used to get you to your destination.

Entropy can also be envisioned as a measure of disorganization, so another way to state the second law is that self-contained systems tend to lose organization over time. For example, if you leave a glass of water on a desk when the classroom is closed up for summer break, you would be walking away from an organized system, with water compartmentalized within the glass. Over time, water in the room will become less organized, with molecules evaporating from the glass and mixing randomly with the air in the room. You could return the system to its former organized state by pumping all the air through a chilled condenser and collecting the water back into the glass, but this would require the input of lots of energy from outside the system. In a similar way, ecosystems generate and maintain the organization of living biomass, but this is possible only because of constant energy input from the sun.

Check your progress:

An incandescent lightbulb gets very hot to the touch, but a fluorescent bulb gets only a little warmer than the surrounding air. Mindful of the second law, explain the source of this heat, and compare the efficiency of the two kinds of lighting.

Answer: A lightbulb transforms electrical energy to light energy. The second law states that some of this energy is inevitably lost in the form of heat. An incandescent bulb is less efficient than a fluorescent bulb, generating more heat and less light per watt of electricity it consumes.

The laws of thermodynamics inform our understanding of ecosystem structure and function. Figure 2 shows, in highly schematic form, the flow of energy through an idealized terrestrial food chain. After some light is reflected back into the sky, much of the solar energy entering a plant is used up in **transpiration**, which removes water from the leaves, pulling replacement fluids up through the stem. Plants use some of the remaining solar energy to synthesize high-energy organic compounds like sugar and ATP. For this reason, photosynthetic organisms are collectively called **primary producers**. The total amount of energy captured by photosynthesis across the whole ecosystem per unit time is called **gross primary productivity**. After plants have captured energy, they must then use a share of these photosynthetic products to support their own life processes. Respiration at night, and the energetic cost of maintaining non-green plant parts, must be entered on the debit side of the energy ledger. Whatever is left, called **net primary productivity**, accumulates as energy in plant biomass, which may become new tissue in a living plant, humus in the soil, or food for an animal. After animals have consumed their share of the total plant biomass, any remaining energy that accumulates in organic material is called **net ecosystem productivity**.

In aquatic systems, algae are important photosynthetic organisms, and productivity occurs in the epilimnion. A conventional way to measure productivity directly at representative depths in a lake is to divide a water sample into two bottles: one of clear glass and the other painted black. Dissolved oxygen is measured at the outset of the experiment, then the sample bottles are sealed and resuspended at the same depth on a line attached to a tethered float. After 24 hours, the bottles are pulled up to the surface and dissolved oxygen is measured again. In the dark bottle, the change in oxygen concentration represents oxygen used in respiration only, since there was no light to power photosynthesis. In the light bottle, the change in oxygen represents net productivity, since both respiration and photosynthesis have occurred in this sample. To calculate productivity, we use the simple equation

Gross Photosynthesis – Respiration = Net Photosynthesis

Since the dark bottle gives us a way to measure respiration, and the light bottle tells us net photosynthesis, we can rearrange the equation to get gross photosynthesis as follows:

Net Photosynthesis + Respiration = Gross Photosynthesis

For example, suppose initial readings were 5 mg/l oxygen, and after incubation we measured 3 mg/l in the dark bottle and 6 mg/l in the light bottle. We would know respiration used 5 – 3 = 2 mg/l. Net photosynthesis would be 6 – 5 = +1 mg/l as measured in the light bottle, and gross photosynthesis must have been 1 net + 2 respiration = 3 mg/l gross photosynthesis in the light bottle.

To convert oxygen generated in photosynthesis to energy, we use the chemical formula

$$6\,CO_2 + 12\,H_2O \rightarrow C_6H_{12}O_6 + 6\,O_2 + 6\,H_2O$$

For every 6 moles of O_2 generated in photosynthesis, 1 mole of sugar is added (at least temporarily) to the biomass of the ecosystem. This translates to 192 grams of oxygen for every 180 grams of sugar. Since the caloric content of sugar is 4.2 kcal/g, each gram of oxygen attributed to gross photosynthesis represents $(180/192)\,g \times 4.2\,kcal/g = 3.9\,kcal$ of energy captured by photosynthetic algae in the lake.

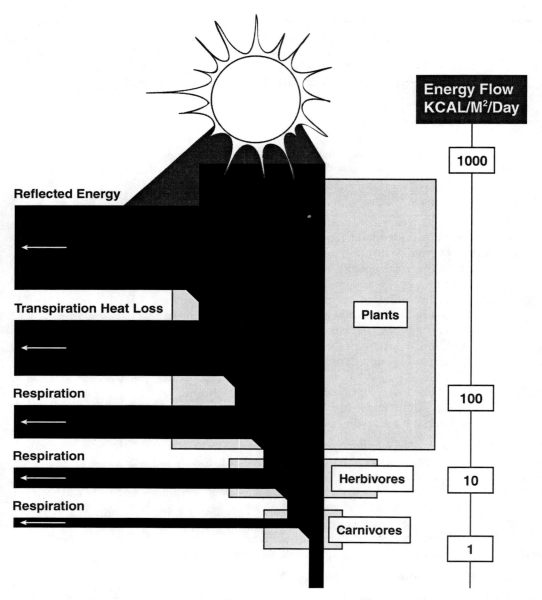

Figure 2   Energy flow in ecosystems conforms to the second law of thermodynamics. Thickness of black "pipe" represents energy in kcal/m2/day, flowing down from the sun through three steps in a food chain. Energy lost as heat is shown on the left. The logarithmic scale on the right demonstrates roughly 90% energy loss at each trophic level. Gray boxes represent standing biomass. (Concept based on the work of H.T. Odum, reprinted in Kemp *et al.*, 2004.)

Animals that eat plants are called **herbivores**. Since they represent the first link in the food chain after plants, herbivores are also called **primary consumers**. **Carnivores** are meat-eating animals. Since they consume other consumers, carnivores are also called **secondary consumers**. Larger carnivores eat smaller carnivores, so we can identify additional steps in the food chain as tertiary consumers, quaternary consumers, and so on. Each step in this sequence is called a **trophic level**. Note that available energy declines by about 90% as it passes through a trophic level. The extent of second-law energy loss varies, depending on the type of biological community, but the "ten percent rule" for energy conversion to the next trophic level is a convenient principle to guide our thinking about energy flow.

You can visualize the food chain as an energy pyramid, with total energy available to each trophic level roughly 10% as much as the level just below it (Figure 3). By the time we get to the top carnivores, there is not much energy left. This is why large predators at the top of the food chain must range over a large land area to harvest the food they need. To put it another way, the base of their food pyramid must be very large in order to support one pair of hawks or mountain lions on the top tier.

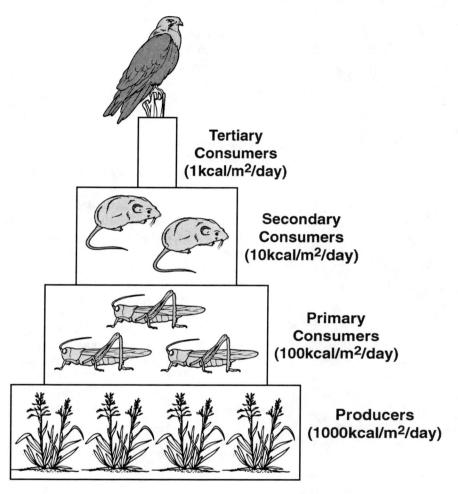

Tertiary Consumers (1kcal/m²/day)

Secondary Consumers (10kcal/m²/day)

Primary Consumers (100kcal/m²/day)

Producers (1000kcal/m²/day)

Figure 3 An energy pyramid demonstrates the second law of thermodynamics. Each trophic level receives about 1/10 as much energy as the level below it. (Numbers indicate orders of magnitude for energy flow. Boxes and numbers of organisms are not to scale.)

The energy pyramid explains why some kinds of toxic agents become more concentrated as they move through a food chain. This **biological concentration** of toxins was discovered by accident when a water-insoluble pesticide called DDT was widely sprayed on forests, farmlands, and marshes to control insect pests.

The problem, first publicized by Rachel Carson in her classic *Silent Spring*, arises from the fact that DDT is an artificially designed organic compound not metabolized by living cells. Since it is soluble in lipids rather than in water, DDT is not readily excreted by animals. Instead, it accumulates in the fat deposits of an organism's body. As a result, most of the DDT an animal has ever eaten remains in its tissues. If those contaminated animals provide food for a predator, the predator's every meal includes all the DDT accumulated over the prey's lifetime. It is as if all the other biomolecules in food were boiled away by digestion and respiration, leaving a concentrated residue of DDT behind. As a result, concentrations of DDT rise with each step in the trophic pyramid. DDT sprayed on a pasture would be concentrated by a factor of 10 in consumer biomass, by 10×10 in secondary consumers, by $10 \times 10 \times 10$ in tertiary consumers, etc. It is no wonder that top carnivores like the osprey (Figure 4) suffered ill effects of DDT poisoning in sufficient numbers early on to alert biologists to the problem of biological concentration.

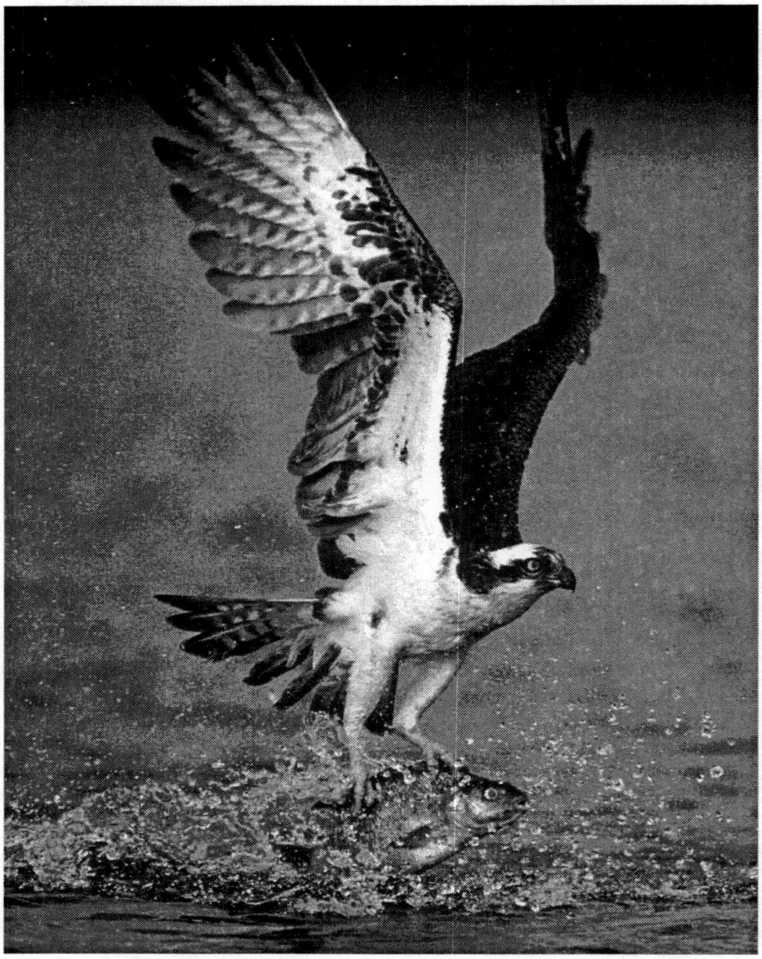

Figure 4   As top carnivores in coastal environments, ospreys were among the first organisms affected by DDT biologically magnified in the aquatic food chain.

Check your progress:

List an example of an organism that occupies each of these trophic levels:
Producers
Consumers
Secondary consumers
Tertiary consumers

Hint: Choose a plant or alga as a producer, an herbivore as a consumer, a small carnivore as a secondary consumer, and a top carnivore as a tertiary consumer.

Ecologist Howard Odum pioneered comprehensive efforts in the late 1950s to measure energy flow and material cycling at an ecosystem level. He chose Silver Springs in Florida as a model system because its spring-fed waters provide stable temperatures and a constant influx of mineral nutrients throughout the year. Accumulation of biomass at each trophic level was carefully monitored, and the energy content of organic materials was determined by burning dried plant or animal samples in controlled conditions to assess their energy content. Odum's results (Figure 5) set a standard for research in what is now called **systems ecology.**

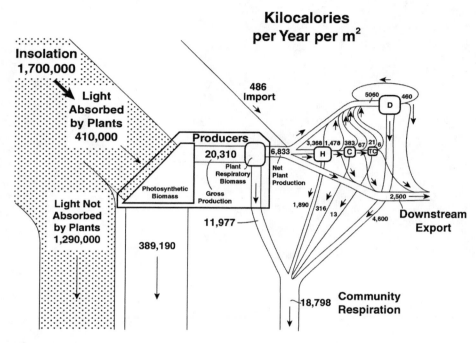

Figure 5   Howard Odum's energy flow diagram from the Silver Springs study. Trophic stages for consumers are represented as H = herbivores, C = carnivores, TC = top carnivores, and D = decomposers. As reprinted in Kemp and Boynton, 2004.

One useful concept that emerged from studies of this kind is **ecological efficiency,** or E_t. We define E_t as productivity at trophic level t (in biomass or energy per unit time) divided by the productivity of the next lower level. To express efficiency as an energy ratio, we use the following calculation:

$$E_t = P_t / P_{t-1}$$

E_t = ecological efficiency at trophic level t
P_t = net productivity at trophic level t
P_{t-1} = net productivity at trophic level t–1
Productivity can be measured either in kcal energy or in grams of biomass.

As an example, suppose a pine forest were infested with an outbreak of pine looper caterpillars (Figure 6). If we assume these caterpillars have about the same caloric content per gram of tissue as the pine needles they are eating, and if trees produced 200 g needles per square meter each season, while caterpillars feeding on those needles produced 14 g of insect biomass per square meter, the ecological efficiency for the herbivores would be 14/200 = 0.07, or 7%.

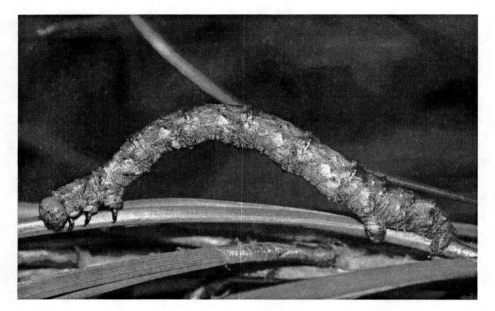

Figure 6   Northern pine looper caterpillars feed on pine needles.

Check your progress:

Ecological efficiency of carnivorous mammals is usually a little lower than ecological efficiency of reptilian carnivores at the same trophic level. How might this be explained?

Answer: Basal metabolic rate is higher in mammals. They burn more calories at rest, so they do not convert as many of their food calories to biomass.

Not all plant material is consumed by herbivores, and not all animals are consumed by carnivores. Some plant material dies before it is eaten. Some wild animals die of old age. Leaves cover the forest floor in the fall, and mature algae cells drift down to the bottom of a pond. Herbivore digestion is incomplete, so animal manure contains a lot of unused plant biomass. Most of this dead material is consumed by **detritivores** such as bacteria, fungi, and many kinds of invertebrates in the **decomposer** community. If you have observed a hay infusion or fruit flies in the laboratory, you are already familiar with organisms in this ecological category. In Howard Odum's Silver Springs study, detritivores included bacteria and scavengers such as crayfish. They are illustrated in his biomass pyramid as a slender column, taking some of its energy from each of the trophic levels in the food chain (Figure 7).

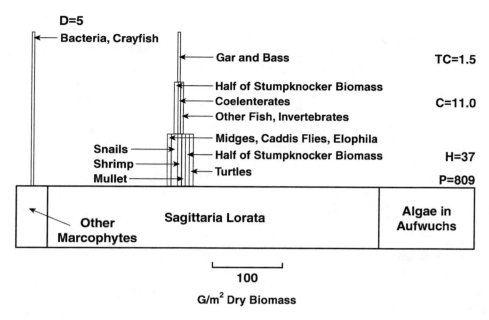

Figure 7 Odum's pyramid of biomass from his study of Silver Springs. Trophic stages are represented as P = producers, H = herbivores, C = carnivores, TC = top carnivores, and D = decomposers. (From Howard Odum, 1957, as re-drawn in Kemp and Boynton, 2004.)

The importance of detritivores in an ecosystem depends on the portion of plant material that goes uneaten by herbivores. In aquatic systems, short-lived algae are producers at the base of the food chain. A typical algae cell can double itself every day, but populations do not expand exponentially because most of the cells are consumed by **zooplankton** within hours of their formation. The **standing crop** of algae biomass that we could harvest at any point in time is small in comparison to the high primary productivity of the aquatic system. Trees, in contrast, may produce biomass more slowly than algae in a pond, but they protect a much larger proportion of their cells from immediate herbivory. Tree biomass accumulates in large plant bodies, so a mature forest has a huge standing crop of uneaten plant material. This means that detritivores have a lot more "leftovers" to consume in a forest than in a pond. In a forest, the bacteria, fungi, and invertebrate decomposers in fallen logs and leaf litter make up a much larger ecosystem component than you could find consuming the meager organic residue in a typical freshwater ecosystem.

To understand how a lower rate of production can result in a larger standing biomass, think of productivity as your salary and biomass as the size of your bank account. You probably know "algae people" who make a lot of money, but spend it just as fast, never saving anything. You probably also know "tree people" who put a little of every paycheck into savings so that their net worth accumulates over time. In the same way that a small paycheck can generate a large bank account, a forest gradually amasses a large standing crop by protecting its assets in the form of wood, roots, and leaves over decades of time. For this reason, it is necessary to distinguish between a pyramid of biomass, showing the amount of organic material present at each trophic level, and a pyramid of energy, showing how many kilocalories flow through each level on an annual basis. The second law dictates that the pyramid of energy must become significantly smaller at each step, but the pyramid of biomass can have a larger or smaller ratio of producers to consumers, depending on their relative life spans and energy storing potential. A good example of variation in biomass pyramids is supplied by Carlos Duarte and colleagues in a 2000 study of plankton in the Mediterranean (Figure 8). At low nutrient levels, the pyramid of biomass can be inverted because biomass of slow-growing algae never gets a chance to accumulate. By changing the concentration of dissolved nutrients, Duarte *et al.* altered the relative sizes of trophic levels in the biomass pyramid, even though energy always flows in the same pattern of decreasing energy availability through the food chain.

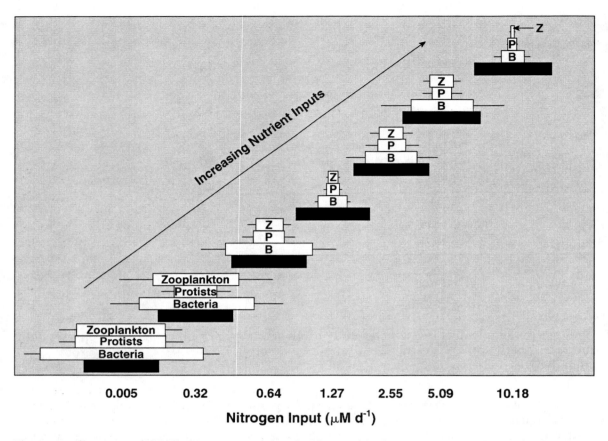

Figure 8 Duarte *et al.* (2000) demonstrated that the shape of the biomass pyramid in a planktonic community can be changed by adding inorganic nutrients to the water. Black bars represent producer biomass.

Check your progress:

Given the "ten percent rule," how can producer biomass be less than consumer biomass in an ecosystem?

Answer: Biomass is the result of energy flow over a period of time. If consumer biomass is larger, it is because consumers are living longer than producers in this community, and accumulating biomass over a longer period of time. Their "bank account" is larger, even though their "salary" is smaller.

METHOD A: PRODUCTIVITY OF PLANKTON

[Laboratory activity]

Research Question

What are the magnitudes of gross vs. net productivity in a plankton community?

Preparation

This laboratory method establishes a simple two-species plankton community. The single-celled alga *Chlorella* is chosen to represent freshwater phytoplankton, and *Daphnia pulex* to represent zooplankton. Stock cultures of both are readily available. Order enough *Daphnia* for each laboratory group to use 40 individuals. To culture *Chlorella* in the laboratory, remove labels and rinse plastic 2-liter soda bottles: you will need one bottle for every five laboratory groups. Fill the bottle 3/4 full with 1500 ml of commercial spring water or dechlorinated tap water, and add 5 g 20-20-20 soluble fertilizer to each bottle. Inoculate the bottle with *Chlorella*. As a control, fill another soda bottle 3/4 full of water, add 5 g fertilizer, and maintain it at the same temperature. Shake well, screw on caps, and incubate bottles lying on their sides at room temperature about 50 cm from a 4-tube fluorescent light bank or in a partially shaded part of a greenhouse for about a week. When the water in the *Chlorella* bottle looks green, it is ready to use. Make sure algae suspensions are shaken well before dispensing in smaller containers to students.

For oxygen measurements, obtain water testing kits reading oxygen in ppm, which can be translated to mg/l. Alternatively, you may wish to use a meter with dissolved oxygen probe for faster analyses. Incubation can be conducted in a greenhouse, in an environmental chamber, or under fluorescent lights. If you put algae cultures in a greenhouse, partially shade them with cheesecloth or other translucent material to avoid the photoinhibition algae experience in direct sunlight. If using an environmental chamber, simulate local summer temperature and day length. (A day/night regime of 16 hours of light and 8 hours of darkness, with a temperature of 25° C, is a reasonable simulation of summer in mid-U.S. latitudes.) A fluorescent light fixture about 50 cm from the cultures will provide adequate light for algae growth.

Materials (per laboratory team)

6 wide-mouth specimen bottles with screw caps, 50 ml volume

3 sheets (about 30 cm square) aluminum foil

Dissolved oxygen test kit or meter with dissolved oxygen probe

150 ml *Chlorella* culture

Daphnia culture, with at least 40 individuals

150 ml of control water without algae

3 beakers, 50 ml size

Thermometer

Compound microscope

Slides, cover slips

Large-bore dropper for transferring *Daphnia*

Markers for labeling culture bottles

2 Pasteur pipettes, with bulb

(Optional) photometer or light meter

Procedure

1. Slowly pour a sample of *Chlorella* culture, without mixing in additional air, into a small beaker and perform a test for dissolved oxygen. When performing an oxygen test, always use a thermometer to make sure the tested samples are at the same initial temperature. Record your results in the Data Table for Method A in the pre-incubation column for all four bottles containing *Chlorella*. Then do the same for a sample of control water, recording dissolved oxygen in the pre-incubation column for these two samples.

2. Label four of the 50-ml sample bottles "*Chlorella*—Light," "*Chlorella*—Dark," "*Chlorella* + *Daphnia*—Light" and "*Chlorella* + *Daphnia*—Dark." Fill all four bottles to the brim with *Chlorella* culture. To each of the two bottles labeled "*Daphnia*," add 20 individual *Daphnia* from your stock culture, using a large-bore pipette to avoid harming them. Label the remaining two sample bottles "Control—Light" and "Control—Dark," and fill these two bottles with algae-free control water. Screw all six caps on tightly.

3. Wrap the three bottles labeled "Dark" in aluminum foil. Make sure the foil covers all the glass so that no light can enter the dark bottles.

4. Place the six samples in an environmental chamber, a greenhouse, or under a fluorescent light bank at ambient temperature. If your tops seal well and light is from above, lay the bottles on their sides to allow more light to reach the algae. Record the temperature and note day length if using an environmental chamber. If you have a light meter or photometer, measure light intensity next to your samples, and record this value.

5. Place a drop of the remaining *Chlorella* culture on a glass slide, cover the drop with a cover slip, and observe under high magnification with a compound microscope. Draw a typical *Chlorella* cell on the data page. If you have not already done so in a previous laboratory, place a single *Daphnia* on a slide without a cover slip and draw it as well.

6. After incubation of at least one day, and not more than three days, measure dissolved oxygen again in each bottle. Note the number of days the cultures have been sealed in the sample bottles, and record your results in the data table. The dark bottles containing organisms should have less oxygen than they did in the initial measurement, because without light, these communities have been engaged in respiration but not photosynthesis. In the light bottles, both photosynthesis and respiration have occurred, so their oxygen levels should be higher.

7. Calculate net photosynthesis, community respiration, and gross photosynthesis for each pair of bottles as described in the introduction. If your samples were incubated for more than one day, divide these values by the number of days incubated to get daily rates. Record your results in the combined cells in the three right-hand columns in the data table.

8. Compare your own results with means of the entire class, and interpret your results by answering Questions for Method A.

Data Table for Method A

EXPERIMENTAL CONDITIONS	DISSOLVED O$_2$ BEFORE INCUBATION (mg O$_2$/l)	DISSOLVED O$_2$ AFTER INCUBATION (mg O$_2$/l)	NET PRIMARY PRODUCTION (mgO$_2$/l/day)	COMMUNITY RESPIRATION (mg O$_2$/l/day)	GROSS PRIMARY PRODUCTION (mgO$_2$/l)
Control Light					
Control Dark					
Chlorella Light					
Chlorella Dark					
Chlorella + *Daphnia* Light					
Chlorella + *Daphnia* Dark					

Incubation Conditions:

Light intensity:_____   **Day length:** _____

Temperature: _____   **Days incubated:** _____

Drawing of algae	Drawing of *Daphnia*

Questions for Method A

1. Define the difference between gross primary productivity and net primary productivity. Explain how you measured each of these values in the pair of bottles containing *Chlorella* culture alone.

    _____

    _____

    _____

    _____

    _____

2. Using figures from the Introduction, calculate the amount of energy algae are capturing in gross photosynthesis in your two sample cultures on a daily basis.

    _____

    _____

    _____

    _____

    _____

3. In the pair of bottles containing *Daphnia*, what was the effect of zooplankton on gross primary productivity? on respiration? on net productivity? Did these figures match your expectations?

    _____

    _____

    _____

    _____

    _____

4. Why was the plain water control necessary? Did either control show any difference in oxygen concentration during incubation? If so, how does this affect interpretations of your other measurements?

    _____

    _____

    _____

    _____

    _____

5. What would the shape of the trophic pyramid look like in your cultures containing both *Chlorella* and *Daphnia*? How would you measure ecological efficiency of *Daphnia*?

    _____

    _____

    _____

    _____

    _____

METHOD B: PYRAMID OF BIOMASS FOR PLANKTON

[Laboratory activity]

Research Question

What is the structure of the biomass pyramid in a sample of plankton?

Preparation

This laboratory exercise analyzes a previously collected sample of planktonic organisms. You will need to purchase only one hand-held plankton sampling net to collect plankton from freshwater or marine habitats for analysis by the class. A tow net with 5" to 8" diameter mouth and an attached collecting bottle works well. Select a plankton net with fine mesh, 20 micrometer size, to collect the smaller phytoplankton species. (WildCo Wildlife Supply and Forestry Suppliers carry fine-mesh plankton samplers.) Continue tossing the net until the sample looks turbid, then transfer to a glass sample bottle. A large fishing float attached to the line about 3" from the net is helpful in keeping the net off the bottom. Cast out from a dock or shore and retrieve the net by hand to get a plankton sample. Even in cool weather, you can usually collect algae and zooplankton (Figure 9). Although this procedure calls for only enough data to describe a single biomass pyramid, you may wish to take samples at different locations or at different times of year for a more detailed study.

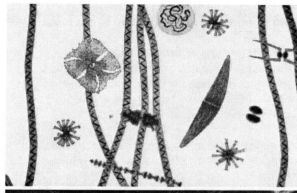
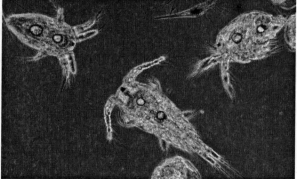

Figure 9   Plankton samples contain a variety of species.

To preserve plankton, make up a solution of Formalin-Acetic Acid (FAA) by mixing equal volumes of 37% formalin with glacial acetic acid. Add 1 ml (20 drops) of FAA to each 50 ml of phytoplankton sample that you collect. Store preserved samples in the dark for longer preservation. A preserved sample should be useable for this laboratory for several years. Thoroughly mix your samples and divide them into 10-ml vials if desired for convenient allocation to laboratory groups.

Materials (per laboratory team)

Compound microscope with ocular micrometer (mechanical stage preferable)

Preserved plankton sample (10 ml)

Pasteur pipette, or dropper, with bulb

Glass slide, cover slips

Calculator

Informational materials on phytoplankton and zooplankton

Procedure

1. Shake your sample vial to suspend preserved plankton. Transfer a drop to a glass slide using a pipette or dropper.
2. Place the slide on the mechanical stage of your microscope, and focus on the plankton. Move the slide to a point near the upper-left corner of the cover slip, and scan across the slide until you encounter an organism. Identify the organism, and place it in a trophic level classification. All algae are primary producers. Most protozoans are primary consumers. Larger micro-invertebrates such as *Daphnia* or copepods can be identified as secondary consumers. Tertiary consumers such as fish fry are rarely collected in plankton samples.
3. Find the appropriate section of the Data Table for Method B for this organism's trophic level, and enter its name or description on the first line of that section. Estimate the microorganism's length, width, and height using the ocular micrometer. Since measurements are comparative, you do not need to calibrate the micrometer unless directed to do so by your instructor. Just make sure to measure all organisms on the same scale. Height estimates will be approximate, but you should get a sense whether the organism is cylindrical or flattened, for example, by using the fine focus. Enter these measurements in the data table.
4. Continue on across the slide, classifying and measuring each new organism you encounter. Make sure you enter algae among the primary producers, protists among the primary consumers, and larger invertebrates among the secondary consumers. After measuring a type of organism once, you do not need to measure each additional one you find of similar size. Record an average size, and simply count additional individuals of the same type, making tally marks in the data table as you go.
5. When you finish scanning all the way across the cover slip, use the other knob on the mechanical stage to drop down one field of view, and scan back across the sample in the other direction. Continue until you have counted plankton species in the entire drop, which is 1/20 ml of the sample.
6. After you have counted and measured the organisms in your sample, add up the total number of each type you found. Then multiply the number of individuals × length × width × height to get total volume of this kind of organism in your sample. Record this total, expressed in cubic micrometer units, in the right-hand column of the data table.
7. Add total volume of producers, recording this total at the bottom of the first section in the data table. Repeat for total volume of primary consumers and total volume of secondary consumers. Since plankton are neutrally buoyant, volume is proportional to wet biomass in these organisms. Illustrate your results by drawing a pyramid of biomass on the Results for Method B graph.
8. Interpret your results by answering Questions for Method B.

Data for Method B:
Plankton Counts at Three Trophic Levels

PRIMARY PRODUCERS							
SPECIES NAME OR DESCRIPTION	L	W	HT.	MEAN VOL.	TALLY MARKS	TOTAL NUMBER COUNTED	TOTAL BIOMASS VOLUME

TOTAL VOLUME OF PRODUCERS:

PRIMARY CONSUMERS							
SPECIES NAME OR DESCRIPTION	L	W	HT.	MEAN VOL.	TALLY MARKS	TOTAL NUMBER COUNTED	TOTAL BIOMASS VOLUME

TOTAL VOLUME OF PRIMARY CONSUMERS:

SECONDARY CONSUMERS							
SPECIES NAME OR DESCRIPTION	L	W	HT.	MEAN VOL.	TALLY MARKS	TOTAL NUMBER COUNTED	TOTAL BIOMASS VOLUME

TOTAL VOLUME OF SECONDARY CONSUMERS:

Results for Method B:
Pyramid of Biomass for Plankton Sample

SECONDARY CONSUMERS	
PRIMARY CONSUMERS	
PRODUCERS	

←——— **UNITS OF VOLUME** ———→

Observations:

_____

_____

_____

_____

_____

_____

_____

_____

_____

_____

_____

_____

_____

_____

_____

Questions for Method B

1. How would you describe the relationships among trophic levels in this study? Is this what you expected to find? Explain.

_____

_____

_____

_____

_____

2. Reference to Figure 8 demonstrates that biomass pyramids in plankton communities can be inverted; that is, with producer biomass smaller than consumer biomass. How is this possible, given the second law of thermodynamics?

_____

_____

_____

_____

_____

3. Is diversity roughly equivalent among the three trophic levels, or are some levels more species-rich than others? Propose one or two hypotheses for this observation.

_____

_____

_____

_____

_____

4. Why are decomposers so poorly represented in the plankton community?

_____

_____

_____

_____

5. Assume a fish farmer is trying to raise fish strictly on the aquatic food chain, without supplementing their food supply. If the farmer has two equal-sized ponds, one stocked with carp feeding exclusively on algae and the other with bass feeding at the fifth tier of their aquatic food chain, how many kilograms of carp could be harvested each year for each kilogram of bass? (Use $E_t = 0.1$ for each trophic level.)

_____

_____

_____

_____

_____

METHOD C: ESTIMATING ECOLOGICAL EFFICIENCY OF LEAF MINERS

[Laboratory/campus, late summer or early fall]

Research Question

What is the ecological efficiency of leaf miners?

Preparation

Leaf miners are very common herbivores that consume the soft tissue inside leaves. Several insect groups, including flies and beetles, are represented by species in this niche. Oak, Holly, and Chrysanthemum plants are frequent hosts. Hatching from eggs oviposited on or within leaves, the larval leaf miner chews a tunnel that gets wider as the insect grows. The tunnel is easily visible through the transparent epidermis of the leaf (Figure 10).

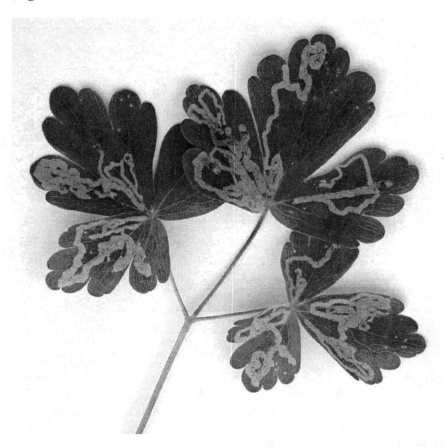

Figure 10   A leaf miner leaves evidence of its dietary history in a winding trail through the leaf.

Since these insects eat little or nothing as adults, their entire dietary history is apparent in the winding trail they leave behind them in the leaf. Leaf miners thus present an excellent opportunity to calculate ecological efficiency of an herbivore. Biomass produced by the herbivore can be estimated as volume of the mature larva or pupa. Plant biomass consumed is measured by the volume of the tunnel. The ratio of leaf miner biomass/plant biomass eaten is a measure of ecological efficiency of the herbivore, as explained in the Introduction. Since leaf miners live in an essentially two-dimensional world, the areas as seen from a top view of both the insect and the tunnel can be used to calculate the efficiency ratio.

If you can find affected plants on campus, students can collect their own leaves for analysis. Leaves with leaf miner larvae or pupae still inside are needed for the calculation. Leaves can be pressed, preserving both the leaf and the dried insect, and used for more than one class. An alternate approach is to have students search for pictures similar to Figure 10 on the Internet, and do their analysis based on enlarged prints of the photographs.

Materials (per laboratory team)

Dissecting microscope with ocular micrometer

Leaves with leaf miner larvae or pupae inside

Calculator

Ruler, marked in mm

Thread (30 cm length)

Procedure

1. Using a calibrated ocular micrometer, measure length and width of the leaf miner. Calculate the area of the top surface of the leaf miner by multiplying length × width. Enter your area estimate in the Data Table for Method C. (If using enlarged photographs, use a ruler to measure length and width of the larva image.)
2. Measure the length of the leaf miner's tunnel. For small specimens, use the highest power of your dissecting scope. Measure the width of your microscope's field of view by placing a ruler on the stage. Then trace the course of the miner's tunnel, noting "landmarks" at the edge of each visual field and moving the slide to advance one field at a time. Multiply the number of visual fields by the number of mm in a field, and you have the length of the tunnel. For larger specimens, (and for photos) you can do this by laying a thread over the course of the tunnel, and then stretching the thread out to measure with a ruler. Record tunnel length, in mm, in the data table.
3. Measure and record the width of the tunnel at the location of the mature larva. To calculate the area of the tunnel, as seen from the top, you can assume the tunnel is shaped like a long skinny triangle, with the current location of the insect at its base, and the place where the miner's egg hatched at its point. Since a triangle's area is one-half the base times the height, you can multiply the length of the tunnel by one-half the maximum width to get an approximate area.
4. Divide the area of the miner by the area of its eaten food to calculate an ecological efficiency ratio. Remember that both numerator and denominator of this fraction contain a depth measurement equal to the leaf thickness. Since the same depth measurement is in the numerator and the denominator, they cancel, so we will not have to measure the thickness of the leaf.
5. If possible, compare ecological efficiencies for more than one kind of miner or for more than one host species. Photocopy the data page as needed to extend your study to include more specimens.
6. Interpret your data by answering Questions for Method C.

Data Table for Method C

SAMPLE NO.	MINER WIDTH	MINER LENGTH	MINER AREA	TUNNEL MAX. WIDTH	TUNNEL LENGTH	TUNNEL AREA = ($\frac{1}{2}$ W) × L	ECOLOGICAL EFFICIENCY
1							
2							
3							
4							
5							
6							
7							
8							

Questions for Method C

1. Relate the concept of ecological efficiency, as measured in this exercise, with the trophic pyramid illustrated in Figure 3. What would the trophic pyramid look like for leaves and leaf miners?

_____

_____

_____

_____

_____

2. You calculated ecological efficiency in this exercise by comparing biomass of an insect to the biomass it consumed. What kind of measurements would you need to base your efficiency calculation on kcal of energy in the insect vs. kcal of energy in the leaf tissue it ate?

_____

_____

_____

_____

_____

3. How would you expect ecological efficiency of a leaf miner to compare with efficiency of an adult leaf-eating beetle flying from branch to branch and chewing on the same kinds of leaves? Explain.

_____

_____

_____

_____

_____

4. Explain how the second law of thermodynamics applies to ecological efficiency of leaf miners.

_____

_____

_____

_____

_____

5. Do you think a leaf miner qualifies as an herbivore or a parasite? On what basis would you make a distinction between these categories?

_____

_____

_____

_____

_____

FOR FURTHER INVESTIGATION

1. Use the light-bottle, dark-bottle technique of Method A to measure gross primary production and net community productivity for a field-collected sample of plankton. How do results compare with your artificial plankton community?
2. Collect plankton samples from different depths by spacing the net at different distances from a float attached to the line. Do you see differences in phytoplankton densities above and below a thermocline, as explained in Chapter 16?
3. Use the key words "secondary plant compounds" and "tannins" to find out how plants have evolved defenses against leaf-eating species. How might these chemical defenses affect ecological efficiency?

FOR FURTHER READING

Carson, Rachel. 1962. *Silent Spring*. Houghton Mifflin, N.Y.

Duarte, Carlos M., Susana Agustíl, Josep M. Gasol, Dolors Vaqué, and Evaristo Vazquez-Dominguez. 2000. Effect of nutrient supply on the biomass structure of planktonic communities: an experimental test on a Mediterranean coastal community. *Marine Ecology Progress Series* 206: 87–95.

Kemp, W. M. and W. R. Boynton. 2004. Productivity, trophic structure, and energy flow in the steady-state ecosystems of Silver Springs, Florida. *Ecological Modelling* 178:43–49.

Martin, Jennifer. 2001. *Marine Biodiversity Monitoring: Protocol for Monitoring Phytoplankton*. Department of Fisheries & Oceans Biological Station, St. Andrews, New Brunswick Canada. http://www.eman-rese.ca/eman/ecotools/protocols/marine/phytoplankton/intro.html

Micscape Magazine. 2000. Pond Life Identification Kit. http://www.microscopy-uk.org.uk/index.html?http://www.microscopy-uk.org.uk/pond/

Needham, J. G. and P. R. Needham. 1989. *A Guide to the Study of Freshwater Biology*. McGraw-Hill, New York.

Soils

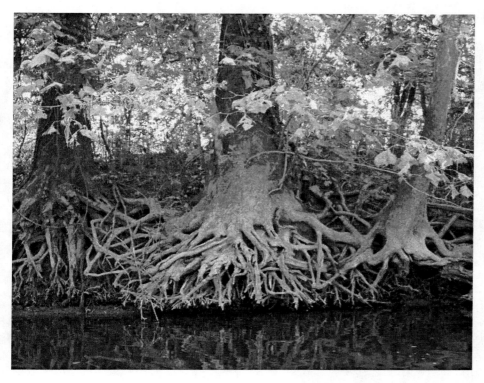

Figure 1   Tree roots fight a losing battle against soil erosion along the banks of the White River in Indiana.

INTRODUCTION

Soil is a natural resource easily ignored until it is gone. Water flowing across the surface of the ground after a heavy rain mobilizes soil particles and dissolved nutrients, especially where soils have been disturbed by agriculture, mining, or construction, and carries them into rivers and streams. Along stream banks, soil erosion constantly moves sediments out of terrestrial and into aquatic ecosystems. Trees growing along river banks retard soil loss, but extensive human engineering of waterways for improved agricultural drainage exacts a steep environmental cost. When flow rates are artificially increased by digging deeper and straighter stream channels, tree roots can no longer hold the embankments, and erosion takes another load of soil into the river every time it rains (Figure 1). The unfortunately common practice of stripping protective vegetation from the **riparian zone** along streams exacerbates this problem, as does harvesting too many trees from hillsides within the watershed. In alluvial bottomlands, moving water eats away at soils that were deposited by historically slower-moving river systems over a vast expanse of geologic time. Many hectares of productive farmland can be lost in a few short years of poor management. The silt and nutrients washed into streams have negative consequences for the aquatic system as well. Rivers are muddied, silt buries bottom-dwelling invertebrates and fish eggs, and overnourished algae bloom only to decompose, stealing life-sustaining oxygen from the water. Even after a river enters the ocean, marine organisms flee or die from freshwater effluent laden with eroded soils, agricultural chemicals, and untreated wastewater (Figure 2). At the mouth of the Mississippi River, a "dead zone" bigger than Lake Ontario develops every summer in the Gulf of Mexico, and it continues to expand as we flush more and more of our ultimate source of agricultural wealth into the sea.

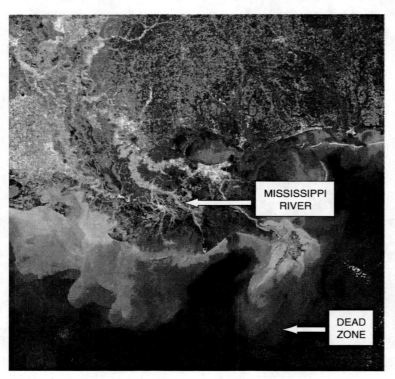

Figure 2   Sediments cloud ocean waters in a "dead zone" of hypoxia at the mouth of the Mississippi River.

In the Great Plains, plant communities dominated by native grasses built up and protected deep, rich prairie soils until much of the region was converted to row-crop agriculture in the 1800s. Replacing native perennials with annual crop plants such as wheat left the soil exposed to the weather much of the year. When crops failed during an extended drought in the 1930s, the bare soil dried to a powder and began to move on the wind. Dust storms choked people and animals, covered up what was left of the vegetation, and displaced rural populations throughout a "dust bowl" that extended from Texas to Minnesota (Figure 3). Impressed with the gravity of this disaster, the U.S. government developed an extensive system of advisory support, financial incentives, and agricultural restrictions to control soil erosion. Contour plowing, cover crops, and windbreaks became common conservation practices. As we came to understand the negative effects of erosion on aquatic systems, the federal government took steps to reduce sediment runoff into streams. Lumbering practices in national forests were altered to protect watersheds, and construction engineers were required to manage sediment runoff more effectively. Although conservation practices have improved, the total area of land impacted by farming, forestry, and development continues to expand. Soil erosion remains a global concern, especially in the developing world, where every shovelful of soil on every hectare of farmland is needed to support a growing human population.

Check your progress:

Describe five human activities that accelerate the rate of soil erosion.

Answer: Exposing soil to wind in dry regions, channelizing streams, disturbing riparian vegetation, harvesting too many trees from steep slopes, and disturbing soil during construction

As Conservationist Aldo Leopold pointed out over half a century ago, sound land management begins with an understanding of the role of soils in sustaining natural communities. Soils are the interface between the **biotic** and **abiotic** components of a terrestrial ecosystem. Here bedrock is weathered to release minerals taken up and incorporated into organic molecules by plants. Here dead leaves decompose, converting what was biotic back to abiotic material. Here bacteria fix nitrogen from the atmosphere, sheltered within the roots of their host legumes. Here water is sequestered between particles of silt and clay, minerals are leached from humus, and soil organisms stir and transform the ingredients of life.

These chemical and biological interactions produce a characteristic **soil profile**. Road cuts or embankments are good places to see how the soil is structured in your area (Figure 4). You can also use a soil sampler to extract a core of soil for analysis in an area of interest (Figure 5). Because different processes occur at different depths, soil develops in layers, called **soil horizons** (Figure 6). Lying on top of the soil is a layer of litter (dead leaves and other plant material) and "duff" (plant material degraded by soil organisms). Since this layer is composed primarily of organic material, it is called the O horizon. Below this is a layer of topsoil, called the A horizon. Mineral soil is enriched with decomposing organic material in this layer. Humic acids, resulting from the breakdown of plant material, give the A horizon a dark color. Plant roots grow through this layer, and earthworms burrow through it, consuming leaf mold and speeding up the process of decomposition by bacteria and fungi.

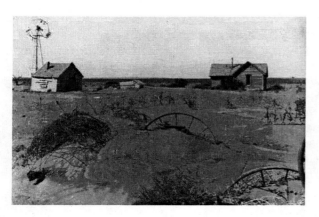

Figure 3 Unusually dry summers and poor soil conservation practices led to devastating wind erosion during the dust bowl years of the 1930s.

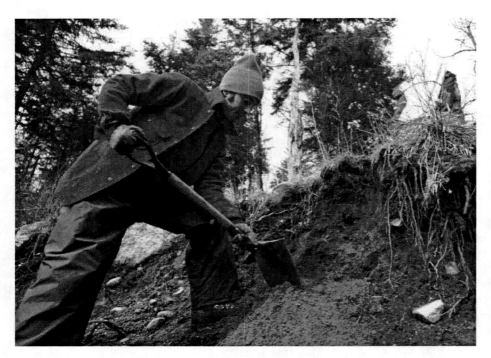

Figure 4 A scientist examines a soil profile in Ontario.

Beneath the topsoil is a layer of subsoil called the B horizon. This layer has little organic matter, and tends to resemble the underlying rock in its chemical makeup. Fine particles in this layer bind positively charged ions washed down from above, including calcium [Ca^{++}], ammonium [NH_4^+], and potassium [K^+]. Iron and aluminum ions leached out of the upper layers are also recaptured here, their oxidized forms creating horizontal bands of red or yellow within the B horizon. The zone of maximal leaching at the bottom of the A horizon is sometimes given a separate classification, the E horizon. The E stands for **eluviation**, which refers to materials dissolving in water and moving down through the soil. **Illuviation**, the opposite process, refers to deposition of dissolved substances as they are recaptured in the subsoil.

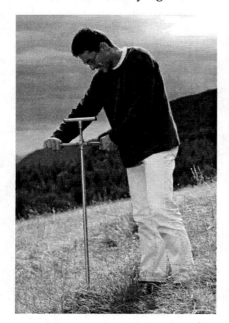

Figure 5 A sampler is pushed into the ground to extract a soil core for analysis.

Under the subsoil lies the C horizon, where bedrock weathers and breaks up into small particles over time. This rocky layer is called "parent material" because it gives rise to the mineral components of the soil. In glaciated regions or coastal plains, parent material may be made up of loose geologic deposits rather than bedrock. The type of rock under the soil makes a large difference in its resultant characteristics. Limestone-based soils are rich in calcium and other minerals, and the calcium carbonate in limestone buffers pH, making these soils neutral or slightly alkaline. Sandstone-based soils lack buffering capacity, so they tend to be more acidic. Granite, a common form of igneous rock, also lacks buffering capacity, but tends to weather very slowly, so soils on granite tend to be shallow, with a limited B horizon.

Check your progress:

Name four major soil horizons and briefly describe processes occurring in each.

Answer: O Horizon: litter accumulation
A horizon: decomposition of organic matter and leaching of nutrients
B Horizon: recapture of dissolved ions as they pass through mineral soil
C horizon: weathering of parent material

Soil Profile

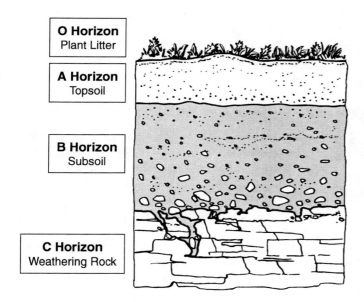

O Horizon
Plant Litter

A Horizon
Topsoil

B Horizon
Subsoil

C Horizon
Weathering Rock

Figure 6 A soil profile is made up of distinctive layers, or horizons. Decomposing plant material (O Horizon) adds humus to a layer of topsoil rich in nutrients (A Horizon). Below this is a layer of subsoil (B Horizon), whose clay particles recapture ions leaching out of the topsoil. Weathering parent rock (C Horizon) adds minerals and particles to soil as it gradually breaks down.

Soil particles come in many sizes, which are classified for convenience as clay, silt, or sand. Clay particles are the smallest, defined as smaller than 0.002 mm. Silt particles are of intermediate size, between 0.002 and 0.05 mm. Sand particles are largest, from 0.05 to 2 mm. Anything larger than 2 mm in diameter is classified as gravel. Soil containing a mixture of sand, silt, and clay particles is called loam. The size of the soil's particles determines its capacity to hold water, which is ecologically very important. Three critical measures of water in the soil are saturation capacity, field capacity, and wilting point. **Saturation capacity** refers to the amount of water a soil contains when all the spaces between soil particles are filled with water. Sand has the highest saturation capacity, because its relatively large particles cannot be packed as tightly together as other soil types, so there is more room for water in between the grains of sand. Silt has an intermediate saturation capacity, and clay has very little, since its tiny particles fit closely together, without much space left for water.

Field capacity measures the amount of water remaining in the soil after the force of gravity has pulled all it can down through the soil column. Because water adheres to soil and to itself, drained soil still contains water clinging to soil particles against the pull of gravity. Field capacity is a more ecologically important measure of soil water than saturation capacity, because soils do not remain saturated unless they lie below the water table. After water drains down through the soil after a rain, field capacity measures how much water is actually left to support plant life. To measure field capacity, wet soil is allowed to drain, and then weighed. The sample is then dried in an oven and weighed again. The difference between the wet weight and dry weight represents the grams of water that were in the drained soil. This water weight is divided by the dry weight and multiplied by 100% to calculate field capacity. A good way to think of field capacity is to consider how much water, in comparison to its own dry weight, can soil take up and hold against the pull of gravity? Particle size significantly affects field capacity of the soil (Figure 7). The smaller the particles in soil, the greater their surface to volume ratio. A gram of clay therefore has much more surface area among its tiny particles than a gram of sand has among its fewer, larger particles. Clay has the highest field capacity, losing very little water to drainage after saturation. Silt has an intermediate field capacity and sand has a low field capacity. This means that clay soils dry out very slowly after rains, but sandy soils dry out much sooner.

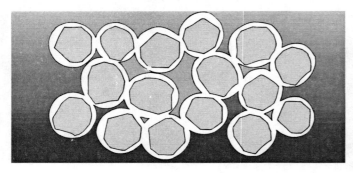

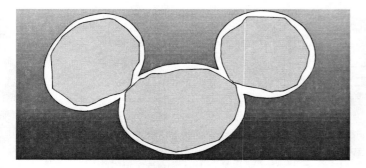

Not all water held in the soil against the pull of gravity is available to plants. Although the higher solute concentration within root tissues creates osmotic potential, which draws water from the surrounding soil, there is a limit to this water movement. The force needed to move water against its tendency to remain in place is measured in pressure units, and is called **water potential**. At a water potential equivalent to −15 atmospheres of suction, water is attracted equally to soil and roots, so no more water movement occurs. At this point, we say the water content of the soil has dropped to a **wilting point**, because plants start to droop when they can no longer extract soil water. Sand and silt contain almost no water at the wilting point, but tiny clay particles hold much of their water too tightly to be taken up by plant roots.

Figure 7 Small soil particles (top) have higher field capacity than large soil particles (bottom) because the smaller particles have more surface area per unit volume of soil. Water clinging to particles is illustrated in white.

The amount of water actually available to plants is the difference between the field capacity and the wilting point. This difference is not great in sandy soils because they have a low field capacity. It is also not ideal in clay soils, because they have a high wilting point. Silty soils make the most water available to plants because they have both a relatively high field capacity and a relatively low wilting point (Figure 8).

Check your progress:

Why do silty soils make more water available to plants than either sandy or clay soils?

Answer: Sand does not hold as much water against the pull of gravity, and clay holds water so tightly that roots cannot extract all the water held among its particles.

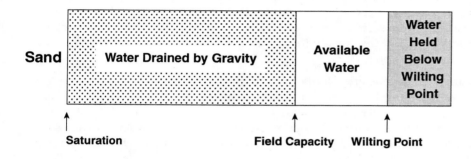

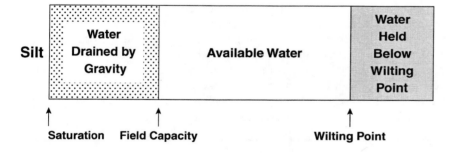

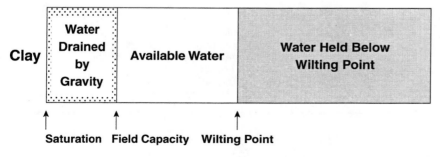

Figure 8 Comparison of available water among three soil types. Silty soils make more water available to plants because of their high field capacity and low wilting point.

Nutrient cycling, a property of all sustainable ecosystems, occurs primarily in the soil. Nitrogen serves as a good case study. It is an especially important nutrient because of its presence in the amino acid residues of proteins, and often is the limiting factor for plant growth. Since the atmosphere is 78% nitrogen gas, this element is available everywhere on the planet. However, the gaseous form of nitrogen (N_2) is very stable. Its two nitrogen atoms are not easily split apart, which must be done as a first step in synthesizing nitrogenous organic compounds. This critical step in the nitrogen cycle, called **nitrogen fixation**, occurs occasionally when nitrogen is oxidized by lightning strikes, but more often through metabolic activity of a few specially adapted microorganisms. Blue-green bacteria like *Anabaena* can capture nitrogen in a wet environment, and *Rhizobium* bacteria do so in root nodules of their host legumes. Since fixation uses a low-energy substrate (N_2) to make a high-energy product (NH_4^+), this chemical transformation uses a lot of energy. According to V. P. Gutschick (1981), it takes approximately 10 grams of sugar to fuel fixation of one gram of nitrogen. To put this in perspective in English units of measure, bacteria would need to consume more than two tons of sugar to convert all 420 pounds of nitrogen gas contained in the air within a 30 × 30 foot classroom into organic nitrogen. It is not surprising, therefore, that nitrogen fixation is frequently dependent on the chemical energy captured by photosynthesis, either inside the cell as we see in *Anabaena*, or through the cooperation of a host plant, as we see in *Rhizobium*.

Once nitrogen is fixed as ammonium, the soil bacteria *Nitrosomonas* and *Nitrobacter* can extract energy for their metabolic needs by oxidizing ammonium ions. Ions of NH_4^+ are converted first to nitrite (NO_2^-), and then to nitrate (NO_3^-). Oxidized nitrogen can be taken up by plants and converted to amino acids with some photosynthetic energy expended for the additional biomolecular construction costs. Amino acids are used by plants and by animals farther up the food chain to build proteins. Organic nitrogen excreted by animals and released by decay of organic matter is converted back to ammonium in a series of energy-releasing reactions called **ammonification**. Enzymes within most cells are capable of this step, so it tends to happen as a consequence of protein digestion. Cycling of nitrogen from ammonium through oxidized nitrogen to organic nitrogen and back to ammonium occurs readily within organisms and in the soil because the energy involved in these steps is comparatively modest. However, there are bacteria that disrupt this cycle by converting nitrates in soil all the way back to nitrogen gas. These organisms, called denitrifying bacteria, are **facultative anaerobes**. In the absence of oxygen, they capture chemical energy by reducing oxidized forms of nitrogen, which escapes from the soil as N_2 gas. Denitrifying bacteria gain back a great deal of the energy that was expended to fix nitrogen in the first place, but the community loses soil nitrogen as a result. Since denitrification occurs in poorly aerated soils, such as marshlands and flooded plains, waterlogged soils tend to be low in available nitrogen. It is no wonder that carnivorous plants such as pitcher plant and Venus' fly trap, which catch insects as a supplementary source of nitrogen, find their niche in boggy habitats.

Check your progress:

Diagram steps in the nitrogen cycle, naming organisms facilitating major steps.

Hint: You should show nitrogen gas converted first to ammonium, then to nitrite, then to nitrate and finally to organic nitrogen. Ammonification and denitrification should be included to complete the nitrogen cycle.

Humans alter the nitrogen cycle by artificially fixing nitrogen and applying tons of soluble nitrogen in the form of ammonium, nitrites, or nitrates to agricultural fields. Because these nitrogen fertilizers are highly soluble, they tend to flow with rainwater down to the water table and across the ground to nearby streams. Since nitrates and nitrites are toxic to humans, and since excess nitrogen overstimulates algae, leading to oxygen depletion as discussed above, managing nitrogen in agro-ecosystems is of paramount importance. It is significant that when the Ecological Society of America planned a series of reports designed to educate the public about important ecological issues, they chose human intervention in the nitrogen cycle as their very first topic (Vitousek *et al.*, 1997).

Ecosystems less impacted by human intervention tend not to overnourish stream water, because decomposition of leaf litter and other organic debris releases nitrogen and other essential nutrients gradually, to be taken up by plants and used over and over again. Fungi and bacteria are the primary decomposers in soils, but their relative importance depends a great deal on the temperature. Which do you think thrives best in cold soils? Think about organic decay inside your refrigerator. A refrigerator set at 50° F will stop almost all bacterial growth, but fungi can grow, albeit slowly, on the neglected carton of cottage cheese left too long on the bottom shelf. Similarly, northern or high-altitude soils are generally too cool to support much bacterial growth, so fungi are the primary decomposers in these ecosystems. Fungi release acid to digest their food, which also retards bacterial growth. Because soils are actually frozen much of the year, decomposition may not keep up with the rate of litter accumulation. Humic acids from these slowly decomposing materials tend to add more acidity. Temperate soils therefore tend to be acidic, and relatively rich in organic matter.

Tropical soils, by contrast, support both fungi and bacteria that quickly break down organic material. Faster plant growth in warmer climates takes up nutrients almost as quickly as they become available. Although the lush vegetation of the rainforest would seem to indicate rich supporting soils, most of the nutrients in warm-climate ecosystems are retained in the biotic parts of the system. A rainforest tree crashing down in a storm decomposes with remarkable speed, contributing the nutrients in its massive body to surrounding trees within just a few weeks of its demise. In rainforest regions, heavy rains can quickly flush free nutrients from the soil. As a result, clearing away tropical forest to create new farm land quite often exposes soils holding few remaining nutrients. One solution to this problem is to cultivate perennial plants in the tropics rather than annuals, for better nutrient retention and soil protection. The plowed fields that yield so much food in temperate climates may not represent ecologically sound agriculture in large regions of the tropics.

Check your progress:

Compare the chemical and biological properties of tropical and temperate soils.

Answer: Organic matter is rapidly decomposed in tropical soils. As a result, these soils tend to retain fewer nutrients than northern soils.

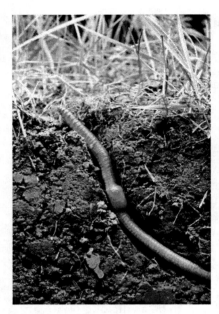

Figure 9 The nightcrawler *Lumbricus terrestris*, lives in permanent vertical burrows, which significantly enhance air and water movement through the soil.

As important as soils are in determining patterns of life on our planet, the reverse is also true. The biological community living in a place exerts lasting effects on the soil. Soil pH in a maple forest, where fallen leaves decompose very quickly, will be measurably higher than the pH of soil in a pine forest in the same climate and on the same parent material. Animals, such as earthworms and burrowing ants (Figure 9), play key roles in aeration, mixing, and pulling organic materials down into the soil. As soil scientists learn more about soil function, we realize that the total soil ecosystem should be considered in management decisions. Pesticides that kill insects above ground also kill soil organisms, with consequences that should not be ignored. Nowhere is it more clear that all the parts of an ecosystem are tied together than in this hidden, but vitally important, ecological realm.

METHOD A: PHYSICAL PROPERTIES OF SOILS

[Laboratory activity]

Research Question

How does particle size affect field capacity of soil?

Preparation

This exercise requires comparison of a soil sample from your campus with samples of clay and of sand (method adapted from Bouyoucos, 1951.) *If using a soil sampler on campus (Figure 5) check with your facilities manager to make sure you are clear of buried pipe, drainage lines, electrical conduit, and data cable.* Push a soil sampler into the ground to a depth of several inches, twist a half-turn, and pull out the soil core. Each laboratory group will need at least 100 g of soil for the two procedures, so repeat core sampling as needed. Alternatively, construction sites on campuses often expose soil banks. If this is the case, a hand spade can be used to collect a sample.

As controls, the soil sample is compared against samples of clay and sand. Moist clay can be ordered from ceramic supply sources. *If using powdered clay or dry sand, avoid inhaling dust, as silicates in sand and clay can cause respiratory problems.* Wetting the material and then air-drying prior to student use is good practice. Also, silica-free sand is available through building supply companies, sold for the purpose of filling sandboxes in playgrounds.

A 0.1 normal solution of sodium hydroxide will be needed to prepare soil samples for the separation of particles. Add 4 g NaOH pellets to 1 liter of water for a laboratory class to share. Although this is not a very strong solution, exercise caution and rinse with water if skin contacts the solution.

A Bouyoucos hydrometer that reads *grams of soil per liter* is essential for this experiment. Bouyoucos hydrometers, also called soil hydrometers, are available from *Hogentogler & Co., Canadawide Scientific,* and from *Analytica.* These glass instruments measure the amount of suspended sediment by floating higher in more dense solutions and lower in less dense solutions. Since heavier particles settle out of a soil suspension first, carefully timed hydrometer readings indicate how much sediment remains after sand and then after silt has fallen out of the suspension. Since water changes density as it warms or cools, hydrometers are calibrated to be used at a particular temperature, generally 21° C. Fill a liter flask for each lab group with tap water ahead of time, and allow the water to equilibrate to room temperature.

For the second procedure, students will need access to a laboratory sink to drain flowerpots and a drying oven or warm, well-ventilated location to dry samples. A drying oven set at 105° C will dry samples overnight, but air drying for a week between laboratory sessions yields fairly good results.

Materials (per laboratory team)

For Procedure 1

Large mortar and pestle

0.1 normal NaOH solution

1-liter flask with water at room temperature

Thermometer, to check water temperature

Soil sample (50 g)

Small bucket or plastic bin

Wash bottle, filled with tap water

Spatula or plastic spoon

Long stirring rod

Thermometer, to check water temperature

1-liter graduated cylinder

Magnetic stirring platform

Stirring bar, shorter than diameter of graduated cylinder

Bouyoucos hydrometer

Access to balance, accurate to 0.1 g

Clock or lab timer

For Procedure 2

Three 3" plastic flower pots with drainage holes in the bottom

3 aluminum weighing trays, or 3 squares (6" each) of aluminum foil

Paper toweling

Samples of campus soil, clay, and sand (50 g each)

Access to balance, accurate to 0.1 gram

Access to drying oven

Procedure 1: Estimating sand, silt, and clay components of campus soil

1. Weigh out 50 grams of air-dried soil. Place sample in mortar cup, add enough NaOH solution to cover the soil, and grind with pestle for 5 minutes to separate all soil particles.
2. Your hydrometer is calibrated for use in water of a particular temperature. (Commonly, this is 21° C.) Make sure the water in your liter flask is of the correct temperature. If not, add warm or cool water to adjust it, and stir well before beginning your test.
3. Place a stirring bar in the bottom of the graduated cylinder, add 500 ml water, and turn on the stirrer. The speed should be adequate to create a vortex in the water, but not so high that the stirring bar skips around in the cylinder.
4. With the magnetic stirrer running, use the spatula to scoop soil into the cylinder. Then use the wash bottle to rinse soil off the spatula into the cylinder. Finally, rinse the mortar cup into the cylinder. Make sure the stirring bar keeps spinning as you add soil. If it stops, use a long stirring rod to keep the sediments afloat.
5. Fill the graduated cylinder up to the 1 liter mark with water. Stir thoroughly. When the soil "milkshake" is completely blended, place the hydrometer carefully into the suspension (Figure 10). When it stops bobbing up and down, turn off the magnetic stirrer and mark the time. Note how the hydrometer begins to sink as sand settles out and the density of the suspension decreases. After 2 minutes and 40 seconds, read the level of the suspension on the neck of the hydrometer. Mark this on the Data Sheet for Method A-1 as the "silt plus clay" reading.

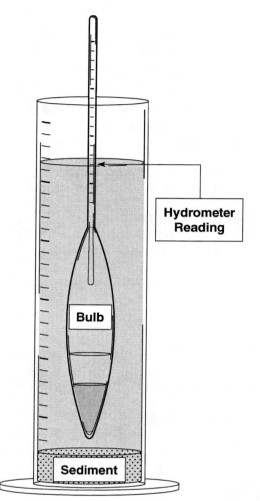

Hydrometer Reading

Bulb

Sediment

6. You now have two hours to wait for your next reading. This would be an ideal time to begin the tests of field capacity (Procedure 2).

7. After two hours, take another hydrometer reading. At this point, the silt will have settled out, so this reading tells you how much clay remains suspended in the water. (Longer settling time is required in some hydrometer methods, but two hours gives a good estimate.) Record your "Clay" reading in the data table.

8. Observe the pattern of sediments in the bottom of the graduated cylinder. Can you see layers of sediment, with larger particles at the bottom and smaller ones at the top? Record your observations at the bottom of the results page.

9. Calculate portions of sand, silt, and clay as directed on the Calculation Page for Method A-1.

10. Interpret your results by answering Questions for Method A.

Figure 10 Soil hydrometer method. As sediments fall out of suspension, the density of the mixture in the graduated cylinder becomes less dense, so the hydrometer floats lower in the water. Read the scale on the hydrometer stem where it breaks the surface of the suspension. Units are in grams of soil per liter.

Procedure 2: Measuring field capacity of soil samples

1. Line three flowerpots with a layer of paper toweling in the bottom. Place about 50 grams of sand or sandy soil in one pot, 50 grams of clay soil in a second, and 50 grams of your campus soil sample in a third.
2. Saturate the three samples completely with water. Set them in a sink or in a bucket to allow the pots to drain for 15 minutes. When the pots stop dripping, the soil is at field capacity.
3. If you do not have aluminum weighing trays, make a tray of aluminum foil by folding a 12×12 sheet in quarters, then folding up the edges to hold soil. Label each weighing tray, one for sand, one for clay, and one for your soil sample. Weigh each aluminum tray and record these weights in the Data Table for Method A-2.
4. Using a spoon or spatula, scoop as much of the drained soil as possible into the appropriate weighing tray. Weigh the tray with wet soil, subtract the weight of the tray, and record "wet weight" for this sample in the data table. Repeat for the other samples.
5. Place aluminum weighing trays with soil in a drying oven overnight, set at 105° C and with a ventilation fan running. Alternatively, let your samples air-dry for a week.
6. Weigh the tray with dried soil, subtract the weight of the tray, and record "dry weight" for this sample in the data table. Repeat for the other samples.
7. Complete the Calculations for Method A-2, and compare the field capacities of your three samples.
8. Interpret your results by answering Questions for Method A.

Data Table for Method A-1:
Hydrometer Readings

TIME ELAPSED SINCE SOIL BEGAN SETTLING	BOUYOUCOS HYDROMETER READING (grams/liter)	MATERIAL REMAINING IN SUSPENSION
0 minutes	50	sand + silt + clay
2 minutes, 40 seconds		silt + clay
2 hours		clay

Calculations for Method A-1:
Percent Sand, Silt, and Clay

PARTICLE TYPE	GRAMS OF PARTICLES IN 50-GRAM SAMPLE	PERCENT COMPOSITION = grams/50 g × 100%
SAND	(sand + silt + clay) − (silt + clay) =	%
SILT	(silt + clay) − (clay) =	%
CLAY	(clay) =	%

Description of Sediment Layers in Cylinder

_____

_____

_____

_____

_____

_____

Data Table for Method A-2:
Results for Three Soil Samples

DATA FOR SAND	WT. OF ALUMINUM WEIGHING TRAY	WT. OF TRAY WITH SAND	WT. OF SAND
WET WEIGHT			
DRY WEIGHT	_____		

DATA FOR CAMPUS SOIL	WT. OF ALUMINUM WEIGHING TRAY	WT. OF TRAY WITH SOIL	WT. OF SOIL
WET WEIGHT			
DRY WEIGHT	_____		

DATA FOR CLAY	WT. OF ALUMINUM WEIGHING TRAY	WT. OF TRAY WITH CLAY	WT. OF CLAY
WET WEIGHT			
DRY WEIGHT	_____		

Calculations for Method A-2
Field Capacity

$$\text{Field capacity} = \frac{(\text{wet weight of soil}) - (\text{dry weight of soil})}{(\text{dry weight of soil})} \times 100\%$$

	SAND SAMPLE	CAMPUS SOIL SAMPLE	CLAY SAMPLE
WET SOIL WEIGHT			
DRY SOIL WEIGHT			
FIELD CAPACITY	%	%	%

Questions for Method A

1. Based on your hydrometer readings, how would you describe the soil on your campus? Sandy, silty, mostly clay, or loamy? Given what you know about the geology and topography of your location, is this the soil composition you would expect?

   _____

   _____

   _____

   _____

2. From your observations of sediments accumulating in the bottom of the cylinder, what kinds of water movement in a river would keep sand suspended long enough to be transported downstream? Silt? Clay? Can you explain why silt, sand, and clay tend to be deposited in different locations along a river system?

   _____

   _____

   _____

   _____

3. Based on the composition of your soil, what hypothesis would you make about its field capacity, in comparison to sand at one extreme and clay at the other? Did your actual measurement of field capacity conform to this expectation? Explain.

   _____

   _____

   _____

   _____

4. How might the frequency of irrigation on your lawns in summer be related to the field capacity of the soil?

   _____

   _____

   _____

   _____

5. How might you design an experiment to measure the wilting point of your campus soil? Can you guess, from the hydrometer data, whether the wilting point would be comparatively high or comparatively low? Explain.

   _____

   _____

   _____

   _____

METHOD B: SOIL pH IN TWO MICROHABITATS

[Outdoor activity]

Research Question

Does the type of plant cover affect soil chemistry?

Preparation

This exercise involves field testing pH, comparing microhabitats on your campus. A portable pH meter with soil probe is the easiest way to take multiple measurements. Soil pH measurement depends on some free water in the soil, so plan this exercise at a time of year when the soil is not completely dry. Depending on the trees and shrubs on your campus, you may have several kinds of microhabitats to choose from. Evergreen shrubs such as juniper or *Taxus* and evergreen trees such as spruce or pine affect pH if their needles are allowed to decompose where they fall. If leaf litter is completely removed by your grounds-keeping staff, effects of plants on the soil will be harder to discern. Be aware also that fertilizers affect pH by adding salts to the soil. It is wise to check with facilities management to find out if any fertilizer applications are planned, and to allow several rains to remove free salts after fertilizer application before doing this exercise.

Materials (per laboratory team)

Portable pH meter with soil probe

Soil thermometer (if meter does not also record temperature)

Procedure

1. In consultation with your instructor, choose a tree or shrub that you suspect may affect soil pH. If this species is represented by several specimens on your campus, decide on a sampling plan that will distribute sample sites around several plants.
2. A lawn area nearby will serve as your control plot. Alternate readings between your shrub/tree sites and your lawn sites.
3. To take a reading, push the soil probe into the ground, taking care to sample at the same depth each time. Give the meter a minute to generate a reliable reading, and write down the pH in the appropriate column of the Data Table for Method B. As you are taking each reading make note of the depth of leaf litter and any other details you see associated with this site. Add these observations to the right-hand column in the data table. Record the temperature, either by reading directly from your meter or with a separate measurement using a soil thermometer, and record that number as well. Repeat your measurements for 10 tree/shrub sites and 10 lawn sites.
4. Because pH is a logarithmic scale, these data are not likely to be normally distributed. To test differences in pH between tree/shrub and lawn sites, it is therefore best to use a **non-parametric** statistical test. In Calculations for Method B, follow instructions for a Mann-Whitney U test.
5. Interpret your data by answering Questions for Method B.

Data Table for Method B:
Temperature and pH Readings

LAWN SITES (CONTROL GROUP)		
SITE #	pH	TEMP.
1-a		
2-a		
3-a		
4-a		
5-a		
6-a		
7-a		
8-a		
9-a		
10-a		

TREE/SHRUB SITES (TREATMENT GROUP)		
SITE #	Ph	TEMP.
1-b		
2-b		
3-b		
4-b		
5-b		
6-b		
7-b		
8-b		
9-b		
10-b		

Calculations for Method B:
The Mann-Whitney U-Test

pH VALUES FROM LAWNS

LOWEST   (Rank in order)   HIGHEST
⇩   ⇩

pH VALUES FROM TREE/SHRUB SITES

LOWEST ⇨

HIGHEST ⇨

U value: [   ]   Critical value: [   ]   Conclusion: [   ]

336

1. In the Mann-Whitney U-Test table, first enter the 10 pH values for lawns in the unshaded cells across the top, ranking them in order from lowest on the left to highest on the right.
2. In the unshaded cells down the left-hand side, enter the 10 pH values for tree/shrub sites, ranking them from lowest at the top to highest at the bottom.
3. For each of the shaded cells in the body of the table, compare the lawn pH value at the column heading with the tree/shrub pH value at the row heading for that cell. If the lawn pH above is higher than the tree/shrub pH at the left, write a + sign in that cell. If the lawn pH is lower, write a − sign. If both are equal, write ½ .
4. Count plus signs for the entire table, scoring each ½ marked cell as half a plus sign. Now count minus signs for the entire table, scoring each ½ as half a minus sign. Compare the number of + and the number of − signs counted. Whichever number is greater is the Mann-Whitney U value. (See example below.)
5. The null hypothesis for this test is that the two sites do not differ in pH. The critical value for this test, with 10 columns and 10 rows, is 77. Higher U values mean greater significance. If the Mann-Whitney U value is greater than 73, you have demonstrated a difference in pH between the two microhabitats at a significance level of $p = 0.05$. If the U value is less than 77, the pH values do not differ significantly between the sites.

Sample Table

pH VALUES FROM LAWNS

pH VALUES FROM TREE/SHRUB SITES	6.3	6.4	6.7	6.9	7.2	7.2	7.4	7.5	7.6	7.8
5.9	+	+	+	+	+	+	+	+	+	+
6.1	+	+	+	+	+	+	+	+	+	+
6.1	+	+	+	+	+	+	+	+	+	+
6.3	½	+	+	+	+	+	+	+	+	+
6.5	−	−	+	+	+	+	+	+	+	+
6.6	−	−	+	+	+	+	+	+	+	+
6.8	−	−	−	+	+	+	+	+	+	+
6.9	−	−	−	½	+	+	+	+	+	+
7.0	−	−	−	−	+	+	+	+	+	+
7.2	−	−	−	−	½	½	+	+	+	+

The number of + signs, and hence the U value, is 80. This exceeds the critical value of 77. In this hypothetical example, tree/shrub sites are significantly more acidic than shrub sites.

Questions for Method B

1. The Mann-Whitney U method tests the null hypothesis that differences in pH among the sites are due to sampling error. Did you reject or accept this null hypothesis? Explain your conclusion.

_____

_____

_____

_____

2. Did you notice any differences in temperature between the sites under trees or shrubs vs. the lawn sites? Aside from the immediate effects of temperature on pH assessment, how might a cooler temperature affect soil chemistry? (Hint: Think about soil organisms.)

_____

_____

_____

_____

3. Did you notice variation in leaf litter depth among your tree/shrub sites? Do your pH and temperature readings suggest that litter depth might be an important factor? Explain.

_____

_____

_____

_____

4. Suppose in this exercise your results showed a mean difference in pH of the two kinds of sites, but the Mann-Whitney test yielded a U value of 70. Can you conclude with certainty that pH is the same in these two habitats? Can you conclude that there is a real difference? How might you resolve any unanswered questions?

_____

_____

_____

_____

5. Acid rain, caused by air pollutants returning to earth in the form of sulfuric or nitric acid, lowers the pH of the soil. Why does rain of pH 4.5 cause more damage in some ecosystems and less in others?

_____

_____

_____

_____

METHOD C: NUTRIENT CAPTURE BY SOILS

[Laboratory activity]

Research Question

Does soil texture affect elution and recapture of nitrate ions?

Preparation

This exercise is based on movement of nitrate ions through soil. This is a critical issue for agriculture, since nitrates are commonly applied as fertilizer and loss through the soil column means higher crop production costs. It is also a water quality issue, since nitrates and nitrites that percolate through soil end up in groundwater and surface waters to the detriment of human and ecosystem health. Because nitrates are commonly evaluated in water quality tests, kits for nitrate assay are available at a range of prices and sophistication. Choose a kit that measures nitrates in the 5–50 ppm range. You may want to use the same kit for water quality analysis in an outdoor activity.

Clay, sand, and campus soil can be obtained as described in Method 1. *If powdered soils are used, take care to avoid inhaling dust.* Wetting the soils and letting them air dry is a good precaution. An optional, and interesting, addition to the exercise is to compare a piece of intact sod to the loose soil samples. A hand trowel can be used to cut a small circle of sod from intact turf. Trim the sod with a sharp knife to fit the Buchner funnel. Weigh the sod, and remove soil from the bottom until it weighs 50 grams. Place the sod on top of a layer of filter paper in the funnel, and compare elution rates through sod with elution rates through loose soils. You may wish to do one demonstration with sod for the entire laboratory.

Potassium nitrate is a strong oxidizing agent, and should be handled with care in dry form. Make 500 ml of 0.05 Normal solution per laboratory group. Alternatively, potassium nitrate can be purchased as a 0.1 N solution and diluted by half for this exercise.

Materials (per laboratory team)

Kit for testing nitrates in water samples (5–50 ppm sensitivity)

3 Buchner funnels (ceramic or polypropylene), 5–7 cm diameter

3 sheets filter paper to fit Buchner funnels

3 flasks (250 ml each) for collecting eluted solution

Separatory funnel (100 ml or larger), glass or polypropylene

Ring stand

350 ml potassium nitrate solution (0.05 N)

50 g sample of sand

50 g sample of clay soil

50 g sample of campus soil

Marking pen or wax pencil

Procedure

1. Place a Buchner funnel in each of the three flasks, and put a circle of filter paper in the bottom of each funnel.
2. Weigh 50 g of sand and place this sample on top of the filter paper in the first funnel. Similarly, prepare a 50 g sample of clay and a 50 g sample of campus soil, placing them in the other two funnels. Mark the three flasks "sand," "clay," and "campus," indicating the type of soil in the funnel in each flask.

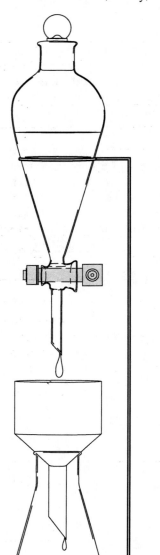

3. Fill the separatory funnel with 100 ml of 0.05 N potassium nitrate (KNO_3). Position it in the ring stand so that the tip of the funnel is just a little higher than the top of your Buchner funnels as they sit in their flasks. (See Figure 11.)
4. Adjust the stopcock on the separatory funnel so that it drips steadily onto the soil surface. As it flows through the soil, you should collect eluted material in the flask. After the 100 ml of solution has all run into the first soil sample, set this sample aside to continue eluting through the soil.
5. Position the second Buchner funnel and its flask under the separatory funnel. Refill the separatory funnel with 100 ml more of potassium nitrate solution, and drip this through your second soil sample. Repeat for the third sample.
6. After all the Buchner funnels have stopped dripping, use a graduated cylinder to measure how much of the solution passed through the soil. Enter your results in the Data Table for Method C.
7. Use a water quality test kit to assess how much nitrate nitrogen is present in the water that ran through each soil sample. Perform a control analysis on the unused potassium nitrate solution, so you know what level of nitrate entered the soil. Record your results in the data table.
8. Analyze your results by answering Questions for Method C.

Data Table for Method C:
Effects of Aerobic and Anaerobic Incubation on Soil Nutrients

SOIL TYPE	VOLUME OF SOLUTION ELUTED	NITRATE CONCENTRATION (PPM)
SAND	81 ml	10
CLAY	71 ml	10
CAMPUS SOIL	(—	5
CONTROL (No soil exposure)	Not applicable.	20

Figure 11   Buchner funnel apparatus for testing nitrate elution through soils.

Questions for Method C

1. Which type of soil retained the greatest volume of solution? Explain this result, based on your understanding of particle size in each soil type.

_____ Clay or compus soil _____ loose. _____

_____

_____

_____

2. Which kind of soil recaptured nitrate as it passed through the soil column? Explain why you think this result was obtained.

_____ Compus soil ___ out. _____

_____

_____

_____

3. Why do soil conservation agencies strongly recommend getting a soil test before applying fertilizers on farm fields?

_____ To make sure the soil would have enough nitrogen. Agencies would want to make sure the soil would be able to hold the fertilizers with nitrogen longer. _____

_____

4. Although septic sewer lines go to a wastewater treatment plant in most communities, water entering storm drains is usually diverted into nearby streams or rivers. In areas of moderate to high rainfall, groundwater also feeds surface streams. If too much nitrogen fertilizer were applied to lawns on your campus, what are the consequences for organisms and people living downstream from you?

_____ Its going to stream across the river _____ water _____

_____

_____

_____

5. Discuss advantages and disadvantages of "organic" fertilizer, applied in the form of animal manure, as opposed to potassium nitrate as a means to enhance soil nitrogen levels. Consider both the farmer's perspective and the perspective of the greater community.

_____ organic fertilizer are considered "nasty" - smell bad, _____

_____ horse - unsanitary _____

_____

_____

FOR FURTHER INVESTIGATION

1. Collect soils from a large transect across a river valley near your campus. Analyze soil particle composition using the Bouyoucos hydrometer method, and plot silt content as a function of elevation. You may also wish to compare plant communities on different soils analyzed in your survey.
2. Compare pH under different kinds of trees and shrubs on your campus. Do some species have a greater impact on soil chemistry than others?
3. Try incubating soil in a jar, covered by 10 cm of water. Test soil nitrates and nitrites in the soil before and after incubation. As a control, do the same experiment with soil sterilized by autoclaving or by heating in a 350-degree oven for 2 hours. Do live organisms make a difference in the process of denitrification?

FOR FURTHER READING

Bouyoucos, G. H. 1951. A Recalibration of the Hydrometer for Making Mechanical Analysis of Soils. *Agron. J.* 43: 434–438.

Gutschick, V. P. 1981. Evolved Strategies in Nitrogen Acquisition in Plants. *American Naturalist* 118: 607–637.

Leopold, Aldo. 1949. *A Sand County Almanac.* Oxford University Press, N. Y.

Sugden, Andrew, Richard Stone, and Caroline Ash. 2004. Soils, the Final Frontier. Introduction to special edition on soils. *Science* 304:1613.

Vitousek Peter M., John Aber, Robert W. Howarth, Gene E. Likens, Pamela A. Matson, David W. Schindler, William H. Schlesinger, and G. David Tilman. 1997. Human Alteration of the Global Nitrogen Cycle: Causes and Consequences. *Issues in Ecology I. Ecological Society of America.* http://www.esa.org/science/Issues/FileEnglish/issue1.pdf

Island Biogeography

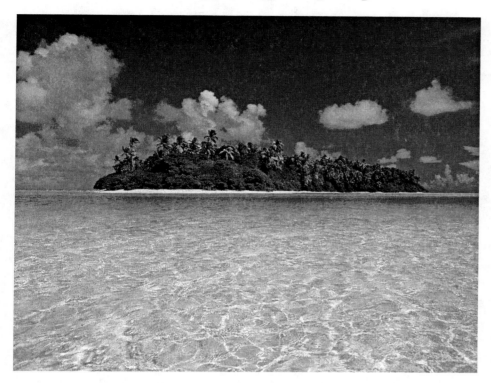

Figure 1   A tropical island presents opportunities for ecological research.

INTRODUCTION

Field research is rewarding, but always challenging, and sometimes bewildering. The ecologist attempting to measure one variable typically encounters a hundred more thrown in for good measure by the complex amalgam of chance and causality we call living nature. Population fluctuations, interactions with other species, weather patterns, human interference, and many more unforeseen factors impinge on the ecologist's best-laid experimental plans. When ecologically significant forces are acting all around us, how can we pin down the cause of a significant ecosystem change, such as coral bleaching or amphibian extinction? How can we establish a "control ecosystem" to contrast with our observations of the natural world? Simplicity and replication, the twin pillars of experimental science, are not as easily attained in ecology as in physics or biochemistry. When we discover a natural system that lends itself to controlled investigation, field researchers are understandably excited by the opportunity. This is why islands, with their well-defined boundaries, isolation from interference, and simplified biological communities, have played such an important role in the development of ecological thought (Figure 1).

Ecologists Robert MacArthur and E. O. Wilson saw opportunity in islands as natural laboratories for investigating community structure. Drawing on their extensive experience exploring biodiversity on island chains around the globe, they realized islands provided a proving ground for their developing conception of biotic communities as dynamic systems, not just static collections of species.

Through comparisons of islands, MacArthur and Wilson could gather repeatable measurements of ecological processes to find how each influences the resulting flora and fauna. Their seminal 1967 book, called *The Theory of Island Biogeography,* begins with the observation that the number of species on an island is related to its area. On a graph displaying each variable on a logarithmic scale, the relationship can be drawn as a straight line. This **species–area relationship** has since been demonstrated in many kinds of organisms on many kinds of island clusters (for example, see the distribution of bats on Caribbean islands in Figure 2). The empirically derived expression for the species–area relationship is as follows:

Species–area relationship:

$$S = C\,A^z$$

Taking the log of both sides: $\qquad\qquad \log S = \log C + z \log A$

S = the number of species present
C = a constant that varies with the taxonomic group
A = the area of the island
Z = a constant, roughly equal to 0.3 for island habitats

Species-Area Curve for Caribbean Bats

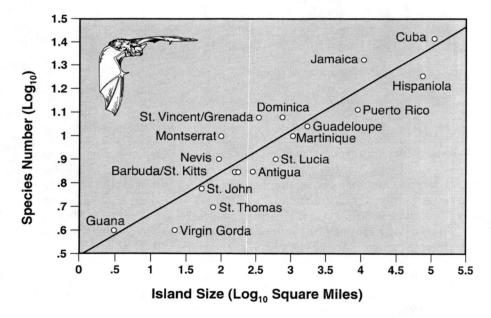

Figure 2 Speciesarea relationship for bats on Caribbean islands. (From Scott Pedersen. 2005. http://biomicro.sdstate.edu/pederses/caribres.html)

Note that taking the logarithm of both sides transforms the equation to linear form. To visualize the biology behind this formula, it is instructive to note that a tenfold increase in the area of an island produces an approximately twofold increase in its species count (Figure 3).

Species–Area Relationship

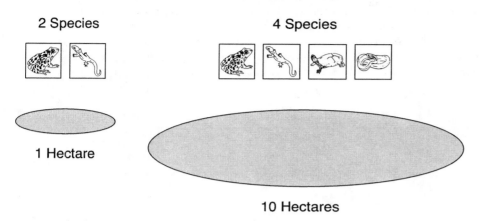

2 Species

4 Species

1 Hectare

10 Hectares

Figure 3   An island ten times as large can support twice as many species.

To explain this empirically derived species–area relationship, MacArthur and Wilson theorized that species numbers on islands represent a state of equilibrium—a delicate balance between local extinction on one side of the ecological teeter-totter and immigration across the water on the other. Island size, they reasoned, should have little influence on immigration rates, but a lot to do with extinction. Therefore, as island size increases, extinction rates should slow and the balance should shift toward greater biodiversity (Figure 4).

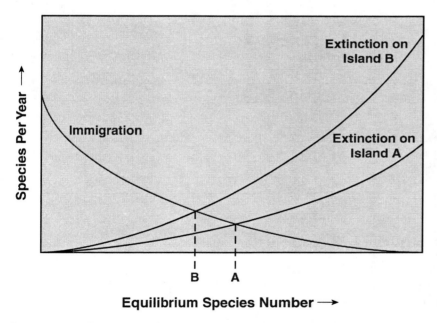

Figure 4   The Area Effect. In MacArthur and Wilson's model, a larger island (A) would have a lower rate of extinction, and would thus have a higher equilibrium species number than a smaller island (B).

Distance from the mainland should have the greatest impact on immigration, so all other things being equal, an island farther from sources of immigrants should have fewer species than an island closer to shore (Figure 5). Comparative data support this part of the theory as well. Easter island, remotely located in the South Pacific, has only 47 species of native higher plants, according to biogeographer Jared Diamond (2004). The flora of Catalina, an island of roughly equivalent size only 42 km off the coast of California, has more than ten times as many native plant species. The higher flow of immigrant species to Catalina pushes its equilibrium number higher, even though Catalina's rate of extinction is expected to be roughly the same as Easter's. MacArthur and Wilson concluded that size and location both influence the balance between immigration and extinction on islands.

Check your progress:

Why would the number of species already on an island affect the rate at which new immigrants successfully establish themselves?

Hint: Think about niche space.

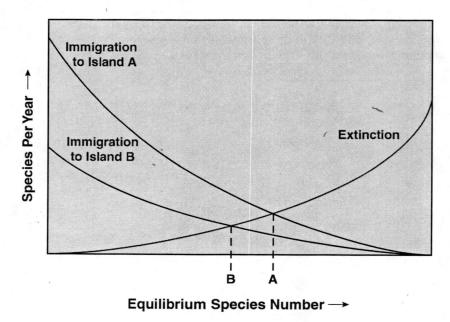

Figure 5 The Distance Effect. In MacArthur and Wilson's model, an island nearer the mainland (A) would receive immigrants at a higher rate, and would thus have a higher equilibrium species number than an island of the same size located farther from shore (B).

While still a graduate student working with E. O. Wilson, Daniel Simberloff saw an opportunity to test these theories in the small mangrove islands that dot the shoreline of southern Florida (Figure 6). Simberloff and Wilson first censused all the arthropods living in the canopy of several mangrove islands in Florida bay. This was no small task. Mangrove thickets are notoriously difficult to walk through, and arthropods are so diverse that identification to species requires considerable expertise. Through persistence and collaborative taxonomic work, Simberloff and Wilson established solid baseline data on the invertebrate fauna of their miniature islands. These data, according to the theory, represented equilibrium species numbers determined by the islands' sizes and locations.

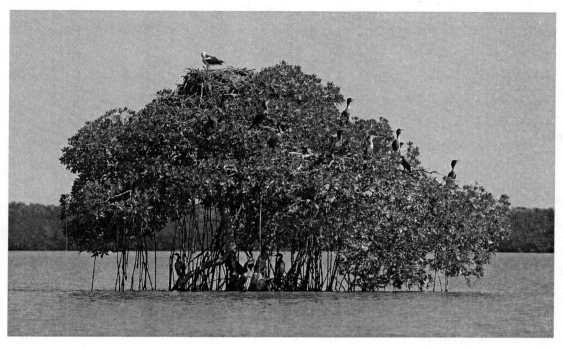

Figure 6   A mangrove island off the coast of Florida provides nesting sites for birds, and a permanent home for many small arthropod species. Simberloff and Wilson (1970) removed invertebrates (but not birds) from four islands and documented their recolonization.

Simberloff and Wilson then manipulated their experimental system. They blanketed and fogged four of the mangrove islands, completely eliminating all their resident invertebrate species. The researchers then carefully documented recolonization of the islands with repeated follow-up visits. After two years, all but the most remote island had returned to their former equilibrium species numbers (Figure 7). Interestingly, recolonized islands supported a somewhat altered list of species, even though total species numbers were about the same as the original census figures. The study's conclusion was that biogeographic principles do operate on island communities, regardless of the kinds of species that happen to occur in a particular place.

Check your progress:

Why was the Simberloff–Wilson study of mangrove islands deemed so important by ecologists, given that the species–area curve had already been discovered by comparing species numbers on oceanic islands?

Answer: Comparative studies can show correlations between variables, but a controlled experiment provides more convincing evidence of causal relationships.

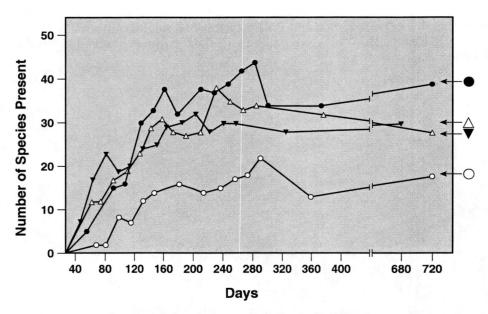

Figure 7 Simberloff and Wilson's survey results documenting recolonization of four mangrove islands. Two years after all insects were removed from the islands, biodiversity had recovered to nearly their original species numbers (indicated by arrows at right), with the exception of the most distant island from shore (open circles). (After Simberloff and Wilson, 1970.)

Island biogeography theory has been substantially refined and modified in the 40 years since its introduction, but it remains central to our understanding of community dynamics. Ecologists quickly realized that the same theory explaining immigration and extinction on oceanic islands would also apply to other kinds of isolated habitat. For example, consider a marmot living in the Southwestern United States (Figure 8). Marmots are adapted to the kinds of cold, rocky habitats found at northern latitudes or high altitudes. During periods of glaciation thousands of years ago, marmots were able to migrate south across much of North America. When the climate warmed up, marmot populations retreated to the tops of mountains, where they remain isolated today. For marmots, the Southwest consists of "sky islands" of alpine habitat surrounded by a "sea" of inhospitable lowlands (Figure 9). Given enough time, communities of mammals adapted to alpine habitats on Southwestern mountain ranges conform to the same kinds of species–area relationships that terrestrial animals exhibit on oceanic islands (Brown 1971). Similarly, a chain of lakes can be considered an archipelago for fish, and a patch of forest is an island for tree-nesting birds.

Because human activities have seriously fragmented habitats around the world, island biogeography theory is especially relevant to conservation biology. To an increasing degree, parks and wilderness preserves are becoming scattered islands of natural habitat in a landscape so altered by human activity that it no longer supports native species. Whether we consider fragmentation of tropical forest in Bolivia (Figure 10) or native prairie reduced to bits and pieces in the American corn belt, we find immigration between habitat patches has become increasingly difficult for species facing local extinction on shrinking remnants of their former continental ranges. Guided by application of island biogeography theory, conservationists stress the importance of wildlife corridors between existing parks to enhance rates of population exchange, and larger blocks of preserved land in recognition of the species–area relationship. Debates about preserving a single large or several small preserves have largely focused on the applicability of biogeography theory to particular environments. Island biogeography not only gives us opportunities to understand the history of natural communities, but also helps us find ways to protect biodiversity for the future.

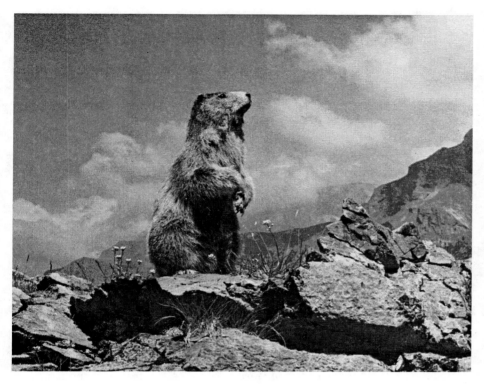

Figure 8   A marmot is a medium-sized mammal confined to alpine habitats.

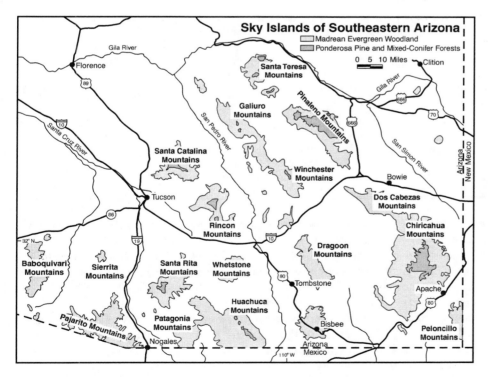

Figure 9   "Sky islands" are illustrated as shaded areas on a map of Southeastern Arizona. (From C. J. Bahre, 1998.)

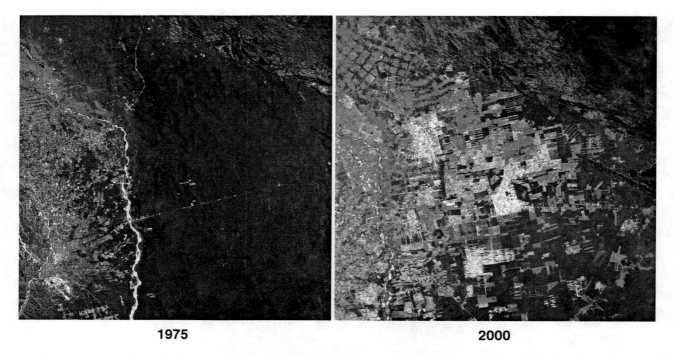

1975 **2000**

Figure 10   Habitat fragmentation revealed by satellite images taken in 1975 (left) and 2000 (right) of an area originally covered in tropical dry forest east of Santa Cruz de la Sierra, Bolivia. A formerly continuous forest (dark area) has been reduced to small habitat islands.

Check your progress:

Why are tunnels constructed under highways for wildlife migration an increasingly important strategy for maintaining biodiversity?

Answer: Highways divide the landscape into habitat islands. If migration across the highway is limited, the species–area relationship reduces biodiversity through elevated extinction in the lands remaining between roads.

Speciation also has a significant influence on the makeup of island communities, but on a different scale of time. Whereas immigration and extinction can transform a community in tens or hundreds of years, evolution at the level of species occurs over thousands or millions of years. When isolated for a very long time from the mainland gene pool, island populations change via **genetic drift** and **natural selection**. Both Charles Darwin and Alfred Russel Wallace came away from extensive collecting trips through islands realizing that isolation and speciation go hand in hand. Island species may arrive by happenstance, but many of them experience predictable changes as they adapt to an insular environment. For example, the capability of flight that undoubtedly helped bring birds to islands in the first place tends to be lost in the absence of mainland predators. The endemic Hawaiian goose, called the nene, is a weak flier in comparison to other species of geese (Figure 11). Size, too, may be subject to rapid evolutionary change. Large mammals such as the elephant show a tendency toward reduced size when permanently marooned on islands, while small rodents tend to become larger over evolutionary time. (For a detailed and accessible discussion of evolution on islands, see Quammen, 1997.)

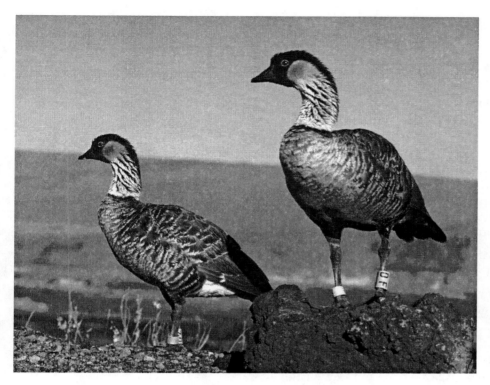

Figure 11 Nene, the endemic Hawaiian goose, is distinct from mainland species.

Whether or not they develop "island" peculiarities, long-isolated populations develop genetic differences, which may be sufficient to block renewed gene flow if these organisms are later reintroduced to the mainland. By definition, a population no longer able to breed with the ancestral type is a new species. This so-called **allopatric** model of speciation is apparent in the various stages of genetic difference found between island and mainland populations today. Since physical isolation commonly precedes genetic isolation, it is likely that most of the earth's species were once residents of islands, separated by water or by discontinuous habitat from others of their kind, at some critical juncture in their evolutionary past.

Check your progress:

Based on the allopatric speciation model, what role could habitat islands such as mountaintops play in developing biodiversity?

Answer: A population stranded on a mountaintop for a sufficient duration accumulates genetic differences, which prevent interbreeding with ancestral populations, and so becomes a separate species.

METHOD A: BIOGEOGRAPHY SIMULATION GAME

[Laboratory]

Research Question

How do island size and distance from immigration sources influence the equilibrium between immigration and extinction?

Preparation

In this simulation exercise, egg cartons simulate islands, and ping-pong balls represent species. Remove the hinged lids from cardboard or plastic egg cartons, leaving only the cupped base portion. Dozen-sized egg cartons are needed for the large islands. Half-dozen–sized cartons can be used for the small islands, or you can cut some dozen-sized cartons in half. A hard surface 8' long, either on the floor or on long benches, is required to bounce the balls into the egg cartons to simulate species becoming established on islands.

This simulation works best with four people in each group.

Materials (per laboratory team)

1 dozen-sized egg carton (with lid removed)

1 half-dozen–sized egg carton (with lid removed)

16 ping-pong balls

1 pair of dice, of different colors (e.g., a red die and a green die)

Small plastic cup for shaking dice

Felt-tip markers to match dice colors (e.g., a red and green marker)

Masking tape and meter stick (can be shared with other groups)

Procedure

1. Number the six cups at one end of the large egg carton 1 through 6 by writing numbers with a colored marker on the inside of each depression where an egg would sit. Number the six cups at the other end 1 through 6 with the other colored marker. These numbered cups represent niches for species living on an island (see Figure 12). Be aware that calling these cups "niches" is an oversimplification. Since a niche is not just a physical space, think of each cup as a unit of habitat containing sufficient resources to sustain a population of one species.
2. Number the cups in the small egg carton 1 through 6 with any color.
3. Place the large (dozen-sized) egg carton on a hard floor surface. This represents a large island. Use masking tape to mark the position of the mainland, one meter away. Alternatively, place the large egg carton one meter from the edge of a bench or table.
4. Designate four people on your team as a) colonization simulator, b) extinction simulator, c) ping-pong ball catcher, and d) data recorder.

Egg Carton Simulates Large Island. Balls Represent Resident Species.

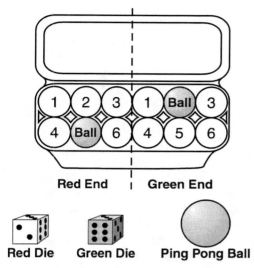

Red End | **Green End**

Red Die   **Green Die**   **Ping Pong Ball**

Figure 12 Apparatus for biogeography simulation game. An egg carton represents an island with 12 "niches" available for colonization. Ping-pong balls bounced into the "island" represent colonizing species. Red and green dice are used to decide which species will become locally extinct in each round of play.

5. *Simulate colonization of a large island.* Taking five ping-pong balls in hand, the colonization simulator stands on the mainland (behind the tape line on the floor or at the edge of the table) and tries to bounce ping-pong balls into the niche spaces on the "island." The only rule is that the ball must bounce off the floor at least once before it lands in a cup. The ping-pong ball catcher helps round up the balls that do not go into a cup, returning them to the colonization simulator for the next round. Balls that land on top of the island but do not settle into a "niche" in one of the cups have not become "established," and must be removed.

6. After the five-ball colonization trial, the extinction simulator shakes the dice in the plastic cup, draws one die out at random, and tosses it. The color and number of the die indicates one "niche" on the island. (For example, if the green die comes up with #3, then look at the #3 cup on the green end of the island.) If this "niche" is empty, extinction is zero for this round. If this "niche" is occupied, remove the ball that sits in that place. One "extinction event" has occurred. (A piece of tape wrapped sticky-side-out around your finger can help remove balls from their "niches" more easily.)

7. At the end of one round of colonization and extinction, the recorder writes down the following information in Data Table 1 for Method A: a) how many species existed on the island at the beginning of this round (which will be 0 the first time), b) how many successful immigration events occurred out of the five attempts, c) how many individuals exist on the island after colonization, and d) how many extinction events (zero or one) occurred in this round.

8. Repeat steps 5 through 7 for 30 rounds, simulating five colonization attempts followed by an extinction trial in each round. Record data after each round.

9. *Simulate colonization of a small island.* Replace the large egg carton with the half-dozen–sized egg carton. Remove one of the dice from the extinction simulator's plastic cup. Repeat steps 5 through 7 as before, with the exception that the extinction simulator throws the same die each time, and removes any "species" that exist in the indicated "niche." Continue for 30 iterations, recording your results in Data Table 2 for Method A.

10. *Simulate colonization of a distant island.* If you have time, try to simulate colonization of the large island at a distance of *2 meters* away from the "shoreline" where the colonization simulator stands. Simulate 30 rounds of colonization and extinction as before, recording your results in Data Table 3 for Method A.

11. Pool data from the first (large island) simulation. Begin by counting how many colonization attempts were made on islands containing zero established species. Look down through *Column 1* in your own Data Table 1 to find all cases in which the initial species number is zero. Multiply the number of cases by five to determine how many total colonization attempts were made to colonize islands with zero initial colonists. Write this number in the first line of Column 1 in Data Table 4. Next, for all the cases you have identified, add up all the "successful colonization events on islands with 0 species" from Data Table 1, and record this sum in Column 2 of Data Table 4. The idea here is to calculate a success rate for all attempts made on islands with 0 colonists.

12. Repeat step 11 for all the cases you can find in Data Table 1 in which the island has 1 species at the beginning of a simulation round. Enter the sums for total attempts and total successes in Data Table 4. Repeat for cases in which the island already had 2, 3, 4, 5, 6, 7, 8, 9, 10, and 11 species at the beginning of a round, filling out the first and second columns of Data Table 4. We can assume the rate of immigration onto islands already containing 12 species is 0, since there are no niches left to colonize on a full island.

13. Combine your data with all the other groups in your class, summing total attempts and total successes for each initial species condition for the class as a whole. Record these totals in the third and fourth columns of Data Table 4. Then divide (total successes)/(total attempts) to calculate the rate of immigration onto islands for the class as a whole. When you have completed this step, you should be able to demonstrate that the success of immigration is negatively related to species already on the island.

14. Pool class data for extinction rates in a similar fashion. First, recognize that the numbers in the third column of Data Table 1 are the numbers present when an extinction trial is conducted. We can assume the rate of extinction is zero when no species are on the island. Look down through Column 3 to find all cases in which 1 species is present. Write the total number of these cases in Column 1 of Data Table 5. Then add up the number of extinction events that actually occurred in these cases, from the corresponding lines in Column 4. Record this sum in Column 2 of Data Table 5.

15. Repeat step 14 for cases with 2, 3, 4, 5, 6, 7, 8, 9, 10, and 11 species present at the beginning of the extinction trial. Record your results, filling in the first two columns of Data Table 5.

16. Combine your data with all the other groups in your class, summing total number of extinction trials and total extinction events on islands at each initial species number. Record these totals in the third and fourth columns of Data Table 5. Then calculate the rates of extinction for the whole class by dividing (total number of extinction events)/(total number of trials) at each species density. Record these fractions in the fifth column of Data Table 5. We can assume that the rate of extinction for islands with 12 species present is 1.0, since the die will indicate the removal of one of the 12 balls every time when the island is completely full.

17. *Plot the class immigration rates,* with initial species number on the x-axis and rate of colonization on the y-axis, on the graph labeled Results for Method A: Immigration and Extinction Curves, Based on Class Totals.

18. *Plot the class extinction rates,* with initial species number on the x-axis and rate of extinction on the y-axis, on the same graph with the immigration curve. Examine the graph. The immigration line should have a negative slope, showing decreasing rates of successful colonization as the number of species on the island increases. The extinction curve should have a positive slope, showing increasing rates of extinction as more and more species fill up the island. The x value that lies beneath the point of intersection of the two lines is the predicted equilibrium value for species on the large island. Compare your graph with Figure 4.

19 Plot the total species number on the large island, listed in the first column of Data Table 1, against time, measured in trial numbers. Trial number should go on the x-axis and number of species on the island on the y-axis. Compare your graph with Figure 7. Make similar plots for your results from the small island experiment and the distant island experiment. Compare the stability of equilibria, and the equilibrium species numbers from the three experiments. Record your thoughts about these three experiments.

20. Analyze your results by answering Questions for Method A.

Data Table (1) for Method A:
Large Island Simulation

TRIAL #	COLUMN 1 INITIAL NUMBER OF RESIDENT SPECIES	COLUMN 2 NUMBER OF SUCCESSFUL COLONIZATION EVENTS	COLUMN 3 # SPECIES AFTER IMMIGRATION (ADD COLUMNS 1 AND 2)	COLUMN 4 NUMBER OF EXTINCTION EVENTS
1	0			
2				
3				
4				
5				
6				
7				
8				
9				
10				
11				
12				
13				
14				
15				
16				
17				
18				
19				
20				
21				
22				
23				
24				
25				
26				
27				
28				
29				
30				

Data Table (2) for Method A:
Small Island Simulation

TRIAL #	COLUMN 1 INITIAL NUMBER OF RESIDENT SPECIES	COLUMN 2 NUMBER OF SUCCESSFUL COLONIZATION EVENTS	COLUMN 3 # SPECIES AFTER IMMIGRATION (ADD COLUMNS 1 AND 2)	COLUMN 4 NUMBER OF EXTINCTION EVENTS
1	0			
2				
3				
4				
5				
6				
7				
8				
9				
10				
11				
12				
13				
14				
15				
16				
17				
18				
19				
20				
21				
22				
23				
24				
25				
26				
27				
28				
29				
30				

Data Table (3) for Method A:
Distant Island Simulation

TRIAL #	COLUMN 1 INITIAL NUMBER OF RESIDENT SPECIES	COLUMN 2 NUMBER OF SUCCESSFUL COLONIZATION EVENTS	COLUMN 3 # SPECIES AFTER IMMIGRATION (ADD COLUMNS 1 AND 2)	COLUMN 4 NUMBER OF EXTINCTION EVENTS
1	0			
2				
3				
4				
5				
6				
7				
8				
9				
10				
11				
12				
13				
14				
15				
16				
17				
18				
19				
20				
21				
22				
23				
24				
25				
26				
27				
28				
29				
30				

Data Table (4) for Method A:
Team & Class Immigration Results

Initial number of resident species	Column 1: Number of colonization attempts by your group	Column 2: Successful colonization events by your group	Column 3: Class total: number of attempts	Column 4: Class total: number of successes	Mean Rate of Immigration: (Divide column 4 by column 3)
0					
1					
2					
3					
4					
5					
6					
7					
8					
9					
10					
11					
12		0		0	

Data Table (5) for Method A:
Team & Class Extinction Results

Initial number of resident species	Column 1: Number of extinction trials by your group	Column 2: Number of extinction events in your group	Column 3: Class total: number of extinction trials	Column 4: Class total: number of extinction events	Mean Rate of Extinction: (Divide column 4 by column 3)
0		0		0	
1					
2					
3					
4					
5					
6					
7					
8					
9					
10					
11					
12					1.00

Results for Method A:
Immigration and Extinction Curves
Based on Class Totals

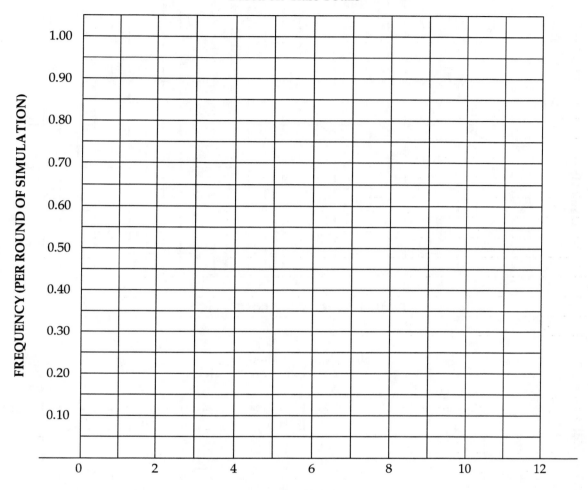

NUMBER OF SPECIES ON THE ISLAND

```
------ IMMIGRATION CURVE
——— EXTINCTION CURVE
```

Estimate the equilibrium species number for the large island, based on population size at which extinction and immigration lines intersect:

_____

Results for Method A:
Changes in Species Number on Large Island

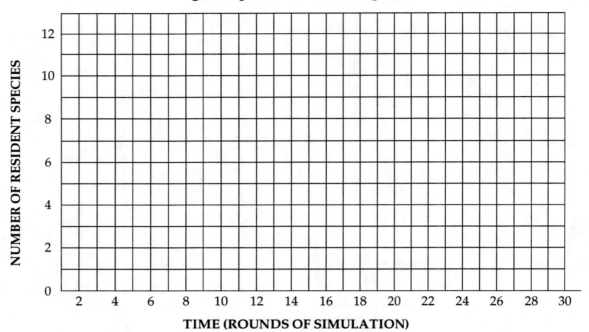

Results for Method A:
Changes in Species Number on Small Island

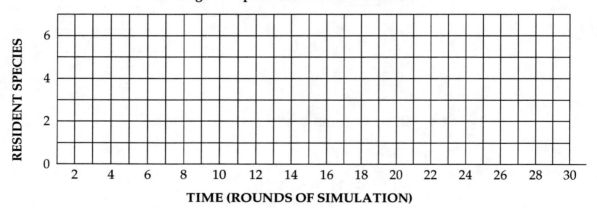

Results for Method A:
Changes in Species Number on Distant Island

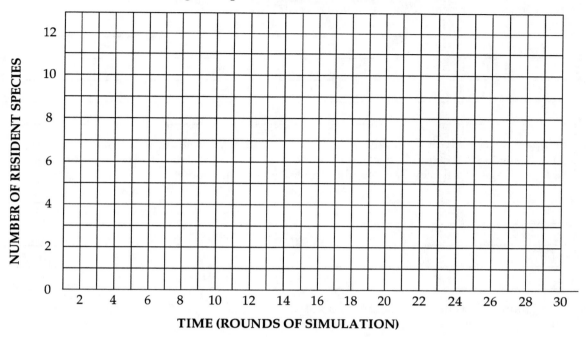

Observations:

_____

_____

_____

_____

_____

_____

_____

_____

_____

_____

_____

_____

Questions for Method A

1. Compare your immigration and extinction curves with Figure 4. Did your observed immigration and extinction curves resemble the theoretical curves? Explain.

_____

_____

_____

_____

_____

2. Compare the hypothetical equilibrium state derived from your immigration and extinction curves with the mean species numbers you actually observed near the end of the large island simulation. Did your large island achieve an equilibrium state near the predicted number? Explain.

_____

_____

_____

_____

_____

3. Each group had a different colonization simulator, so the accuracy of tossing balls onto the island could vary from group to group. Is it possible that migration to islands from the mainland might also vary from one situation to another? Propose several ecological factors other than distance that might affect successful colonization.

_____

_____

_____

_____

_____

4. How did the small island results compare with the large island results? Could this result have been predicted by the species–area formula? Explain.

_____

_____

_____

_____

_____

5. If you had time to conduct a distant island simulation, comment on your findings. If not, what would you expect the results of this simulation to demonstrate?

_____

_____

_____

_____

_____

METHOD B: SPECIES–AREA RELATIONSHIP FOR BIRD COMMUNITIES

[Mapping or computer activity]

Research Question

Do resident birds in regional parks and preserves exhibit a species–area curve?

Preparation

This activity requires data collection from species checklists and paper maps or digital maps. A list of 10–15 parks or wildlife preserves near your campus will be useful as a starting point. It is desirable to include a large range of park sizes, from small city parks to large state or national parks. The procedure focuses on forested areas, but undisturbed desert, marsh, or prairie habitats may be more appropriate for some regions. Preselecting parks that are surrounded by impacted habitat will provide clearer results. Maps of local parks and wildlife preserves are usually available on request, and may be used to measure the park's forested area. Alternatively, digital topographic maps are available on-line and in CD-ROM format. Digital mapping software has the advantage of coming with area calculation functions. The U.S. Geological Survey and Topozone (http://www.topozone.com) maintain sites for maps of any location in the United States. Natural Resources Canada (http://maps.nrcan.gc.ca/topo_e.php) offers topographic maps of Canada.

Checklists of resident birds are developed by many parks. On-line checklists can be obtained from state ornithological groups, and from clearinghouse sites such as the Northern Prairie Wildlife Research Center's 2005 *Bird Checklists of the United States*, found at http://www.npwrc.usgs.gov/resource/othrdata/chekbird/bigtoc.htm.

Materials (per laboratory team)

List of regional parks or other forested sites to be included in this survey

Topographic maps (paper or digital) for each site

A checklist of birds found at each site

Ruler (or software) for determining map areas

Calculator with $\log_{10}$ function

Procedure

1. Obtain a list of regional parks or refuges from your instructor. Write site names into the first column of the Data Table for Method B or C. For each site, consult a topographic map and find boundaries of the forested area, which is typically shaded green. Estimate the area of forest habitat, using the map's grid lines and the map scale. Use either km^2 or mi^2, but be consistent. If contiguous forested land outside the park boundary appears free of artificial disturbance, include these areas in the calculation of forest area as well. Record the estimated area of each site in the second column of the data table.
2. Consult a bird checklist for each site, counting the number of resident species. If the checklist identifies rare or transient birds, do not include them in your species count. These species have not succeeded in the establishment phase of colonization. Record the number of resident species in the third column of the data table.

3. Use a calculator to determine $\log_{10}$ of each area and $\log_{10}$ of each species number that you generated in steps 1 and 2. Record these log calculations in the fourth and fifth columns of the data table.

4. In Results for Method B or C, plot $\log_{10}$ of area on the x-axis vs. $\log_{10}$ of species number on the y-axis. If you see a trend line, use a ruler to draw the best straight line through your points. If you have access to regression software, test the significance of a nonzero slope.

5. Calculate the slope of the best line through your points, either with linear regression or by calculating (log species)/(log area). Enter this number in the box at the bottom of the graph. The slope of the log-log plot is equal to the constant z from the species–area equation.

6. Record comments, and analyze your results by answering Questions for Method B or C.

METHOD C: SPECIES–AREA RELATIONSHIP FOR ARTIFICIAL ISLANDS

[Campus activity]

Research Question

Do invertebrates hiding under objects on the ground exhibit a species–area curve?

Preparation

A month or more before the laboratory begins, create habitat islands of five sizes by cutting a plywood sheet as shown in Figure 13. Place the "islands" on the ground in a relatively undisturbed part of the campus where killing the grass or other plants under the sheets will not matter. Several replicates are desirable, but the number of plywood sheets you will need depends on the size of the class. The same set of "islands" could be used for more than one section if insects are set free after the laboratory to recolonize the islands. With a waterproof marker or pencil, give each "island" a unique number for site identification.

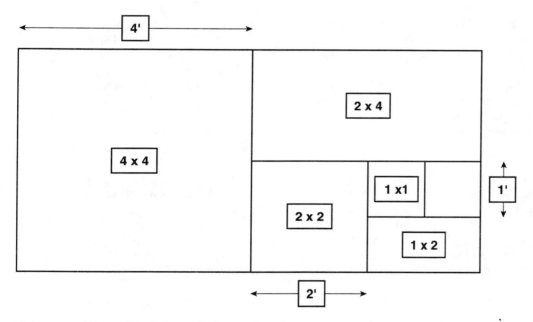

Figure 13   Cut a 4' × 8' sheet of plywood as shown to make five sizes of "islands" for Method C.

Pitfall traps consisting of collecting jars buried flush with the ground under the plywood sheets and filled $\frac{1}{2}$ full with isopropyl alcohol can be used to collect colonizing invertebrates, but students may instead collect and count live invertebrates using forceps and small vials. Species may be identified on-site without making a collection if students are given some help with field identification. Instruct students to be careful in collecting scorpions, centipedes, and some kinds of spiders by hand.

Materials (per laboratory team)

Five collecting jars, approximately 50 ml, with isopropyl alcohol preservative

Wax pencil or marker for labeling vials

Meter stick

Forceps

Calculator with $\log_{10}$ function

Procedure

1. Working as a team, you will be assigned one set of five different-sized plywood "islands" as your sampling area.
2. Note the identification number on each of your "islands" and record these site numbers in the first column of the Data Table for Method B or C.
3. Measure the length and width of your "islands" in cm. Calculate area of each "island" in cm^2, and record these numbers in the second column of the data table.
4. Carefully turn over one of the "islands." *Take care when turning over plywood—venomous spiders, scorpions, and snakes often hide under lumber.* It is best to lift the opposite side of the sheet, keeping the plywood between you and any large organism trying to escape. Count the numbers of species you see under the plywood island. Include vertebrates such as mice if they are present, but most of the organisms will be invertebrates such as isopods, centipedes, millipedes, or ground beetles. Using forceps, you may wish to collect one of each species for taxonomic identification. Repeat this procedure for each of the plywood islands in your study area.
5. Use a calculator to determine $\log_{10}$ of each area and $\log_{10}$ of each species number that you generated in step 4. Record these log calculations in the fourth and fifth columns of the data table.
6. For the purpose of replication, pool your data with two other groups to include data from 15 "islands" in your data table.
7. In Results for Method B or C, plot $\log_{10}$ of area on the x-axis vs. $\log_{10}$ of species number on the y-axis. If you see a trend line, use a ruler to draw the best straight line through your points. If you have access to regression software, test the significance of a nonzero slope.
8. Calculate the slope of the best line through your points, either with linear regression or by calculating (Δlog species)/(Δlog area). Enter this number in the box at the bottom of the graph. The slope of the log-log plot is equal to the constant z from the species–area equation.
9. Record comments, and analyze your results by answering Questions for Method B or C.

Data Table for Method B or C

SITE NAME	AREA (km² or cm²)	SPECIES #	LOG₁₀ AREA	LOG₁₀ SPECIES
1.				
2.				
3.				
4.				
5.				
6.				
7.				
8.				
9.				
10.				
11.				
12.				
13.				
14.				
15.				

Observations:

_____

_____

_____

_____

_____

_____

_____

_____

_____

_____

_____

_____

_____

_____

Results for Method B or C:
Log$_{10}$ Area vs. Log$_{10}$ Species Number

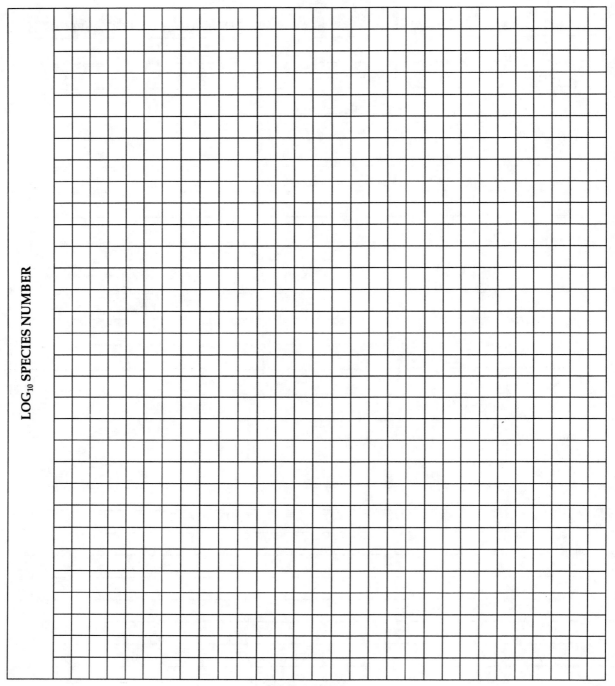

LOG$_{10}$ SPECIES NUMBER

LOG$_{10}$ AREA

Estimate of slope = Δ(log species)/ Δ(log area) = z =

Questions for Method B or C

1. How comparable are habitat islands in this study to oceanic islands? Do you think the organisms counted in your study could move easily between habitat islands, or not?

_____

_____

_____

_____

_____

2. Are all organisms included in your counts equally constrained by habitat island boundaries? How does this correspond to species on oceanic islands?

_____

_____

_____

_____

_____

3. Did your graph show a significant relationship between species and area? Explain.

_____

_____

_____

_____

_____

4. Look at the points that fell farthest above or below the line on the graph. On consulting your park maps or the position of the plywood islands, does distance from sources of colonizers play any role in creating these outliers?

_____

_____

_____

_____

_____

5. If islands promote speciation, can it be argued that habitat fragmentation by humans is speeding up the process of species formation? Will this counterbalance accelerated extinction due to habitat loss? Explain.

_____

_____

_____

_____

_____

FOR FURTHER INVESTIGATION

1. Calculate an extinction curve for the small island in the biogeography simulation game, and plot this curve on the same graph you prepared for the large island. How do the two curves compare? Can you explain the consequence of this simulation result in biological terms?
2. Measure the area of your own campus and compile a bird checklist, observing resident birds in late spring as well as winter months to include summer migrants. Where does your campus fall on the graph of log (forested area) vs. log (species number) from Method B?
3. Try testing the distance effect by placing plywood islands of the same size at different distances from a source of immigration, such as a patch of woods. Do more distant habitat islands reach equilibrium more slowly? Do they reach a lower equilibrium number of species?

FOR FURTHER READING

Brown, James H. 1971. Mammals on mountaintops: non-equilibrium insular biogeography. *American Naturalist* 105:467–478.

Diamond, Jared M. 2004. *Collapse: how societies choose to fail or succeed*. Viking, N. Y.

MacArthur R. H. and E. O. Wilson. 1967. *The theory of island biogeography*. Princeton University Press, Princeton, N. J.

Northern Prairie Wildlife Research Center. 2005. *Bird Checklists of the United States*. http://www.npwrc.usgs.gov/resource/othrdata/chekbird/bigtoc.htm

Powledge, F. 2003. Island biogeography's lasting impact. *BioScience* 53: 1032–1038.

Quammen, David. 1997. *The song of the dodo: island biogeography in an age of extinctions*. Simon & Schuster, N. Y.

Simberloff, D. S. and E. O. Wilson. 1970. Experimental zoogeography of islands: a two year record of colonization. *Ecology* 51: 934–937.

Simberloff, D. S. 1974. Equilibrium theory of island biogeography and ecology. *Annual Review of Ecology and Systematics* 5:161–182.

Simberloff, D. S. 1976. Experimental zoogeography of islands: effects of island size. *Ecology* 57(4):629–648.